Handbook of Supportive Care in Cancer

BASIC AND CLINICAL ONCOLOGY

Editor

Bruce D. Cheson, M.D.

National Cancer Institute
National Institutes of Health
Bethesda, Maryland

1. Chronic Lymphocytic Leukemia: Scientific Advances and Clinical Developments, *edited by Bruce D. Cheson*
2. Therapeutic Applications of Interleukin-2, *edited by Michael B. Atkins and James W. Mier*
3. Cancer of the Prostate, *edited by Sakti Das and E. David Crawford*
4. Retinoids in Oncology, *edited by Waun Ki Hong and Reuben Lotan*
5. Filgrastim (r-metHuG-CSF) in Clinical Practice, *edited by George Morstyn and T. Michael Dexter*
6. Cancer Prevention and Control, *edited by Peter Greenwald, Barnett S. Kramer, and Douglas L. Weed*
7. Handbook of Supportive Care in Cancer, *edited by Jean Klastersky, Stephen C. Schimpff, and Hans-Jörg Senn*

ADDITIONAL VOLUMES IN PREPARATION

Paclitaxel in Cancer Treatment, *edited by William P. McGuire and Eric K. Rowinsky*

Handbook of Supportive Care in Cancer

edited by

Jean Klastersky
Institut Jules Bordet
Université Libre de Bruxelles
Brussels, Belgium

Stephen C. Schimpff
University of Maryland Medical System
and University of Maryland Medical Center
Baltimore, Maryland

Hans-Jörg Senn
Kantonsspital
St. Gallen, Switzerland
and Basel University Medical School
Basel, Switzerland

Marcel Dekker, Inc. New York • Basel • Hong Kong

Library of Congress Cataloging-in-Publication Data

Handbook of supportive care in cancer / edited by Jean Klastersky, Stephen C. Schimpff, Hans-Jörg Senn.
p. cm. — (Basic and clinical oncology ; 7)
Includes bibliographical references and index.
ISBN 0-8247-9272-6 (alk. paper : hardcover)
1. Cancer—Palliative treatment. 2. Cancer—Complications—Treatment. I. Klastersky, J. (Jean) II. Schimpff, Stephen C. III. Senn, Hans-Jörg. IV. Series.
[DNLM: 1. Neoplasms—therapy. W1 BA813W v. 7 1995 / QZ266 H236 1995]
RC271.P33H36 1995
616.99'406—dc20
DNLM/DLC
for Library of Congress 94-41531
CIP

The publisher offers discounts on this book when ordered in bulk quantities. For more information, write to Special Sales/Professional Marketing at the address below.

This book is printed on acid-free paper.

MARCEL DEKKER, INC.
270 Madison Avenue, New York, New York 10016

Current printing (last digit):
10 9 8 7 6 5 4 3 2

Printed in the United States of America

Series Introduction

The current volume, *Handbook of Supportive Care in Cancer,* is the seventh in the Basic and Clinical Oncology series.

Many of the advances in oncology have resulted from close interaction among various disciplines within the field of medicine and related specialties. This volume follows and expands on this concept to illustrate the success of this relationship as demonstrated by new developments in the supportive care of the cancer patient. These advances have led to both improvements in outcome and a reduction in toxicity from our therapies, in part related to the appropriate use of hematopoietic growth factors and antibiotic support. There has also been a recognition of the importance of areas such as pain control, psychosocial oncology, and quality of life.

As editor of the series, my goal is to recruit volume editors who have not only established reputations based on their outstanding contributions to oncology, but also an appreciation for the dynamic interface between the laboratory and the clinic. To date, the series has consisted of monographs on topics that are of a high level of current interest; *Handbook of Supportive Care in Cancer* certainly fits into that category as a most important addition to the series.

Volumes in progress focus on the use of purine analogs in cancer therapy, the role of paclitaxel, and controversies in breast cancer. I anticipate that these volumes will provide a valuable contribution to the oncology literature.

Bruce D. Cheson

Preface

It is expected that the number of people afflicted with cancer will increase substantially over the next decades. However, it is not expected that significant progress in presently available antineoplastic therapies will take place rapidly enough to substantially alter their prognostic outlook. This is especially true for the vast number of middle-aged and elderly cancer patients with epithelial neoplasias, for whom truly curative therapeutic options are not, and in all likelihood will not be, available during the years to come. Even if the present boom in molecular biology and preclinical gene-therapy projects in the laboratory leads to real progress at the clinical level, it will take many years for significant prognostic gains to "pay off" in community oncology practice.

In other words, more patients in the near future will be receiving present-day, mostly intensive antineoplastic therapies from surgeons, radiotherapists, and medical oncologists, and at least half of them will finally die from various life-threatening complications of their ultimately "incurable" disease. These patients will often pass through a more or less prolonged phase of chronic cancer characterized not only by the manifestations of the illness itself, but by repeated episodes of side effects from various therapies. The emotional burden of the potentially fatal outcome, preceeded by episodes of mostly partial and transient remissions, as well as the progressive deterioration of physical and social capabilities, are additional reasons for concern. This reality, faced by too many of our adult cancer patients, is why we developed this text, *Handbook of Supportive Care in Cancer.*

Supportive care is difficult to define. It is the totality of medical, nursing, psychosocial, and rehabilitative support that our patients need from the onset of their disease through various active therapeutic phases for long-term cure—or until death. The scope of supportive care is therefore inevitably very wide and heterogeneous, as it encompasses care of cancer manifestations, prevention and management of therapeutic side effects, and psychological and spiritual support, in the broadest sense.

Supportive care is part of the management of cancer and other presently incurable diseases, such as chronic neurological diseases, AIDS, and so on. One could argue that *basic* supportive care is part of any general practitioner's, and at least practicing oncologist's, medical armamentarium: every internist and medical oncologist treats infections and other complications or manifestations of cancer or its therapies, diagnoses hypercalcemia, and provides pain therapy and some kind of psychosocial assistance.

Given the importance of supportive care (in many instances more than specific antineoplastic therapy itself), extensive clinical research and specialized teaching are necessary for its improvement and success, and require motivated specialists involved in active investigation, professionalization, and teaching of its various areas.

These areas are extremely heterogeneous and, as such, extremely challenging! Supportive care branches out to many subspecialties of the traditional medical and nursing care system and encompasses a broad and highly interesting variety of facets, such as those discussed in this book.

Supportive care differs considerably from palliative care, although these fields may overlap, and semantics may play a role. Palliation of symptoms, by either active prevention or therapeutic intervention, is certainly a main goal of any supportive care strategy. However, the term *palliative care*, as used today by its proponents and in the literature, is normally reserved for the approach to the terminal, and especially dying, patient. Thus, palliative care addresses only the "terminal" aspect (although clearly an important one) of the broad umbrella of supportive care, which is concerned with the optimal well-being of the cancer patient in all stages of this usually long and complicated disease.

Such a definition carries many practical difficulties, as it brings under a "common hat" many different specialties that differ considerably in approach, technique, and health care personnel. The infectious disease specialist might not be interested in pain control, and the nurse providing stomach care might not necessarily be attentive to research on bisphosphonates in patients with osteolytic bone metastases. Nevertheless, all these approaches are applicable to a patient with neoplastic disease, be it limited or extensive, early or late, curable or not! A common—interdisciplinary and multiprofessional—forum is thus necessary to bridge these various aspects, all of which have one common aim: comprehensive supportive care in cancer.

Early attempts to bring together on a multiprofessional level those who are interested in oncological supportive care have been made through various international meetings during the last eight years in Switzerland, Belgium, and the United States. These meetings have been attended by hundreds of doctors, oncology nurses, and other health care workers interested in cancer patients' well-being. References to the publication of the main lectures of these "pioneer" meetings are given in this book.

Another constructive step was taken in 1991 by creating a new interdisciplinary society, the Multinational Association of Supportive Care in Cancer (MASCC). MASCC aims to provide the common ground on which people with different expertise and interest meet with the basic goal of improving supportive care in cancer through mutual education and common research. MASCC plans to achieve its goals by organizing annual supportive care symposia (the last ones in February 1993, in St. Gallen, Switzerland, and in March 1994, in New Orleans), where specialized and also more general information will be exchanged at an international, multiprofessional level. MASCC has also created its own official journal, *Supportive Care in Cancer*, which is open to important contributions from any field of supportive care in oncology.

Finally, the board of the young and dynamic MASCC society and several additional international experts felt the need to publish an authoritative handbook on supportive care in cancer. This textbook should complete the educational structures already available for scientific and professional interaction and cooperation in this essential field of cancer medicine. The chapters were provided by internationally known experts, who have attempted to cover all relevant aspects of supportive care in cancer, mainly from the viewpoint of medical oncology and oncology nursing.

The text is designed to be comprehensive in scope, yet didactic and directly useful to the health care practitioner. We have attempted to make it useful for oncologists, surgeons, and general physicians, as well as for nurses, psychologists, social workers, pharmacists, or other providers who work daily with cancer patients. We have covered the most frequent and life-threatening problems in greater detail (e.g., infection, metabolic derangements), and given attention to areas often not addressed (e.g., sexual adjustments to cancer and its therapy).

It is our hope, and that of all the dedicated authors of this handbook, that our message cuts across the traditional professional boundaries of specialized care in cancer, in order to truly optimize comprehensive supportive care for all cancer patients.

Jean Klastersky
Stephen C. Schimpff
Hans-Jörg Senn

Contents

Contributors

Jean-Jacques Body, M.D., Ph.D. Associate Professor, Department of Medicine, Institut Jules Bordet, Université Libre de Bruxelles, Brussels, Belgium

D. Bron, M.D., Ph.D. Associate Professor, Department of Hematology, Institut Jules Bordet, Université Libre de Bruxelles, Brussels, Belgium

Albano Del Favero Associate Professor, Institute of Internal Medicine I, University of Perugia, Perugia, Italy

M. Dicato, M.D. Head, Department of Hematology-Oncology, Centre Hospitalier de Luxembourg, Luxembourg

C. Duhem, M.D. Department of Hematology-Oncology, Centre Hospitalier de Luxembourg, Luxembourg

Kenji Eguchi, M.D. Head, Department of Internal Medicine, National Cancer Center Central Hospital, Tokyo, Japan

David S. Ettinger, M.D. Professor, Department of Medical Oncology, Johns Hopkins Oncology Center, Baltimore, Maryland

Ronald Feld, M.D., F.R.C.P.C. Deputy Chief, Department of Medicine, Ontario Cancer Institute, Princess Margaret Hospital, Toronto, Ontario, Canada

Rebecca S. Finley, Pharm. D., M.S. Associate Professor, Department of Pharmacy Practice and Science, University of Maryland School of Pharmacy, and University of Maryland Cancer Center, Baltimore, Maryland

James G. Gallagher, M.D., Ph.D. Clinical Professor of Medicine, Jefferson Medical College, Philadelphia, and Department of Hematology-Oncology, Geisinger Clinic, Danville, Pennsylvania

Arnold Ganser, M.D., Ph.D. Senior Lecturer, Division of Hematology, Department of Medicine, Johann-Wolfgang Goethe University, Frankfurt, Germany

Agnes Glaus, R.N., M.Sc. Head Nurse, Medizinische Klinik C, Kantonsspital, St. Gallen, Switzerland

Gertrude Grahn, Ph.D., RNT Senior Lecturer, Care Research Unit, Lund University, Lund, Sweden

Stuart A. Grossman, M.D. Associate Professor of Oncology, Medicine, and Neurosurgery, and Director, Neuro-Oncology, Johns Hopkins Oncology Center, Baltimore, Maryland

Jerzy G. Hildebrand, M.D., Ph.D. Professor, Department of Neurology, Hôpital Erasme, Université Libre de Bruxelles, Brussels, Belgium

Anders Hyltander, M.D., Ph.D. Department of Surgery, Sahlgrenska University Hospital, Göteborg, Sweden

Debra Broadwell Jackson, Ph.D., R.N., E.T. Professor, Department of Health Science, Clemson University College of Nursing, Clemson, South Carolina

Jean Klastersky, M.D., Ph.D. Chief, Department of Medicine, and Professor of Medicine, Oncology, and Physical Diagnosis, Institut Jules Bordet, Université Libre de Bruxelles, Brussels, Belgium

J. Norelle Lickiss, M.D., F.R.A.C.P., F.R.C.P.E. Associate Professor, Royal Prince Alfred Hospital, Sydney, New South Wales, Australia

Kent Lundholm, M.D., Ph.D. Professor, Department of Surgery, Sahlgrenska University Hospital, Göteborg, Sweden

Ursula S. Ofman, Psy.D. Clinical Psychologist, Psychiatry Service, Memorial Sloan-Kettering Cancer Center, New York, New York

C. Daniel Overholser, Jr., D.D.S., M.S.D. Professor and Chairman, Department of Oral Medicine, School of Dentistry, and Associate Professor of Oncology, School of Medicine, University of Maryland at Baltimore, Baltimore, Maryland

Darius Razavi, M.D. Head, Psycho-Oncology and Rehabilitation Unit, Service de Médecine Interne et Laboratoire d'Investigation Clinique H. J. Tagnon, Institut Jules Bordet, Université Libre de Bruxelles, Brussels, Belgium

F. Ries, M.D. Physician, Department of Hematology-Oncology, Centre Hospitalier de Luxembourg, Luxembourg

Fausto Roila, M.D. Vice-Director, Division of Medical Oncology, Policlinico Hospital, Perugia, Italy

Rolf Sandström, M.D. Department of Surgery, Sahlgrenska University Hospital, Göteborg, Sweden

Stephen C. Schimpff, M.D. Executive Vice President, University of Maryland Medical System, and Professor of Medicine, Oncology, and Pharmacology, University of Maryland Medical Center, Baltimore, Maryland

Louis E. Schroder, M.D. Associate Professor, Division of Hematology-Oncology, Department of Internal Medicine, University of Cincinnati Medical Center, Cincinnati, Ohio

Daniel A. Scott, M.D. Head, Clinical and Field Evaluation, Enteric Diseases Program, Naval Medical Research Institute, Bethesda, Maryland

Jean-Paul Sculier, M.D. Chief of Intensive Care, Department of Medicine, Institut Jules Bordet, Université Libre de Bruxelles, Brussels, Belgium

William J. Slichenmyer, M.D. Senior Clinical Fellow, Department of Medical Oncology, Johns Hopkins Oncology Center, Baltimore, Maryland

Friedrich Stiefel, M.D. Palliative Care Unit, Department of Hematology-Oncology, Kantonsspital, St. Gallen, Switzerland

Martin H. N. Tattersall, M.D., M.Sc. Professor of Cancer Medicine, University of Sydney, Sydney, New South Wales, Australia

Bert Thürlimann, M.D. Department of Internal Medicine C, Division of Oncology-Hematology, Kantonsspital, St. Gallen, Switzerland

Maurizio Tonato, M.D. Director, Division of Medical Oncology, Policlinico Hospital, Perugia, Italy

David A. Van Echo, M.D. Clinical Director, University of Maryland Cancer Center, and University of Maryland, Baltimore, Maryland

Nicholas J. Vogelzang, M.D. Professor of Medicine, Section of Hematology-Oncology, University of Chicago, Chicago, Illinois

David G. Warr, M.D., F.R.C.P.C. Staff Physician, Department of Medicine, Ontario Cancer Institute, Princess Margaret Hospital, Toronto, Ontario, Canada

1

Therapy of Infections in Cancer Patients

Jean Klastersky
Institut Jules Bordet, Université Libre de Bruxelles, Brussels, Belgium

I. APPROACH TO FEVER IN CANCER PATIENTS

Fever has long been associated with malignancy and remains a common problem in cancer patients. With the advent of cytotoxic therapy, fever in the cancer patient has been closely linked with infection, especially when the patient is granulocytopenic. Because fever can be the only sign of infection in neutropenic patients, it appearance commands a series of diagnostic and therapeutic measures, to be taken empirically, that is, without precise knowledge of the nature and cause of the infection (1). This approach is quite different from that usually recommended to deal with fever in nonneutropenic patients; under these more current circumstances, it is important, first, to decide whether fever is caused by infection or another process; then, the site of the infection the offending pathogen are sought through a series of microbiological techniques. Finally, when a precise clinical and microbiological diagnosis is available, the choice of therapy can be made on rational grounds. Of course, depending on the acuteness of the disease, these diagnostic steps can be accelerated, and occasionally, presumptive therapy is also prescribed in nonneutropenic patients.

If the diagnostic work-up is negative and fever persists for more than 7 days, it is customary to speak about fever of unknown origin (FUO). A series of other diagnostic considerations, as discussed later, is then considered.

The pattern of fever is usually unimportant for making a causal diagnosis; in cancer patients, as in those without malignancies, fever is usually the consequence of infection; as a matter of fact, in patients with neoplasms, series of factors predisposes these patients to infection and decreases their resistance to it.

Fever can be caused by the cancer itself, however, through tumor-related necrosis, hemorrhage, or pyrogens; this is definitely a less common cause of pyrexia than infection, with the possible exception of certain tumors, such as Hodgkin's lymphoma. Because the direct causal relationship between the tumor and the fever is rarely obvious, these pyrexias are often considered FUOs (2).

Finally, fever in cancer patients can be caused by any disease, unrelated to infection or cancer, that can affect noncancer patients; here also, if the causal relationship is unclear, the differential diagnosis of FUOs is to be undertaken; moreover, one must stress that cancer patients are often exposed to various medical interventions that can be responsible, directly or not, for fever (Table 1).

A. Fever Caused by Infection

Here we distinguish between fever that occurs during neutropenia and that in nonneutropenic patients. Acute fever in nonneutropenic cancer patients, if clinical signs suggest infection, should not be managed differently from that in patients without cancer, with special attention to a possible relief of cancer-caused obstruction of natural passages. There are several examples of such infections caused by obstructions, including pneumonia in bronchial cancer and cholangitis in pancreatic carcinoma. Obstruction is also frequently responsible for relapses of infection after successful therapy. Various techniques are available for relief of such obstructions: laser for ear, nose, and throat (ENT) or bronchial tumor, tube or stint in cystic duct or ureters, and others.

Table 1 Fever in Cancer Patients

Infection
Bacterial
Fungal
Viral
Protozoal
Tumor
Necrosis
Hemorrhage
Pyrogens
Obstruction → infection
Other causes
Unrelated to cancer
Related to the tumor or its therapy

In neutropenic patients, the pyrexial episode requires prompt intervention on an empirical basis, as discussed later. Neutropenia and fever should be clearly defined using such criteria as those employed by the Immunocompromised Host Society (3). One example of fever is an oral temperature >38.5°C once or >38°C on two or more occasions during a 12 h period. The major risk for acute bacterial infections occurs when the polymorphonuclear leukocytes (PMN) <500/mm^3. However, patients presenting with >500 but <1000 PMN/mm^3 and whose counts are anticipated to fall below 500/mm^3 within 24–48 h because of antecedent therapy are also at risk. Any analysis should separately evaluate patients with <100 PMN/mm^3.

Neutropenia predisposes to severe and rapidly progressing infection by bacterial and fungal pathogens; it also interferes with the usual clinical manifestations of sepsis. Therefore, empirical therapy has become an accepted practice and has been designed to cover the most likely pathogens, namely gram-negative rods, and especially *Pseudomonas aeruginosa* in the earliest studies. Of course, besides these "microbiologically defined infections," in some patients no microbiological or clinical cause for the infection is found (unexplained fever); in others, only clinical clues lead to a presumptive diagnosis of infection (clinically defined infection). The criteria for these categories have been established (3) and are widely accepted. In Table 2, the proportion of microbiologically documented and clinically defined infections and that of unexplained fevers is indicated, as observed in recent European Organization for Treatment and Research of Cancer (EORTC) trials.

As can be seen in Table 3, during the past two decades, we have witnessed a progressive reduction in gram-negative infections and a gradual rise in gram positives, namely those caused by *Staphylococcus epidermidis* and the streptococci.

Although gram negatives represent today only 31% of the pathogens responsible for sepsis in granulocytopenic patients, these infections can be fulminant:

Table 2 Infection Documentation in International Antimicrobial Therapy Cooperative Group (IATCG) Trials VIII and IX

Microbiologically defined	
Bacteremia	314(24%)
Bacterial-nonbacteremic	61(5%)
Viral	12(1%)
Fungal	23(2%)
Mixed	8(0.5%)
Clinically defined	332(26%)
Unexplained fever	493(38%)
Fever not related to infection	47(3.5%)
Total	1290

Table 3 Microbiological Nature of Febrile Neutropenia: Single-Organism Bacteremia in EORTC Trials

	I (1973–1978)	II (1978–1980)	III (1980–1983)	IV (1983–1986)	V (1986–1988)	VIII (1989–1991)
Single-organism bacteremias/ number of febrile episodes (%)	145/453 (32%)	115/419 (27%)	141/582 (24%)	219/872 (25%)	213/749 (28%)	151/694 (22%)
Gram-negative bacteremias (%)	103 (71%)	74 (64%)	83 (59%)	129 (59%)	78 (37%)	47 (31%)
Gram-positive bacteremias (%)	42 (29%)	37 (36%)	58 (41%)	90 (41%)	135 (63%)	104 (69%)

that is, if *P. aeruginosa* is involved. Empirical therapy of febrile neutropenia thus takes a broad-spectrum coverage against gram negatives. If neutropenia is severe and expected to be prolonged, a combination of a cephalosporine with an aminoglycoside is superior to single-drug therapy (4); the EORTC group recently successfully used ceftazidime or ceftriaxone with amikacin. Because the aminoglycoside carries a risk of ototoxicity and/or nephrotoxicity, especially when other toxic agents are used, it should not be continued beyond 48–72 h unless microbiological data strongly support its use.

The question of whether the gram positives should be covered from the start is as yet unsettled. Most studies used vancomycin or teicoplanin. Some authors claim that staphylococcal infections are quite indolent and carry a very low mortality rate and thus do not require empirical therapy before their microbiological documentation; others have stressed the high morbidity and serious mortality (±15%) of streptococcal infections (5) and recommend either prophylaxis or empirical therapy under circumstances in which streptococcal infection is a major threat.

Fungal infection can be documented in 5% of patients as the cause of the initial febrile neutropenia; this figure has not changed much over the years. It is obvious that bacterial and fungal sepsis can coexist and that the bacteremia may overshadow the more difficult to document fungal infection; the latter manifests itself as a persisting or recurring fever after the eradication of bacteremia by empirically prescribed antibiotics. This explains why it has become accepted to administer empirically amphotericin B to those granulocytopenic patients who remain febrile after a few days of broad-spectrum antimicrobial therapy and in whom no bacteria can be documented (6). As neutropenia persists, the risk of fungal infection increases; many fevers in patients with prolonged neutropenia are caused by fungi.

Viral infection is uncommonly diagnosed in neutropenic patients without concomitant immunosuppression as occurs after bone marrow transplantation. Herpes simplex virus causes fever quite early after bone transplantation, during the neutropenic episode; in most centers involved in bone marrow transplantations, prophylactic acyclovir is administered to prevent these infections (7). Cytomegalovirus (CMV) causes infection that, in cancer patients at least, most often manifests itself as a diffuse interstitial pneumonitis; these infections usually occur once the patient is no longer neutropenic although still severely immunosuppressed. Fever under these circumstances, especially if associated with pulmonary symptoms, is an indication for bronchoalveolar lavage (BAL) and subsequent therapy based on the findings; if BAL is not available or feasible, CMV and *Pneumocystis carinii* should both be covered with ganciclovir and co-trimoxazole (sulfamethoxazole and trimethoprime), respectively. Actually, in many centers handling bone marrows transplanted patients, it has become customary to perform BAL 30 days after the transplant even in asymptomatic patients and, if positive for CMV, to treat the patient at that point (8). An overall algorithm for the management of febrile neutropenia is presented in Table 4.

Table 4 Guidelines for the Diagnostic and Therapeutic Approach to Febrile Episodes in Granulocytopenic Patients[a]

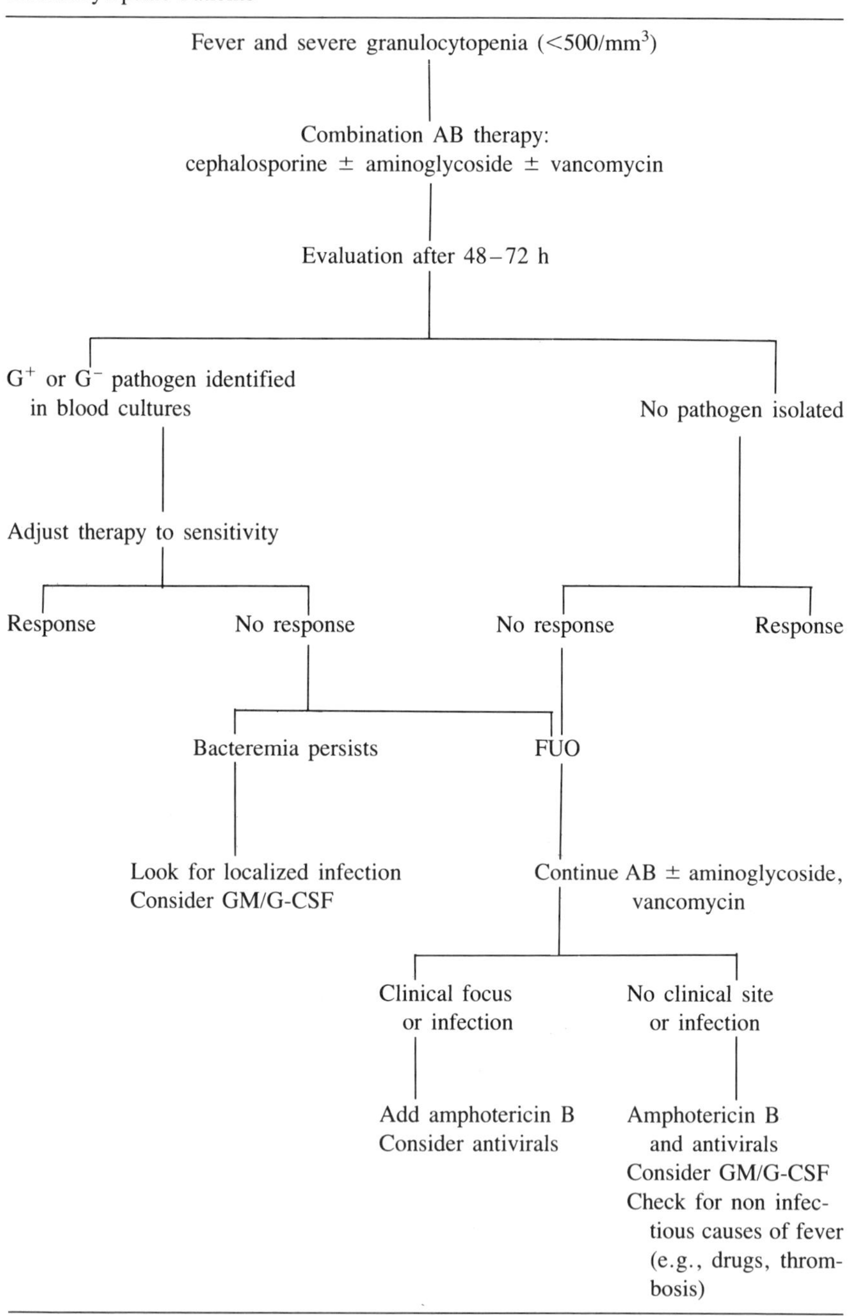

[a]AB, antibiotic; G$^+$, gram positive; G$^-$, gram negative.

B. Fever Caused by Cancer

Neoplasms are reported as an important cause of fever in most reviews (2,9); however, all are not caused by the neoplasm itself, since the tumor predisposes directly or indirectly to local or systemic infection, which is actually the real cause of fever in most cases. Obstruction and neutropenia are among the most important cancer-related or cancer treatment-related factors that predispose to infection.

Fever caused by the tumor itself was rarely found in neutropenics, among a pediatric and young adult patient population, most of whom had leukemia or lymphoma. On the other hand, in the same study, the underlying malignancy could be implicated in 25% of fevers in nongranulocytopenic solid tumor patients. This was especially notable in patients with Ewing's sarcoma and neuroblastoma (10).

Two studies were reported on FUO in cancer patients, most of whom were not neutropenic throughout the course of pyrexia. In one study, among 36 patients, 18 patients had infections, and in the other 18 patients only the neoplasm appeared to be responsible for the fever (11); in the other report, in 47 patients, infection caused the fever in 27 (57%) and pyrexia was attributed to the cancer itself in 18 (38%) (12). The data are summarized in Table 5. It can be seen that in patients with underlying lymphomas, the tumor was responsible for prolonged

Table 5 Noninfectious Febrile Episodes Caused by the Underlying Cancer

Lymphoma	18/26 (69%)	
Hodgkin's disease		12/18
Non-Hodgkin's lymphoma		6/8
Leukemia	5/29 (17%)	
Acute lymphocytic		3/7
Acute granulocytic		2/13
Chronic lymphocytic		0/4
Chronic granulocytic		0/5
Solid tumors	13/28 (46%)	
Breast		7/12 (58%)
Head and neck[a]		2/5
Lung		0/4
Gynecological tract[b]		2/3
Rhabdomyosarcoma		1/1
Melanoma		0/1
Kidney		1/1
Prostate		0/1

Source: From References 11 and 12.
[a]Cancer of larynx, 3; esophagus, 1; thyroid, 1.
[b]Cancer of cervix, 1; vulva, 1; uterus, 1.

fever in 69% but was the cause for only 17% among the leukemics, who were usually neutropenic.

A variety of solid tumors were also responsible for FUO; the number in each category are small, and no firm conclusions can be made. It is nevertheless interesting to note that fever caused by the tumor was found in 7 of 12 patients with breast cancer (58%) but in only 2 of 9 of those with pulmonary or head and neck tumors (22%). Tumor-associated fever was reported with some frequency in breast cancer (0.7%) and was found to be associated with progressive and widely disseminated disease; it disappeared in patients whose neoplasia responded to therapy.

A striking feature of the patients with neoplastic fever in the two series already mentioned was also the extension and progressive nature of the underlying neoplasm: all the lymphomas presented visceral involvement or new nodes; all the cases of leukemia were in relapse or during the first evolutive stage; and solid tumors were widely metastatic and were often associated with extensive liver metastases.

Liver involvement as a cause of neoplastic fever was reported in the past; the mechanism of the production of fever by liver metastases is unknown, however.

Why lymphomas, renal carcinoma, and some other tumors produce fever is unclear; although it is often stated that inflammation and necrosis of tumors explain the pyrexia in most patients with neoplastic fever, it appears that such an explanation is not valid in many patients. In particular, in Hodgkin's disease, neoplastic fever is usually seen in patients with nodular sclerosis lymphoma. Nevertheless, fever is probably mediated in these cases by the same cytokines as in other pyrexias. Endogenous pyrogen (interleukin-1) production has been suspected in febrile patients with Hodgkin's disease; how and why these substances are produced remain to be discovered.

It is quite difficult to be certain that a fever is caused only by a neoplasia; the diagnosis rests, in most cases, on the absence of demonstration of an infection or other pyrogenic process. Clinical characteristics may be useful to separate between infectious and neoplastic fevers; the infected patient is often ill, or even toxic, with chills, tachycardia, and possible hypotension. In fever related to neoplasia, chills and tachycardia are lacking or minimal; the patient may feel quite well and be unaware of the pyrexia, which is often intermittent. These criteria are not sufficient in most cases, however, to make a firm diagnosis.

Although the rapidity of microbiological diagnosis of infection is constantly improving, it still may take time, and as a matter of fact, many febrile patients with cancer, especially if neutropenia is present, are treated presumptively with antibiotics for a hidden infection.

Others have proposed the use of antiinflammatory agents to make the differential diagnosis between infectious and neoplastic causes. Aspirin and acetaminophen have little effect on fevers caused by a malignant tumor. On the other hand, it has been reported that indomethacin dramatically and completely eliminates such fevers. More recently, naproxen was found very effective for such purposes; a prompt and complete lysis of fever was obtained in 20 patients within 12 h, and was maintained with adequate doses (13). Based on these observations, the "naproxen test" (three doses of 375 mg naproxen at 12 h intervals) has been proposed for the diagnosis of neoplastic fever; it should result in complete lysis of pyrexia, and the patient should experience sustained normal temperature while receiving naproxen. However, the claim that fevers caused by infections, allergic drug reactions, and/or collagen diseases do not respond to naproxen should be supported by prospective and comparative studies on adequate numbers of patients. It is clear that naproxen and other similar agents can control fever in patients for which no other cause than the tumor itself can be found. Whether this effect is really specific and thus can be used as a diagnostic tool remains to be proven.

C. Noninfectious Nonneoplastic Causes of Fever in Cancer Patients

Persistent fevers, which are related neither to infection nor to cancer, usually belong to the variety of FUOs. The spectrum of FUO has not changed significantly over the last 40 years. Besides infections and neoplasms, which are the two most common causes of FUO, multisystemic diseases (systemic lupus erythematosis, Still's disease, temporal arteritis and other vasculitis, granulomatous diseases, and others) account for 10–20% of the cases in several studies (2,9). Drug-related fevers and factitious pyrexias are reported in 1–3 and 3–5%, respectively.

Miscellaneous causes are found in approximately 15% of patients; this is a complex group of rare diseases that can be occasionally associated with persistent fevers, including aortic or arterial aneurysm, emboli, atrial myxoma, thrombophlebitis, familial Mediterranean fevers, and allergic reactions (Table 6).

No diagnosis is reported in 10–25% of the cases; in this respect, it is important to emphasize that fevers of uncertain etiology that persist for extremely prolonged periods of time carry a different type of differential diagnosis (14). FUO of more than 1 year duration is rarely caused by infection or lymphoma, but it is associated more often with granulomatous disease, such as granulomatous hepatitis, Crohn's disease, or a hidden neoplasm, such as colonic carcinoma.

Studies that specifically considered the problem of fever in cancer patients that was unrelated to cancer or infection found that such a situation was not a major diagnostic problem. Among 47 patients with undiagnosed fevers, we found only 2 patients whose pyrexia was not related to infection or the tumor itself; 1 had a pulmonary fibrosis from busulfan administration and 1 had multiple pulmonary emboli (12). In another study, in 36 patients with cancer and

Table 6 Causes of FUOs (%)

	1961	1973	1982	1984	1992
Infection	36	34	30	31	23
Neoplasm	20	19	31	18	7
Multisystemic disease	17	10	10	14	21
Drug related	1	1	0	0	3
Factitious	3	3	3	4	3
Miscellaneous[a]	15	9	8	10	17
No diagnosis	9	25	16	22	26
Total numbers	100	80	105	133	199

Source: From References 2 and 9.
[a]For example, aneurysm, emboli, Crohn's disease, atrial myxoma, Mediterranean fever, and thyroiditis.

prolonged fever, all fevers could be explained by infection or the tumor itself (11).

Acute fevers that are not directly related to the tumor or caused by infection appear to be more common in cancer patients. In a prospective study of 1001 febrile episodes in patients with cancer, Pizzo et al. found that nearly 50% of such episodes, at least in nongranulocytopenic cancer patients, were unrelated to infection or to the underlying malignancy. They believed that the most common designation for these episodes was that associated with administration of chemotherapy (10). Since most patients received combination chemotherapy, the responsible drug(s) were difficult to assign. In addition, a few febrile episodes were related to transfusions. That study was performed in children and young adults with cancer; it is possible that in older patients, similar febrile episodes could have been related to a broader spectrum of diseases or events; however, no objective data are available (Table 7).

D. Protracted Fevers in Cancer Patients

Persistent fever (FUO) after recovery from granulocytopenia in acute leukemia was found to be 15% among 168 patients; fungal infections were the most common cause (9 of 26 patients) (15). A common late infection during the course of protracted granulocytopenia, as seen in aggressively treated hematological patients, is hepatosplenic candidiasis. These patients have prolonged fevers that do not respond to antibiotics; they are usually in the process of recovering from prolonged and severe neutropenia. Quite characteristic are the multiple hepatic and splenic abscesslike lesions (ultrasound and/or computed tomographic, CT, scan) from which the microorganisms can occasionally be cultured (16). As

Table 7 Distribution of Febrile Episodes Following Initial Evaluation According to the Patient's Granulocyte Count

	Fever	
	Without granulocytopenia	With granulocytopenia
Total episodes	208	793
Infectious	17%	52%[a]
Noninfectious	70%[b]	—
Unexplained	13%	48%

Source: Adapted from Pizzo et al. (10).
[a]Of these, 27% were microbiologically documented.
[b]Of these, 16% were cancer, 46% chemotherapy, 1% transfusion, and 7% post-operative.

already mentioned, others have studied prolonged fevers of uncertain origin in cancer patients, some of whom, but not all, were granulocytopenic. Luft et al. (11) found that 18 of 36 patients with FUO had fever caused by infection; of the 12 patients whose infection could be microbiologically documented, 9 were caused by fungi. Klastersky et al. (12) found infection as the cause of prolonged fever of uncertain etiology in 27 of 47 cancer patients; fungal infections were documented in 5.

These findings are summarized in Table 8. Although such a retrospective analysis implies some simplifications, it can be seen that abscesses and pneumonias were the most common clinical presentations. Abscesses were mainly intraabdominal and associated with cancer, surgery, and rectal or disseminated infections. Gram-negative bacilli predominated, but cultures often revealed mixed infections with gram positives, bacteroides, and occasionally herpes simplex virus (HSV).

Pneumonia was the next most common cause of prolonged fever in cancer patients; of 17 cases, 7 were caused by fungi 1 and by CMV, and in the others, the diagnosis was not microbiologically documented. This leaves the possibility that some of these pneumonias were not caused by infectious agents or were caused by pathogens that are difficult to isolate, such as viruses, fungi, or protozoans.

It should be pointed out that some series reviewed here were evaluated before the extensive practice of bone marrow transplantation and before the advent of modern diagnostic tools, such as the CT scan, magnetic resonance imaging, and various sophisticated microbiological procedures. Nevertheless, the frequency of fungal infection in cancer patients with protracted fevers is high enough to recommend the empirical use of antifungal agents when bacterial, viral, or protozoal infections have been reasonably ruled out (Table 9). This applies mainly

Table 8 Persistent Fever in Cancer Patients

	Bacteria			Fungi			Viruses				
Sites of infection	G^+	G^-	TB	*Candida* sp.	*Aspergillus* sp.	Others	HSV	CMV	Others	Presumed infections	Total
Endocarditis or catheter related	4										4
Disseminated infection		1		3		3[a]					7
Abscesses	2	12	1[b]	2			1[c]			4	22
Pneumonia				1	5	1		1		9	17
Urinary tract infection		1		1							2
Gastrointestinal (GI) infection		1							1[d]	4	6
Meningitis						1[e]					1
ENT infection							1			1	2
Arthritis-osteomyelitis	1					1[f]					2
Total	7	15	1	7	5	6	2	1	1	18	63

[a]Histoplasmosis (disseminated).
[b]Tuberculous (TB) pericarditis.
[c]Herpetic perirectal cellulitis.
[d]Non-A, non-B heptatitis
[e]Cryptococcal meningitis.
[f]Sporotrichosis (arthritis).
Source: Adapted from References 11, 12, and 15.

Table 9 Fever in Nonneutropenic Cancer Patients Without Clinical Documentation

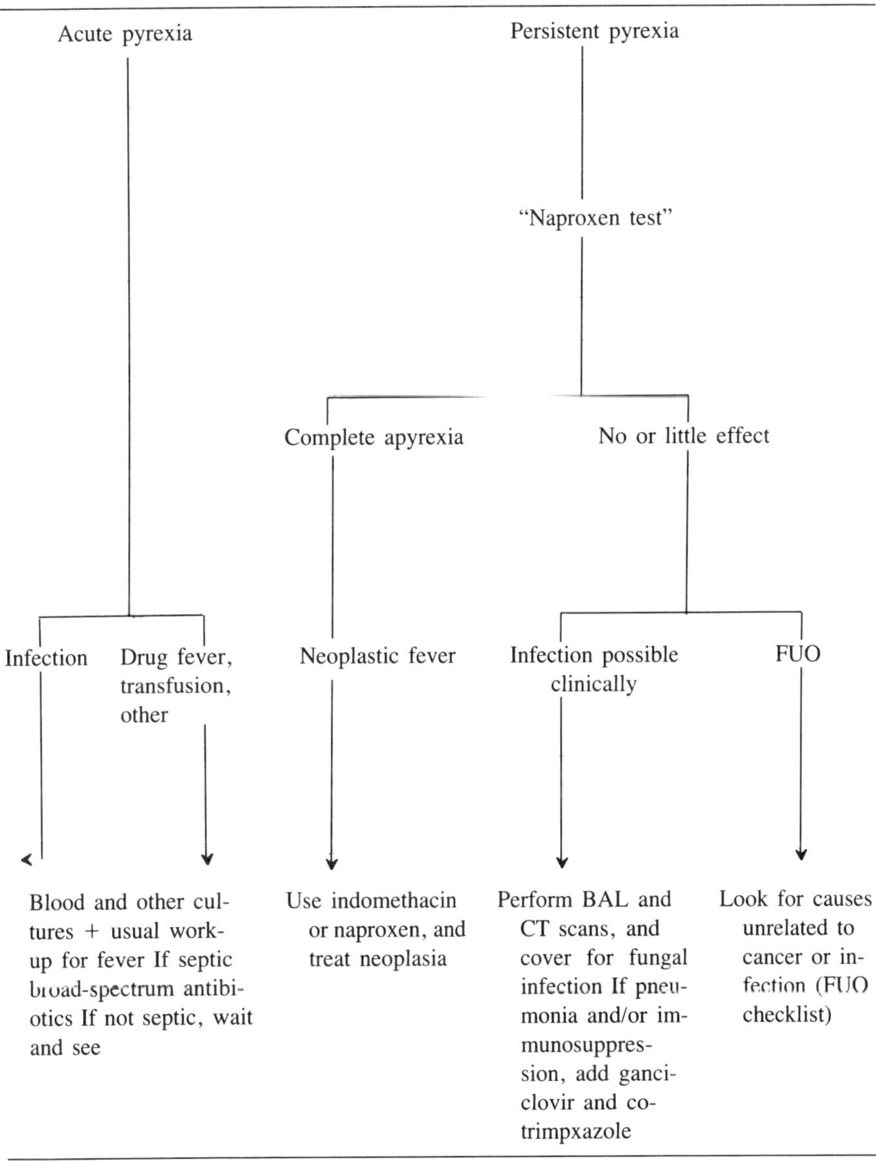

to cases without clinical or radiobiological documentation; if a likely focus for infection (abscess or pneumonia) is detected, it should be aggressively approached to look for a specific diagnosis.

E. Role of Colony-Stimulating Factors in Cancer Chemotherapy

Granulocyte colony-stimulating factor (G-CSF) and granulocyte-macrophage colony-stimulating factor (GM-CSF) are hematopoietic growth factors now available commercially for use in patients. The predominant effects of G-CSF are to stimulate the survival, proliferation, differentiation, and function of neutrophil granulocyte precursors and/or mature cells. GM-CSF acts not only on cells of the neutrophil lineage but also on cells of the eosinophil and monocyte-macrophage lineages. The distinctive properties of each agent were recently reviewed (17,18).

The hematological effects of G-CSF and GM-CSF alone in cancer patients were recently reviewed (19) and provide a basis for understanding their effects when used in conjunction with chemotherapeutic agents. An illustration of the hematological effects of postchemotherapy CSF come from a U.S. study of G-CSF given in a preventive manner, commencing the day after a 3 day chemotherapy regimen for small cell lung cancer and continuing for 14 days (20). The effects of shortening the duration of neutropenia and elevating the nadir neutrophil level persisted throughout six cycles of chemotherapy.

Similar effects of preventive postchemotherapy with GM-CSF on neutrophil levels after chemotherapy have been described. GM-CSF also elevates eosinophil levels during leukocyte recovery. Platelet levels have appeared reduced in some studies of postchemotherapy GM-CSF, but this has not clearly been of clinical significance.

Although these effects on neutrophil levels are expected to correlate with reduced risk of infection, it is important to demonstrate that these hematological effects of CSFs indeed translate into clinical benefits. This is because it is likely that, in addition to neutrophil numbers, other aspects of neutrophil function that CSFs modulate, such as their state of activation and mobility, are also important in determining whether there is overall clinical benefit or detriment. Differences in local practices regarding prophylactic antibiotic usage, indications for admission of the febrile neutropenic patient, use of oral antimicrobial agents for the empirical treatment of febrile neutropenic patients, and policies for cessation of parenteral antibiotics and hospital discharge of these patients may also be important.

The clinical benefits of preventive G-CSF were demonstrated in a randomized placebo-controlled double-blind study. G-CSF reduced the incidence of febrile neutropenic events in cycle 1 and over six cycles by approximately 50%, and GM-CSF has also been evaluated in preventive schedules of administration. The results of these studies have been complicated by the fact that GM-CSF itself induces fever, which can be difficult to prospectively distinguish from the fever of infection.

Delayed preventive schedules of G-CSF administration were as effective in supporting neutrophil recovery as longer schedules, but the clinical applications of this approach have not been tested in large randomized blinded studies. With GM-CSF, one study found a delayed schedule to be inferior in supporting neutrophil levels. Concurrent administration of CSF and chemotherapy may paradoxically augment rather than reduce the myelotoxicity of some chemotherapeutic agents by inducing cycling of hematopoietic cells; this has been reported with both G-CSF and GM-CSF. The effects of preemptive CSF administration have not been fully evaluated, but it is possible that abrupt CSF withdrawal may temporarily stop CSF-stimulated hematopoietic cells from cycling, thereby protecting them from the myelotoxic effects of some chemotherapeutic agents. The value of a rescue G-CSF schedule, in which G-CSF administration is commenced at the time of onset of a febrile neutropenic episode along with empirical antibiotics, has been the subject of an Australian study, for which the results should soon be available.

II. BLOOD-BORNE INFECTIONS

A. Bacteremias Caused by Common Pathogens

Bacteremia is still the most common type of infection related to neutropenia in cancer patients; it is usually caused by common bacteria, such as the gram-negative enteric rods and *P. aeruginosa*. The clinical signs and symptoms, with the exception of fever, may be inconspicuous, and the initial site of infection is often not obvious because of the granulocytopenia, which reduces inflammatory reactions. The usual work-up for blood-borne infections, namely bacteremia, is summarized in Table 10.

The bacteremia can progress rapidly, especially if *P. aeruginosa* is involved, into vasomotor collapse and death; actually, *P. aeruginosa* kills at least 50% of infected neutropenic patients within 48 h after its first clinical manifestations if no effective therapy is prescribed on a presumptive basis. These observations constitute the rationale for the concept of empirical therapy in febrile neutropenic cancer patients.

A decade ago, gram-negative rod bacteremia was the most frequent serious infection in neutropenic patients with cancer. *Escherichia coli*, *Klesbsiella* species, and *P. aeruginosa* were the most common organisms, and overall, gram-negative rods were responsible for more than two-thirds of the bacteremic episodes in these patients. As already mentioned (Table 3), more recently gram-positive cocci have emerged as important agents of bacteremia in neutrope-

Table 10 Diagnostic Microbiological Work-up of Bacteremia, Fungemia, and Viremia in Immunocompromised Cancer Patients

	Remarks
Methods of proven efficacy	
Aerobic broth blood cultures (two to three samples at 30 minute intervals, 5 days of observation)	High volume and resin are better (at higher cost) Longer observation required for rare fastidious bacteria and *Histoplasma caspulatum*
Lysis-centrifugation blood culture	Best for yeasts and mycobacteria (high cost)
Anaerobic broth blood cultures	Restrict to high-risk patients (GI, gynecological, head and neck); aerobic bottle detects *Bacteroides fragilis* group and clostridia
Quantitative blood cultures through central catheter + peripheral vein samples (catheter-related infections)	For coagulase-negative staphylococci only (controversial for other pathogens)
Buffy coat culture for CMV (shell-vial) and direct immunofluorescence detection of CMV in polymorphonuclear leukocytes	In bone marrow and organ transplant patient (heavy workload)
Viral cultures in urine	
Blood culture of *Toxoplasma gondii*	
Methods of (yet) unproven efficacy	
Anitgen or characteristic metabolite detection for *Candida* and *Aspergillus* in serum	Low sensitivity
Antigen detection in urine (*Candida*)	Low sensitivity
PCR detection of *Candida* in whole blood	Few commercial kits

nic patients. Possibly, the mucositis associated with intensive chemotherapy or viral infections, the increasing use of Hickman or Broviac intravascular catheters and/or the administration of quinolone antibiotics as prophylactic agents make gram-positive cocci now responsible for most episodes of bacteremia in neutropenic patients.

Most gram-positive isolates in the past were either *Staphylococcus aureus* or *S. epidermidis*. In the past few years, other gram-positive cocci, including viridans streptococci, *Streptococcus mitis*, *Streptococcus pyogenes*, *Streptococcus pneumoniae*, and *Enterococcus* species, have emerged as major pathogens in bacteremic episodes. In the most recent EORTC trial in 747 patients, gram-positive cocci accounted for 64% of single-organism bacteremias. Although bacteremias caused by gram-positive cocci are clearly increasing in this population, the mortality associated with these organisms remains low (especially for *S. epidermidis* infections) and empirical therapy directed specifically at gram-positive bacteria is not recommended by most investigators unless there is a special incidence of breakthrough bacteremia or resistant organisms in a given institution. Others have reported serious morbidity and significant mortality from streptococcal bacteremia in neutropenic patients and recommend prophylaxis or early therapy.

The overall therapeutic strategy for the management of bacteremia has been already touched upon in the section on febrile neutropenia. As already stated, empirical therapy with broad-spectrum antibiotics is required in neutropenic patients with fever, 20–30% of whom eventually prove to be bacteremic. Once the microbe is isolated, therapy can be based on its sensitivity to antimicrobials. It has been shown that the bactericidal activity in the serum (SBA) is predictive of the outcome of gram-negative bacteremia in granulocytopenic patients (21); neutropenics require higher levels of SBA than nonneutropenic patients: a 1:16 active dilution is necessary to predict a 80% response rate during granulocytopenia, but a 1:8 dilution suffices in other patients. Thus, in theory, if a high SBA is achieved, the type of therapy, whether single drug or a combination, and the nature of the antimicrobial(s) used may be unimportant. However, the value of SBA does not reflect the rate of bacterial killing and, on the other hand, synergism, and thus multiple-drug therapy has been shown significant for the outcome of gram-negative bacteremia in severely neutropenic patients. In addition, our group has shown that full therapy with ceftazidime plus amikacin was superior to ceftazidime combined with a short (three doses) course of amikacin in patients with gram-negative bacteremia; the benefit of combination therapy, in this study, was confined to patients with severe and protracted neutropenia (4). These observations parallel those on synergism, in which benefit could be demonstrated only in patients with severe granulocytopenia. It is possible that the benefit of combination therapy is related to synergism, resulting in both increased SBA and more rapid killing. In patients with less severe neutropenia, or when granulocytopenia is expected to be of short duration, single-drug therapy is probably appropriate if the isolated pathogen is sensitive to it.

Of course, the use of aminoglycosides implies the risk of nephro- and ototoxicity, which is increased if other potentially toxic drugs (e.g., cyclosporine, amphotericin B, and vancomycin) are used at the same time. These situations require close supervision of the renal function and antibiotic serum levels; it also take clinical judgment in individual patients in deciding which risk is greatest. Most investigators probably agree to treat bacteremia caused by *P. aeruginosa* with combination therapy in all patients. Such an attitude may also appear sensible for other gram-negative bacillary bacteremias, as long as the patient remains severely neutropenic and/or until the clinical condition clearly stabilizes.

As far as gram-positive infections are concerned, once again, the in vitro sensitivity of the isolated pathogen commands the therapy to be prescribed. For *S. epidermidis*, which represents ±25% of the isolates, most strains are sensitive only to vancomycin or teicoplanin, which are the drugs of choice. There are no clear indications that one drug is superior to the other or that major differences in toxicity exist. However, most of the streptococci are sensitive to penicillin G and to many penicillin-related drugs. Thus, if no hypersensitivity exists, therapy is not a problem for infections caused by these organisms; nonetheless, if the patient is allergic to penicillins, vancomycin or teicoplanin remains the optimal choice. The drugs and their dosage, as used in the EORTC studies, are indicated in Table 11.

There are limited data on restrictive adjustments of therapy, once the offending pathogen is known. Most investigators agree that, if a patient is on both anti–gram-positive (vancomycin or teicoplanin) and anti–gram-negative coverage, the former can be discontinued if a gram-negative pathogen is isolated.

On the other hand, under the same conditions, if a gram-positive organism is isolated, one hesitates to discontinue anti–gram-negative coverage. Older studies showed that early discontinuation of such therapy in patients who remain febrile and granulocytopenic can lead to fulminant bacterial infection upon discontinuation of empirical therapy even if initially taken blood cultures remained negative (22). Of course, anti–gram-negative therapy can be simplified at that point, and in most cases, a single drug (ceftazidime, ceftriaxone, or imipenem) appears sufficient as a companion antibiotic to the anti–gram-positive coverage; the latter can be adapted to the nature and sensitivity of the isolated microorganism.

The algorithm shown in Table 12 will probably be helpful in most cases of

Table 11 Drugs Used at the Institut Jules Bordet and/or in the EORTC Protocols for the Management of Infections in Neutropenic Patients

Ceftazidime (Glazidim)	2 g three times per day IV
Imipenim (Tienam)	500 mg four times per day IV
Amikacin (Amikin)	20 mg/kg/day (maximum 1.5 g/day) in one dose
Ceftriaxone (Rocephin)	4 g once per day IV
Piperacillin-Tazobactam (Tazocin)	4 g four times per day IV
Vancomycin (Vancocin)	1 g/12 h
Amphotericin B (Fungizone)	1.2 mg/kg/day
Fluconazole (Diflucan)	200–400 mg/day
Acyclovir (Zovirax)	500 mg three times per day
Ganciclovir (Cymevene)	5 mg/kg/8 h
G-CCF (Neupogen)	5 gamma/kg/day

Table 12 Modification of Empirical Therapy According to Microbiological Results

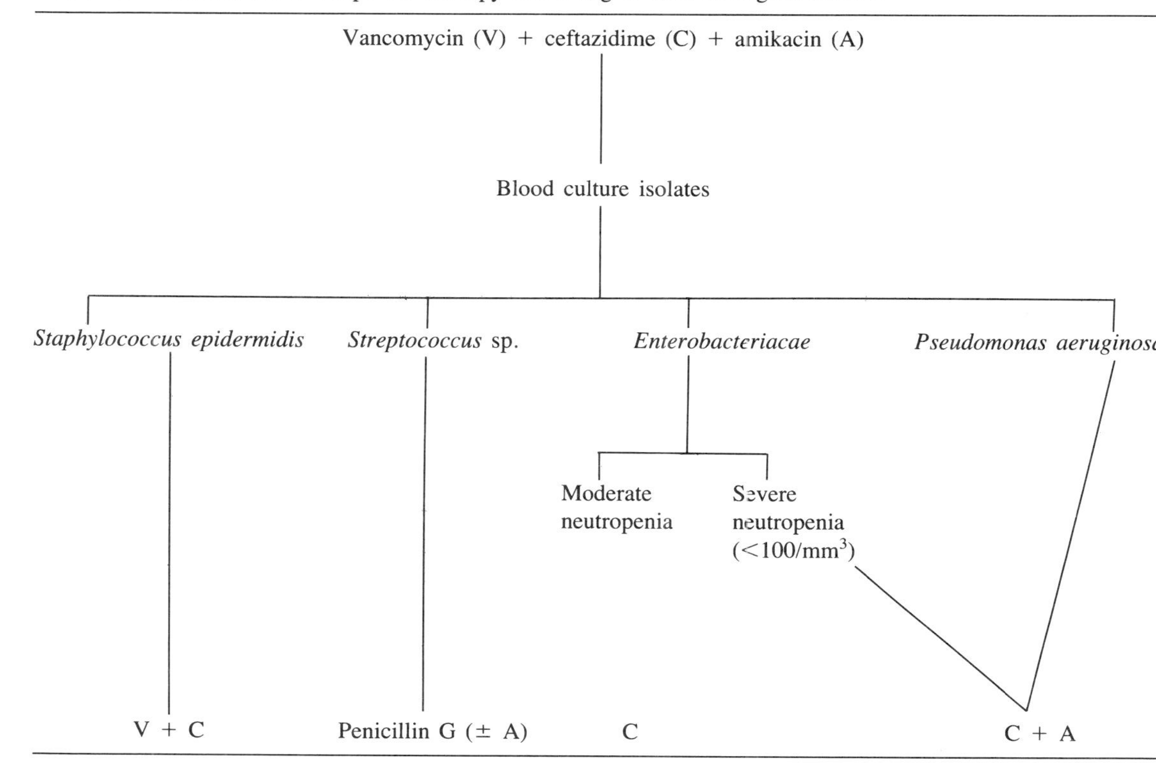

documented bacteremias occurring in neutropenic patients. It does not take into account the case of bacteremia caused by unusual microorganisms with unexpected sensitivities; in addition, the physician must consider the changes in susceptibility of more usual pathogens that often occur as the result of antibiotic pressure.

B. Bacteremias Caused by Opportunistic Pathogens

Isolated humoral immunity dysfunction has been associated with infections caused by encapsulated bacteria. Patients with multiple myeloma and hypogammaglobulinemia are more susceptible to *Pneumococcus* and *Haemophilus influenzae* infections. *Salmonella* infections are more severe in patients with impaired cellular immunity. This includes patients of extreme age, with malnutrition, malignancy, or acquired immune deficiency syndrome (AIDS), and those receiving corticosteroids or other immunosuppressive therapy. The incidence of salmonellosis over the past 16 years in our cancer patients was 0.8% of admissions. The number of cases per year ranged between 2 and 8, and all were sporadic cases. Although hematological malignancy accounted for 5–10% of admissions, 65% of *Salmonella* infections occurred in this category; major predisposing factors in cancer patients are the antineoplastic chemotherapy, antacids, and corticosteroids. Overall bacteremia occurs in 65% of cases, as opposed to 9% in the normal host. Despite in vitro susceptibility, third-generation cephalosporine therapy results in a high rate of failure, and fluoroquinolones constitute actually the first choice for salmonellosis.

Corynebacterium jekeium is a lipophilic saprophyte of the skin with a preferential colonization of the rectal, inguinal, and axillary areas. Colonization is associated with underlying malignancy, mainly hematological, long duration of hospitalization, and broad-spectrum antibiotic treatment. Septicemia develops in granulocytopenic patients with indwelling catheters. Infected perianal fissure and cellulitis of bone marrow biopsy or insertion of catheter sites have been reported as primary sources of septicemia. Secondary cutaneous lesions, rashes, necrotic lesions, or abscesses of soft tissue have also been described. *C. jekeium* is characterized by its high degree of resistance to antibiotics, such as penicillins and cephalosporines, but it is susceptible to glycopeptides; removal of the infected catheter and treatment with vancomycin constitute the optimal management of these infections.

Rothia dentocariosa, *Capnocytophaga* species, and *Eikenella corrodens* are part of the mouth flora. Bacteremia in granulocytopenic patients with oral mucositis or ulcerations has been reported with these organisms.

In the past 5 years, several other bacteria have emerged as new causes of infection in neutropenic and nonneutropenic patients with cancer. *Xanthomonas maltophilia* is increasing as a cause of nosocomial infections in these patients and may be resistant to multiple antibiotics; trimethoprim-sulfamethoxazole and some of the new fluoroquinolones may be effective. *Pseudomonas putrefaciens* (*Alteromonas putrefaciens*) is a nonglucose-fermenting gram-negative rod known to cause otitis media and to infect leg ulcers; this organism was recently described as a cause of fulminant sepsis in a neutropenic patient with metastatic carcinoma.

Leuconostoc species, which are gram-positive cocci with high-level vancomycin resistance, were recently described as a cause of bacteremia in patients with underlying diseases, including leukemia and human immunodeficiency virus infection. *Leptotrichia buccalis*, an anaerobic gram-negative rod, has been reported as a cause of bacteremia in patients with advanced malignancies who have oral mucosal ulceration or inflammation; this organism is usually susceptible to penicillins, cephalosporines, tetracyclines, clindamycin, and metronidazole.

C. Bacteremias Associated with Catheters

Since the 1980s, indwelling intravenous silastic catheters have become used increasingly in the management of cancer patients. As foreign bodies, however, they provide a source of both infectious and noninfectious complications. Although the incidence of catheter-associated infections varies among different studies, the risk for developing a bacteremia, whenever a patient has a catheter, appears to be increased severalfold among both neutropenic and nonneutropenic patients. The coagulase-negative staphylococci are the most common cause of catheter-associated bacteremia, but *S. aureus*, *Bacillus* sp., corynebacteria, and gram-negative organisms (especially *Acinetobacter* sp. and *Pseudomonas* sp.) can also cause these infections. *Candida* sp. and *Mycobacterium fortuitum* are two additional opportunistic causative agents of catheter-related bacteremia in cancer patients.

For the neutropenic cancer patient with an indwelling catheter who develops a bacteremia, it is often possible to treat the infection without removing the catheter. This is particularly true when the infection is caused by coagulase-negative staphylococci, but even patients with gram-negative infections can be successfully treated. The anticiotic(s) should be rotated to include all ports and lumina, bacause the infection can be restricted to only one of these and treatment failure can otherwise occur (23). However, several caveats must be noted. Certain bacterial organisms (e.g., *Bacillus* sp.) may not be eradicated even when they are sensitive to the antibiotics being delivered, and thus, when these are isolated, it is generally necessary to remove the device. The presence of candidemia is an indication for catheter removal because failure to do so is associated with a higher incidence of systemic sequelae. Patients with tunnel infections, whether caused by bacteria, mycobacteria, or fungi, virtually always require the removal of the device and systemic antibiotics to treat the infection. Patients with simple exit site infections, on the other hand, can gernerally be treated with vigorous hygiene and antibiotic therapy.

Although several noncontrolled studies have suggested that using subcutaneously implanted devices may have a lower risk for infection than the externalized (i.e., Hickman-Broviac) catheters, a prospective randomized study comparing these two types of devices performed at the National Cancer Institute failed to confirm any difference in the incidence of infectious or noninfectious complications between these types of devices. Thus, which type of catheter to place is a function of patient preference and the type of therapy to be delivered. It is hoped that improvements in catheter design will result in surfaces that block the attachment of microorganisms and thus reduce these infectious complications.

D. Fungemias

The evaluation of the incidence of candidiasis is very difficult in immunocompromised patients. Studies from Sloan-Kettering and M. D. Anderson reported 12 candidiasis per 100 leukemia admissions; candidemia represented 5–7% of all positive blood cultures in several cancer centers. One of the more recent autopsy series reported 25% of fungal infections in leukemia and bone marrow transplant recipients, 58% being attributed to *Candida* sp.

Acute hematogenous candidiasis is the most common presentation, and the majority of cases are caused by *Candida albicans*, although in some institutions it is being supplanted by *Candida tropicalis*. *Candida krusei* emerged recently, and the role of fluconazole has been pointed out by many investigators; however, colonization by that species has been reported before the use of fluconazole, and *C. krusei* infections can occur in patients who did not receive fluconazole. This indicates that fluconazole is not the only factor responsible for the increasing incidence of *C. krusei*. *Candida parapsilosis* is associated with total parenteral nutrition. *Candida guillermondii*, *Torulopsis glabrata*, and *Candida lusitaniae* may infrequently cause fungemia, and multiple candidal fungemia is uncommon. Laboratory tests are disappointing; blood cultures are positive in only one-third of autopsy-proven candidiasis; therefore, even a single blood-positive culture should be taken into account in neutropenic patients. Indeed, mortality is not lower than in patients with three or more positive blood cultures. Serological tests have low sensitivity, although the recent detection of D-arabinitol (arabitol) seems to be promising, as demonstrated in an animal model of disseminated candidiasis.

Surveillance cultures have a positive predictive value for *C. tropicalis* but not for other *Candida* species. For all these reasons, recognition of clinical manifestations is very important: persistence or relapse of fever despite broad-spectrum antibiotics in neutropenic patients, hypotension, myalgia, and development of small red maculopapular cutaneous lesions are indicative of acute hematogenous candidiasis. Its major acute complication is endophthalmitis; orbital pain, blurred vision, scotomata, photophobia, and loss of vision are the major symptoms, and lesions similar to Roth's spots, with extension to the vitreous, are very suggestive. *Candida* endophthalmitis requires vitrectomy and local instillation of 5–10 μg amphotericin B.

Chronic disseminated candidiasis is another important complication of fungemia that usually goes undetected until recovery from neutropenia. Early manifestations are relapse of fever and increase in alkaline phosphatase. Hepatic, splenic, renal, and pulmonary abscesses can be demonstrated by CT scan. Diagnosis is confirmed by histological demonstration of fungi on liver biopsy, but culture of biopsy tissue often remains negative.

Amphotericin B is the therapy of choice for fungemia caused by *Candida* other than *C. lusitaniae*; the daily dose ranges from 0.5 to 1 mg/kg. Fluconazole at 6 or 12 mg/kg is indicated for *C. lusitaniae* infections but could probably be used for the infections caused by the other sensitive *Candida* sp. as well (24).

For chronic disseminated candidiasis, liposomal amphotericin B and fluconazole appear better tolerated and less toxic than amphotericin B; therapy must often be prolonged for weeks or months (Table 13).

Malassezia furfur (*Pityrosperum orbiculare*) is a lipophilic cutaneous saprophyte that has caused fungemia in debilitated patients with total parenteral nutrition. Supplementation of conventional media with olive oil is necessary for the growth of this fungus, although blood culture retired through the catheter of parenteral nutrition contain sufficient amounts of fatty acids to allow the fungus to grow in vivo. Removal of the infected catheter, discontinuation of parenteral nutrition, and treatment with amphotericin B are important measures in neutropenic cancer patients; fatal cases with pulmonary involvement have been reported.

Trichosporosis, caused mainly by *Trichosporon beigelii*, is very similar to candidiasis. Clinically undistinguishable cutaneous lesions may occur but evolve into necrotic ulcers. Renal involvement seems to be more frequent, with subsequent rapid renal failure. Cryptococcal antigen test is positive in trichosporosis at a low titer level (<1:32) and may be a clue to the diagnosis. Most of the cases reported in neutropenic patients have been fatal because *Trichosporon* is resistant in vitro to amphotericin B. Experience with triazoles alone or combined with amphotericin B or 5-flucytosine is still too limited. Other unusual opportunistic yeasts responsible for fungemia in neutropenic patients have been reported increasingly during the last decade. These include *Geotrichum*, *Hansenula*, and *Rhodotorula*. A handful of cases are reported, and the epidemiological, clinical, and prognostic factors are not well defined. Most cases had removal of involved catheters and received amphotericin B therapy.

Protothecosis, an algal infection, was reported recently in a child with Hodgkin's disease; *Prototheca wickerhamii* mixed with *T. glabrata* was isolated in blood culture taken through a Hickman catheter.

Table 13 Therapy For Fungal Infections[a]

	First choice	Alternative	Comments
Candidiasis			
Acute hematogenous candidiasis	Ampho B + 5-FC (0.5–1 mg/kg/day)	Ampholiposomes or fluconazole	Total dose of Ampho B 1–1.5 g
Chronic disseminated candidiasis	Fluconazole (6–12 mg/kg)	Ampholiposomes	
Endophthalmitis	Vitrectomy with local Ampho B (5–10 mg)	Fluconazole	
Invasive aspergillosis	Ampho B (1–1.5 mg/kg/day)	Itraconazole, 400 mg/day	Total dose of Ampho B 2 g
Cryptococcus	Ampho B + 5 FC (0.5 mg/kg/day + 100 mg/kg/day)	Fluconazole or itraconazole	6 weeks followed by maintenance therapy
Mucormycosis	Surgical debridement or excision + Ampho B (1 mg/kg/day)		Total dose of Ampho B 2 g
Histoplasmosis, coccidioidomycosis	Itraconazole (400 mg/day)	Ketoconazole (400 mg/day)	Maintenance therapy required
blastomycosis	Ampho B (1 mg/kg/day)	Itraconazole (400 mg/day)	
Pseudoallescheriosis	Miconazole (80–90 mg/kg/day IV)		
Trichosporosis, fusaridiosis		Amphiliposomes or fluconazole or combination therapy, Ampho B + fluconazole	
Sporotrichosis	Itraconazole (400 mg/day)	Ampho B (1 mg/kg/day)	

[a]Ampho B, amphoterian B; 5-FC, 5-flucytosine.

III. OPPORTUNISTIC PNEUMONIAS

A. Bacterial Pneumonias

Pulmonary infections are frequent among immunocompromised patients. Granulocytopenic patients may lack symptoms of infection, such as cough and sputum production, and more than one-third do not present rales or consolidation signs; about 50% of neutropenic patients with bacterial pneumonia present with a bacteremia; this is the most reliable way to establish the microbiological diagnosis and orient therapy. Most patients with bacterial pneumonia complicating severe neutropenia require empirical therapy similar to that described for febrile neutropenia and blood-borne infections. The combination of gram-negative bacteremia and pneumonia makes the prognosis worse compared to that for bacteremia alone.

Bacterial pneumonia in neutropenic patients is caused by the same spectrum of pathogens involved in bacteremias. As a matter of fact, the symptoms and signs of systemic sepsis often overshadow the specific pulmonary manifestations. Therapy should be instituted empirically, as in suspected bacteremia, taking into account that bacterial pneumonia during severe neutropenia carries a poor prognosis.

The incidence of tuberculosis has increased during the last decade in relation to the AIDS epidemic. Because the diagnosis is often delayed, transmission of the disease to the immunocompromised patient is possible, although in cancer patients, reactivation of a long-dormant disease is more frequent. Patients with Hodgkin's disease, lung cancer, leukemia, head and neck cancer, and stomach cancer appear to have an increased risk of tuberculosis. Most of the cases are suspected on routine chest x-ray with apical pulmonary infiltrates and cavitation. Rarely, tuberculosis may present with disseminated granulomas and be confused with metastasis. Miliary tuberculosis is very rare and tends to occur among leukemic patients.

A 6 month course of therapy is adequate in immunocompromised patients, with pyrazinamide being given for the first 2 months of therapy. Pulmonary infection caused by mycobacteria other than tuberculosis is very rare and occurs in association with chronic pulmonary disease and lung cancer.

Nocardiosis, mainly due to *Nocardia asteroides*, is an uncommon pulmonary infection in cancer patients. Traditionally it has been associated with lymphoma and leukemia, but has also been reported in patients with solid tumors. The radiographic appearance of pulmonary nocardiosis is variable and includes solitary or multiple cavitary lesions, diffuse bronchopneumonia, reticulonodular infiltrates, and empyema. Upper lobes are commonly involved. Nodular subcutaneous lesions and cerebral abscesses may be associated with nocardial pneumonia and should alert one about the possibility of this diagnosis. Intravenous (IV) sulfonamides at a dose of 6–8 g/day or trimethoprim-sulfa methoxazole

(TMP-SMX) at a dose of 480 mg (TMP) and 400 mg (SMX) twice daily, either IV or orally, is the therapy of choice. Diagnosed early and treated adequately, nocardiosis usually has a favorable outcome.

Legionellosis accounts for about 6% of nosocomial pneumonias and 3% of community-acquired pneumonias. A frequency of 13% was reported among bone marrow transplant recipients, and overall, a greater acquisition of legionellosis has been documented in immunocompromised patients. In some institutions, it has been associated with contaminated cooling tower reservoirs and hospital potable water. High fever with relative bradycardia and extrapulmonary manifestations, such as nausea, diarrhea, headache, and changes in mental status, constitute the principal characteristics of the disease. Radiological findings are variable and include unilobar or multilobar consolidation, lung abscess, and empyema. Laboratory studies may reveal hyponatremia, hypophosphatemia, abnormal liver tests, proteinuria, and microscopic hematuria. *Legionella* is diagnosed by culture of sputum or bronchoalveolar lavage on semiselective charcoal-yeast medium or direct fluorescent antibody test and by serum antibody and urinary antigen detection. If untreated, mortality from legionellosis is high in immunosuppressed patients. Erythromycin combined with rifampicin or fluoroquinolones combined with rifampicin constitutes the therapy of choice.

B. Fungal Pneumonias

Invasive aspergillosis, mainly caused by *Aspergillus fumigatus* and *Aspergillus flavus*, is one of the most common fatal infections in neutropenic cancer patients. The risk of infection increases in proportion to the duration of neutropenia. The two major sites of infection are the lungs and the paranasal sinuses. The clinical manifestations include persistent or recurrent fever, despite broad-spectrum antibiotics, pleuritic chest pain, and dry cough. Dyspnea and hypoxemia appear late and are indicative of extensive invasion and poor prognosis. Nasal discharge, epistaxis, and facial swelling and tenderness indicate sinus involvement. Chest CT scans are superior to standard x-rays and should be performed early. Radiological patterns include solitary nodular lesion, multiple nodular lesions, triangular peripheral infiltrates with tendency to cavitation, and diffuse pulmonary infiltrates. Dissemination to the major organs has been reported, the most common and often fatal being to the central nervous system (CNS), which occurs in 10–15% of cases. Many epidemics of invasive aspergillosis have been described in relation to building construction around hospitals (25). Prevention of aspergillosis consists in isolation of the patient in a protected environment. Amphotericin B at 1 mg/kg/day IV, for a total dose of 2 g, is the therapy of choice. Mortality is the highest among bone marrow recipients, more than 80% (26).

Mucormycosis produces clinical manifestations similar to those of aspergillosis. It is less frequent, with a more fulminant course, and survival is exceptional, despite amphotericin therapy.

Coccidioidomycosis, histoplasmosis, and blastomycosis are restricted to geographically well-defined areas in northwestern America and Africa. A history of travel or stay in these endemic areas is important because long-dormant infection of the lungs can be reactivated during immunosuppression. For immunocompromised patients with severe disease, amphotericin B remains the therapy of choice (Table 14).

Fusariosis and pseudoallescheriosis can produce opportunistic pneumonia very similar to aspergillosis and mucormycosis, with some principal differences: cutaneous maculopapular lesions are more frequent and may produce necrotic ulcers. *Fusarium* and *Pseudallescheria boydii* can be isolated blood; both organisms are resistant to amphotericin B. Fluconazole has been proposed for *Fusarium* infections.

The diagnosis of pulmonary aspergillosis and other similar fungal infections is very difficult; one should have a high degree of diagnostic suspicion in patients who are predisposed to these complications. Today, high-resolution chest computed tomographic scanning combined with microbiological examination of the product of BAL probably represents the best chance for precise diagnosis.

C. Pneumonia Caused by Protozoans

P. carinii pneumonia (PCP) is an increasing opportunistic infection in cancer patients with impaired cellular immunity, namely those with lymphoma, leukemia, immunosuppressive therapy, and bone marrow transplantation. Presenting symptoms include dyspnea, fever, and dry cough; blood gases reveal hypoxemia. Chest x-ray classically shows diffuse interstitial pulmonary infiltrates, and pneumatoceles have been reported. Pneumothorax has been described increasingly in relation to pentamidine inhalation. BAL is a safe and sensitive procedure for establishing the diagnosis (27). PCP in cancer patients is best treated with trimethoprim-sulfamethoxazole at a daily dose of 20 mg/kg/day of TMP and 100 mg/kg/day of SMX in four divided doses, for a total duration of 14 days. Pentamidine at 4 mg/kg/day, diluted in 250 ml of 5% dextrose and infused over 60 minutes, constitutes an effective alternative to TMP-SMX, although the side effects are more severe, including arrythmia, hypotension, hypoglycemia, hypocalcemia, and azotemia. Aerosolized pentamidine has no systemic toxicity, but its use is decreasing because of a high rate of early relapse and a high frequency of extrapulmonary pneumocystosis (28). For mild and moderate PCP, oral administration of TMP-dapsone seems to be safe and effective. Relapse after a first episode of PCP is not uncommon in cancer patients, and secondary prophylaxis may be indicated for patients who are supposed to remain severely immunosuppressed; this is the case after allogeneic bone marrow transplantation.

Table 14 Clinical Characteristics and Specific Therapy of Fungal Opportunistic Pneumonia

	Clinical patterns	Recommended therapy
Aspergillus sp.	Acute onset, chest pain, cutaneous ulcerations (rare), CNS absecesses; nodular x-ray in filtrates unique or multiple, with halo sign or cavitation	Amphotericin B: 1 mg/kg/day IV up to 2 g total dose
Mucorales	Acute onset and fulminant course, palate necrotic ulcer; ecthyma gangrenosum-like or nodular cutaneous lesions (disseminated); x-ray findings similar to aspergillosis	Amphotericin B: 1 mg/kg/day IV up to 2 g total dose
Coccidioides sp.	Travel to endemic area important, acute progressive pneumonia and miliary dissemination	Amphotericin B: 1–1.5 mg/kg/day IV up to 2–2.5 g total dose
Histoplasma capsulatum	Hepatospenomegaly, patchy infiltrates or miliary dissemination; chest x-ray may be normal	Amphotericin B (as for *Coccidioides*); ketoconazole or itraconazole 400 mg/day orally; can be given for moderate disease
Fusarium	Similar to aspergillosis, with more frequent cutaneous ulcerations; both can be isolated from blood	Both invariably resistant to amphotericin B; no standard therapy for *Fusarium*; miconazole 60–90 mg/kg/day IV of for 6 weeks therapy of choice of pseudoallerscheriosis

Rhodococcus equi is a pathogen of farm animals, causing suppurative pulmonary lesions in horses, pyometra in cattle, and suppurative adenitis in swine. Patients with severe deficiency in cellular immunity, such as lymphoma, transplant recipients, or AIDS or those receiving immunosuppressive therapy and who are in contact with farm animals, are at risk of pneumonia with *R. equi*, which mimics mycobacterial infections with cavitary lesions in the upper lobes. The overall mortality is 20%. The organism is mainly an intracellular parasite and should be treated with an antibiotic that can penetrate the cells. Combination of erythromycin and rifampicin seems to be the therapy of choice, and long duration is recommended (29).

D. Viral Pneumonias

Cytomegalovirus pneumonia occurs in about 15% of bone marrow transplant recipients. The risk persists until day 120 after transplantation and is maximal around day 60. Seronegative recipients transplanted with bone marrow from seropositive donors are at high risk of CMV pneumonia. Cough, fever, and diffuse pulmonary infiltrates are the common presenting manifestations. CMV interstitial pneumonia may be part of a clinical syndrome including pancytopenia, hepatitis, and gastrointestinal ulcerations. The mortality from CMV pneumonia has decreased from 90% before ganciclovir to about 25%. The presence of CMV in a BAL specimen and/or a CMV-positive buffy coat obtained on day 35 were significant factors associated with CMV pneumonia. These investigations are now performed routinely on days 30–35 after bone marrow transplantation in most units, and recent studies suggest that ganciclovir should be given as soon as CMV is detected. Newer methods, such as antigen detection and polymerase chain reaction (PCR), have significantly shortened the delay in diagnosis (30).

Ganciclovir is given at the dose of 5 mg/kg thrice daily IV for 2 weeks, followed by maintenance therapy with 5 mg/kg once daily, 5 days weekly until day 120. CMV immune globulin continues to be used, although its efficacy for prophylaxis and treatment is controversial (Table 15).

Adenovirus pneumonia was reported in 5% of bone marrow transplant recipients; it is usually bilateral and interstitial, and pleural effusion has been described in 20% of cases. Disseminated adenovirus infection with fatal hepatic necrosis has been described in cancer patients. Conjunctivitis may be a clue to the diagnosis. Adenovirus has been associated with hematuria in bone marrow transplant recipients.

Herpes simplex virus and herpes zoster-varicella (HZV) pneumonias have become rare in immunocompromised patients since the introduction of acyclovir. Previously, HSV pneumonia was mainly reported in allogeneic bone marrow transplant recipients; mucocutaneous lesions preceded the onset of pneumonia in

Table 15 Clinical Characteristics and Specific Therapy of Opportunistic Pneumonia

	Clinical patterns	Recommended therapy
Pneumocystis carinii	Subacute onset, dyspnea, interstitial infiltrates	TMP-SMX (20 and 100 mg/kg) IV per day for 14 days or pentamidine, 4 mg/kg/day IV, TMP-dapsone, 300 mg and 25 mg four times per day orally
Rhodococcus equi	Animal contacts, caviary lesions of upper lobes	Erythromycin + rifampicin
Strongyloides stercoralis	Urticaria and pruritus, gastrointestinal symptoms, eosinophilia may be lacking in 50% of immunosuppressed patients, diffuse alveolar infiltrates	Thiabendazole, 25 mg/kg twice per day IV for 7–15 days
CMV	Subacute onset, BMT recipients, hypoxia, interstitial pneumonia	Ganciclovir, 5 mg/kg three times per day IV, *or* foscarnet, 60 mg/kg IV three times per day
HSV and VZV	Subacute onset, mucosal and cutaneous lesions may precede pneumonia, interstitial, focal, and multifocal	Acyclovir, 10–125 mg/kg three times per day IV for 10 days
Adenovirus	Subacute conjunctivitis, hematuria, diffuse interstitial, pleural effusion	No therapy
RSV	Subacute onset, upper respiratory symptoms, bilateral diffuse infiltrates	Ribavirin

more than 90% of cases. Focal or multifocal pneumonia can occur secondarily to contiguous spread of infection in patients with endotracheal intubation, and diffuse interstitial pneumonia was described as a part of disseminated HSV infections.

VZV pneumonia usually develops 1–6 days after the onset of exanthema. In one recent series, which evaluated 73 immunocompromised patients with disseminated HZV in a comparative trial of acyclovir and vidarabine, pneumonia occured in only 1 patient. Immunocompromised patients can develop severe or fatal pneumonia caused by the respiratory syncytial virus (RSV), and mortality as high as 66% has been reported among bone marrow transplant (BMT) recipients. Ribavirin seemed to have a beneficial effect in the management of patients in a recent outbreak.

IV. INFECTIONS OF THE DIGESTIVE TRACT

A. Infectious Diarrheas

The digestive tract, with its rapidly proliferating mucosa and its load of bacteria, is often the source of bacteremia in neutropenic patients. In addition, it is the natural site of a series of specific gastrointestinal infections, some of which are more common in cancer patients because of neutropenia, immunodepression, or both (31).

E. coli and *Salmonella* sp. are common causes of infectious diarrhea; the spectrum of clinical disease includes fever, nausea, vomiting, and abdominal cramps. Severe infections and deaths can occur in immunocompromised patients. Bacteremia has been reported in 30% of cancer patients with *Salmonella* infection but in less than 5% of others with this infection; *Salmonella typhimurium* is an especially common cause of serious infection in cancer patients.

Aeromonas hydrophila has been described as a gastrointestinal pathogen in immunosuppressed patients with hematological malignancies or hepatic disease, especially in those who were neutropenic. Although *Aeromonas* enteritis is usually mild and self-limited, it can cause fulminant bloody diarrhea in immunocompromised patients.

Cancer patients are also at increased risk of *Clostridium difficile* colitis because antibiotic administration is common and because of the higher rate of colonization in oncology units. *C. difficile* infection in cancer patients usually presents as a typical pseudomembranous colitis with severe diarrhea, abdominal pain, and fever. It usually responds promptly to vancomycin or metronidazole but can be fatal if untreated. *C. difficile* colitis has been described in cancer patients following chemotherapy without exposure to antibiotics.

Other bacteria are rarely reported as a cause of infectious diarrhea in cancer patients. Namely, *Mycobacterium tuberculosis* and *Mycobacterium avium-intracellulare*, which cause febrile hepatosplenomegaly, adenopathy, and abdominal pain in AIDS patients, are rarely seen in cancer patients (32).

Although the lower digestive tract is often involved in neutropenic patients who develop disseminated candidiasis, most of these patients do not develop symptoms suggestive of enteritis. Colonization of the digestive tract by *Candida* sp. most likely serves as the primary site for disseminated candidiasis, and oral fungal prophylaxis reduces the frequency of *Candida* infections in controlled studies of neutropenic patients. Other fungi are only anecdotally reported in association with enteritis in cancer patients.

Cytomegalovirus is rather commonly associated with enteritis and/or ulceration of the digestive tract in immunosuppressed patients with AIDS; it is a rare cause of digestive tract disease in cancer patients but has been reported as a cause of gastroenteritis in bone marrow transplant recipients.

Similarly, parasitic infections, such as giardiasis, cryptosporidiosis, isosporidiasis, strongyloidosis, and amebiasis, are commonly seen in AIDS patients but have been rarely reported in cancer patients.

B. Infectious Mucositis

Thrush is a common complication in all kinds of debilitated patients, including those with cancer, whether neutropenic and/or immunodepressed. It causes complaints of dysphagia and/or odynophagia. The infection may extend from the oral mucosa into the esophagus or upper respiratory tract and often results in anorexia and weight loss from decreased food intake. Esophageal infection can be demonstrated by a radiograph of the esophagus and is confirmed by endoscopy and biopsy. The combination of oral candidiasis and esophageal symptoms is highly specific and sensitive for candidal esophagitis. Under these circumstances, an empirical trial of systemic therapy with ketoconazole or fluconazole may obviate the need for endoscopy in many patients. Of course, esophagitis may be present without thrush and must be differentiated form herpes, cytomegalovirus, and reflux esophagitis; in these cases, endoscopic evaluation with biopsy is the definitive diagnostic procedure.

Some patients with candidal mucositis respond to topical antifungal therapy, but most neutropenic and/or immunosuppressed patients require systemic therapy with amphotericin B or one of the imidazoles (ketokonazole or fluconazole). Local therapy and systemic oral therapy with imidazoles is effective for the prevention of oral and esophageal candidal infection.

With documentation of a viral infection, acyclovir and ganciclovir are indicated for herpes simplex and cytomegalovirus esophageal infections, respectively.

C. Noninfectious Causes of Diarrhea and Mucositis

Most malignancies can have a direct effect on the gastrointestinal system. Tumors of the gastrointestinal tract itself, including head and neck, esophageal, stomach, small bowel, and colorectal cancer, obviously can cause problems of malnutrition, obstruction, ulceration, bleeding, or perforation. In addition to the gastrointestinal primary lesions, a number of tumors, including melanoma, breast cancer, ovarian cancer, lymphoma, and leukemia, can involve the gastrointestinal tract. Infiltration by these malignancies can cause the problems noted earlier and can also be responsible for protein-losing enteropathies, malabsorption, and secondary infections of the gastrointestinal tract, such as perirectal abscesses with leukemia.

Some tumors induce diarrhea by active secretion of secretagogues; this is the case in pancreatic cholera and carcinoid syndrome; somatostatin and its synthetic analog have been reported effective under these conditions.

Surgical resections and radiotherapy can alter the function of the digestive tract. Nausea, vomiting, and diarrhea are frequently acute side effects of irradiation to the small bowel. One may also see delayed transit time, increased intestinal secretions with dilated loops of small bowel, and malabsorption of glucose, fat, and protein. Late effects include ulceration and a reduction in intestinal caliber and elasticity.

Nausea and vomiting are perhaps the most common manifestations of gastrointestinal toxicity of chemotherapeutic agents. This complication occurs with almost every major class of compounds; violent and prolonged nausea and vomiting may occur after administration of cisplatin, 5-azacytidine (azacitidine), streptozotocin, dacarbazine, and others.

Stomatitis, which includes cheilosis, glossitis, pharyngitis, and other mucosal toxicities of the alimentary canal, is also seen with a number of chemotherapeutic agents. Ulceration of the stomach and/or duodenum is a well-known complication of administration of corticosteroids.

Constipation and adynamic ileus are two of the major toxic effects of vincristine administration. Diarrhea can be severe with actinomycin D, 5-fluorouracil, and cisplatin administration.

D. Perianal Infections

The perianal area is a common site of bacterial infection, especially in patients with acute monocytic leukemia, during episodes of neutropenia. The main symptoms are pain and fever; the lesions usually spread rapidly and often progress to necrosis, leaving major sequelae if not treated early; bacteremia caused by *P. aeruginosa* and/or *E. coli* is often documented. Radiotherapy has been recommended but is usually ineffective.

The role of surgery is controversial: extensive operative procedures are made difficult by concomitant thrombocytopenia. In most patients therapy consists of broad-spectrum antibiotics and analgesics.

E. Neutropenic Enterocolitis: Typhlitis (Appendicitis)

Neutropenic enterocolitis, formerly also termed typhlitis, is a rare but well-recognized gastrointestinal condition occurring during therapy of acute leukemia, lymphoma, aplastic anemia, and certain solid tumors. It is characterized by bowel wall inflammation and edema that can progress to necrosis, usually in the terminal ileum, cecum, or right colon. Profound neutropenia secondary to chemotherapy has been considered the hallmark of the disease and a major etiologic factor in its development; antitumor agents may also play a role in this disease. Once the process begins, organisms invade the injured bowel wall, aggravate the damage, and invade the bloodstream; bacteremia caused by multiple gram-negative rods is frequent.

The most common presenting signs and symptoms are fever, abdominal pain, and watery diarrhea. The abdomen is distended and tender, and x-ray demonstrates evidence of paralytic ileus with thickening of the bowel wall.

Care of these patients should be individualized. Nonoperative treatment with bowel rest, decompression, nutritional support, and broad-spectrum antibiotics is recommended initially. Operative intervention is recommended for those with perforation or those whose condition deteriorates. The overall mortality is very high, in excess of 50% (33).

F. Abdominal Surgery

The onset of abdominal pain in the setting of neutropenia can be caused by a variety of intraabdominal processes, and surgeons are frequently called to evaluate and treat these complications.

At this time, clear-cut guidelines do not exist for the treatment of acute abdominal pain in neutropenic patients. Pain usually can be diffuse or localized; it can be associated with nausea, diarrhea, vomiting, constipation, jaundice, and/or abdominal distension. This last sign was associated with increased mortality in some series. No symptom or sign is pivotal in the decision for or against surgical intervention; clinical and/or radiological evidence of a surgically treatable disease should prompt surgical intervention, but the approach should be very thorough to avoid needless operations. Otherwise, it is often recommended to treat those patients conservatively, because neutropenic enteropathy is responsible for the majority of cases. As indicated in Table 16, which is based on three publications about abdominal pain in neutropenic patients, necrotizing enteropathy was diagnosed in 81 of 169 neutropenic patients (48%) who presented with a painful acute abdomen. Hepatic disease, often related to drug administration, and severe constipation were each responsible for this presentation in 6% of the cases; the other causes represented a wide spectrum of diseases, of which none represented more than 5% (34–36).

Spontaneous intestinal and colonic perforation occurs more frequently in patients receiving corticosteroids with or without chemotherapy. Malignancy can be histologically documented at the site of perforation in about 50% of these patients. Operation may also needed for obstructing carcinomatosis of the gastrointestinal, pancreatic, biliary, or urinary tract. In advanced disease, these operations do not always prevent recurrence of the obstruction; laparotomy is justified if performance status is compatible with a reasonable quality of life.

V. NEUROLOGICAL MANIFESTATIONS

A. Opportunistic Infections of the Central Nervous System

Infections of the nervous system are rare in patients with cancer, accounting for about 1% of neurological events; however, it is important to recognize these complications because some may be treated successfully.

The distribution of microorganisms causing neurological infections in patients

Table 16 Diseases Responsible for Surgical Intervention in Neutropenic Patients

Necrotizing enteropathy	81	48.0
Hepatic disease	11	6.5
Constipation-ileus	10	6.0
Appendicitis	7	4.0
Perforated colon	7	4.0
Perforated stomach	6	3.5
Cholecystitis	6	3.5
Gastric hemorrhage	4	2.3
Retroperitoneal hemorrhage	4	2.3
Neoplastic infiltration	4	2.3
Graft-versus-host disease	4	2.3
Perforated stomach	3	1.7
Peritonitis	3	1.7
Perforated ileum	2	1.2
Hemorrhage in tumor	2	1.2
Lymphadenitis	2	1.2
No disease	2	1.2
Eseophagitis	2	1.2
Pneumonia	2	1.2
Incarcerated hernia	1	0.6
Hemorrhage in ileum	1	0.6
Hemmorhage in colon	1	0.6
Splenic infarction	1	0.6
Pseudomembranous colitis	1	0.6
Total	169	100

with cancer is different from that found in the general population. In fact, the agents responsible for the infections of the nervous system in cancer are similar to those found in other pathological conditions in which immunity is depressed, suggesting that immunodepression is an important factor in the pathogenesis of nervous system infections in patients with malignant tumors.

A second important factor predisposing patients with cancer to neurological infections is neutropenia. Finally, another predisposing circumstance for central nervous system infection is head and spine surgery.

The type of the underlying disease and its associated defect in host defense mechanisms allow, with a high degree of accuracy, prediction of the responsible organism of CNS infection. Table 17 summarizes the principal clinical features of CNS opportunistic agents.

Neutropenia can predispose to bacterial meningitis with the usual pathogens

Table 17 Central Nervous System Infection in Patients with Cancer

Infection and usual causative agents	Clinical clues	Laboratory findings
Meningitis		
Streptococcus pneumoniae	Meutropenia, splenectomy, fever, ±nuchal rigidity, headache post-surgery (head and neck)	Minimal pleocytosis if neutropenic, gram-positive diplococci on smear, positive culture, positive CIE in CSF or urine, blood cultures positive, CSF protein ↑, glucose ↓
Neisseria meningitidis	Neutropenia, splenectomy, fever, rash, headache, arthralgias, ±nuchal rigidity, rapid progression	Minimal pleocytosis, gram-negative diplococci on smear, positive culture, CIE positive in CSF, blood cultures positive, CSF protein ↑, glocuse ↓
Pseudomonas aeruginosa, Ehterobacteriaceae	Neutropenia, leukemia, fever, headache, minimal neurological findings, minimal defects in mentation or level of consciousness, ecthyma gangreonsum	Minimal pleocytosis, gram-negative rods on smear, positive culture of CSF and blood
Listeria monocytogenes	Immunosuppression, T lymphocyte defects, ±CNS signs, fever, headache, ±nuchal rigidity, minimal personality change, cranial nerve palsy	Mononuclear or polymorphonuclear pleocytosis, CSF protein ↑, glucose ↓, or normal + gram stain of CSF sediment (30%), positive CSF culture
Cryptococcus neoformans	Immunosuppression, low-grade fever, minimal nuchal rigidity, mild headache, ±cranial nerve palsy, personality change, insidious onset	Lymphocytic pleocytosis, positive CSF Gram stain or india ink preparation, positive culture (large volumes), positive latex agglutination in CSF or serum

Meningoencephalitis		
Toxoplasma gondii	Immunosuppression, lymphoma, meningoencephalitis ± focal signs, multiple-organ involvement, rapid progression	Minimal pleocytosis (lymphocytes), IgM-IFA specific antibody rise, Sabin-Feldman dye test ≥ 1:1000
Varicella-zoster virus, herpes simplex virus	Immunosuppression, skin lesions	Brain biopsy positive, positive vesicle culture
Brain abscess		
Aspergillus, Mucor sp.	Neutropenia, immunosuppression, nasopharyngeal involvement, ±brain abscess, sudden onset of major neurological findings postneurosurgery, pulmonary infection	Mild lymphocytic pleocytosis, CSF protein, glucose ± culture
Nocardia asteroides	Immunosuppression, T lymphocyte defects, pulmonary infection, subcutaneous abscesses, focal neurological signs	Biopsy of brain abscess, culture at other sites of infection

CIE; CSF, cerebrospinal fluid; IFA.

(*S. pneumoniae* and *Neisseria meningitidis*) but also with gram-negative bacilli. This is a very rare event: meningitis has not been documented in more than 2000 consecutive patients with febrile neutropenia studied by the EORTC Cooperative Group. Bacteremia can usually be documented along with the meningitis during neutropenia. Diagnosis may be difficult: neutropenic patients often lack the usual clinical signs and symptoms of infection because of the reduced inflammatory reaction. In severely neutropenic patients, pleocytosis within the cerebrospinal fluid may be minimal. Therapy requires high doses of effective antimicrobials; third-generation cephalosporines (ceftazidime and ceftriaxone) and imipenem penetrate well into the cerebrospinal fluid; in gram-negative bacillary meningitis, intrathecal injection, via lumbar puncture or intraventricularly, of aminoglycosides might be considered.

In patients with cellular immunity defects, *Listeria monocytogenes*, *Toxoplasma gondii*, *Cryptococcus neoformans*, and *N. asteroides* are opportunistic agents able to cause meningitis, meningoencephalitis, or brain abscesses. It should be stressed that these infections are relatively rare: 2.7% in Hodgkin's disease, 0.6% for patients with non-Hodgkin's lymphomas, and 2.5% in patients with chronic lymphocytic leukemia. In granulocytopenic patients, *Aspergillus*, *Candida*, and Mucorales should be added to the list of possible causative agents; here, however, the involvement of CNS is usually secondary to hematogenous dissemination or direct extension from the sinuses, especially in aspergillosis and mucormycosis.

Toxoplasma encephalitis, which is extremely common in AIDS patients, is rare in patients with neoplastic disease. Among 25 cancer patients who developed toxoplasmosis between 1972 and 1978 at the Sloan-Kettering Cancer Center (37), 8 had CNS toxoplasmosis; 3 had focal symptoms, and 5 presented with diffuse encephalitis. The majority of these patients had hematological malignancies, mainly Hodgkin's disease, and all these infections were fatal despite therapy. Reactivation of latent infection accounts for the majority of CNS toxoplasmosis cases during immunosuppression.

The only change in cerebrospinal fluid may be moderate elevation of protein; pleocytosis is often absent. The parasite can be demonstrated in centrifuged cerebrospiral fluid by Giemsa staining, and it has been cultured on tissue monolayers used for viral isolation; this method must be compared to the fastidious inoculation of specimens into mice. A fourfold increase in IgG antibody titers and demonstration of local production in the cerebrospinal fluid of toxoplasma IgG antibodies are indicative of active disease. Cerebral CT scan usually demonstrates nodular ring-enhancing lesions, and magnetic resonance imaging can detect lesions not visualized by the CT scan. Stereotactic biopsy may be warranted in some circumstances.

Therapy of CNS toxoplasmosis consists of oral administration of the combination pyrimethamine-sulfadiazine at 50 mg/day and 8 g/day, respectively. The mortality rate is about 70%. Other alternatives under evaluation include the association clindamycin-pyrimethamine or dapsone-pyrimethamine.

C. neoformans is another opportunistic agent that can cause infection of CNS in cancer patients. It is associated mainly with lymphoma (38). Demonstration of budding yeast in cerebrospinal fluid by india ink preparation, isolation on culture, and detection of *Cryptococcus* antigen constitute the principal methods of diagnosis. Combined therapy of amphotericin B (0.5 mg/g/day) with 5-flucytosine (100–150 mg/kg) is the first choice in immunocompromised patients. Duration of therapy should be at least 6 weeks. Therapy with triazoles, such as fluconazole at 400 mg/day, is comparable to that with amphotericin B; early results with oral itraconazole at the dose of 200 mg daily are also encouraging.

L. monocytogenes is a relatively frequent opportunistic pathogen encountered in cancer patients with central nervous system infection. It is a food-borne disease; dairy products, especially raw milk and soft cheeses, meat, eggs, and some vegetables have been incriminated as carriers (39). Meningitis, meningoencephalitis, and, less commonly, brain abscesses have been reported in immunocompromised patients. Bacteremia is usually present patients with central vervous system infection. Because the organisms are present in small numbers in the cerebrospinal fluid, direct Gram stain may be negative.

High-dose ampicillin alone or in combination with an aminoglycoside is usually recommended. Duration of therapy should be at least 2 weeks. Isolated reports have shown that TMP-SMX is also an effective therapy and may constitute a good alternative for patients allergic to penicillin.

Mortality for patients with *L. monocytogenes* central nervous system infections varies from 30 to 62% (Table 18).

Progressive multifocal leukoencephalopathy (PMLE) is a demyelinating disease caused by the human polyomavirus JC virus (JCV). In cancer patients, PMLE has been mainly associated with Hodgkin's disease and chronic lymphocytic leukemia. The classic triad of hemianopsia, hemiparesis, and dementia, associated with subcortical hypodensities without contrast enhancement on CT scan, and the presence of IgG antibodies to JCV in a patient with cellular immunodeficiency should alert the physican to the possibility of PMLE. Brain biopsy is the most reliable and accurate method for the diagnosis. The prognosis is poor because no active antiviral drug is available (40).

B. Noninfectious Causes of CNS Disease in Cancer Patients

Neurological complications are exceedingly common in cancer patients; CNS lesions can be documented at postmortem examination in about 30% of patients with cancer. As already stated, infections represent only a small fraction of these events (± 1%). The principal situations that can mimick neurological infectious diseases are metastatic disease, cerebrovascular disorders, meningeal carcinoma-

Table 18 Therapy of Neurological Opportunistic Infections

Agent	Therapy
Listeria monocytogenes	Ampicillin, 3 g four times per day IV, + gentamicin, 1 mg/kg three times per day IV, or TMP-SMX, 480–2400 mg/day IV
Toxoplasma gondii	Pyrimethamine-sulfadiazine, 50 mg, 8 g/day orally for 5 weeks; alternatives: Clindamycin-pyrimethamine or dapsone-pyrimethamine
Cryptococcus neoformans	Amphotericin B, 0.7–1 mg/kg IV, + 5-fluorocytosine, 100 mg/kg/day; alternatives: fluconazole, 6–12 mg/kg/day orally or IV; itraconazole, 5 mg/kg/day orally
JCV	No therapy available
Aspergillus, *Mucor*	Amphotericin B, 1 mg/kg; consider surgery if feasible
HSV	Acyclovir, 10 mg/kg IV every 8 h for 10–14 days; alternative therapy, vidarabine

tosis, epidural spinal compression, chemotherapy-induced encephalopathy, and paraneoplastic syndromes (Table 19).

With modern imaging techniques, the differential diagnosis between brain metastases and abscesses is usually quite simple. Among cerebrovascular complications in patients with cancer, septic embolism was found in 13% of the patients with leukemia or lymphoma and in 5% of those with solid tumors. Other causes for cerebrovascular disease in those patients were cerebral hemorrhage and cerebral infarction related to intravascular coagulation, nonbacterial intravascular endocarditis, and venous thromboses of the sinus or large cortical veins.

Meningeal carcinomatosis can have an indolent course, similar to that of

Table 19 Neurological Complications in Cancer Patients and Their Possible Infectious Disease Counterparts

Brain metastases	Brain abscesses, granulomas
Cerebrovascular diseases	Septic embolus, vascultitis
Meningeal carcinomatosis	Chronic meningitis (cryptococcal)
Epidural compression	Epidural abscess
Drug-induced encephalopathy	Encephalitis (PMLE, toxoplasmosis)
Paraneoplastic syndromes	Encephalitis (PMLE, toxoplasmosis)

chronic meningitis caused by *C. neoformans*; the pleocytosis can be absent and hypoglycorrachia present in both diseases, and microbiological exclusion of possible infection must be performed.

Drug-induced encephalopathy (ifosfamide, 5-fluorouracil, cytosine arabinoside (cytarabine), and others) and paraneoplastic syndromes (limbic, brain stem, and bulbar encephalitis) are rare complications that can mimick chronic encephalopathy of infectious causes, namely progressive multifocal leukoencephalopathy and toxoplasmic infection. Once again, these possibilities should be ruled out by adequate imaging and microbiological investigations.

VI. CUTANEOUS INFECTIONS IN CANCER PATIENTS

Cutaneous effects of malignancy can appear as a result of several different processes. Eruptions may be produced by tumor spread or intracutaneous metastases, by tumor humoral products, by idiopathic reactions to the tumor, by tumor-induced diminution of body defenses, or by concomitant disorders resulting from the same genetic predisposition that promoted the neoplastic process.

Radiotherapy of any tumor can produce massive cellular lysis and erythema multiforme. Local radiotherapy can also induce alopecia and subsequent radiodermatitis with its own oncogenic problems. Cancer chemotherapy drugs can produce the side effects of alopecia, mucosal damage, pigmentation, exfoliation, and, in some instances, allergic eruptions. Other drugs produce radiation damage recall, increased sensitivity to ultraviolet light, or recall of previous erythematous ultraviolet-induced cutaneous damage, as well as idiosyncratic reactions: marrow suppression, unusual pigmentation, and even xerosis.

One serious dilemma appearing during cancer therapy is the appearance of a generalized, erythematous, morbiliform, or maculopapular eruption in an ill patient. The differential diagnosis is usually fourfold: sepsis, cutaneous tumor invasion, graft-versus-host syndrome from bone marrow or blood product transfusion, or drug allergy. In febrile patients, sepsis is the most imminent worry. A biopsy specimen of the skin should be sent for histology and smears with special stains and for attempted culture of fungi, bacteria, and viruses. All nonessential drugs (especially allopurinol) should be discontinued, but specific tumor treatment should be continued until an adequate diagnosis can be made.

Skin lesions, an important clue to the cause of septicemia, result from several main processes: disseminated intravascular coagulation and coagulopathy, direct vascular invasion and occlusion by bacteria or fungi, immune vasculitis and immune complex formation, emboli from endocarditis, and vascular effects of toxins. Vascular invasion by bacteria may result in a severe inflammatory reaction, as in meningococcemia, or in a minimal reaction, as in ecthyma gangrenosum. Gram-strained smears of scrapings from the base of skin lesions,

Table 20 Selected Types of Cutaneous Lesions Caused by Opportunistic Organisms Infecting Immunocompromised patients

Erythematous macules	Vesicles, bullae
Plaques	Hemorrhagic lesions
Papules, nodules	Ecthyma gangrenosum
Pustules	Cellulitis
Abscesses	Toxic epidermal necrolysis
Subcutaneous nodules, panniculitis	

a frequently neglected procedure, is an important diagnostic adjunct. Skin biopises are particularly important in the diagnosis of infections caused by *Candida* (41).

The gross morphological appearance of skin lesions caused by infection in the immunocompromised patient is not very helpful in making an etiological diagnosis (Table 20). Thus, to take advantage of the skin as an "early warning system" of serious infection, skin biopsies for culture and histological examination should be carried out in any immunocompromised patient with an unexplained skin lesion (42).

REFERENCES

1. Klastersky J. Empiric antimicrobial therapy for febrile granulocytopenic cancer patients: lessons from four EORTC trials. Eur J Cancer Clin Oncol 1988; 24(Suppl I):S35–S45.
2. Petersdorf RG, Beeson PB. Fever of unexplained origin: report on 100 cases. Medicine (Baltimore) 1961; 40:1–30.
3. Pizzo PA, Armstrong D, Bodey G, et al. The design, analysis, and reporting of clinical trials on the empirical antibiotic management of the neutropenic patient. Report of a consensus panel. J Infect Dis 1990; 161:397–401.
4. EORTC International Antimicrobial Therapy Cooperative Group. Ceftazidime combined with a short or long course of amikacin for empirical therapy of gram negative bacteremia in cancer patients with granulocytopenia. N Engl J Med 1987; 317:1692–1698.
5. Awada A, Van der Auwera P, Meunier F, Daneau D, Klastersky J. Streptococcal and enterococcal bacteremia in patients with cancer. Clin Infect Dis 1992; 15:33–48.
6. EORTC International Antimicrobial Therapy Cooperative Group. Empiric antifungal therapy in febrile granulocytopenic patients. Am J Med 1989; 86:668–672.
7. Saral R. Acyclovir prophylaxis of herpes simplex virus infections. A randomized doubleblind controlled trial in bone marrow transplant patients. N Engl J Med 1981; 305:63–67.
8. Schmidt GM, Horak DA, Niland JC, et al., City of Hope-Stanford Syntex CMV Study Group. A randomized, controlled trial of prophylactic ganciclovir for

cytomegalovirus pulmonary infection in recipients of allogeneic bone marrow transplants. 1991; 324:1005–1011.

9. Knockaert DC, Vanneste LJ, Vanneste SB, Bobbaers HJ. Fever of unknown origin in the 1980s: an update of the diagnosis spectrum. Arch Intern Med 1992; 152:51–55.
10. Pizzo AP, Robichaud KJ, Wesley R, Commers JR. Fever in the pediatric and young adult patient with cancer: a prospective study of 1001 episodes. Medicine (Baltimore) 1982; 61:153–165.
11. Luft FC, Rissing JP, White A, Brooks GF. Infections or neoplasm as causes of prolonged fever in cancer patients. Am J Med Sci 1976; 272:65–74.
12. Klastersky J, Weerts D, Hensgens C, Debusscher L. Fever of unexplained origin in patients with cancer. Eur J Cancer 1973; 9:649–656.
13. Chang JC, Gross HM. Neoplastic fever responds to the treatment of an adequate dose of naproxen. J Clin Oncol 1985; 3:552–558.
14. Wolff SM, Fauci AS, Dale DS. Unusual etiologies of fever and their evaluation. Annu Rev Med 1975; 26:277–281.
15. Talbot GH, Provencher M, Cassileth PA. Persistent fever after recovery from granulocytopenia in acute leukemia. Arch Intern Med 1988; 148:129–135.
16. Kauffman CA, Bradley SF, Ross SC, Weber DR. Hepatosplenic candidiasis: successful treatment with fluconazole. Am J Med 1991; 91:137–141.
17. Gasson JC. Molecular physiology of granulocyte-macrophage colony-stimulating factor. Blood 1991; 77:1131–1145.
18. Demetri GD, Griffin JD. Granulocyte colony-stimulating factor and its receptor. Blood 1991; 78:2791–2808.
19. Lieschke GJ, Burgess AW. Granulocyte colony stimulating factor and granulocyte-macrophage colony-stimulating factor (Parts 1 and 2). N Engl J Med 1992; 327:28–55, 99–106.
20. Crawford J, Ozer H, Stoller R, et al. Reduction by granulocyte colony-stimulating factor of fever and neutropenia induced by chemotherapy in patients with small cell lung cancer. N Engl J Med 1991; 325:164–170.
21. Sculier JP, Klastersky J. Significance of serum bactericidal activity in gram negative bacillary bacteremia in patients with or without granulocytopenia. Am J Med 1984; 76:429–435.
22. Pizzo PA, Robichaud RJ, Gill FA, et al. Duration of empiric antibiotic therapy in granulocytopenic cancer patients. Am J Med 1979; 68:194–200.
23. Reed WP. Intravenous access devices for supportive care of patients with cancer. Curr Opin Oncol 1991; 3:634–642.
24. Gerson SL, Talbot GH, Hurwitz S, et al. Prolonged granulocytopenia: the major risk factor for invasive pulmonary aspergillosis in patients with acute leukemia. Ann Intern Med 1984; 100:345–351.
25. Pannuti CS, Gingrich RD, Pfaller MA, Wenzel RP. Nosocomial pneumonia in adult patients undergoing bone marrow transplantation: a 9-year study. Clin Oncol 1991; 9:77–84.
26. Arnow PM, Sadigh M, Costas C, Weil D, Chudy R. Endemic and epidemic aspergillo- sis, hospital epidemiology, diagnosis, and treatment. J Infect Dis 1991; 164:988–1002.

27. Varthalitis I, Meunier F. *Pneumocystis carinii* pneumonia: the pathogen, the diagnosis and recent advances in management. Int J Antimicrob Agents 1991; 1:97–108.
28. Raviglione MC. Extrapulmonary pneumocystosis: the first 50 cases. Rev Infect Dis 1990; 12:1127–1138.
29. Harvey RL, Sunstrum JC. *Rhodococcus equi* infection in patients with and without human immunodeficiency virus infection. Rev Infect Dis 1991; 13:139–145.
30. Bensinger WI. Supportive care in marrow transplantation. Curr Opin Oncol 1992; 4:614–623.
31. Rubinoff MJ, Field M. Infectious diarrhea. Annu Rev Med 1991; 42:403–410.
32. Bodey GP, Fainstein V, Guerrant R. Infections of the gastrointestinal tract in the immunocompromised patient. Annu Rev Med 1986; 37:271–281.
33. Wade DS, Nava HR, Douglass HO. Neutropenic enterocolitis. Clinical diagnosis and treatment. Cancer 1992; 69:17–23.
34. Starnes HF, Moore FD, Mentzer S, et al. Abdominal pain in neutropenic cancer patients. Cancer 1986; 57:616–621.
35. Wade DS, Douglass HJ, Nava HR, Piedmonte M. Abdominal pain in neutropenic patients. Arch Surg 1990; 125:1119–1127.
36. Glenn J, Funkhouser WK, Schneider PS. Acute illnesses necessitating urgent abdominal surgery in neutropenic cancer patients; description of 14 cases and review of the literature. Surgery 1989; 105:778–789.
37. Hakes TB, Armstrong D. Toxoplasmosis: problems in diagnosis and treatment. Cancer 1983; 52:1535–1540.
38. Kaplan MH, Rosen PP, Armstrong D. Cryptococcosis in a cancer hospital: clinical and pathological correlated in forty-six patients. Cancer 1977; 39:2265–2274.
39. Farber JM, Peterkin PI. *Listeria monocytogenes*, a food-borne pathogen. Microbiol Rev 1991; 55:476–511.
40. Major EO, Ameniya K, Tornatore CS, Houff SA, Berger JR. Pathogenesis and molecular biology of progressive multifocal leukoencephalopathy, the JC virus-induced demyelinating disease of the human brain. Clin Mircobiol Rev 1992; 5:49–73.
41. Kingston ME, Mackey D. Skin clues in the diagnosis of life-threatening infections. Rev Infect Dis 1986; 8:1–11.
42. Wolfson JS, Sober AJ, Rubin RH. Dermatologic manifestations of infections in immunocompromised patients. Medicine (Baltimore) 1985; 64:115–133.

2

Prevention of Infection in Cancer Patients

Daniel A. Scott
Naval Medical Research Institute, Bethesda, Maryland

Stephen C. Schimpff
University of Maryland Medical System, and University of Maryland Medical Center, Baltimore, Maryland

I. INTRODUCTION

Implementing appropriate strategies to prevent infection in any immunocompromised patient begins with an assessment of the type of immune defect(s) from which they suffer. This then helps define the types of infections that pose the greatest risk to that patient. The major types of immune defects that clinicians encounter can be divided into six broad categories: (1) granulocytopenia, (2) deficiencies of cellular immunity, (3) deficiencies of humoral immunity, (4) obstruction of a normal lumen by tumor or fibrosis, (5) central nervous system dysfunction, and (6) damage to normal anatomical barriers, such as the skin or mucosal surfaces. Although approaches to preventing infection vary with each type of immune defect and the severity of the defect in a given patient, four general approaches can be applied to all patients: (1) attempt to improve the patient's immune defect(s), (2) reduce acquisition of potential pathogens, (3) suppress organisms with which the patient is already colonized that are likely to cause infection later, and (4) reduce or avoid procedures that disrupt normal anatomical barriers.

II. GRANULOCYTOPENIA

The risk of infection varies inversely with the absolute granulocyte count. Infection rates begin to rise between 500 and 1000 cells/μl and to increase markedly below 100 cells/μl, with the majority of bacteremias occurring in this group. The predominant infections seen early in the course of neutropenia are bacterial (Table 1). Gram-negative rods were formerly the major pathogens, but for a variety of reasons the numbers of gram-positive infections, particularly *Staphylococcus* spp. and α-hemolytic streptococci, have increased dramatically over the past two decades. Fungi, such as *Candida* spp. and *Aspergillus flavus* and *Aspergillus fumigatus*, also are important pathogens particularly with more prolonged granulocytopenia. Efforts to prevent infection in these patients encompass each of the four approaches and are discussed here.

A. Improve Host Defense Mechanisms

Decreasing the duration and severity of neutropenia is the best approach; however, favorable responses to cytotoxic drugs are correlated with the ability

Table 1 Factors Predisposing to Infection Among Patients with Cancer

Granulocytopenia (e.g., acute leukemia), usually with associated damage to body barriers (especially alimentary canal mucosa, respiratory tract ciliary function, and integument); common organisms:
Gram-negative bacilli: *Pseudomonas aeruginosa*, *Klebsiella pneumoniae*, and *Escherichia coli*
Gram-positive cocci: *Staphylococcus aureus*, *Staphylococcus epidermidis*, and α-hemolytic *Streptococcus* species
Yeasts: *Candida* spp., *Torulopsis glabrata*
Fungi: *Aspergillus* spp., *Mucor*
Cellular immune deficiency (e.g., lymphoma); common organisms:
Bacteria: *Listeria monocytogenes*, *Salmonella* spp., *Mycobacterium* spp., *Nocardia asteroides*, and *Legionella pneumophila*
Viruses: varicella-zoster, herpes simplex, and cytomegalovirus
Fungi: *Cryptococcus neoformans*, *Histoplasma capsulatum*, and *Coccidiodes immitis*
Protozoa: *Pneumocystis carinii* and *Toxoplasma gondii*
Helminth: *Strongyloides stercoralis*
Humoral immune dysfunction (e.g., multiple myeloma); common organisms: *Streptococcus pneumoniae* and *Haemophilus influenzae*
Obstruction to natural passages (e.g., solid tumors)
Common sites: respiratory tract, biliary tract, and urinary tract
Common organisms: locally colonizing
Central nervous system dysfunction (e.g., brain tumors)
Common sites: pneumonitis and urinary tract infection
Common organisms: locally colonizing
Infections associated with medical procedures
Procedures: intravascular catheters, urinary catheters, and respiratory assist devices
Common organisms: locally colonizing

Source: From Ref. 46.

to give maximum doses of chemotherapeutic agents, which naturally result in increased side effects, including bone marrow suppression. Early attempts focused on granulocyte transfusions. These have been shown in small controlled trials to prevent gram-negative bacteremia and to improve the survival of infected patients with persistent neutropenia (1–4). Schiffer, in a review of granulocyte transfusions, suggests that some of the reasons for poor responses that caused this technique to be largely abandoned were the generally low doses of leukocytes used and the lack of attention to the problem of alloimmunization (5). Transfusions must be given on a daily basis, which places a great logistical strain on blood banks and taxes the donor pool. He describes good results using leukocytes from chronic myelogenous leukemia patients because of the high doses that can be achieved and their content of early cells that continue to divide for several days but have not caused problems with a graft-versus-host response. Another potential approach, which to our knowledge has not been tried, would be to treat a related single donor with a colony-stimulating factor, giving rise to high leukocyte count and peripheral progenitor cells. Another problem with leukocyte transfusions, which can be minimized with current techniques for screening donors, is the risk of transmitting such infections as cytomegalovirus (CMV), other viruses, or, more rarely, parasitic pathogens, such as toxoplasmosis. Our recommendation at this time is not to use granulocyte transfusions on a prophylactic basis but to consider them a treatment modality for patients with life-threatening infection who respond poorly to known appropriate antibiotics in the face of persistent neutropenia.

The cloning and expression of the recombinant myeloid colony-stimulating factors (CSF), granulocyte CSF (G-CSF) and granulocyte-macrophage CSF (GM-CSF), have led to a whole new approach to chemotherapy-induced neutropenia. They can stimulate the recovery of neutrophil counts (6) and may have beneficial effects on phagocyte function (7). The usual approach to these cytokines has been to utilize them to allow more aggressive cancer chemotherapy, perhaps even avoiding the need for autologous bone marrow transplantation in some instances. G-CSF has been shown in a randomized, double-blind, placebo-controlled trial to decrease the incidence of severe neutropenia, infection, antibiotic requirements, and period of hospitalization in patients receiving standard chemotherapy for small cell lung cancer (8). GM-CSF has shown promise in uncontrolled trials, but no controlled data are available. These cytokines have been used in the setting of bone marrow transplantation to speed recovery following engraftment. Peters and colleagues, working with breast cancer patients in autologous bone marrow transplantation (ABMT), have shown that GM-CSF begun immediately after marrow reinfusion led to a substantially shortened period of neutropenia (9). They later found that G-CSF gave similar results and that the period of absolute neutropenia, which had been unaffected by posttransplant CSF administration, could be shortened by infusion of peripheral blood progenitor cells. These cells are collected by leukopheresis before bone marrow transplant after pretreatment with either GM- or G-CSF (10). This has led to fewer adverse events, including less time in the intensive care unit, a shorter hospital stay, and a reduction in total cost from about $100,000 to approximately $75,000 per transplant episode (W.P. Peters, personal communication). Decreased morbidity has also been seen using GM-CSF after ABMT for lymphoid neoplasias (11).

Use of these cytokines in allogeneic bone marrow transplantation has been more cautious because of the fear that they may increase the incidence or severity of graft-versus-host disease or precipitate relapses in patients with myeloid leukemias (12). Increased graft-versus-host disease was not seen in early studies of GM-CSF in patients with graft failure (13), and GM-CSF has been shown to speed neutrophil recovery in recipients of marrow from HLA-identical siblings (14). A beneficial effect was not seen in patients who received methotrexate as part of their post-transplant immunosuppressive regimen compared to patients who received prednisone and cyclosporine.

Despite the various studies of these agents, there is still a need to perform appropriate prospective, randomized controlled trials to determine the best and the most logical approaches to cytokine use for infection prevention. Based upon the available data, however, the following recommendations seem appropriate. Clearly they are useful in the setting of autologous bone marrow transplantation for reducing the nadir and the duration of granulocytopenia. Second, they are appropriate for patients receiving aggressive therapy that would be likely to cause more than a week of significant granulocytopenia. We define *significant* as certainly < 500 polymorphonuclear leukocytes (PMN)/μl, and perhaps a level $< 200/\mu$l, because almost all serious infections occur only in patients who have < 200 PMN/μl.

The best approach to granulocytopenia is to avoid it altogether. At present, most chemotherapeutic agents kill dividing cells. This accounts for their preference for rapidly dividing tumor cells but also their significant effects on bone marrow and rapidly dividing mucosal cells. The development of monoclonal antibodies has led to the study of tumor-specific monoclonals as chemotherapeutic agents and as carrier molecules delivering chemotherapeutic agents, radioactivity, or toxins directly to tumor cells. Immunoglobulins bound to such toxins as *Pseudomonas* exotoxin A and the plant toxin ricin are known as immunotoxins and have shown promise in several areas (15,16). Perhaps this type of targeted approach will lead to effective chemotherapy strategies that do not induce granulocytopenia.

B. Reduce Acquisition

The concept is to reduce acquisition of new organisms, because it has been demonstrated that more than 50% of the infections in this patient population are caused by organisms acquired by the patient during hospitalization (17). The major routes of acquisition are the hands of health care workers, food, water, and the air. Hand washing is the most basic technique but is frequently overlooked by health care workers. Even in the midst of a recent study of the efficacy of different hand-washing agents when the professional staff was being observed, they took advantage of only approximately 40% of hand-washing opportunities (18). Although hand washing with any product is probably better than none, Doebbeling et al. found chlorhexidine significantly reduced nosocomial infections compared with the combined use of soap and alcohol. Chlorhexidine is currently the agent of choice and should be made readily available throughout hospital wards.

Gram-negative bacilli are acquired principally from food and, to a lesser degree, from water and hands. If the major cause of serious infection from acquired organisms are gram-negative rod infections, then the major sources must be dealt with, namely food and water. Remington and Schimpff summarized the findings of others in an editorial entitled "Please Don't Eat the Salads," in which they point out that a simple approach to a low microbial content diet can be quite effective (19). The importance of properly cooking meat was recently reemphasized by a large outbreak of disease at a fast-food restaurant secondary to *Escherichia coli* O157:H7 in undercooked hamburger. *Candida* can also be acquired from food products, including many fruits and unpasteurized fruit juices.

Most city water supplies are reasonably satisfactory, provided the faucet aerator at the end of the piping system has not become laden with organic debris that can support the growth of gram-negative rods, such as *Pseudomonas aeruginosa* or *Serratia marcescens*. Significant gram-negative contamination has also been linked to nosocomial sources, such as an ice machine.

Some bacterial pathogens, such as *Staphylococcus aureus*, can be acquired via aerosol. In these cases there is usually a point source, such as a patient with staphylococcal pneumonia, and the problem is best handled by isolating the source patient. *Aspergillus* can also be acquired via the air, and here the problem is more difficult because the spores are ubiquitous. Outbreaks have been associated with new construction or renovation, for example. In this situation care must be taken to ensure a clean air supply before beginning work. Laminar airflow rooms or other prophylactic measures may be required, especially for patients expected to have prolonged neutropenia. The old "standard" approach to reverse isolation, which generally included gowns, gloves, mask, and frequently booties and hats, with no attention to food, water, or air, was ultimately proved by Nauseef and Maki to be of no utility (20). However, laminar airflow rooms can be effective in assuring adequate air filtration for patients at high risk of infection by airborne-related organisms, such as *Aspergillus* (21). Even here, however, there may be other techniques for air filtration that can be more simply utilized than placing the patient in the isolation setting. A portable laminar airflow unit was as effective as a wall unit in preventing infection in one study from Japan (22).

C. Suppression of Potential Pathogens

1. Skin

Cutaneous infections are common in granulocytopenic patients, particularly at sites where the skin has been interrupted by invasive procedures. It has been suggested that daily bathing with such agents as chlorhexidine may decrease the incidence of infection. The axilla and perianal area are at particularly high risk, and twice daily swabbing with povidone-iodine during the period of granulocytopenia has been shown to decrease infections (23); chlorhexidine should be equally effective.

2. Periodontium

Periodontal infections are frequent during periods of granulocytopenia (see Chapter 5). The oral mucosa is also a likely source of α-hemolytic streptococcal bacteremia. A program of professional and personal dental care, with plaque removal, repair of any caries, and teeth extraction when necessary, as well as daily brushing and flossing, is prudent. Despite concerns to the contrary, pretherapy prophylaxis by a dental professional followed by regular brushing and flossing does not lead to bleeding or bacteremia but rather reduces acute flare-ups of chronic periodontitis during granulocytopenia (see Chapter 5).

3. Oral Viral Infections

Herpes simplex virus is latent in most adults and is commonly recognized as a severe oral or esophageal infection in the first 20 days following bone marrow transplantation (24). Acyclovir has been found to be nearly 100% effective as prophylaxis among these patients (25). Although severe herpes simplex oral infections are seen in patients with leukemia or other patients with cancer receiving intensive chemotherapy, it has been said that the frequency and severity are much less than in bone marrow transplant patients. Bustamante and Wade at the University of Maryland Cancer Center have now developed data that demonstrate that acute myelocytic leukemia patients receiving induction therapy have frequent herpes simplex oral infections (66% reactivation rates in seropositive patients), which in turn can be substantially prevented by the use of acyclovir (26). It is important to recognize that the oral infection frequently encountered has a bacterial component or even a component caused by *Candida albicans* or *Candida tropicalis*. This is similar to the observation of *Candida* esophagitis: that is, if one evaluates these patients early in their course, one finds that the initial lesion is often caused by herpes simplex, which in turn allows invasion by bacteria and then by *Candida*. Prevention of the initial viral lesion in turn helps to prevent the superinfection with bacteria and fungi.

4. Antibacterial Prophylaxis

Several different antibiotic strategies have been found to try to prevent bacterial infections. An early approach was to use a combination of oral nonabsorbable antibiotics, such as gentamicin, vancomycin, and nystatin (21). This was shown to reduce the incidence of infection, particularly gram-negative bacteremia; however, the regimens were expensive and poorly tolerated and resistant isolates were soon detected. Trimethoprim-sulfamethoxazole (TMP-SMX) was undergoing studies to prevent *Pneumocystis carinii* pneumonia and was coincidentally found to decrease the incidence of bacterial infection as well (27). The toxicities seen with TMP-SMX, such as prolongation of marrow suppression, development of resistant isolates, and possibly increased fungal infections, along with the lack of efficacy against *P. aeruginosa*, led to trials of the newly developed fluoroquinolones norfloxacin and ciprofloxacin (28–30). These have been effective in preventing gram-negative infections and are better tolerated than other regimens, but they have been associated with an increase in gram-positive infections and if used frequently will certainly lead to the development of resistant gram-negative organisms. Vancomycin has been shown to prevent infections with gram-positive organisms effectively, but with reports of vancomycin-resistant enterococci and coagulase-negative staphylococci, for which there is no other therapy, it does not seem prudent to use vancomycin in this manner (31). If used as prophylaxis, these antibiotics should be reserved for those patients with profound, persistent neutropenia (which we define for these purposes as <100 PMN/μl for more than 10 days), who are at particularly high risk of bacteremia.

5. Antifungal Prophylaxis

Fungal infections remain a significant problem in neutropenic patients, and therapy of established disease is less than optimal. Therefore, several methods of prophylaxis have been investigated. Initial attempts focused on oral nonabsorbable polyenes, such as nystatin. Doses ranging from 2 to 30 million units/day produced disappointing results (32). Combining nystatin with oral amphotericin B did not add to its efficacy (33). Clotrimazole troches are effective in some groups but not in patients with leukemia, which probably means that they are not effective in a combined setting of severe neutropenia and mucosal damage when antibiotic therapy has further shifted the oral flora toward yeasts (34). Flucytosine is not considered an option for prophylaxis because of bone marrow suppression (5-flucytosine is partially converted to 5-fluorouracil) and the rapid development of resistance (35).

Fluconazole is a new bistriazole that is well absorbed and widely distributed in the body and has a wide spectrum of antifungal activity. In neutropenic animal models of disseminated candidiasis, it works best when given before infection or very early in the course (36). In a randomized, double-blind placebo-controlled trial in bone marrow transplant patients, fluconazole clearly decreased the number of invasive fungal infections (Table 2) (37). There was no change in overall mortality; however, the mortality attributed to fungal infection was decreased in the fluconazole group. There was also a significant increase in the mean alanine aminotransferase level in the fluconazole patients. In this trial there was a slight increase in colonization with *Candida krusei* in the fluconazole group, and this organism was responsible for all three episodes of candidemia in the fluconazole group. Others reported a marked increase in the number of infections with *C. krusei* when fluconazole prophylaxis was instituted in their bone marrow transplant patients (38). In adults undergoing chemotherapy for acute leukemia, fluconazole decreases colonization with *Candida* spp., except *C. krusei*, and decreases superficial fungal infections (39). However, it does not significantly decrease the number of invasive fungal infections, the use of amphotericin B, or mortality. At this time fluconazole prophylaxis should be used with caution. It has not been shown to decrease amphotericin B use, and as was seen in animals with ketoconazole, there is the possibility that it may decrease the effectiveness of subsequent amphotericin B. Nevertheless, its use is common today because it seems to be better than any other available approach.

Systemic prophylactic amphotericin B has been advocated by some authors (40), but this has not been well studied. Perfect et al. (41) studied a regimen of 0.1 mg/kg/day of intravenous amphotericin B versus placebo in autologous bone marrow transplant patients. They found a decrease in candidal colonization but no differences in the number of fungal infections, number of patients advanced to high-dose amphotericin B, or overall mortality. More encouraging results have been reported by Rousey et al. (42), by whom a decrease in invasive aspergillosis was observed, but historical controls were used, which makes these data less than ideal.

Amphotericin B administered as a nasal spray has been studied at the University of Maryland Cancer Center (43). It was effective in decreasing nasal colonization with *Aspergillus* but did not decrease the number of *Aspergillus* infections or the requirement for systemic amphotericin B. Culture-positive

Table 2 Definite Cases and Deaths Ascribed to Fungal Infection

	Fluconazole	Placebo
Total infections	5[a,b]	28
Total deaths	1[a]	10

[a]Includes three *Candida krusei* and two *Aspergillus* and Mucorales.
[b]$p < 0.001$ compared with placebo.
Source: Ref. 37.

Aspergillus sinusitis was decreased, but the overall incidence of clinically apparent sinusitis was the same in both groups, and this may merely reflect the difficulty in recovering *Aspergillus* in the presence of the nasal spray.

At the present time, the use of intravenous or intranasal prophylactic amphotericin cannot be recommended. Further trials are required to define better the role, if any, of prophylactic amphotericin B, either the standard desoxycholate or new preparations, such as liposomal amphotericin.

D. Reduce or Avoid Invasive Procedures

Using invasive diagnostic procedures and monitoring devices only when absolutely necessary and continuously reevaluating the need for such devices is the best way to avoid infectious complications. If urinary catheters are used, essentially all of them will become colonized and represent a risk for infection. There is little in the way of specific care that will prevent colonization, although maintaining a closed system is of some benefit. Short-term antibiotic prophylaxis may be appropriate in some situations but does not prevent infection for long.

For intravenous catheters, the data on prevention differ with the type of catheter. The most common types of venous access in cancer patients are the long-term, tunneled central venous catheters, such as the Hickman-Broviac. These are placed in the operating room under sterile conditions, and the major issues simply involve using appropriate sterile technique for flushing the ports and infusing solutions. If percutaneously placed central venous catheters are used, they should be placed under strict sterile conditions with a broad sterile field and protective attire, the skin should be cleansed with chlorhexidine, and catheters should be changed only because of signs of infection (44,45). Routine changes, especially over a guide wire, do not decrease the rate of infections and may increase the complication rate (45).

Infection prevention must be considered even when antibiotics are being used for treatment. Many antibiotics, such as those commonly used for empirical therapy (e.g., ticarcillin and piperacillin), suppress the enteric microbial flora because of their hepatoenteric circulation. This suppression reduces colonization resistance and makes it easier for an acquired organism to colonize. It has therefore been argued that, because anaerobes rarely cause infection during granulocytopenia, one should use agents for empirical therapy that do not suppress anaerobes (e.g., ceftazidime, which has no anaerobic activity, or imipenem, which has no hepatoenteric circulation).

III. CELLULAR IMMUNE DYSFUNCTION

Defects in cellular immunity lead to infection with an entirely different array of pathogens from those seen with granulocytopenia. Typically they are intracellular organisms and are found in patients with lymphomas or lymphocytic leukemias and after bone marrow transplant on long-term suppressive therapy, particularly those being treated for graft-versus-host disease. The organisms include those listed in Table 1 (46). The issues surrounding prevention can be approached in the same way as for those with granulocytopenia.

A. Improve Host Defenses

Currently there are no methods of improving cellular immunity in general, analogous to techniques used for raising granulocyte counts. There have been attempts to transfer immune cells for specific diseases, such as CMV infection, but this is an exception. The use of vaccines is another possible approach. In general, live virus vaccines, such as yellow fever, oral polio, and oral typhoid vaccine, should be avoided in patients with cellular immune defects. The exception may be the Oka/Merck attenuated varicella vaccine that will likely soon be licensed for use in the United States (47). Primary varicella infection is associated with a high risk of morbidity and mortality in immunocompromised children and adults. The vaccine has been shown to protect both healthy children and children with acute leukemia in remission, although side effects were quite common in the immunocompromised patients (48–50). Ideally, the vaccine should be given before the most acute period of immunosuppression. This strategy can be applied to patients scheduled to undergo solid organ transplants and bone marrow transplants and perhaps lymphoma patients, but this luxury does not exist in patients with newly diagnosed acute leukemia. Another approach is to vaccinate family members who are susceptible to varicella with the hope of reducing acquisition of primary infection in the immunocompromised child. The major concern is possible spread of the vaccine strain to the immunocompromised patient. In a study of 30 children with cancer and 37 healthy siblings who were vaccinated, no cases of varicella were attributable to the vaccine strain in either group (51). It appears that to transmit the vaccine a rash must develop, which is very rare in normal hosts. It is unclear as yet whether the vaccine will have an affect on reducing herpes zoster, a major problem for bone marrow transplant patients, postradiation lymphoma patients, and others.

B. Reduce Acquisition

With the recent increase in tuberculosis (TB) cases, particularly multidrug-resistant *Mycobacterium tuberculosis*, preventing infection is of paramount importance. TB is transmitted by aerosol, with infection rates of 5% for contacts of smear-negative cases and reaching 80% for close contacts of smear-positive cases. Prevention of nosocomial transmission involves housing patients with respiratory infections on separate wards, respiratory isolation, control of ventilation systems, and possibly the use of ultraviolet lights to kill viable bacteria.

As noted previously, *Aspergillus* is also transmitted via air, but the spores are ubiquitous, not transmitted via infected patients. Special care must be taken when any construction or renovation takes place: this can be the source of increased numbers of spores. As noted, laminar flow rooms or other air filtration techniques may be required for patients at high risk, such as autologous bone marrow transplant patients.

Disseminated toxoplasmosis can produce devastating neurological disease and fatalities in immunocompromised patients. Transmission is via consumption of cysts found in infected tissue from virtually any animal or mature oocysts excreted in the stool of members of the cat family only. Transfusion of blood or leukocytes or organ transplantation can also transmit the disease. New infections can be prevented by avoiding contact with cat feces, thoroughly cooking all meat, washing hands after contact with raw meat, and washing all fruits and vegetables. Although there are few data, some recommend not using blood from seropositive donors for transfusion to immunosuppressed hosts (52).

It was recently demonstrated that epidemic listeriosis could be traced to contaminated foods (53), and now recent evidence has shown that the majority of sporadic cases are also food borne (54,55). In a case-control study, an increased risk of infection was associated with soft cheeses, food from delicatessen counters, and eating undercooked chicken. The U.S. Centers for Disease Control, Food and Drug Administration, and Food Safety and Inspection Service recommend that high-risk individuals avoid soft cheeses (Mexican style, Brie, feta, Camembert, and blue-veined cheese), recook leftover or ready-to-eat foods, such as hot dogs, thoroughly before eating, and avoid or thoroughly cook foods from delicatessen counters (56).

C. Suppression of Potential Pathogens

Treatment of some latent infections or antimicrobial prophylaxis can prevent disease in some circumstance. Isoniazid (INH) should be given for 12 months to those with depressed cellular immunity and a positive purified protein derivative (PPD) test (defined as ≤ 5 mm induration in this population). Since cellular immune depression may lead to false negative PPD results, a proxy may be needed, such as a Gohn (primary) complex on chest radiograph. If there has been contact with a known case or INH or multidrug-resistant TB, an alternative agent, such as rifampin, or combination therapy may be appropriate. There are few data to show that any agent other than INH works for prophylaxis, and the approach to an individual patient should be based on sensitivities of the isolate from the index case and consultation with an expert in the field.

P. carinii pneumonia can be prevented by administration of trimethoprim-sulfamethoxazole (27). Alternative regimens include aerosolized pentamidine, although this is more expensive and has been associated with upper lobe and extrapulmonary disease in acquired immunodeficiency syndrome patients, and dapsone with or without trimethoprim. TMP-SMX has the additional advantage that it may provide prophylaxis against recrudescent toxoplasmosis in seropositive patients. Toxoplasmosis can be effectively prevented by a regimen of pyrimethamine and sulfadiazine, which has been recommended for the seronegative recipients of seropositive solid organs, such as hearts, in whom the risk of disease is very high. Other indications for this regimen are less clear.

Strongyloides stercoralis has the ability to complete its entire life cycle within the human host and can therefore produce a syndrome of hyperinfection affecting the gastrointestinal tract and lungs and even disseminate to the central nervous system and other sites. Disseminated disease carries a high mortality and is extremely difficult to treat. This can be easily prevented by treatment with thiabendazole for 3 days before beginning any immunosuppressive therapy. Suggested methods of diagnosis include stool samples, duodenal aspirates, and sputum Papanicolaou smears, but diagnosis can be difficult and it may be prudent to treat any patient with a significant exposure history empirically (e.g., previous residence in Puerto Rico, Central America, or other high-risk areas).

Several members of the herpesvirus family, herpes simplex, varicella-zoster virus, and CMV, are important pathogens in this population. As discussed, herpes simplex virus can be prevented by treatment with acyclovir and varicella addressed by use of the vaccine. There is no known prevention for herpes zoster. CMV has been a very difficult pathogen because of the high morbidity and mortality associated with invasive disease and its resistance to currently available antiviral agents. Autologous bone marrow transplant recipients who are seropositive or who receive a seropositive marrow are at particularly high risk. Intravenous immunoglobulin and acyclovir may have some benefit, but studies are conflicting and more recent studies have focused on ganciclovir (GCV), which does not require phosphorylation by viral thymidine kinase and is thus more active against CMV, which lacks this enzyme (57). Two studies have shown that allogeneic bone marrow transplant patients who are followed prospectively with surveillance cultures and are then treated with GCV have a significant decrease in invasive CMV disease and death (58,59). One problem with this approach is that not all patients develop positive cultures before invasive disease. Two recent studies evaluated GCV given prophylactically to seropositive recipients of allogeneic bone marrow transplants (60,61). Both showed significantly decreased CMV infection and a decrease in the incidence or severity of CMV disease. The study in which disease was significantly decreased also used acyclovir (for herpes simplex prophylaxis) during the period of neutropenia before engraftment. In all these studies, significant neutropenia was seen, which frequently required stopping the GCV and, in the study by Goodrich et al., was associated with an increase in bacterial infection (60). A phase I–II study of foscarnet shows it to be safe, except when given with cyclosporine and amphotericin B because of its nephrotoxicity, in bone marrow transplant (BMT) patients, and it appeared to prevent CMV infection and disease (62). It is clear that some type of prophylactic therapy for CMV is required in seropositive BMT patients. Because of their different toxicities, it may be that the best approach combines ganciclovir before and after the transplant with foscarnet given during the period of neutropenia. Another interesting approach being pursued by Riddel et al. at the Fred Hutchinson Cancer Research Center is the establishment of CMV immunity by the "adoptive transfer" of antigen-specific T cells (63,64). They iso- lated and propagated in vitro $CD8^+$ cytotoxic T cells from CMV-seropositive bone marrow donors and then showed that these can establish CMV immunity in BMT recipients. These data are exciting and may represent an approach for the future.

IV. Humoral Immune Dysfunction

Among cancer patients, this type of defect is seen mainly in patients with multiple myeloma, chronic lymphocytic leukemia, and late after BMT in the course of chronic graft-versus-host disease. The main pathogens unique to this defect are encapsulated bacteria, such as *Streptococcus pneumoniae* and *Haemophilus influenzae*.

A. Improve Host Defenses

Treatment of the underlying disease may result in improvement of the immune defect, but these diseases are not curable at this time, so this provides only temporary benefit, if any. Replacement with intravenous immunoglobulin has been shown to decrease the number of bacterial infections in IgG-deficient patients with chronic lymphocytic leukemia (65). In allogeneic bone marrow transplant patients, it decreases the incidence of interstitial pneumonia, bacterial infections, and acute graftversus-host disease (66). However, a recent placebo-controlled study using intravenous (IVI) immunoglobulin for autologous bone marrow transplant patients showed no decrease in infection, and the IVI group had a significantly higher number of deaths caused by a higher incidence of hepatic venoocclusive disease (67).

Capsular polysaccharide vaccines are available for *S. pneumoniae* and *Neisseria meningitidis* types A, C, Y, and W135, and a conjugated capsular vaccine is now available for *H. influenzae* type B. These should be given; however, there is little evidence that they are effective because these patients do not respond with adequate if any normal antibody reaction.

B. Suppress Potential Pathogens

The only potential role for suppressive antimicrobial therapy is in children with splenectomies in whom long-term oral penicillin has been shown to decrease the incidence of bacterial infections. Some have suggested this approach in BMT patients, but the data are unclear; vaccination in these patients plus immune serum globulin seems more appropriate.

V. OBSTRUCTION OF NATURAL PASSAGES

Solid tumors may impinge on the lumen of a variety of organs, such as bronchial obstruction by bronchogenic carcinoma, obstruction of the urinary tract secondary to cervical or prostatic carcinoma, eustachian tube by nasopharyngeal carcinoma, or biliary obstruction secondary to pancreatic or biliary duct carcinoma. In all these examples stasis leads to colonization and then infection with the normal flora found in the region of the obstruction. Relief of the obstruction via surgery, radiation therapy, mechanical stents, percutaneous drainage, or some combination of these is the key to the treatment and prevention of infection in these patients. Many of these patients are debilitated, and they should also receive standard vaccinations, such as the influenza and pneumococcal vaccines.

VI. DAMAGE TO NORMAL ANATOMICAL BARRIERS

Damage to mucosal barriers is frequently seen with aggressive chemotherapy in which the normal mucosa of the gastrointestinal tract and respiratory tract are damaged. Here, meticulous hygiene and treatment or prevention of any concomitant infections, such as herpetic mucositis or candidiasis, are important.

Bridging normal defenses via the placement of intravenous, arterial, or urinary catheters or endotracheal tubes frequently leads to infection. As discussed previously, the removal of any of these devices at the earliest possible time and meticulous care will help prevent infection.

Normal barriers can also be interrupted secondary to nervous system dysfunction, leading to aspiration or incontinence of urine or feces. This may be caused by primary central nervous system tumors, metastatic disease to the brain or spinal cord, or paraneoplastic syndromes. Treatment of the underlying disease to try to reverse any dysfunction and meticulous nursing care may help prevent infection.

REFERENCES

1. Alavi JB, Root RK, Djerassi I, et al. A randomized clinical trial of granulocyte transfusions for infection in acute leukemia. *N Engl J Med* 1977; 295:706–711.
2. Herzig RH, Herzig GP, Graw RG Jr, et al. Successful granulocyte transfusion therapy for gram-negative septicemia. A prospectively randomized controlled study. *N Engl J Med* 1977; 296:701–705.
3. Strauss RG, Connett JE, Gale RP, et al. A controlled trial of prophylactic

granulocyte transfusions during initial induction chemotherapy for acute myelogenous leukemia. *N Engl J Med* 1981; 305:597–638.

4. Clift RA, Sanders JE, Thomas ED. Granulocyte transfusions for the prevention of infection in patients receiving bone-marrow transplants. N Engl J Med 1978; 298:1052–1057.
5. Schiffer CA. Granulocyte transfusions: an overlooked therapeutic modality. *Transfusion Med Rev* 1990; 4:2–7.
6. Lieschke GJ, Burgess AW. Granulocyte colony-stimulating factor and granulocyte-macrophage colony-stimulating factor. *N Engl J Med* 1992; 327:99–106.
7. Roilides E, Walsh TJ, Pizzo PA, Rubin M. Granulocyte colony-stimulating factor enhances the phagocytic and bacterial activity of normal and defective human neutrophils. *J Infect Dis* 1991; 163:579–583.
8. Crawford J, Ozer H, Stoller R, et al. Reduction by granulocyte colony-stimulating factor of fever and neutropenia induced by chemotherapy in patients with small-cell lung cancer [see comments]. *N Engl J Med* 1991; 325:164–170.
9. Brandt SJ, Peters WP, Atwater SK, et al. Effect of recombinant human granulocyte-macrophage colony-stimulating factor on hematopoietic reconstitution after high-dose chemotherapy and autologous bone marrow transplantation. *N Engl J Med* 1988; 318:869–876.
10. Peters WP. Use of cytokines during prolonged neutropenia associated with autologous bone marrow transplantation [see comments]. *Rev Infect Dis* 1991; 13:993–996.
11. Nemunaitis J, Rabinowe SN, Singer JW, et al. Recombinant granulocyte-macrophage colony-stimulating factor after autologous bone marrow transplantation for lymphoid cancer. *N Engl J Med* 1991; 324:1773–1778.
12. Armitage JO. The use of granulocyte-macrophage colony-stimulating factor in bone marrow transplantation. *Semin Hematol* 1992; 29:14–18.
13. Nemunaitis J, Singer JW, Buckner CD, et al. Use of recombinant human granulocyte-macrophage colony stimulating factor in graft failure after bone marrow transplantation. *Blood* 1990; 76:245–253.
14. Nemunaitis J, Buckner CD, Appelbaum FR, et al. Phase I/II trial of recombinant human granulocyte-macrophage colony-stimulating factor following allogeneic bone marrow transplant. *Blood* 1991; 77:2065–2071.
15. Cobb PW, LeMaistre CF. Therapeutic use of immunotoxins. *Semin Hematol* 1992; 3(Suppl 2):6–13.
16. Pai LH, Pastan I. Immunotoxin therapy for cancer. *JAMA* 1993; 269:78–81.
17. Schimpff SC, Young VM, Greene WH, Vermeulen GC, Moody MR, Wiernik PH. Origin of infection in acute nonlymphocytic leukemia. Significance of hospital acquisition of potential pathogens. *Ann Intern Med* 1972; 77:707–714.
18. Dobbeling BN, Stanley GL, Sheetz CT, et al. Comparative efficacy of alternative hand-washing agents in reducing nosocomial infections in intensive care units. *N Engl J Med* 1992; 327:88–93.
19. Remington JS, Schimpff SC. Please don't eat the salads. *N Engl J Med* 1981; 304:433–435.
20. Nauseef WM, Maki DG. A study of the value of simple protective isolation in patients with granulocytopenia. *N Engl J Med* 1981; 304:448–453.

21. Schimpff SC, Greene WH, Young VM, et al. Infection prevention in acute nonlymphocytic leukemia. Laminar air flow room reverse isolation with oral, nonabsorbable antibiotic prophylaxis. *Ann Intern Med* 1975; 82:351–358.
22. Hasegawa H, Horiuchi S. Application of simplified bioclean apparatuses for treatment of acute leukemia. *Jpn J Clin Oncol* 1983; 13(Suppl 1):133–142.
23. Murillo J, Schimpff SC, Brouillet MD. Axillary lesions in patients with acute leukemia: evaluation of a preventive program. *Cancer* 1979; 43:1493–1496.
24. Wade JC, Newton B, McLaren C. Intravenous acyclovir to treat mucocutaneous herpes simplex virus infection after marrow transplantation. *Ann Intern Med* 1982; 96:265.
25. Wade JC, Newton B, Flourney N, et al. Oral acyclovir for prevention of herpes simplex reactivation after marrow transplantation. *Ann Intern Med* 1984; 100:823–828.
26. Bustamante CI, Wade JC. Herpes simplex virus infection in the immunocompromised cancer patient. *J Clin Oncol* 1991; 10:1903–1915.
27. Hughes WT, Kuhn S, Chaudhary S, et al. Successful chemoprophylaxis for *Pneumocystis carinii* pneumonitis. *N Engl J Med* 1977; 297:1419–1426.
28. Dekker AW, Rozenberg-Arska M, Verhoef J. Infection prophylaxis in acute leukemia: a comparison of ciprofloxacin with trimethoprim-sulfamethoxazole and colistin. *Ann Intern Med* 1987; 106:7–12.
29. Karp JE, Merz WG, Hendricksen C, et al. Oral norfloxacin for prevention of gram-negative bacterial infections in patients with acute leukemia and granulocytopenia: a randomized, double-blind, placebo-controlled trial. *Ann Intern Med* 1987; 106:1–7.
30. GIMEMA Infection Program. Gruppo Italiano Malattie Ematologiche Maligne dell'Adulto. Prevention of bacterial infection in neutropenic patients with hematologic malignancies. A randomized, multicenter trial comparing norfloxacin with ciprofloxacin. *Ann Intern Med* 1991; 115:7–12.
31. Attal M, Schlaifer D, Rubie H, et al. Prevention of gram-positive infections after bone marrow transplantation by systemic vancomycin: a prospective, randomized trial. *J Clin Oncol* 1991; 9:865–870.
32. Wade JC, Schimpff SC, Hargadon MT, Fortner CL, Young VM, Wiernik PH. A comparison of trimethoprim-sulfamethoxazole plus nystatin with gentamicin plus nystatin in the prevention of infections in acute leukemia. *N Engl J Med* 1981; 304:1057–1062.
33. Hann IM, Prentice HG, Corringham R, et al. Ketoconazole versus nystatin plus amphotericin B for fungal prophylaxis in severely immunocompromised patients. *Lancet* 1982; 1:826–829.
34. Owens NJ, Nightingale CH, Schweizer R, Schauer PK, Dekker PT, Quintiliani R. Prophylaxis of oral candidiasis with clotrimazole troches. *Arch Intern Med* 1984; 144:290–293.
35. Drouhet E, DuPont B. Evolution of antifungal agents: past present and future. *Rev Infect Dis* 1987; 9(Suppl 1):S4–S14.
36. Walsh TJ, Lee J, Aoki S, et al. Experimental basis for use of fluconazole for preventive or early treatment of disseminated candidiasis in granulocytopenic hosts. *Rev Infect Dis* 1990; 12(Suppl 3):S307–S317.

37. Goodman JL, Winston DJ, Greenfield RA, et al. A controlled trial of fluconazole to prevent fungal infections in patients undergoing bone marrow transplantation. *N Engl J Med* 1992; 326:845–851.
38. Wingard JR, Merz WG, Rinaldi MG, Johnson TR, Karp JE, Saral R. Increase in *Candida krusei* infection among patients with bone marrow transplantation and neutropenia treated prophylactically with fluconazole [see comments]. *N Engl J Med* 1991; 325:1274–1277.
39. Winston DJ, Chandrasekar PH, Lazarus HM, et al. Fluconazole prophylaxis of fungal infections in patients with acute leukemia. Results of a randomized placebo-controlled, double-blind, multicenter trial. *Ann Intern Med* 1993; 118:495–503.
40. Tam JY, Blume KG, Prober CG. Prophylactic fluconazole and *Candida krusei* infections [letter]. *N Engl J Med* 1992; 326:891.
41. Perfect JR, Klotman ME, Gilbert CC, et al. Prophylactic intravenous amphotericin B in neutropenic autologous bone marrow transplant recipients. *J Infect Dis* 1992; 165:891–897.
42. Rousey SR, Russler S, Gottlieb M, et al. Low-dose amphotericin B prophylaxis against invasive *Aspergillus* infections in allogeneic marrow transplantation. *Am J Med* 1991; 91:484.
43. Cushing D, Bustamante C, Devlin A. Aspergillus infection prophylaxis: amphotericin-B nose spray, a double-blind trial. In *Interscience Conference on Antimicrobial Agents and Chemotherapy*. 1991; Abstract 737.
44. Maki DG, Ringer M, Alvarado CJ. Prospective randomized trial of povidone-iodine, alcohol, and chlorhexidine for prevention of infection associated with central venous and arterial catheters. *Lancet* 1991; 338:339–343.
45. Cobb DK, High KP, Sawyer RG, et al. A controlled trial of scheduled replacement of central venous and pulmonary-artery catheters. *N Engl J Med* 1992; 327:1062–1068.
46. Pizzo PA, Schimpff SC. Strategies for the prevention of infection in the myelosuppressed or immunosuppressed cancer patient. Cancer Treat Rep 1983; 67:223–234.
47. Gershon AA, LaRussa P, Hardy I, Steinberg S, Silverstein S. Varicella vaccine: the American experience. J Infect Dis 1992; 166(Suppl 1):S63–S68.
48. Hardy IB, Gershon A, Steinberg S, LaRussa P. NIAID Collaborative Varicella Vaccine Study Group. The incidence of zoster after immunization with live attenuated varicella vaccine. A study in children with leukemia. *N Engl J Med* 1991; 325:1545–1550.
49. Gershon AA, Steinberg SP, LaRussa P, et al. Immunization of healthy adults with live attenuated varicella vaccine. *J Infect Dis* 1988; 158:132–137.
50. Weibel R, Neff BJ, Kuter BJ, et al. Live attenuated varicella virus vaccine: efficacy trial in healthy children. *N Engl J Med* 1984; 310:1409–1415.
51. Remington JS, McLeod R. Toxoplasmosis. In: Gorbach SL, Bartlett JG, eds. Infectious Diseases, 1st ed. Philadelphia: WB Saunders, Harcourt Brace Jovanovich, 1992:1328–1342.
52. Diaz PS, Au D, Smith S, Amylon M, Link M, Arvin AM. Lack of transmission of the live attenuated varicella vaccine virus to immunocompromised children after immunization of their siblings. *Pediatrics* 1991; 87:166–170.

53. Linnan MJ, Mascola L, Lou XD, et al. Epidemic listeriosis associated with Mexican-style cheese. *N Engl J Med* 1988; 319:823–828.
54. Schuchat A, Deaver KA, Wenger JD, et al. Role of foods in sporadic listeriosis. I. Case-control study of dietary risk factors. *JAMA* 1992; 267:2041–2045.
55. Pinner RW, Schuchat A, Swaminathan B, et al. Role of foods in sporadic listeriosis. II. Microbiologic and epidemiologic investigation. *JAMA* 1992; 267:2046–2050.
56. Nightingale SL. Efforts to prevent foodborne listeriosis. *JAMA* 1992; 268:180.
57. Schmidt GM. Prophylaxis of cytomegalovirus infection after bone marrow transplantation. *Semin Oncol* 1992; 19:20–26.
58. Goodrich JM, Mori M, Gleaves CA, et al. Early treatment with ganciclovir to prevent cytomegalovirus disease after allogeneic bone marrow transplantation. *N Engl J Med* 1991; 325:1601–1607.
59. Schmidt GM, Horak DA, Niland JC, Duncan SR, Forman SJ, Zaia JA. A randomized, controlled trial of prophylactic ganciclovir for cytomegalovirus pulmonary infection in recipients of allogeneic bone marrow transplants; the City of Hope-Stanford-Syntex CMV Study Group [see comments]. *N Engl J Med* 1991; 324:1005–1011.
60. Goodrich JM, Bowden RA, Fisher L, Keller C, Schoch G, Meyers JD. Canciclovir prophylaxis to prevent cytomegalovirus disease after allogeneic marrow transplant. *Ann Intern Med* 1993; 118:173–178.
61. Winston DJ, Ho WG, Bartoni K, et al. Ganciclovir prophylaxis of cytomegalovirus infection and disease in allogeneic bone marrow transplant recipients. Results of a placebo-controlled, double-blind trial. *Ann Intern Med* 1993; 118:179–184.
62. Reusser P, Gambertoglio JG, Lilleby K, Meyers JD. Phase I–II trial of foscarnet for prevention of cytomegalovirus infection in autologous and allogeneic marrow transplant recipients. *J Infect Dis* 1992; 166:473–479.
63. Riddell SR, Watanabe KS, Goodrich JM, Li CR, Agha ME, Greenberg PD. Restoration of viral immunity in immunodeficient humans by the adoptive transfer of T cell clones. *Science* 1992; 257:238–241.
64. Riddell SR, Reusser P, Greenberg PD. Cytotoxic T cells specific for cytomegalovirus: a potential therapy for immunocompromised patients. *Rev Infect Dis* 1991; 13(Suppl 11):S966–S973.
65. Cooperative Group for the Study of Immunoglobulin in Chronic Lymphocytic Leukemia. Intravenous immunoglobulin for the prevention of infection in chronic lymphocytic leukemia. A randomized, controlled trial. *N Engl J Med* 1988; 319: 902–907.
66. Sullivan KM, Kopecky KJ, Jocom J, et al. Immunomodulatory and antimicrobial efficacy of intravenous immunoglobulin in bone marrow transplantation [see comments]. *N Engl J Med* 1990; 323:705–712.
67. Wolff SN, Fay JW, Herzig RH, et al. High-dose weekly intravenous immunoglobulin to prevent infections in patients undergoing autologous bone marrow transplantation or severe myelosuppressive therapy. A study of the American Bone Marrow Transplant Group. *Ann Intern Med* 1993; 118:937–942.

3

Bleeding and Coagulation Problems

M. Dicato, F. Ries, and C. Duhem
Centre Hospitalier de Luxembourg, Luxembourg

I. INTRODUCTION

The time-honored coagulation cascade as an attempt to explain hemostasis by sequential conversion of clotting factors into their respective active proteins is at present considered inadequate. The complexity of multiple systems sequentially and simultaneously must be explained differently.

More emphasis is being placed on the role of tissue factor, endothelial exposure, and the cell surface thrombin binding thrombomodulin, which is converted into a protein C activator. Antithrombin III (ATIII), protein S, and especially protein C with thrombin interplay result in multiple feedback mechanisms of activation of classic clotting factors V and VIII and negative feedback mechanisms to thrombin itself.

Certainly not all mechanisms of procoagulant and anticoagulant activity are identified. For example, it is interesting to note how there has been a shift of emphasis in the explanation of thrombosis from the classic cascade and ATIII involvement to protein C and its activation by thrombin.

This understanding will probably allow us in the near future to predict not only propensity to thrombosis, but also prophylaxis and treatment duration in common thrombotic events. Note that the usual coagulation tests, such as prothrombin and (activated) partial thromboplastin time, do not detect abnormalities in these pathways. A recently published, remarkable study revealed an autosomal dominant trait of resistance to activated protein C, responsible for nearly half of cases of venous thrombosis (1).

Normal hemostasis is a fine-tuned equilibrium between procoagulant and anticoagulant factors involving multiple interrelated cascades and spanning wide fields of clinical and laboratory medicine. Hemostatic problems in oncological patients are complex because they involve multiple physiological events simultaneously, including disease- or drug-induced bone marrow failure with pancytopenia, inadequate clotting factor production as a result of malnutrition or liver failure, drug-related hemostatic disorders, peripheral blood cell consumption, fibrinolysis, hypercoagulable states, infection, and many others, such as leukostasis and dysproteinemia.

Each of these aspects must be addressed separately and, at the same time, be integrated in a complex setting. Often only one or a few aspects are apparent and others are clinically less obvious although part of the same general underlying mechanism. The leukemic patient with sepsis and severe pancytopenia often presents with the entire spectrum of bleeding problems and sometimes also disseminated intravascular coagulation. On the other hand, the solid tumor patient will have (to a lesser extent) hemorrhagic, but more often thrombotic problems.

The availability of hematopoietic growth factors, high-dose chemotherapy, autologous bone marrow transplantation, and peripheral blood stem cell collection has increased the number of solid tumor patients liable to go into profound pancytopenia and who present with the same management problems as the classic leukemic patient.

For more extensive biological details on coagulation and for technical details on transfusion, please refer to the classic hemostasis and transfusion medicine textbooks (e.g., Refs. 2 and 3). For a book on supportive care in cancer, the specific neoplasia-related aspects and the more common problems of hemostasis are addressed in this chapter.

II. BLEEDING PROBLEMS

Hemorrhage is very common in cancer patients. The awareness and the advent of preventive measures, however, have markedly decreased the incidence of hemorrhagic deaths in acute leukemia, for instance, from over 60% to less than 10% over the past 40 years (4,5).

In leukemia and in intensive chemotherapy, profound pancytopenia is unavoidable. The anemia is easily alleviated by packed red blood cell transfusions. We have seen a shortening of the duration of severe neutropenia with the widely available granulocyte and granulocyte-macrophage colony-stimulating factors. For severe thrombocytopenia, platelet substitution as of now is still mandatory, but pharmacological means have become available and are currently undergoing clinical trials and will soon be widely available.

A. Thrombocytopenia

1. Platelet Substitution

Thrombocytopenia is an increasing problem as treatment for cancer has become more intensive over the past years and, even more, with the advent of cytokines and peripheral blood stem cell collection and support. For a short time platelet substitution is successful, but in the long-term platelet support situation, induced alloimmunization is found in a substantial number of patients and its management is a difficult and unresolved issue. It is therefore important to try to avoid or at least decrease the incidence of induced alloimmunization and its consequence of refractoriness to platelet transfusion. Several aspects have been and still are explored in this field. Over the past years, several (6,7) but not all (8) studies have indicated that the use of single-donor platelet preparations and the practice of leukocyte depletion will minimize alloimmunization. Older studies have suggested that there is a relation between the frequency rather than the amount of cellular blood exposure that induces HLA antibody formation (9).

Several studies have compared single-donor to random-donor platelets, and although there are contradictions, many physicians favor single-donor prearations with the hope of decreasing alloimmunization. The issue of selecting, especially in refractory patients, random, single, or HLA-matched donors is not settled, either, but non–HLA-matched donors are certainly easier to obtain—and at a lower cost—in most settings. An interesting study (10) showed recently that by using a cross-match assay that has become available over the past few years, an adequate prediction of refractoriness can be made, which is superior to HLA matching especially in alloimmunized patients. Previously, however, a randomized study comparing HLA-compatible to single-donor apheresis platelets showed no difference between the two groups (11). When feasible in our department, we favor random single-donor platelets, and most patients are able to provide a few donors—family or others.

Leukocyte depletion has been correlated in most studies with a decrease in alloimmunization, especially when using the lowest possible white blood cell (WBC) contamination. The combined use of the more recent apheresis machines with better performing filters has decreased the amount of WBC contamination per platelet collection. Obviously, red blood cell substitution should also be as low as possible in leukocytes. Another potential clinical benefit of reduction in WBC in blood components is prevention of febrile reactions and cytomegalovirus (CMV) transmission. In a large study (12), no CMV transmission was noted in 184 patients with usage of filters, but 75 of 303 control patients had positive CMV conversion. Filter usage most likely will reduce other viral transfusions, including herpes, Epstein-Barr virus, hepatitis B and C, parvovirus B19, and human T cell lymphotrophic virus types I and II. It follows that it is of paramount importance to avoid sensitization of patients by previous blood products.

Another approach to decrease alloimmunization is to use ultraviolet radiation (UVR) on platelets (13). UVR decreases the ability of lymphocytes to stimulate or respond to mixed lymphocyte cultures, and UV-irradiated macrophages have been shown to have a poor antigen presentation. UVR-treated platelets are able to shorten the bleeding time and improve the platelet count and have a hemostatic effect in thrombocytopenic situations. The light sources, the bags used, and the way the platelets are prepared are important. Because the existing data are encouraging, larger controlled studies should evaluate the appropriateness of this technique.

Another issue is to determine when platelets should be given. To correct a prolonged bleeding time in a profoundly thrombocytopenic but otherwise stable patient, a platelet count $> 40{,}000/\mu l$ must be attained; however, bleeding problems in stable patients with a count between 20,000 and $40{,}000/\mu l$ are not frequent. Many clinicians use a threshold $< 20{,}000$ to start platelet transfusion. The reference for this is a study by Gaydos et al. in 1962 (4). In that study, however, the authors could not establish a threshold above which there was no bleeding. A more recent study by Gmur et al. (5) provided a workable hypothesis using random single-donor platelets with the schedule outlined in Table 1.

2. *Pharmacological Management of Thrombocytopenia*

The need for cytokines to reduce hematological chemotherapy toxicity is driven by the growing evidence that the dose intensity of administered cytotoxic agents may determine the effectiveness of some chemotherapeutic regimens.

Table 1 Proposal for Single-Donor Platelet Transfusions

Morning platelet count ($\times 10^9$/liter)	Prophylactic platelet transfusion, same day
0–5	In every case
6–10	If fresh minor hemorrhage, body temperature >38°C
11–20	Coagulation disorders and/or heparin, before bone marrow biopsy or spinal tap
>20	Major bleeding complications, before minor surgical procedures: biopsies, central venous catheters, arterial punction, others

One approach to dose intensification is the administration of a single or several courses of high-dose chemotherapy with autologous peripheral blood stem cell rescue. An alternative approach is the use of repeated, closely timed courses of semi-intensive chemotherapy; granulocyte colony-stimulating factor (G-CSF) and granulocyte-macrophage CSF (GM-CSF) have already demonstrated their ability to reduce chemotherapy-induced neutropenia and infections in this setting.

Thrombocytopenia and clinical bleeding have proven to be more intractable problems, and there is an urgent need for hematopoietic growth factors (GFs) that increase the platelet count: such candidate GFs, alone or in combination, would eliminate or at least lessen the degree and/or duration of chemotherapy-induced thrombocytopenia. To date, megakaryocytic lineage-specific GFs have not been identified, and cytokines with in vitro multilineage effects are currently being evaluated in humans for their ability to increase platelet numbers after chemotherapy.

Because of different responses of the megakaryocyte-restricted progenitors and the megakaryocytes themselves to several experimental stimuli, the concept has arisen that the regulation of platelet production is at least two-sided, with separate control of progenitor proliferation and megakaryocyte maturation (14). A number of peptides have been described that regulate the proliferation of megakaryocyte progenitors in vitro but without restriction to this lineage. Interleukin-3 (IL-3) and GM-CSF both have megakaryocyte colony-stimulating activity (14), and stem cell factor (SCF, or kit-Ligand) is capable of enhancing megakaryocyte proliferation in combination with other GFs (15). Erythropoietin (Epo) may also augment in vitro proliferation (14). Recently, the existence of a unique cytokine specific to the megakaryocytic lineage (so-called Meg-CSF) and exhibiting proliferative stimulation on progenitors was demonstrated, but the molecule remains to be purified and cloned (16).

Megakaryocyte maturation has traditionally been thought to be regulated by a megakaryocyte-restricted factor, designated thrombopoietin. To date, there is no definitive evidence for a single "thrombopoietin" molecule. In contrast, several GFs can promote megakaryocyte maturation—IL-6 (14), IL-11, leukemia-inhibitory factor (LIF) (17), and oncostatin M—all lacking lineage specificity.

Characterized cytokines that promote megakaryocyte processes are listed in Table 2. It is noteworthy that inhibitors of megakaryocytic development have been described, too, which, like the growth-promoting cytokines, are devoid of lineage specificity. They are mainly transforming growth factor β, IL-4, interferon, and platelet factor 4 (14).

Both proliferation- and maturation-enhancing cytokines are currently being investigated for their ability to augment platelet numbers in animal models and in humans.

Table 2 Cytokines Promoting Megakaryocytopoiesis

Cytokine	Primary effect[a]	Platelet count[b]
SCF	P	NC[c]
IL-3	P	I[c]
GM-CSF	P	V[c]
IL-3 + GM-CSF	P + M	V[c]
PIXY	P + M	I[c]
IL-6	M	I[c]
LIF	M	I
IL-11	M	I
Epo	P + M	NC[c]

[a]Primary effect: the presumed preponderant influence is indicated. P, proliferative stage; M, maturation stage.
[b]Platelet counts: in vivo effects of the purified cytokine used in normal animal or human.
[c]Clinical trials. NC, no change; I, increased; V, variable.

1. IL-3. Several phase I trials (18–21) have been studying the effect of this pleiotropic cytokine on thrombocytopenia resulting from combination chemotherapy for diverse malignancies, including small cell lung cancer (18,19), ovarian cancer (20), and other advanced malignancies (21). Despite different administration modalities, the results of these studies were all consistent with a significant stimulation of thrombopoiesis by IL-3. Moreover, the late onset and long-lasting effect of the response of thrombopoiesis to IL-3 treatment is in line with stimulation at the megakaryocyte progenitor level. The accompanying increase in plasma IL-6 levels reported by some authors (18,19) could have a causal implication in the thrombopoietic effect, too.
2. IL-3 and GM-CSF. A shortened treatment course of IL-3 sequentially followed by GM-CSF after combination chemotherapy for advanced malignancies of diverse origin failed to induce any significantly accelerated platelet recovery (except in heavily pretreated patients) (22). Recently, two phase I clinical trials using the genetically engineered GM-CSF/IL-3 fusion protein PIXY 321 have been performed to alleviate hematological toxicity after chemotherapy, and significant effects on granulopoiesis and thrombopoiesis could be observed (23,24).
3. SCF. Stem cell factor has little intrinsic megakaryocyte colony-stimulating activity when used alone, and indeed, phase I clinical trials of SCF have not shown any significant effect on thrombopoiesis (25). This GF is known to synergize with IL-3 in augmenting megakaryocyte colony growth in

vitro, and clinical trials combining the administration of these two cytokines in sequence or simultaneously to stimulate platelet production could yield successful results.

4. IL-6. IL-6 belongs to a group of cytokines, including LIF, IL-11, and oncostatin M, that promote megakaryocyte maturation and share a common receptor component, designated gp130. IL-6 is currently being studied in phase I and II clinical trials, the results of which strongly suggest a thrombopoietic effect of this cytokine (26–28).
5. Clinical trials have also begun with IL-11, and the potential thrombopoietic effect of LIF is currently being evaluated in primate models.
6. Although a number of studies have shown that Epo is capable of enhancing in vitro megakaryocytopoiesis, it has little influence on the platelet count when administrated alone in the human.

Cytokines with pure megakaryocyte colony-stimulating and/or thrombopoietin-like properties able to improve thrombocytopenia after classic or high-dose chemotherapy as G-CSF and GM-CSF have done for chemotherapy-induced neutropenia are yet to be identified. While awaiting progress from basic research, recent and still ongoing clinical trials are investigating the best schedule of known cytokines, alone or in combination, in this setting. To date, postchemotherapeutic administration of IL-3 or IL-6 has proved to be significantly effective in increasing platelet num- ber, but the sequential association of IL-3 and GM-CSF has been disappointing.

All cited studies report the administration of potentially thrombopoietic cytokines after standard dose chemotherapy; these induce moderate thrombocytopenia and thus may not be sensitive enough to test the efficacy of the GFs, these last being always appreciated on the basis of platelet number because, at this level of thrombocytopenia, any reduction in bleeding episodes or platelet transfusions cannot be observed (except Ref. 18). Whether these cytokine-induced alterations of coagulation and platelet function are clinically beneficial also remains unknown.

Further trials investigating cytokine combinations (e.g., SCF + IL-3, IL-3 + IL-11 or + LIF, and triple association) will be interesting approaches to the treatment of chemotherapy-related thrombocytopenia.

Because of the lack of any definitive conclusion emerging from these studies, the use of cytokines to lessen cytotoxin-induced thrombocytopenia should at present be limited to clinical investigations. In daily practice, a symptomatic attitude remains indicated, consisting of platelet transfusions for thrombocytopenia, as indicated elsewhere in this chapter.

B. Disseminated Intravascular Coagulation

Disseminated intravascular coagulation (DIC) is a syndrome observed in various, usually severe disorders of many different fields, especially associated with major infection, tissue breakdown, and release from injured tissue of procoagulant material. The symptoms of DIC are caused by uncontrolled production by thrombin of fibrinogen and its degradation produces (FDP) by plasmin. The relative balance between coagulation and fibrinolysis is disturbed, and an excess of each of its aspects is observed clinically, with exaggerated coagulation and thrombosis on the one hand and excessive fibrinolysis and bleeding on the other. The corresponding clinical picture in a given patient is thrombosis and bleeding at the same time. This leads to the consumption of clotting factors and proteinase inhibitors. Liver function is important in the clearance of thrombin and plasmin and the replacement of various consumed factors. The acute-phase reactants fibrinogen and α_2-antiplasmin induce additional excess bleeding and thrombosis, respectively. Because the clotting and fibrinolytic cascades are overfunctioning and FDPs have at the same time procoagulant and anticoagulant activity, most general laboratory tests of hemostasis are abnormal, with a prolonged prothrombin time, (partial) thromboplastin time, and thrombin time and the presence of FDPs. Measurement of the last is the most sensitive test, and the most widely used are the latex agglutination test and, more recently, the cross-linked FDP, D-dimer. Fibrinogen and platelets, being consumed, are usually decreased. In the occasional patient in whom mostly plasminogen activation is present, there may be a clinical picture of fibrinolysis with bleeding and the presence of FDPs and a low fibrinogen as a result of consumption but a normal platelet count with a low α_2-antiplasmin activity.

DIC can be observed as an acute clinical event when coagulation and fibrinolysis are activated by the massive release of procoagulant and fibrinolytic substances, as in acute leukemia. The clinical picture can be multifaceted, with thrombocytopenia secondary to bone marrow failure, increased platelet turnover in infection, tissue infiltration by cancer cells with release of tissue factors, poor liver clearance, and decreased production of clotting factors as a result of hepatic dysfunction.

On the other hand, in solid tumor the pathophysiological events are less acute and massive, allowing the organism to adapt. The clotting aspects are clinically more apparent, with thrombosis caused by excess procoagulant activity and chronic DIC.

Because DIC is secondary to other pathophysiological events inducing activation of procoagulant and profibrinolytic activity, whenever possible the underlying cause should be treated and, along with it, the consumption coagulopathy as indicated. Blood component replacement for consumed and missing clotting factors can be done with frozen plasma. The addition of heparin is advocated by many clinicians, but its definitive value remains to be proven. Some patients present with a clinical picture of bleeding and thrombocytopenia, and adjunct therapy with an anticoagulant may be hazardous. In patients with thrombosis, low-dose heparin can be given. In contrast, some may use antifibrinolytics, such as ϵ-aminocaproic acid or tranexamic acid, but these agents may induce thrombosis, and can be considered in the patient presenting with the "bleeding" type of DIC.

Low-grade or chronic DIC in cancer medicine usually presents as recurrent thrombosis and is discussed in another section of this chapter.

In acute promyelocytic leukemia, DIC is almost always present as a result of the massive release of profibrinolytic agents from the abnormal cells, the more so with chemotherapy, and hemorrhagic death has been drastically reduced by adjunct therapy with heparin (29). The differentiating agent tretinoin (retinoic acid) has also been successful in reducing this bleeding complication (30).

Liver failure is frequent in the patient with advanced cancer. Synthesis and clearance of hemostatic factors are decreased. Management of these patients is difficult and cannot be standardized because the clinical picture is various and rapidly changing. Intracranial bleeding is frequent, and antifibrinolytic agents may be useful.

C. Vitamin K Deficiency

Protracted anorexia leading to malnutrition is frequent in advanced cancer patients. The resulting vitamin K deficiency is a frequent finding in chronically hospitalized patients, and coagulation abnormalities are often observed (31). Vitamin K substitution is simple and should be given to these patients.

III. THROMBOSIS AND OTHER VASCULAR COMPLICATIONS

The relationship between cancer and thrombosis was first reported by Trousseau in 1865 (32). It is now well recognized that disorders in hemostasis are frequent in patients with malignancy, with thromboembolic events preceding or following the diagnosis of cancer (33–35). In a study of 1400 patients with a diagnosis of venous thrombosis, 6% were found to have cancer (36), and thrombotic events can precede the diagnosis of cancer by months or even years. Occult cancer should always be suspected in patients with recurrent, migratory, superficial thrombosis, as well as in patients lacking classic risk factors for thrombosis (37–41). Approximately 15% of patients with malignancy develop an episode of thrombosis (33,42,43). Thromboembolic problems are a major cause of morbidity and mortality in these patients (33,44). Many factors predispose the cancer patient to venous stasis and thrombosis; these include classic risk factors, such as prolonged periods of bed rest, infection, congestive heart failure, and vascular lesions by catheter manipulations, as well as cancer-specific problems, including cancer cell-related procoagulant activity, vascular compression and invasion by tumors, hyperviscosity problems, and chemo- and hormone therapy-related coagulopathy (33–35,42,43,45).

Thrombosis is considered to result from perturbations of three major interdependent components of the hemostatic system: blood flow, the vessel wall, and the composition of the blood itself. Thrombosis can be considered to represent hemostasis at the wrong time and in the wrong place in the circulation; this can occur when prothrombotic activity overwhelms the normal physiological antithrombotic mechanisms or when physiological antithrombotic systems are defective, with a variable impact on local and systemic factors.

A. Abnormalities of Blood Flow

Cancer patients are frequently confined to prolonged bed rest because of surgery, medical complications, or debilitating cancer, and immobilization can be considered a major risk factor for thrombosis. Venous stasis may cause a delayed clearance of activated coagulation factors, and interaction between platelets and vessel wall can be enhanced (46). Venous stasis may be localized in vascular compression by bulky tumor but may also be part of a general phenomenon in congestive heart failure precipitated by chronic illness or cardiotoxic chemotherapy. Additional problems, such as hypoxia, anemia, dehydration, and infection, may play a role. Hyperviscosity and leukostasis, specific problems impairing coagulation and microcirculation, occur primarily in monoclonal gammopathies and myeloproliferative disorders and are discussed elsewhere.

B. Abnormalities of the Vessel Wall

Apart from local compression by bulky tumor, direct tumor invasion of a vessel wall can contribute to enhance local thrombotic phenomena, primarily by interfering with the thromboresistant properties of the normal vessel wall and by the local release of procoagulant factors (47–50).

C. Platelets and Cancer

Secondary thrombocytosis is frequently found in cancer patients (51), but a direct relation between an increase in circulating platelets and an increased frequency of thrombosis is not clear.

Increased platelet-aggregating activity has been demonstrated in cell lines, human tumors, and tumor extracts (52–56). Mechanisms for increased platelet-aggregating activity include tumor-induced thrombin generation, ADP production, and activation of arachidonate metabolism (57–62) in normal platelets. In myeloproliferative disorders, abnormal platelets present increased as well as decreased aggregation.

D. Tumor Cell Procoagulant Activity

From the many published data about tumor cell procoagulant activity, only two factors appear to play a major role in the clinical setting: tissue factor and cancer procoagulant (34,45,63).

Tissue factor is the normal cellular activator of coagulation and has been found in many cancer cell lines and tumor tissue preparations. This factor is a receptor for factor VII and activated factor VII and is at the same time an activator site of unactivated factor VII. Tissue factor-factor VIIa complex is the real coagulation activator, leading to activation of factors IX and X. Factor Xa together with factor Va forms a prothrombinase complex, generating thrombin and thus leading to conversion of fibrinogen to fibrin. Tissue factor appears to be an important activator of the coagulation system in malignant disease. A truncated tissue factor (a second soluble form) has also been described in malignancy with a possible relevance for hypercoagulability in cancer patients (63).

Cancer procoagulant is a proteinase from malignant cells that activates the coagulation system by directly activating factor X. This protein appears to be rather specific for undifferentiated cells; its expression is found in undifferentiated cancer cells, chorionic tissue, and undifferentiated fetal tissues and is repressed in normal tissue and differentiated cancer cells (63). Cancer procoagulant activity has been shown to parallel the course of leukemia, as measured on bone marrow aspirates, before, during, and after remission.

Note that coagulation activation can take place in at least two different environments, the extravascular, extracellular environment of the tumor and the vascular bed. In both systems, factor Xa can bind to membrane-bound Va and prothrombin and to the tumor cell or to platelets or macrophages to form the prothrombinase complex. Thrombin generation leads to the conversion of fibrinogen to fibrin, which can be formed either on the tumor cell membrane or at the vascular level. The net impact of the release of procoagulants from tumor is to facilitate intravascular activation of the coagulation system, leading to disseminated intravascular coagulation and deep vein thrombosis. At the same time, fibrin formation around tumor cells seems to play an essential role in cell growth support and adhesion, as well as in antiimmune defense.

E. Thrombogenic Abnormalities of the Endothelium

The normal vascular endothelium generates numerous molecules that regulate interactions of circulating blood cells and plasma factors. Maladaptive modulations of these endothelium-dependent regulatory pathways can occur in the context of local vascular injury as well as with diffuse infectious and inflammatory processes mediated by various toxins and cytokines (65–67).

Impaired endothelial expression of thromboprotective factors can be seen in various conditions. The most frequently affected factors are prostacyclin (prostaglandin I_2, PGI2), nitrous oxide (endothelially derived relaxing factor), thrombomodulin, heparin-like glycosaminoglycans, tissue plasminogen activator (tPA), and endothelial ADPase. The production of some of these factors can be influenced by drugs (reduced PGI_2 production with antiinflammatory drugs), by atherosclerotic lesions (reduced production of nitrous oxide and thrombomodulin), diffuse infravascular coagulation (inactivation complexing of heparin-like modules by platelet factor 4 secreted from activated platelets), infection, and inflammation [downregulation of tPA production by IL-1, tumor necrosis factor (TNF), and endotoxins].

On the other hand, enhanced endothelial expression of prothrombotic factors can be found; the most frequently incriminated molecules are tissue factor, plasminogen activator 1 and 2, and von Willebrand's factor. Inflammation as mediated by several drugs, toxins, and cytokines can induce an increased release of some or all of these factors.

Finally, the stimulated endothelium expresses specific adhesion molecules that bind to receptors on stimulated peripheral leukocytes, further mediating inflammation. These adhesion molecules are E-selectin, P-selectin, intracellular adhesion molecules 1 and 2, vascular cell adhesion molecules, and leukocyte-activating cytokines, including IL-1, TNF, IL-8, and platelet-activating factor. Most of these factors are upregulated by inflammatory stimuli, and some can interact directly with hemostasis (P-selectin-mediated platelet-neutrophil interactions) or indirectly after attachment and vascular transmigration of mononuclear cells that produce prothrombotic factors.

Several cancer-specific as well as nonspecific therapeutic interventions have been recognized as causing thrombotic complications in cancer patients, sometimes exacerbated by the underlying systemic prothrombotic state.

F. Intravenous Catheter

Cancer patients are frequently treated with infusion of various drugs, blood products, and intravenous feeding using diverse catheter systems and may have invasive investigations by arterial and venous catheterization. Venous thrombosis induced by catheters can be related to various physical, chemical, and microbial causes, including vascular injury from cannulation, use of hyperosmolar substances, microparticulate compounds, irritating action of certain drugs and electrolytes, and catheter infection (34). A relationship exists between the time an indwelling catheter is in place and the occurrence of thrombophlebitis (68). The incidence of thrombosis is also increased in the cannulation of small veins and veins with reduced blood flow (69). In this setting, the presence of a mediastinal tumor can predispose to subclavian or superior vena caval catheter-related thrombosis. Another predisposing factor is the type and schedule of chemotherapy (70). Subclavian vein thrombosis has been described in up to 40%

of patients with long-term venous access by external Hickman catheters (71) and in 16% of patients with totally implanted systems (72). Thrombosis at this site may be difficult to recognize, sometimes being asymptomatic and sometimes announced only by nonspecific chest, neck, or shoulder pain; classic signs include venous dilatation and edema of the ipsilateral arm and venous collaterals in the pectoral and shoulder region. Venography provides a definitive diagnosis.

Catheter-related thrombophlebitis can best be prevented by avoiding the administration of concentrated, irritating solutions through peripheral veins, particularly in the case of a continuous infusion given over a few days. Removal of thrombogenic microparticulate components from infusion fluids by in-line filtration has been shown to reduce the incidence of infusion-related phlebitis and its further complications (73); small amounts of heparin may also be useful as a prophylactic measure (74). Aseptic techniques during catheter manipulations are mandatory, and attention should be paid to the use of less traumatizing catheters and needles.

G. Heparin

Heparin-associated immune thrombocytopenia, related to the source and purification of heparin, is a classic cause of arterial and venous thrombosis (75–78). Because cancer patients are frequently treated with heparin, this problem may arise occasionally.

Heparin-associated thrombocytopenia occurs independently of heparin dose and typically appears 5–10 days after the start of heparin therapy (77); this complication can also develop after intravenous (IV) flushes of a catheter with heparin; this problem appears to be immune mediated, with the presence of heparin-dependent antibodies against platelets leading to platelet aggregation and degranulation (76). The clinical syndrome typically includes an apparently paradoxical development of either arterial or venous thrombosis in thrombocytopenic patients, presumably caused by in vivo platelet aggregation and, possibly, immune-mediated endothelial injury (78).

If this complication is suspected, heparin administration should be stopped and alternative measures for anticoagulation or fibrinolysis should be considered, depending upon the clinical situation.

H. Chemotherapy

In cancer patients suffering from diverse conditions predisposing to thrombotic events, the causal relationship between specific chemotherapeutic agents and thromboembolism is frequently difficult to establish. Several studies have reported an increased incidence, mostly of deep vein thrombosis and pulmonary embolism in patients receiving polychemotherapy for metastatic disease (thrombosis in 18% of patients) (79), as well as early-stage breast cancer (5–7%

incidence of thrombosis) (80). In a controlled trial of adjuvant chemotherapy compared with no treatment, more thrombotic events have been observed in the chemotherapy group (81). In a recent report on breast cancer patients, venous complications have been more frequent with chemohormone therapy (tamoxifen) than with the same chemotherapy regimen alone (2.8 versus 0.8%) in premenopausal patients; in postmenopausal patients, the incidence of thrombotic problems was higher in the chemohormone therapy group compared with tamoxifen only and with no treatment (8.0 versus 2.3 versus 0.4%). A higher incidence of arterial thrombosis was also reported in premenopausal patients on combined chemohormone therapy compared with chemotherapy alone (1.6 versus 0%) (82).

A thrombotic microangiopathy has been described with various agents, including combination therapy with cisplatin, bleomycin, and vinca alcaloids (83,84) and, more frequently, mitomycin (85). The syndrome, closely resembling thrombotic thrombocytopenic purpura and the hemolytic-uremic syndrome, includes signs of microangiopathic hemolytic anemia, renal failure, thrombocytopenia, and pathological formation of microthrombi of fibrin in the renal microcirculation as well as in arterioles of other organs and tissues (86). This life-threatening condition has been treated with staphyloccocal protein A immunoperfusion (87).

Venoocclusive disease of the liver has been observed in patients on high-dose chemotherapy for leukemia (88); its incidence is particularly high in heavily pretreated patients submitted to bone marrow transplantation, including total-body irradiation and high-dose conditioning regimens. This syndrome is characterized by central and sublobular venous occlusion in the liver, with signs of liver congestion, necrosis, and fibrosis; the clinical presentation includes painful hepatomegaly, weight gain, and thrombocytopenia (88–90).

Both thrombotic and hemorrhagic complications, including central nervous system thrombosis, have been reported after asparaginase therapy (91–93). This drug, which acts as a potent protein synthesis inhibitor, can cause deficiencies of factors involved in the coagulation and fibrinolytic process, including fibrinogen, von Willebrand's factor, antithrombin III, and plasminogen (94). In patients presenting with this condition, transfusion of fresh frozen plasma can be helpful, even if only thrombotic events have occurred.

Different complications at the arterial level have been described with various chemotherapy regimens, including vasospasm related to fluorouracil administration (95) and Raynaud's phenomenon with bleomycin, cisplatin, and vinca alcaloid combination regimens (96–98), as well as cerebrovascular ischemia with cisplatin-containing regimens (99,100). Endothelial damage with the release of high-molecular-weight multimers of von Willebrand's factor has been considered a possible explanation for cisplatin-related arterial occlusive complications (101). Pulmonary venoocclusive disease, a complication of chemotherapy, affects the arterial and venous microcirculation of the lungs and shows signs of pulmonary artery hypertension, with muscular arterial wall proliferation, multifocal vasculitis, and venous occlusion (102). Bleomycin has been incriminated in most of the cases described until now; other drugs that have been incriminated are carmustine, high-dose cyclophosphamide, and mitomycin (102). Withdrawal of the incriminated drug and symptomatic treatment of pulmonary hypertension may be helpful (103).

I. Hormone Therapy

Several reports have implicated tamoxifen, an antiestrogen with some estrogen agonist activity, in thromboembolic as well as arterial occlusive complications (104–108). The possible thrombogenic effect of tamoxifen seems to be enhanced by concomitant chemotherapy (82), and the thrombogenic effect seems to be more pronounced in patients with advanced compared with early breast cancer. Preliminary data concerning tamoxifen use as chemoprevention in normal women seem to indicate that the incidence of venous and arterial complications is not increased in this population compared with the no-treatment group (109). Tamoxifen use has been shown to reduce serum levels of antithrombin III (110). A marginal reduction in antithrombin III and protein C was described in a chemoprevention trial (109).

Estrogens, particularly moderate and high-dose diethylstilbestrol as used in early trials for advanced prostate cancer, have been clearly associated with thromboembolic and cardiovascular complications (111). Low-dose estrogen therapy and particularly specific antiandrogen therapy, have reduced this risk in the actual treatment approach.

J. Differentiation Agents

All-*trans*-retinoic acid (ATRA), used as an effective differentiation agent for the treatment of promyelocytic leukemia, has been associated with a reduced risk of early hemorrhagic death as a result of intravascular coagulation but has also been described as a risk factor for thromboembolic (112) and arterioocclusive events (113). This complication could be related to the phase of initial ATRA-induced leukocytosis that is seen in some patients; simultaneous chemotherapy, together with ATRA, should help to prevent this adverse effect.

IV. DIAGNOSIS AND TREATMENT OF THROMBOSIS

As a general principle, the approach to the diagnosis of thromboembolic disease should be the same in cancer patients as in the standard population. In cancer patients the diagnosis can sometimes be less obvious, and the need for complete investigations must be discussed in every situation, according to the prognosis of the underlying disease and the possible therapeutic options.

A. Diagnosis

1. Deep Vein Thrombosis

Many authors recommend first-line noninvasive investigations, such as impedance plethysmography, Doppler ultrasonography, or B-mode ultrasonography (114–122), for diagnosis of deep vein thrombosis of the lower extremities, the most frequent thrombotic problem in cancer patients. All these techniques can be very useful for detection of proximal vein thrombosis, but calf vein thrombosis can be missed. A positive test with one of these techniques generally calls for further investigation with venography; this examination remains the diagnostic reference standard and can provide helpful information about an eventual embolic risk (123,124). A negative test with one of the noninvasive methods allows anticoagulant therapy to be withheld, but a second or even a third control may be needed.

Venography is superseding these other techniques, and we believe that it should be considered a first-line investigation; the procedure can be coupled, if indicated, with the placement of an inferior vena caval filter (125).

2. Pulmonary Embolism

The clinical diagnosis of pulmonary embolism can be very difficult in cancer patients, dyspnea and chest pain being common manifestations of various origins, at least in patients with advanced disease or with thoracic involvement (126). In the postoperative cancer patient, these symptoms can have a more selective meaning, reducing the problems with the differential diagnosis. Overall, even if the clinical suspicion in favor of pulmonary embolism is low, it is potentially dangerous to exclude pulmonary embolism and its therapy on clinical grounds alone.

As a general approach, these patients should undergo chest x-ray, electrocardiography, and arterial blood gas measurement and, as first-line complementary investigation, a perfusion lung scan. If this test is strictly negative, anticoagulant therapy is withheld. In the case of one or several perfusion defects, ventilation lung scanning should be performed, looking for ventilation-perfusion mismatch (127–129). A high probability of embolism based on these tests is generally considered to confer sufficient evidence to justify anticoagulant therapy in the standard situation. If some doubt persists, or if there are relative contraindications for anticoagulation, confirmatory pulmonary angiography should be considered (130–132). Another approach in patients with high clinical suspicion of embolism but with doubtful lung scan results is to investigate first for evidence of deep vein thrombosis and to perform pulmonary angiography only if this investigation is negative. Evidence for deep vein thrombosis, on the other hand, is then considered sufficient for confirmation of pulmonary embolism on clinical grounds and allows initiation of anticoagulation or vena caval filter placement.

3. Upper Limb Vein Thrombosis

In cancer patients, upper extremity vein thrombosis can occur in the context of extrinsic compression or stenosis of the axillary and or subclavian vein by tumor tissue or fibrosis, as well as in relation to catheter-related vessel wall trauma and stasis (133,134); finally, the thrombogenic and sclerosing effect of chemotherapy, as well as the irritative effects from parenteral nutrition, electrolytes, and various other drugs, can play a role (83,135). Differential diagnosis must be made with arm swelling caused by lymphatic obstruction, particularly in the context of locoregional surgery, radiotherapy, and axillary tumor infiltration. Venography must be considered a first-line standard investigation. A locoregional contrast-enhanced computed tomographic (CT) examination can sometimes provide sufficient information and sometimes allows better visualization of an underlying neoplastic or fibrotic process.

4. Migratory Superficial Thrombophlebitis (Trousseau's Syndrome)

The clinical picture of migratory superficial thrombophlebitis is characterized by recurrent thrombophlebitis involving multiple superficial and unusual sites (including arms, forearms, and chest) in patients with absence of apparent predisposing factors (e.g., stasis and bed rest). Classically this syndrome has been related to neoplasia, particularly pancreatic cancer (33). Spontaneous resolution of symptoms in involved areas over a few days has been described, as well as resistance to conventional anticoagulant therapy, particularly of the oral anticoagulant class (136).

5. Nonbacterial Thrombotic Endocarditis

Nonbacterial thrombotic endocarditis, a rare thrombotic complication characterized by aseptic endoluminal cardiac vegetations, has been described in a variety of nonmalignant diseases but is more common in patients with cancer, particularly in the context of mucin-producing adenocarcinomas. This complication may occur in patients with occult, localized neoplasms, as well as in patients with metastatic disease (137–139).

The clinical presentation is dominated by the occurrence of multiple emboli to the brain, spleen, kidney, and heart, leading to signs of infarction or ischemia of these and other peripheral organs (140). Heart murmurs are typically present, and some but not all of these patients have a history of damaged valves. The diagnosis can be confirmed by echocardiography and magnetic resonance imaging of the heart (141).

6. Hepatic Vein Thrombosis and Portal Vein Thrombosis

Hepatic vein thrombosis (Budd-Chiari syndrome) may be caused by a variety of underlying diseases, including malignancy (142–150); in cancer patients this form of thrombosis is most notably associated with myeloproliferative disorders but has also been described in hepatoma and renal cell and adrenal carcinoma. In patients with myeloproliferative disorders, this syndrome can be the first manifestation of the disease and it may occur in the absence of pronounced erythrocytosis or thrombocytosis. The clinical presentation can be acute or insidious, generally including abdominal pain, hepatomegaly, and ascites; sometimes there is distension of superficial abdominal veins and splenomegaly secondary to portal hypertension; jaundice is rare, and liver function tests may be without diagnostic benefit. Liver echography with Doppler sonography, contrast-enhanced CT scanning, and magnetic resonance imaging are useful diagnostic tools. Venography by inferior vena caval and hepatic vein catheterization is the definitive diagnostic procedure.

Portal vein thrombosis may also occur acutely or insidiously; clinical signs include ascites (usually transient, present only during the acute phase), as well as splenomegaly and esophageal varices related to portal hypertension; bleeding of esophagogastric varices may be the first manifestation of this complication (145). Ultrasound examination is generally considered most helpful in establishing the diagnosis, followed by contrast-enhanced CT scan, magnetic resonance imaging, and portal venography.

B. Treatment

1. General Considerations

The first objective of treating patients with venous thromboembolic problems is to prevent death from pulmonary embolism; secondary objectives are to reduce morbidity from the acute event, reduce postphlebitic symptoms, and prevent thromboembolic pulmonary hypertension (146,147) and recurrence. The therapeutic approach to venous thromboembolism includes several therapeutic options: intravenous, subcutaneous, and oral anticoagulant therapy, thrombolysis, inferior vena caval interruption, and, more rarely, surgical thromboembolic deobstruction. The anticoagulant agents (IV heparin, subcutaneous low-molecular-weight heparin, and oral antivitamin K agents) serve primarily to prevent the extension and recurrence of established thrombosis and to prevent recurrent pulmonary embolism by interfering with the normal coagulation process. The thrombolytic agents (streptokinase, urokinase, and tissue plasminogen activator) have the potential for rapid thrombolysis of venous thrombi and pulmonary emboli of recent origin; these agents can be useful in the emergency setting or if there is a need for rapid symptomatic relief in non–life-threatening situations. Interruption of the inferior vena cava by different filter systems allows effective protection from pulmonary embolism; their placement must be considered in the case of high risk for potentially life-threatening embolism and if the use of anticoagulants and/or fibrinolytic agents is contraindicated.

2. Heparin

Heparin may be used for short-term as well as long-term anticoagulation in the therapeutic and prophylactic setting (148–152). The classic method of administration during the acute phase of deep vein thrombosis and thromboembolism is continuous intravenous infusion (149). A generally recommended program includes an initial bolus of 5000 units of heparin intravenously, followed by an infusion of about 1000–1200 units/h; the subsequent dose is adapted to maintain a partial thromboplastin time at 1.5–2 times control (153). A recent trial demonstrated that the duration of initial heparin infusion can be shortened in most cases from 10–14 days to approximately 5 days if adequate oral anticoagulation is given simultaneously with heparin, at least in the standard patient population (154). In cancer patients, long-term outpatient subcutaneous heparin is frequently considered safer than therapy with oral anticoagulants, particularly in patients with cancer-related hypercoagulability and in patients with ongoing chemotherapy who are at risk for thrombocytopenia. Effective anticoagulation in cancer patients is not always possible, and complications may be more frequent compared with the general population (155–157). Patients with liver metastasis or compromised liver function may have reduced synthesis of antithrombin III, implicating an inadequate response to heparin; other patients can develop hemorrhage, especially at tumor-bearing sites (158).

The use of low-molecular-weight heparin (LMW heparin) may offer several advantages in the treatment and prophylaxis of cancer-related thrombosis, with the possibility for outpatient treatment without the need for laboratory monitoring and with a potentially reduced risk of hemorrhage (159,160). Most recently, randomized studies of LMW heparins compared with standard heparin therapy in deep venous thrombosis in the general population provided strong evidence that this therapeutic approach is safe and cost effective; more data are needed in the cancer patient (160).

3. Oral Anticoagulant Therapy

Most patients with deep vein thrombosis treated initially with heparin require continuing anticoagulant therapy to prevent early recurrence of thrombosis (161,162). Coumarinics, the most frequently used agents, have been shown to prevent these recurrences effectively, but their administration needs close laboratory monitoring, particularly until establishment of steady-state levels.

The prothrombin time (PT) test is the most common method for monitoring, being responsive to a reduction in three of the vitamin K-dependent clotting factors, factor II, factor VII, and factor X. Because factor VII has a short half-life, a rapid drop in the prothrombin time can sometimes be observed, while the classic coagulation pathway is still unaffected. Because oral anticoagulants also affect some proteins with thrombolytic activity, such as protein C, whose half-life is short, a paradoxical state of hypercoagulability can sometimes be observed after 2 or 3 days of therapy, before effective reduction in factors II and X. This is why oral anticoagulation should always be given with a 4 day overlap of effective anticoagulation with heparin. To avoid long-term hospitalization, oral anticoagulants, if indicated, can be started within 24 h of first heparin administration (154). The intensity and duration of oral anticoagulant therapy remains a matter of debate (163–165). For patients considered at risk for hemorrhage, a low to moderate reduction in the prothrombin time should not be exceeded; otherwise, it would be cautious to replace oral anticoagulants with low-dose subcutaneous heparin. As far as the duration of the treatment is concerned, recommendations vary markedly from 1 month to 1 year; for patients who have experienced a first episode of deep venous thrombosis, oral anticoagulation for 3 months can be considered a wise compromise, unless there is a high risk of recurrence with a persistent state of hypercoagulability (146).

Recurrent thrombophlebitis, particularly under oral anticoagulation, is not rare in cancer patients. If anticoagulation based on PT measurements has been suboptimal, oral anticoagulants can be reconsidered at a higher dose after initial heparin administration. If thrombophlebitis recurs despite a PT test in the therapeutic range, it seems wise to consider adjusted dose subcutaneous heparin or low-molecular-weight heparin as maintenance treatment. On rare occasions, patients develop further recurrences despite optimal anticoagulation by either method; in these patients placement of an inferior vena caval filter must be considered, but ongoing anticoagulation may be needed to achieve symptomatic control of thrombosis.

4. Thrombolytic Therapy

Thrombolytic agents currently in use, such as streptokinase, urokinase, or tPA, act on the plasmin/plasminogen fibrinolytic system to induce fibrinolysis (166). Because plasmin also hydrolyzes fibrinogen, a systemic lytic state is also induced, correlated with a significant bleeding risk. Compared with the standard patient, supplementary risk factors must be considered in cancer patients: brain tumors and brain metastasis, pericardial metastases, tumor with tendency to bleed, active bleeding of any origin, and recent surgery or biopsy, all factors that contraindicate the use of fibrinolytic agents. Furthermore, cancer patients can have other hemostatic problems, including thrombocytopenia, abnormal platelet function, and disseminated intravascular coagulation, mostly as a result of their underlying disease or therapy. This explains why the use of thrombolytic agents in cancer patients is generally restricted to special settings, such as massive pulmonary embolism with shock or central venous catheter-related thrombosis in patients without specific contraindications (167).

The particular problem of central venous catheter occlusion caused by a clot, limited to the catheter tip, can generally be managed effectively and safely with low-dose local fibrinolysis. Streptokinase or urokinase (5000–10,000 units) or 2 mg recombinant tPA diluted into a volume that will just fill the occluded catheter, instilled and left in place for 1–2 h, usually restores catheter function (168,169); this procedure is very safe and can also be recommended for patients with profound thrombocytopenia. If the clot involves not only the catheter tip but the vessel wall as well, however, this technique is clearly insufficient and the risk of pulmonary embolism can only be avoided with standard anticoagulation or systemically effective fibrinolysis. Placement of the infusion catheter directly in the clot can allow effective resolution of these catheter-related clots, even at moderate dosage (urokinase at 500–2000 U/kg/h) and with few bleeding complications. The median infusion duration for this method is 4 days, and results are best if the thrombus has been clinically present for less than 1 week and is not associated with signs of phlebitis (133).

V. HYPERVISCOSITY, LEUKOSTASIS, AND THROMBOCYTOSIS

A. Hyperviscosity

The hyperviscosity syndrome has been described mostly in monoclonal gammopathies and myeloproliferative disorders. In these conditions, increased blood viscosity induces specific signs and symptoms, most characteristically a triad of bleeding, visual disturbancies, and neurological deficits (170,171). The unique flow characteristics of blood can be altered by both cellular and soluble components. The measurement of viscosity is expressed relative to the viscosity of water and can be performed on whole blood but, in most laboratories, only on plasma or serum. The correlation between measured viscosity and the appearance of clinical symptoms and signs is generally considered rather weak, so that diagnosis depends mostly on clinical suspicion. Because hyperviscosity may lead to severe complications, including death, its diagnosis requires prompt therapeutic intervention.

1. Clinical Manifestations

The classic presentation of hyperviscosity includes bleeding, generally presenting with ecchymoses, epistaxis, and gingival and, more rarely, retinal and gastrointestinal hemorrhage. Visual disturbancies include vision loss, diplopia, and blurred vision. Fundoscopy can show a retinopathy with distended, tortuous, sausage-like appearing retinal veins, described as fundus paraproteinaemicus. The neurological picture includes headache, somnolence, stupor, coma, seizures, dizziness, vertigo, ataxia, hearing loss and sometimes psychiatric presentations (172), and dyspnea.

According to the underlying disease, diverse laboratory abnormalities can be seen, including the presence of a monoclonal immunoglobulin, abnormal coagulation tests (173), pseudohyponatremia (174,175), pseudohypoglycemia (176), cryoglobulinemia (177), plasma hyperviscosity (178), rouleaux formation, increased packed cell volume, and abnormal platelet aggregation tests (172).

According to the soluble or cellular origin of hyperviscosity, two large categories can be discussed: monoclonal gammopathies and polycythemia vera.

2. Monoclonal Gammopathies

The prototype of a malignant disease that induces hyperviscosity is Waldenström's macroglobulinemia, with an incidence of about 10–30% at presentation (172). Hyperviscosity results from high monoclonal IgM concentration and IgM polymer formation. A bleeding diathesis is frequently present, as well as visual and neurological disturbancies. The correlation between absolute IgM level and the degree of hyperviscosity is rather weak and can be a result of the individually variable tendency of the IgM to polymerize and of interactions of the monoclonal protein with other plasma proteins (172).

In multiple myeloma, hyperviscosity has been described in 3–4% of IgG myeloma and 5–10% of IgA myeloma. The symptoms are similar to those described for macroglobulinemia, but hemorrhage is more common in IgA than IgG myeloma with hyperviscosity.

For some monoclonal immunoglobulins the concentration-viscosity relation may be linear; for some others, high viscosity can even occur with a nonlinear relationship at low concentration: this is typically the case for IgG_3 and IgA, which can act as macromolecules as a result of in vivo polymerization (179–183).

Apart from hyperviscosity, monoclonal proteins may interact with coagulation proteins to induce bleeding. Inhibitor activity to factors V, VII, and VIII and the prothrombin complex has been described, as well as reduction in several coagulation factors (173).

Treatment of hyperviscosity and bleeding diathesis of monoclonal gammopathy can be managed with prompt plasmapheresis in the emergency situation, followed by disease-specific cytotoxic therapy (184,185). Plasmapheresis should always be performed if the symptoms or signs of hyperviscosity are present and should be considered if the risk is high, as with significant increases in monoclonal IgM, IgA, and IgG_3. The volume and frequency of plasma exchange depend upon the clinical situation. Plasma exchange (up to 6 liters) may be necessary during the first day in the acute situation, but generally a 3–4 liter exchange is sufficient. A lower volume maintenance program once or twice a week can prevent recurrence while waiting for the effect of the primary, cytotoxic therapy. Because the distribution volume of IgM is lower (80% intravascular) than that of IgG and IgA (40% intravascular), smaller volumes of exchange (2–3 liters/day) may provide effective relief of symptoms in Waldenström's macroglobulinemia. With automated apheresis machines, cellular elements are returned and volume replaced with plasma substitutes. Substitution including fresh frozen plasma may be preferable, particularly if a bleeding diathesis is present (186).

3. Polycythemia Vera

Hyperviscosity caused by increased packed cell volume as occurs in polycythemia vera typically presents with thrombotic complications affecting both the arterial and venous systems (187–189). Arterial thrombosis is predominant at the cerebrovascular and peripheral microvascular level, with signs and symptoms including headache, confusion, vertigo, and stroke, as well as occlusive signs involving fingers and toes, sometimes leading to gangrenous lesions. In the venous circulation, thrombotic complications include superficial and deep venous thrombosis, Budd-Chiari syndrome, and thrombosis of splenic and portal veins.

The role of the frequently elevated platelet count as the pathophysiological cause of these complications in polycythemia vera remains controversial. The essential goal of therapy in the acute situation of polycythemia-related hyperviscosity is to reduce the packed red cell volume by therapeutic bleeding. In patients with symptoms of hyperviscosity, thrombosis, bleeding, or signs of congestive heart failure, with hematocrit values above 0.6, immediate therapeutic apheresis should be performed to lower the hematocrit to below 0.55–0.6. If venisection (phlebotomy) is poorly tolerated, the blood loss can be replaced with physiological solutions. Therapeutic phlebotomy inducing an iron-deficiency state constitutes at the same time standard therapy of the disease and is generally preferable to cytotoxic drugs and radioactive phosphorus because of a reduced risk of leukemogenesis (190–192).

B. Leukostasis

The leukostasis syndrome, mostly discussed in the context of hyperviscosity syndromes, is generally not caused by an increase in whole blood viscosity and should be considered a separate entity (193). Leukostasis occurs in hyperleukocytic leukemias, more commonly in myelocytic than lymphocytic forms. The classic leukostasis syndrome includes dyspnea with respiratory insufficiency, mental status changes with confusion and stupor, visual abnormalities, and a potential for central nervous system hemorrhage (193–195).

These manifestations are caused by the formation of leukocyte aggregates and thrombi, vascular invasion, microcirculation hyperviscosity, and vascular stasis. The syndrome has been mostly described with chronic myelocytic leukemia and acute leukemias, being very rare in chronic lymphocytic leukemia, even at very high lymphocyte counts.

Although no absolute white blood cell level can predict the occurrence of symptoms, patients with granulocyte counts greater than 100,000/ml and lymphocyte counts above 750,000/ml are considered at risk (193).

The optimal therapy for leukostasis should be prompt leukapheresis, a decrease in the white cells by 30–40% generally leading to reversal of the symptoms (196). This can be achieved, on average, with a single procedure. In the acute setting, leukapheresis has an advantage over chemotherapy in giving a quick result without supplemental risk of tumor lysis syndrome or urate nephropathy. It allows the introduction of cytotoxic therapy after initial diagnostic work-up and patient preparation with allopurinol and adequate hydration. Red blood cell transfusion before reduction of the white count should be avoided because of the risk of hyperviscosity (193).

C. Thrombocytosis

Although thrombocytosis is common in cancer patients, symptomatic thrombocytosis is generally limited to patients with myeloproliferative diseases, including essential thrombocythemia, polycythemia vera, chronic myelocytic leukemia, myelofibrosis, and "overlap" myeloproliferative syndromes (197–199). Significant, potentially dangerous thrombocytosis is generally limited to platelet counts above 1,000,000/mm^3, but in some patients complications can occur below these values. Thrombocytosis can present with thrombotic as well as bleeding problems. Bleeding complications are classically of the platelet-vascular type, involving cutaneous and mucosal hemorrhage. Thrombotic complications include deep vein thrombosis and pulmonary embolism but more characteristically also include hepatic vein and portal vein thrombosis, erythromelalgia with burning pain in the extremities, and signs of digital ischemia as well as neurological complications related to cerebrovascular ischemia. Recurrent spontaneous abortions and fetal growth retardation have also been described, probably related to multiple placental infarctions. These complications are recognized with increasing frequency when the platelet count is above 1,000,000/mm^3. Overall, however, the correlation between the degree of thrombocytosis and the risk of hemostatic complications is weak, and indications for therapy according to the platelet count are controversial.

In general, there is little rationale for chronic cytoreductive therapy in asymptomatic patients; however, treatment should be considered in patients with recurrent hemostatic complications, particularly if typical cerebrovascular or digital thrombotic events occur.

If a rapid decrease in the platelet count appears necessary, platelet apheresis should be considered. As far as cytoreductive chemotherapy is concerned, hydroxyurea is probably the most useful agent, providing effective long-term control generally without severe marrow toxicity or serious side effects.

Recombinant interferon-α is also highly effective, generally safe, and rapidly acting at a daily dose of 3×10^6 units subcutaneously, but long-term maintenance therapy is necessary if recurrence of uncontrolled thrombocytosis with related symptoms must be avoided. Side effects are rather frequent and occasionally severe enough to necessitate treatment discontinuation (200,201).

Anagrelide, an orally administered, nonmutagenic drug, has been found to induce a selective platelet reduction in thrombocythemia, probably by suppression of megakaryocytopoiesis with concomitant functional antiplatelet activity. This drug has been shown to be highly effective, even in patients refractory to other treatment modalities, at a dose of 0.5–1 mg four times daily (202).

The use of aspirin and other antiplatelet drugs in thrombocytosis remains controversial and should not be recommended indiscriminately. Because these patients sometimes have abnormal platelet function with bleeding tendencies, serious bleeding complications can be precipitated. On the other hand, patients with recurrent thrombotic complications, particularly of the digital and cerebrovascular ischemia type, will probably benefit from aspirin in combination with platelet-lowering therapy. The decision to treat patients with antiplatelet drugs should therefore be made on an individual basis, depending on the clinical situation, with periodic reassessment according to the evolution of the disease.

REFERENCES

1. Svensson PJ, Dahlback B. Resistance to activated protein C as a basis for venous thrombosis. N Engl J Med 1994; 330:512–522.
2. Colman RW, Hirsch J, Marder VJ, Salzman EW. Hemostasis and Thrombosis, Philadelphia: Lippincott,
3. Mollison PL, Engelfriet CP, Contreras M. Blood Transfusion in Clinical Medicine. Oxford: Blackwell,
4. Gaydos LA, Freireich EJ, Mantel N. The quantitative relation between platelet count and hemorrhage in patients with acute leukemia. N Engl J Med 1962; 266:905–909.
5. Gmur J, Burger J, Schanz U, et al. Safety of stringent prophylactic platelet transfusion policy for patients with acute leukemia. Lancet 1991; 338:1223–1226.
6. Sintnicolaas K, Vriesendorp HM, Sizoo W, et al. Delayed alloimmunization by random single donor platelet transfusions. Lancet 1981; 1:750–753.
7. Gmur J, Von Felten A, Osterwalder B, et al. Delayed alloimmunization using random single donor platelet transfusions: a prospective study in thrombocytopenic patients with acute leukemia. Blood 1983; 62:473–479.
8. Dutcher JP, Schiffer CA, Aisner J, et al. Long-term follow-up of patients with leukemia receiving platelet transfusions: identification of a large group of patients who do not become alloimmunized. Blood 1981; 58:1007–1011.
9. Ferrara GB, Tosi RM, Azzolina G, et al. HLA unresponsiveness induced by weekly transfusions of small aliquots of whole blood. Transplant 1974; 17:194–198.
10. Friedberg RC, Donnelly SF, Boyd JC, et al. Clinical and blood bank factors in the

management of platelet refractoriness and alloimmunization. Blood 1993; 81:3428–3434.
11. Messerschmidt G, Makuch R, Appelbaum F, et al. A prospective randomized trial of HLA-matched versus mismatched single donor platelet transfusions in cancer patients. Cancer 1988; 62:795–801.
12. Klein HG, Dzik WH, Strauss RG, et al. Leukocyte-reduced blood component therapy. ASH Education Program 1992:76–85.
13. Pamphilon DG, Potter M, Cutts M, et al. Platelet concentrates irradiated with ultraviolet light retain satisfactory in vitro storage characteristics and in vivo survival. Br J Haematol 1990; 75:240–244.
14. Hoffman R. Regulation of megakaryocytopoiesis. Blood 1989; 74:1196–1202.
15. Bridell RA, Bruno E, Cooper RJ, et al. Effect of c-kit ligand on in vitro human megakaryocytopoiesis. Blood 1991; 78:2854–2859.
16. Erickson-Miller CL, Ji H, Parchment RE, et al. Megakaryocyte-colony stimulating factor (Meg-CSF) is a unique cytokine specific for the megakaryocyte lineage. Br J Haematol 1993; 84:197–203.
17. Burstein SA, Mei RL, Henthorn J, et al. Leukemia inhibitory factor and interleukin-11 promote maturation of human megakaryocytes in vitro. J Clin Oncol 1992; 153:305–312.
18. Postmus PE, Gietma JA, Damsa O, et al. Effects of recombinant interleukin-3 in patients with relapsed small-cell lung cancer treatment with chemotherapy: a dose-finding study. J Clin Oncol 1992; 10:1131–1140.
19. D'Hondt V, Weynants P, Humblet Y, et al. Dose-dependent interleukin-3 stimulation of thrombopoiesis and neutropoiesis in patients with small-cell lung cancer before and following chemotherapy. J Clin Oncol 1993; 11:2063–2071.
20. Biesma B, Willemse PHB, Mulder NH, et al. Effects of interleukin-3 after chemotherapy. Blood 1992; 80:1141–1148.
21. Lindemann A, Ganser A, Herrman F, et al. Biologic effects of recombinant human interleukin-3 in vivo. J Clin Oncol 1990; 9:2120–2127.
22. Brugger, Frisch J, Schultz G, et al. Sequential administration of interleukin-3 and granulocyte-macrophage stimulating factor following standard-dose combination chemotherapy with etoposide, ifosfamide and cisplatin. J Clin Oncol 1992; 9:1452–1459.
23. Vadhan-Raj S, Rapadopoulos N, Burgess A, et al. PIXY 321 (GMCSF/IL3 fusion protein) chemotherapy induced multilineage myelosuppression in patients with sarcoma. Blood 1992; 80:2490 (Suppl. 1, abstract 987).
24. Jakubowski A, Raptis G, Gilewski T, et al. A phase I/II trial of PIXY 321 (PIX Y) in patients with metastatic breast cancer receiving doxorubicin and thiotepa. Blood 1992; 80:88a (Suppl. 1, abstract 342).
25. Demetri G, Costa J, Hayes D, et al. A phase I trial of recombinant methionyl human stem cell factor (SCF) in patients with advanced breast carcinoma pre- and post-chemotherapy (chemo) with cyclophosphamide (C) and doxorubicin (A) (abstract). Proc Am Soc Clin Oncol 1993; 12:367.
26. Weber J, Yang JC, Topalian SL, et al. Phase I trial of subcutaneous interleukin-6 in patients with advanced malignancies. J Clin Oncol 1993; 11:499–506.
27. Gameren MM, Velenga E, Willemse PHB, et al. The effects of recombinant

interleukin-6 on in vivo hematopoiesis in cancer patients. Blood 1992; 80:249a (Suppl. 1, abstract 985).
28. Demetri GD, Samuels B, Gordon M, et al. Recombinant human interleukin-6 (IL-6) increases circulating platelet counts and C-reactive protein levels in vivo: initial results of a phase I trial in sarcoma patients with normal hematopoiesis. Blood 1992; 80:88a (Suppl. 1, abstract 344).
29. Hoyle CF, Swirsky DM, Freedman L, et al. Beneficial effect of heparin in the management of patients with APL. Br J Haematol 1988; 68:283.
30. Dombret H, Scrobohaci ML, Ghorra P, et al. Coagulation disorders associated with acute promyelocytic leukemia: corrective effect of all trans-retinoic acid treatment. Leukemia 1993; 7:2–9.
31. Alperin JB. Coagulopathy caused by vitamin K deficiency in critically ill, hospitalized patients. JAMA 1987; 258:1916–1919.
32. Trousseau A. Phlegmasia alba dolens. Clin Med Hotel-Dieu Paris (London: New Sydenham Society) 1868; 3:695–727.
33. Sack GH, Levin J, Bell WR. Trousseau's syndrome and other manifestation of disseminated coagulopathy in patients with neoplasms: clinical pathophysiologic and therapeutic features. Medecine (Baltimore) 1977; 56:1–37.
34. Luzzato G, Schafer AI. The prethrombotic state in cancer. Semin Oncol 1990; 17:147–159.
35. Rickles FR, Edwards RL. Activation of blood coagulation in cancer. Blood 1983; 62:14–31.
36. Lieberman JS, Borrero J, Urdaneta E, Wright IS. Thrombo-phlebitis and cancer. JAMA 1961; 177:542–545.
37. Aderka D, Brown A, Zelikovski A, Pinkhas J. Idiopathic deep vein thrombosis in an apparently healthy patient as a premonitory sign of occult cancer. Cancer 1986; 57:1846–1849.
38. Goldberg RJ, Seneff M, Gore J. Occult malignant neoplasm in patients with deep vein thrombosis. Arch Intern Med 1987; 147:251–253.
39. Griffin MR, Stanson AW, Brown ML, et al. Deep venous thrombosis and pulmonary embolism. Risk of subsequent malignant neoplasm. Arch Intern Med 1987; 147:1907–1911.
40. Monreal M, Latoz E, Casals A, et al. Occult cancer in patients with deep venous thromboembolism. A systematic approach. Cancer 1991; 67:541–545.
41. Prandoni P, Lensing AWA, Büller HR, et al. Deep-vein thrombosis and the influence of subsequent symptomatic cancer. N Engl J Med 1992; 327:1128–1133.
42. Sun NCJ, McAfee WM, Hum GJ, et al. Hemostatic abnormalities in malignancy, a prospective study of one hundred eight patients. Am J Clin Pathol 1979; 71:10–16.
43. Soong BC, Miller SP. Coagulation disorders in cancer. Fibrinolysis and inhibitors. Cancer 1970; 25:867–874.
44. Ambrus JL, Ambrus CM, Pickren JW. Causes of death in cancer patients. J Med 1975; 6:61–64.
45. Patterson WP, Ringenberg QS. The pathophysiology of thrombosis in cancer. Semin Oncol 1990; 17:140–146.
46. Shattil SS. Diagnosis and treatment of recurrent venous thromboembolism. Med Clin North Am 1984; 68:577–600.

47. Hedderich GS, O'Connor RJ, Reid EC, et al. Caval tumor thrombus complicating renal cell carcinoma: A surgical challenge. Surgery 1987; 102:614–619.
48. Ritchey ML, Kinard R, Novick DE. Adrenal tumors: involvement of the inferior vena cava. J Urol 1987; 138:1134–1136.
49. Prichett TR, Lieskowsky G, Skinner DG. Extension of renal cell carcinoma into the vena cava: clinical review and surgical approach. J Urol 1986; 135:460–464.
50. Sharifi R, Ray P, Schade SG, et al. Inferior vena cava thrombosis. Unusual presentation of testicular tumor. Urology 1988; 32:146–150.
51. Levin J, Conley CL. Thrombocytosis associated with malignant disease. Arch Intern Med 1964; 114:497–500.
52. Karpatin S, Pearlstein E. Role of platelets in tumor cell metastases. Ann Intern Med 1981; 95:636–641.
53. Marcum JM, McGill M, Bastida E, et al. The interaction of platelet, tumor cells, and vascular subendothelium. J Lab Clin Med 1980; 96:1046–1053.
54. Gasic GJ, Gasic TB, Galanti N, et al. Platelet-tumor cell interactions in mice. The role of platelets in malignant disease. Int J Cancer 1973; 11:704–718.
55. Grignani G, Jamieson GA. Platelets in tumor metastasis: generation of adenosine diphosphonate by tumor cells is specific but unrelated to metastatic potential. Blood 1988; 71:844–849.
56. Bastida E. The metastatic cascade: potential approaches for the inhibition of metastasis. Semin Thromb Hemost 1988; 14:66–72.
57. Gordon SG, Franks JJ, Lewis B. Cancer procoagulant A: a factor X activating procoagulant from malignant tissue. Thromb Res 1975; 6:127–137.
58. Curatolo L, Colucci M, Cambini AL, et al. Evidence that cells from experimental tumours can activate coagulation factor X. Br J Cancer 1979; 40:228–233.
59. Bastida E, Ordinas A, Escolar G, et al. Tissue factor in microvesicles shed from U87MG human glioblastoma cells induces coagulation, platelet aggregation, and thrombogenesis. Blood 1984; 64:177–184.
60. Bastida E, Ordinas A, Jamieson GA. Differing platelet aggregating effects by two tumor cell lines: absence of a role for platelet-derived ADP. Am J Hematol 1981; 11:367–378.
61. Mohanty D, Hilgard P. A new platelet aggregating material (PAM) in an experimentally induced rat fibrosarcoma. Thromb Haemost 1984; 51:192–195.
62. Honn KV, Busse WD, Sloane BF. Prostacyclin and thromboxanes. Implications for their role in tumor cell metastasis. Biochem Pharmacol 1983; 32:1–11.
63. Gordon S. Cancer cell procoagulants and their implications. Hematol Oncol Clin North Am 1992; 6:1359–1374.
64. Scates MS. Diagnosis and treatment of cancer-related thrombosis. Hematol Oncol Clin North Am 1992; 6:1329–1339.
65. Pober JS, Cotran RS. Cytokines and endothelial cell biology. Physiol Rev 1990; 70:427.
66. Harker LA, Mann FG. Thrombosis and cardiovascular disorders. In Fuster V, Verstreate M, eds. Thrombosis and Fibrinolysis. Philadelphia: W. B. Saunders, 1992:1–26.
67. Huber AR, Kinckel S, Todd RF III, Weiss SJ. Regulation of transendothelial neutrophil migration by endogenous interleukin-8. Science 1991; 254:99–101.

68. Bennegard K, Curelaru I, Gustavsson B, et al. Material thrombogenicity in central venous catherization. Comparison between uncoated and heparin-coated, long antebrachial, polyethylene catheters. Acta Anaesthesiol Scand 1982; 26:112–120.
69. Sketch MH, Cale M, Mohiuddin SM, et al. Use of percutaneously inserted venous catheters in coronary care units. Chest 1972; 62:684–689.
70. Lokich JJ, Becker B. Subclavian vein thrombosis in patients treated with infusion chemotherapy for advanced malignancy. Cancer 1983; 52:1586–1589.
71. Lazarus HM, Lowder JN, Herzig RH. Occlusion and infection in Broviac catheters during intensive cancer therapy. Cancer 1983; 52:2342–2348.
72. Lokich JJ, Bothe A Jr, Benotti P, et al. Complications and management of implanted venous access catheters. J Clin Oncol 1985; 3:710–717.
73. Falchuck KH, Peterson L, McNeil BJ. Microparticulate induced phlebitis. Its prevention by in-line filtration. N Engl J Med 1985; 312:78–92.
74. Daniell HW. Heparin in the prevention of infusion phlebitis. JAMA 1973; 226:1317–1321.
75. King DJ, Kelton JG. Heparin-associated thrombocytopenia. Ann Intern Med 1984; 100:535–540.
76. Rizzoni WE, Miller K, Rick M, et al. Heparin-induced thrombocytopenia and thromboembolism in the postoperative period. Surgery 1988; 103:470–476.
77. Stead RB, Schafer AI, Rosenberg RD, et al. Heterogeneity of heparin lots associated with thrombocytopenia and thromboembolism. Am J Med 1984; 77:185–188.
78. Cines DB, Tomaski A, Tannenbaum S. Immune endothelial-cell injury in heparin-associated thrombocytopenia. N Engl J Med 1987; 316:581–589.
79. Goodnough LT, Saito H, Manni A, et al. Increased incidence of thromboembolism in stage IV breast cancer patients treated with a five-drug chemotherapy regimen: a study of 159 patients. Cancer 1984; 54:1264–1268.
80. Weiss RB, Tormey DC, Holland JF, et al. Venous thrombosis during multimodal treatment of primary breast carcinoma. Cancer Treat Rep 1981; 65:677–679.
81. Levine MN, Gent M, Hirsch J, et al. The thrombogenic effect of anticancer drug therapy in women with stage II breast cancer. N Engl J Med 1988; 318:404–407.
82. Sapher T, Torney DC, Gray R. Venous and arterial thrombosis in patients who received adjuvant therapy for breast cancer. J Clin Oncol 1991; 9:286–294.
83. Harrell RM, Sibley R, Vogelzang N. Renal vascular lesions after chemiotherapy with vinblastine, bleomycin and cisplatin. Am J Med 1982; 73:429–433.
84. Jackson AM, Rose BD, Graff LG, et al. Thrombotic microangiopathy and renal failure associated with antineoplastic chemotherapy. Ann Intern Med 1984; 101:41–44.
85. Hamner RW, Verani R, Weinmann EJ. Mitomycin-associated renal failure. Case report and review. Arch Intern Med 1983; 143:803–807.
86. Lesesne JB, Rothschild N, Erickson B, et al. Cancer-associated hemolytic-uremic syndrome: analysis of 85 cases from national registry. J Clin Oncol 1989; 7:781–789.
87. Korec S, Schein PS, Smith FP, et al. Treatment of cancer-associated hemolytic uremic syndrome with staphylococcal protein A immuno-perfusion. J Clin Oncol 1986; 4:210–215.
88. McDonald GB, Sharma P, Matthews DE, et al. Venocclusive disease of the liver

after bone marrow transplantation: diagnosis, incidence and predisposing factors. Hepatology 1984; 4:116–122.

89. Dulley, Kanfer EJ, Appelbaum FR, et al. Venocclusive disease of the liver after chemoradiotherapy and autologous bone marrow transplantation. Transplantation 1987; 43:870–873.
90. Rio B, Andreu G, Nicod A, et al. Thrombocytopenia in venocclusive disease after bone marrow transplantation or chemotherapy. Blood 1986; 67:1773–1776.
91. Priest JR, Ramsay NKC, Steinherz PG, et al. Syndrome of thrombosis and hemorrhage complicating L-asparaginase therapy for childhood acute lymphoblastic leukemia. J Pediatr 1982; 100:984–989.
92. Cairo MS, Lazarus K, Gilmore RL, et al. Intracranial hemorrhage and focal seizures secondary to the use of L-asparaginase during induction therapy of acute lymphocytic leukemia. J Pediatr 1980; 97:829–833.
93. Priest JR, Ramsay NKC, Latchaw RE, et al. Thrombotic and hemorrhagic strokes complicating early therapy for childhood acute lymphoblastic leukemia. Cancer 1980; 46:1548–1554.
94. Pui HC, Jackson CW, Chesney CM, et al. Involvement of von Willebrand factor in thrombosis following asparaginase-prednisone-vincristine therapy for leukemia. Am J Hematol 1987; 25:291–298.
95. Freeman N, Costanza M. 5-Fluorouracil-associated cardiotoxicity. Cancer 1988; 61:36–45.
96. Adoue D, Arlet P. Bleomycin and Raynaud's phenomenon. Ann Intern Med 1984; 100:770.
97. Vogelzang NJ, Bosl GJ, Johnson K, et al. Raynaud's phenomenon: a common toxicity after combination chemotherapy for testicular cancer. Ann Intern Med 1981; 95:228–292.
98. Vogelzang NJ, Torkelson JL, Kennedy BJ. Hypo-magnesemia, renal dysfunction and Raynaud's phenomenon in patients treated with cisplatin, vinblastine and bleomycin. Cancer 1985; 56:2765–2770.
99. Kukla LUJ, McGuire WP, Lad T, et al. Acute vascular episodes associated with therapy of carcinoma of the upper aerodigestive tract with bleomycine, vincristine and cisplatin. Cancer Treat Rep 1982; 66:369–370.
100. Goldhirsch A, Joss R, Markwalder TM, et al. Acute cerebrovascular accident after treatment with cisplatin and methylprednisolone. Oncology 1983; 40:344–345.
101. Licciardello JTW, Moake JL, Rudy CK, et al. Elevated plasma von Willebrand factor levels and arterial occlusive complications associated with cisplatin-based chemotherapy. Oncology 1985; 42:296–300.
102. Lombard CM, Churg A, Winokur S. Pulmonary veno-occlusive disease following therapy for malignant neoplasms. Chest 1987; 92:871–876.
103. Capewell SJ, Wright AJ, Ellis DA. Pulmonary veno-occlusive disease in association with Hodgkin's disease. Thorax 1984; 39:554–555.
104. Lipton A, Harvey HA, Hamilton RW. Venous thrombosis as a side effect of tamoxifen treatment. Cancer Treat Rep 1984; 68:887–889.
105. Nevasaari K, Heikkinen M, Taskinen PJ. Tamoxifen and thrombosis. Lancet 1978; 2:946–947.

106. Hendrick A, Subramanian VP. Tamoxifen and thromboembolism. JAMA 1980; 243:514–515.
107. Fisher B, Costantino J, Redmond C, et al. Clinical trial evaluating tamoxifen in treatment of patients with node-negative breast cancer who have estrogen receptor-positive tumors. N Eng J Med 1989; 320:479–485.
108. Anger AL, Mackie MJ. Effects of tamoxifen on blood coagulation. Cancer 1988; 61:1316–1319.
109. Jones AL, Powles TJ, Treleaven JC, et al. Haemostatic changes and thromboembolic risk during tamoxifen in normal women. Br J Cancer 1992; 66:744–747.
110. Enke RE, Rios CN. Tamoxifen treatment of metastatic breast cancer and antithrombin III levels. Cancer 1985; 53:2607–2609.
111. Blackard CE, Doe RP, Mellinger GT, et al. Incidence of cardiovascular disease and death in patients receiving diethylstilbestrol for carcinoma of the prostate. Cancer 1970; 26:249–256.
112. Runde V, Aul C, Sudhoff T, et al. Retinoic acid in the treatment of acute promyelocytic leukemia: inefficacy of the 13-cis isomer and induction of complete remission by the all-trans isomer complicated by thromboembolic events. Ann Hematol 1992; 64:270–272.
113. Escudier S, Kantarjïan H, Estey R. Thrombosis in acute promyelocytic leukemia (APL) patients treated with all-trans retinoïc acid (ATRA) (Proc ASCO Abstract 1020). J Clin Oncol 1993; 12:310.
114. Forbes CD, Lowe GDO. Clinical diagnosis. In: Hirsh J, ed. Venous Thrombosis and Pulmonary Embolism. Diagnostic Methods, Vol. 18. New York: Churchill Livingstone, 1987:9–19.
115. Hull R, Raskob G, Leclerc J, et al. The diagnosis of clinically suspected venous thrombosis. Clin Chest Med 1984; 5:439–456.
116. Hull R, van Aken WG, Hirsh J, et al. Impedance plethysmography using the occlusive cuff technique in the diagnosis of venous thrombosis. Circulation 1976; 53:696–700.
117. Wheeler HB, Pearson D, O'Connell D, et al. Impedance plebography: technique, interpretation end results. Arch Surg 1972; 104:164–169.
118. Huisman HV, Buller HR, ten Cate CJ, et al. Serial impedance plethysmography for suspected deep venous thrombosis in outpatients. The Amsterdam general practioner study. N Engl J Med 1986; 314:823–825.
119. Hull R, Hirsh J, Carter C, et al. Diagnostic efficacy of impedance plethysmography for clinically suspected deep vein thrombosis: a randomized trial. Ann Intern Med 1985; 102:21–28.
120. Sigel B, Felix WR, Popky LG, et al. Diagnosis of lower limb venous thrombosis by Doppler ultrasound technique. Arch Surg 1972; 104:174–179.
121. Strandness DE, Sumner DS. Ultrasonic velocity detector in the diagnosis of thrombophlebitis. Arch Surg 1972; 104:180–183.
122. Lensing AWA, Prandoni P, Brandjes D, et al. Detection of deep vein thrombosis by real-time B-mode ultrasonography. N Engl J Med 1989; 320:342–345.
123. Rabinov K, Paulin S. Roentgen diagnosis of venous thrombosis in the leg. Arch Surg 1972; 104:134–144.
124. Bettmann MA. Contrast phlebography. In: Hirsh J, ed. Venous Thrombosis and

Pulmonary Embolism. Diagnostic Methods, Vol. 18. New York: Churchill Livingstone, 1987:20–32.

125. Calligaro KD, Bergen WS, Hant MJ, et al. Thromboembolic complications in patients with advanced cancer: anticoagulation versus Greenfield filter placement. Ann Vasc Surg 1991; 5:186–189.
126. Bell WR, Simon TL, Demets DL. The clinical features of submassive and massive pulmonary emboli. Am J Med 1977; 62:355–360.
127. Hull R, Hirsh J, Carter C, et al. Diagnostic value of ventilation-perfusion in patients with suspected pulmonary embolism and abnormal perfusion lung scans. Chest 1985; 88:819–828.
128. Denardo G, Goodwin DA, Ravisini R, et al. The ventilatory lung scan in the diagnosis of pulmonary embolism. N Engl J Med 1974; 282:1334–1336.
129. Williams O, Lyall J, Vernon M, et al. Ventilation-perfusion lung scanning for pulmonary emboli. BMJ 1974; 1:600–602.
130. Hull R, Hirsh J, Carter C, et al. Pulmonary angiography, ventilation lung scanning, and venography for clinically suspected pulmonary embolism with abnormal perfusion lung scan. Ann Intern Med 1983; 98:891–899.
131. Bookstein JJ, Silver TM. The angiographic differential diagnosis of acute pulmonary embolism. Radiology 1974; 110:25–33.
132. Grollman JH, Gyepes MT, Helmer E. Transfemoral selective bilateral pulmonary arteriography with a pulmonary-artery-seeking catheter. Radiology 1970; 96:202–204.
133. Fraschini G, Jadeja J, Lawson M, et al. Local infusion of urokinase for the lysis of thrombosis associated with permanent central venous catheters in cancer patients. J Clin Oncol 1987; 5:672–678.
134. Hung SS. Deep vein thrombosis of the arm associated with malignancy. Cancer 1989; 64:531–535.
135. Montemurro P, Lattanzio A, Chetta G, et al. Increased in vitro and in vivo generation of procoagulant activity (tissue factor) by mononuclear phagocytes after intralipid infusion in rabbits. Blood 1985; 65:1391–1395.
136. Bell WR, Starksen NF, Tong S, et al. Trousseau's syndrome. Devastating coagulopathy in the absence of heparin. Am J Med 1985; 79:423–430.
137. Deppish LM, Fayemi AO. Nonbacterial thrombotic endocarditis. Clinicopathological correlations. Am Heart J 1976; 92:723–729.
138. Ondrias F, Slugen I, Valach A. Malignant tumors and embolizing paraneoplastic endocarditis. Neoplasma 1985; 32:135–140.
139. Min KW, Gyorkey F, Sato C. Mucin producing adenocarcinomas and nonbacterial thrombotic endocarditis. Cancer 1980; 45:2374–2382.
140. Guinn GA, Ayala A, Liddicoat J. Clinical and therapeutic considerations in nonbacterial thrombotic endocarditis. Chest 1973; 64:26–28.
141. Gomes AS, Lois JF, Child JS, et al. Cardiac tumors and thrombus: evaluation with MR imaging. AJR 1987; 149:895–899.
142. Mitchell MC, Boitnott JK, Kaufman S, et al. Budd-Chiari syndrome: etiology, diagnosis and management. Medicine (Baltimore) 1982; 61:199–218.
143. Valla D, Casadevall N, Lacombe C, et al. Primary myeloproliferative disorder and hepatic vein thrombosis. A prospective study of erythroid colony formation in vitro in 20 patients with Budd-Chiari syndrome. Ann Intern Med 1985; 103:329–334.

144. Murphy FB, Steinberg HV, Shires GT, et al. The Budd-Chiari syndrome: an overview. AJR 1986; 147:9–15.
145. Sherlock S. Extrahepatic portal venous hypertension in adults. Clin Gastroenterol 1985; 14:1–19.
146. Levine M, Hirsh J. The diagnosis and treatment of thrombosis in the cancer patient. Semin Oncol 1990; 17:160–171.
147. Scates SM. Diagnosis and treatment of cancer-related thrombosis. Hematol Oncol Clin North Am 1992; 6:1329–1339.
148. Salzman EW, Deykin D, Shapiro RM, et al. Management of heparin therapy. N Engl J Med 1975; 292:1046.
149. Hull RD, Raskob GE, Hirsh J, et al. A double-blind randomized trial of intravenous versus subcutaneous heparin in the initial treatment of proximal-vein thrombosis. N Engl J Med 1986; 315:1109–1114.
150. Galzier RL, Crowell EB. Randomized prospective trial of continuous or intermittent heparin therapy. JAMA 1976; 236:1365–1367.
151. Mant MJ, O'Brien BD, Thong KL, et al. Hemorrhagic complications of heparin therapy. Lancet 1977; 1:1133–1135.
152. Wilson JR, Lampman J. Heparin therapy: a randomized prospective study. Am Heart J 1979; 97:155–158.
153. Basu D, Gallus A, Hirsh J, et al. A prospective study of the value of monitoring heparin treatment with the active partial thromboplastin time. N Engl J Med 1972; 287:324–327.
154. Gallus AS, Jackman J, Mills W, et al. Safety and efficacy of warfarin started early after submassive venous thrombosis or pulmonary embolism. Lancet 1986; 2:1293–1296.
155. Levine MN, Hirsh J. Hemorrhagic complications of anticoagulant therapy. Semin Thromb Hemost 1986; 12:39–57.
156. Levine MN, Raskob G, Hirsh J. Hemorrhagic complications of long-term anticoagulant therapy. Chest (Suppl) 1989; 95:26–36.
157. Chian A, Woodruff RK. Complications and failure of anticoagulation in the treatment of venous thromboembolism in patients with disseminated malignancy. Aust NZ J Med 1992; 22:119–122.
158. Choucair AK, Silver P, Levin VA. Risk of intracranial hemorrhage in glioma patients receiving anticoagulant therapy for venous thromboembolism. J Neurosurg 1987; 66:357–358.
159. Frickler JP, Vergues Y, Schach R, et al. Low dose heparin versus low molecular weight heparin in the prophylaxis of thromboembolic complications of abdominal oncological surgery. Eur J Clin Invest 1988; 18:561–567.
160. Hull RD, Pineo GF. Treatment of venous thromboembolism with low-molecular weight heparins. Hematol Oncol Clin North Am 1992; 6:1095–1104.
161. Hull RD, Delmore T, Genton E, et al. Warfarin sodium versus low-dose heparin in the long-term treatment of venous thrombosis. N Engl J Med 1979; 301:855–858.
162. Lagerstedt CI, Olsson CT, Fagher BO, et al. Need for long-term anticoagulant treatment in symptomatic calf-vein thrombosis. Lancet 1985; 1:515–518.
163. Hirsh J, Poller L, Deykin D, et al. Optimal therapeutic range for oral anticoagulants. Chest (Suppl) 1989; 95:5–11.

164. Hull R, Hirsh J, Jay R, et al. Different intensities of oral anticoagulant therapy in the treatment of proximal-vein thrombosis. N Engl J Med 1982; 307:1676–1681.
165. Holmgren K, Andersson G, Fagrell B, et al. One month versus six months therapy with oral anticoagulants after symptomatic deep vein thrombosis. Acta Med Scand 1985; 218:279–284.
166. Sasahara AA, St Martin CC, Henkin J, Barker WM. Approach to the patient with venous thromboembolism: treatment with thrombolytic agents. Hematol Oncol Clin North Am 1992; 6;1141–1160.
167. Gray W, Bell W. Fibrinolytic agents in the treatment of thrombotic disorders. Semin Oncol 1990; 17:228–237.
168. Atkinson JB, Baguall HA, Gomperts E. Investigational use of tissue plasminogen activator (t-PA) for occluded central venous catheters. J Parenter Enter Nutr 1990; 14:310–311.
169. Haire WD, Atkinson JB, Stephens LC, Kotaluk GD. Urokinase (UK) vs recombinant tissue plasminogen activator (R-TPA) in thrombosed central venous catheters (CVCs): a double-blind randomized controlled clinical trial. (Proc ASCO abstract 1485). J Clin Oncol 1993; 12:431.
170. Fahey JL, Barth WF, Solomon A. Serum hyperviscosity syndrome. JAMA 1965; 192:120–123.
171. Patterson WP, Caldwell CH, Doll DC. Hyperviscosity syndromes and coagulopathies. Semin Oncol 1990; 17:210–216.
172. Somer T. Rheology of paraproteinaemias and the plasma hyperviscosity syndrome. Baillieres Clin Haematol 1987; 1:695–723.
173. Lackner H. Hemostatic abnormalities associated with dysproteinemias. Semin Hematol 1973; 10:125–133.
174. Nanji AA, Blank DW. Pseudohyponatremia and hyperviscosity. J Clin Pathol 1983; 36:834–835.
175. Vader HL, Vink CLJ. The influence of viscosity on dilution methods: its problems in the determination of serum sodium. Clin Chim Acta 1975; 65:379–387.
176. Haibach H, Wright DL, Bailey LE. Pseudohypoglycemia in a patient with Waldenström's macroglulinemia, an artifact of hyperviscosity. Clin Chem 1986; 32:1239–1240.
177. Meltzer M, Franklin EC. Cryoglobulinemia: a study of twenty-nine patients. IgG and IgM cyroglobulins and factors affecting cryoprecipitability. Am J Med 1966; 40:828–836.
178. Pruzanski W, Watt JG. Serum viscosity and hyperviscosity syndrome in IgG multiple myeloma. Ann Intern Med 1972; 77:853–860.
179. Crawford J, Cox EB, Cohen HJ. Evaluation of hyperviscosity in monoclonal gammapathies. Am J Med 1985; 79:13–22.
180. Lindsley H, Teller D, Noonan B, et al. Hyperviscosity syndrome in multiple myeloma. A reversible concentration-dependent aggregation of the myeloma protein. Am J Med 1973; 54:682–688.
181. Preston FE, Cooke KB, Foster ME, et al. Myelomatosis and the hyperviscosity syndrome. Br J Haematol 1978; 38:517–530.
182. Chandy KG, Stockley RA, Leonard RCF, et al. Relationship between serum

viscosity and intravascular IgA polymer concentration in IgA myeloma. Clin Exp Immunol 1981; 46:653–661.
183. Alker U, Hansson UB, Lindstrom FD. Factors affecting IgA related hyperviscosity. Clin Exp Immunol 1983; 51:617–623.
184. Powles R, Smith C, Kohn J, et al. Method of removing abnormal protein rapidly from patients with malignant paraproteinaemias. BMJ 1971; 2:664–667.
185. Buskard NA, Galton DAG, Goldman JR, et al. Plasma exchange in the long-term management of Waldenström's macroglobulinemia. Can Med Assoc J 1977; 117:135–137.
186. Bensinger WI. Plasma exchange in the management of hematologic malignancies. In: Wiernik PH, Canellos GP, Kyle RA, et al., eds. Neoplastic Diseases of the Blood. New York: Churchill Livingstone, 1985:1013–1023.
187. Pearson TC. Rheology of the absolute polycythemias. Bailleres Clin Hematol 1987; 1:637–664.
188. Barabas AP, Offen DN, Meinhard EA. The arterial complications of polycythaemia vera. Br J Surg 1973; 60:183–187.
189. Kremer M, Lambert CD, Lawton N. Progressive neurological deficits in primary polycythemia. BMJ 1972; 3:216–218.
190. Gerson SL, Lazzarus HM. Hematopoietic emergencies. Semin Oncol 1989; 16:532–542.
191. Berk PD, Goldberg JD, Donovan PB, et al. Therapeutic recommendations in polycytemia vera based on polycytemia vera study group protocols. Semin Hematol 1986; 23:132–143.
192. Berk PD, Goldberg JD, Silverstein MN, et al. Increased incidence of acute leukemia in polycytemia vera associated with chlorambucil therapy. N Engl J Med 1981; 304:441–447.
193. Lichtman MA, Heal J, Rowe JM. Hyperleukocytic leukaemia: rheological and clinical features and management. Bailliere's Clin Haematol 1987; 725–746.
194. Vernant JP, Brun B, Mannoni P, et al. Respiratory distress of hyperleucocytic granulocytic leukemias. Cancer 1979; 44:264–268.
195. Lichtman MA, Rowe JM. Hyperleucocytic leukemia: rheologic, clinical and therapeutic considerations. Blood 1982; 650:279–283.
196. Schiffer CA. Therapeutic cytapheresis. In: Wiernik P, Canellos GP, Kyle RA, et al., eds. Neoplastic Diseases of the Blood. New York: Churchill Livingstone, 1985:999–1012.
197. Miters AJ, Schafer AI. Thrombocytosis and thrombocytemia. Hematol Oncol Clin North Am 1990; 4:157–178.
198. Pearson TC. Primary thrombocytemia: diagnosis and management. Br J Haematol 1991; 78:145–148.
199. Schafer AI. Essential thrombocytemia. Prog Hemost Thromb 1991; 10:69–96.
200. Gisslinger H, Chot A, Scheithauer W, et al. Interferon in essential thrombocytemia. Br J Haematol 1991; 79(suppl. 1):42–47.
201. Sacchi S, Tabilio A, Leoni P, et al. Interferon alpha-2b in the long-term treatment of essential thrombocytemia. Am Hematol 1991; 63:206–209.
202. Anagrelide Study Group. Anagrelide, a therapy for thrombocythemic states: an experience in 577 patients. Am J Med 1992; 92:69–76.

4

Management of Nausea and Vomiting

Maurizio Tonato and Fausto Roila
Policlinico Hospital, Perugia, Italy

Albano Del Favero
Institute of Internal Medicine I, University of Perugia, Perugia, Italy

I. INTRODUCTION

From a cancer patient's point of view, nausea and vomiting are the most distressing complications of chemotherapy, but they can also be caused by a variety of other conditions that one should always consider before beginning antiemetic treatment. Nausea and vomiting affect very negatively the psychological status, nutritional balance, social relationships, and, ultimately, quality of life of the patient. Furthermore, when nausea and vomiting are caused by chemotherapy, and this is the most frequent situation in cancer patients, their intensity and persistence can bring the patient to a refusal of treatment, even if it is potentially curative. Every effort should thus be made to clarify the real cause of nausea and vomiting and to treat these symptoms adequately.

During the last decade, considerable progress has been made in the pharmacological treatment of chemotherapy-induced emesis. This progress was achieved through the recognition of different emetic problems (acute, delayed, and anticipatory emesis) and clarification of some aspects of the neuropharmacology of nausea and vomiting, identification of effective antiemetic agents, used alone or in combination, and the adoption of sound methodology in clinical research. Notwithstanding these advances, emesis remains a critical problem in cancer patients, and basic and clinical research still must go far to achieve the ideal goal, that is, the complete control of such symptoms in every cancer patient.

II. MAIN CAUSES OF NAUSEA AND VOMITING IN CANCER PATIENTS

When nausea and vomiting occur in cancer patients, they are most often a consequence of chemotherapy, especially if it includes such drugs as cisplatin (CDDP) that cause emesis in the majority of patients when used without a valid antiemetic treatment. Before the 1980s, emesis was considered by oncologists an almost unavoidable consequence of cancer chemotherapy, and only a few clinical trials on its prevention were planned and executed. The introduction in clinical practice of CDDP, and its wider use in the treatment of advanced cancer, stimulated studies on antiemetic therapy that have made possible considerable advances in the prevention of chemotherapy-induced emesis.

Radiotherapy is also an important cause of emesis, especially when the upper abdomen is irradiated or when radiotherapy is used as total-body irradiation (TBI), as in the conditioning regimens for bone marrow transplantation.

Surgery and related anesthesia can also be a cause of emesis; recognition of this has prompted a series of studies, generally conducted by anesthesiologists, aimed at defining the best antiemetic treatment.

Treatment of a very common and feared symptom of cancer, pain, can induce nausea and vomiting. The increasingly widespread use of narcotic analgesics in cancer patients raises the problem of adequately treating this side effect.

Other causes of nausea and vomiting that should always be taken into consideration in a cancer patient are generally the disease itself or its complications. For example, intestinal obstruction, liver metastases, increased intracranial pressure from cerebral metastases, and hypercalcemia are very common causes of nausea and vomiting and should always be ruled out before identifying the symptoms as caused by treatment. Other causes of emesis may pertain to the medical management of a disease other than cancer, such as labyrinthitis, pancreatitis, uremia, Addison's disease, diabetic ketoacidosis, and hepatitis.

All these causes of nausea and vomiting of course require specific therapeutic intervention, and most of the time this does not include antiemetics. In the following sections, greater emphasis is given to the treatment of chemotherapy-related nausea and vomiting because this is the most relevant problem and the one in which most progress has been made.

III. PATHOPHYSIOLOGY OF NAUSEA AND VOMITING

The development of nausea and vomiting as a result of chemotherapy can be considered an "inappropriate" response of the body to a stimulus that parallels that caused by contaminated food in a biological context. The triggering of the reflex mechanism of vomiting by different stimuli can be realized through various pathways that explain the different emetic potentials of different antineoplastic drugs and the different antiemetic activity of various therapeutic regimens.

The mechanisms of emetic action of antineoplastic agents have not been well defined. There is general agreement, however, that the act of vomiting is controlled by the vomiting center, located in the lateral reticular formation in the floor of the fourth ventricle. Stimulated by afferent impulses, it coordinates the emetic response. Impulses arrive at the vomiting center from the following areas:

The chemoreceptor trigger zone, located within the area postrema on the fourth ventricle, which can be stimulated by substances contained in either the blood or the cerebrospinal fluid
The gastrointestinal tract via sympathetic and vagal pathways
The higher cortical centers, which transmit psychogenic stimuli
The vestibular apparatus of the middle ear (this does not seem to be important for chemotherapy-induced nausea and vomiting)

The neurotransmitters involved in nausea and vomiting caused by antineoplastic agents have not yet been clearly identified. Various neuroreceptors, however, have been pinpointed in or around the area postrema and in the gastrointestinal tract, including dopaminergic, cholinergic, H_1 and H_2 histaminergic, and opioid, and receptors for serotonin (5-hydroxytryptamine, 5-HT). Among the 5-HT receptors, 5-HT_3 seems to play a determinant role in chemotherapy-induced nausea and vomiting. In fact, in experimental studies in animals, some antiemetic drugs, such as sulpiride or domperidone, which are potent antagonists of dopamine (D_2) receptors, have been shown inefficacious in the prevention of CDDP-induced nausea and vomiting, but the selective 5-HT_3 receptor antagonists induced a high rate of complete protection from vomiting.

The precise site of action of 5-HT_3 receptor antagonists has not yet been identified, but two hypotheses have been formulated. The first, based on animal experimental data, supports a vagal afferent site of antiemetic action, probably in the gut wall. Indeed, chemotherapeutic agents may determine 5-HT release from the enterochromaffin cells in the upper gastrointestinal mucosa. 5-HT, stimulating 5-HT_3 receptors on vagal afferent fibers, acts centrally on the chemoreceptor trigger zone and/or on the vomiting center and induces nausea and vomiting.

The second hypothesis that suggests a central mechanism of action of the 5-HT_3 receptor antagonists is based on the presence of several neurons containing 5-HT and/or a high concentration of 5-HT_3 receptors in the area postrema. The depletion of 5-HT from the area postrema and injection of 5-HT_3 receptor antagonists in the same area inhibit CDDP-induced emesis.

The two hypotheses do not exclude each other, so it is also possible that the antineoplastic agents act on different sites and stimulate different receptors so that a combination of antiemetic agents may produce better results than single drugs.

IV. CHEMOTHERAPY-INDUCED EMESIS: GENERAL CONSIDERATIONS

Three types of chemotherapy-induced emesis can be distinguished: acute emesis, which occurs soon after drug administration, delayed emesis which begins about 24 h after chemotherapy administration and may persist for 6–7 days, and anticipatory emesis, which can occur in anticipation of a subsequent course of treatment if there has been poor antiemetic control during the previous course. Although this is an arbitrary distinction, these types of emesis are probably distinct phenomena from a physiopathological point of view and give rise to different therapeutic problems. The most important factors that can influence the efficacy of a given antiemetic treatment were recently reviewed (1), and they are reported in Table 1. Each factor in itself is an important variable, but the interrelation among factors should also be considered in the evaluation of the risk of chemotherapy-induced nausea and vomiting.

A. Variables Related to Chemotherapy

It is well known that antineoplastic drugs differ quantitatively and qualitatively in their emetogenic potential. It is usual to classify the different antineoplastic agents according to their emetogenic potential, whether high, moderate, or low (Table 2). Although this rating reflects a real difference in the emetogenic

Table 1 Variables Affecting Chemotherapy-Induced Vomiting

Variables related to chemotherapy
Type of drug or combination
Dosage and schedule
Route of administration
Variables related to patient population
Sex
Age
Setting and environment
Previous chemotherapy
History of alcohol intake
Others (emesis during pregnancy, susceptibility to motion sickness)
Variables related to antiemetic treatment
Type of drug or combination
Dosage and schedule
Route of administration
Toxicity

Source: From Reference 1.

Table 2 Emetogenic Potential of Cancer Chemotherapeutic Agents

High	Moderate	Low
Cisplatin	Cyclophosphamide	Methotrexate
Dacarbazine	Cytosine arabinoside (cytarabine)	Mitomycin C
Mechlorethamine	Anthracyclines	Bleomycin
Dactinomycin	Carboplatin	Busulfan
	Nitrosoureas	Chlorambucil
	Procarbazine	Melphalan
		Hydroxyurea
		Etoposide
		Teniposide
		Fluorouracil
		Vinca alkaloids

Source: From Reference 1.

capability of different drugs, it must be interpreted with caution because it relies more on empirical clinical observations than on comparative controlled studies. Moreover, it does not take into consideration that antineoplastic drugs are rarely given alone and that dose, route, and schedule of administration are critical in determining the incidence and intensity of nausea and vomiting. Usually, as the dose of a cytotoxic drug increases so does its emetogenic potential [i.e., with CDDP, cyclophosphamide, cytosine arabinoside (cytarabine), doxorubicin, and methotrexate]; as the infusion time of administration of the same dose becomes longer, nausea and vomiting decrease (i.e., CDDP and doxorubicin). Furthermore, a drug combination is generally thought to be more emetogenic than a single drug, unless each of the agents in the combination is given at less than maximum dose. Other important variables are differences among antineoplastic drugs in onset and duration of nausea and vomiting and tolerance of the emetogenic potential. Some drugs induce nausea and vomiting very early after administration (i.e., mechlorethamine and doxorubicin), others after 2–3 h (i.e., most cytotoxic drugs), and, in a few cases, even later (9–12 h for cyclophosphamide). The reasons for these differences are related to the kinetic characteristics of some drugs (i.e., cyclophosphamide), but for most agents they are generally unknown.

Tolerance to emesis can develop with some drugs if they are administered in multiple doses on consecutive days (i.e., CDDP and possibly dacarbazine), but this is not the case if cycles of chemotherapy are given 3–4 weeks apart.

The most important practical consequences of these variables are that patients treated with similar chemotherapeutic regimens must be studied individually and the type and schedule of antiemetic treatment tailored to their anticipated needs.

B. Variables Related to the Patient Population

Variability in antiemetic responses among patients and in the same patient in subsequent cycles of chemotherapy is a common experience, but only recently have the most important patient-related prognostic factors been defined. Most of these studies have been performed in patients treated with CDDP, and their conclusions should therefore be applied with caution when treating patients with different cytotoxic drugs.

Gender is probably the most important factor in conditioning response to antiemetic treatment. In support of this hypothesis are consistent data from three large double-blind, randomized clinical trials in CDDP-treated patients (2–4), which show that females vomit more than males. In these studies, the intensity of nausea, the mean number of vomiting episodes, and the duration of nausea and vomiting were also significantly greater in females than in males. Gender appears to affect the incidence of nausea and vomiting irrespective of antiemetic treatment, primary cancer site, and other patient-related variables, as shown by multivariate analysis.

Age of the patient is another important variable in predicting the risk of nausea and vomiting: complete protection from vomiting is generally better in older patients (>65 years). It is interesting to note that the toxicity of antiemetic therapy is also influenced by age. Such drugs as metoclopramide, which has anti-dopaminergic action, induce acute dystonic reactions more frequently in younger than in older patients. In a retrospective study on about 500 patients, the incidence of extrapyramidal reactions was only 2% in those over 30 years of age but was 27% in younger patients (5).

It is common knowledge that poorly controlled emesis in previous courses of chemotherapy predisposes a patient to unsatisfactory antiemetic results in subsequent treatments. Furthermore, the efficacy of antiemetic treatment decreases progressively with further antiblastic treatment. Therefore, previous experience with cytotoxic chemotherapy, especially with chemotherapy-induced emesis, is a very important factor in determining whether a patient will suffer nausea or vomiting.

History of alcohol intake also seems to play a role in determining the probability of vomiting; patients with a history of chronic, heavy alcohol intake (more that 100 g per day) experience less CDDP-induced nausea and vomiting than those who are not heavy drinkers. These data should be accepted with caution: a selection bias related to the sex and age of heavy drinkers cannot be excluded. The setting of administration of antiblastic agents should also be considered, because some studies have shown that inpatients are better protected from nausea and vomiting than outpatients. Other prognostic factors favoring emesis, such as susceptibility to motion sickness and emesis during pregnancy, should also be considered.

C. Variables Related to Antiemetic Treatment

Many drugs have been shown to be effective and well tolerated in randomized clinical trials for protection from chemotherapy-induced nausea and vomiting, and these include such classes and agents as drug-blocking dopamine receptors (metoclopramide, phenothiazines, butyrophenones, and domperidone), corticosteroids, central nervous system (CNS)-acting drugs (cannabinoids and benzodiazepines) that can be considered established antiemetics, and the new 5-HT_3 receptor antagonists. These drugs differ in their pharmacokinetic and pharmacodynamic characteristics, but it is doubtful whether these characteristics correlate to their antiemetic efficacy.

Of major importance is the well-known fact that the efficacy of these agents varies according to their dose, route, and schedule of administration. Furthermore, because these classes differ in their mechanisms of action, they have been used in various combinations, with great improvement in efficacy and, in some cases, reduced toxicity.

Several considerations should be kept in mind, however, when planning combination regimens. Each agent should be selected on the basis of firm data on its efficacy and used at optimal doses, route, and schedule of administration. It is important that the regimen combine drugs that have different mechanisms of activity and no overlapping toxicities. A combination can be justified even if the added drug is aimed at lessening the toxic effects of the antiemetic or cytotoxic regimen.

Relative toxicity, ease of administration, and cost are other important variables that should be taken into account.

V. THERAPY OF NAUSEA AND VOMITING IN HIGHLY EMETOGENIC CHEMOTHERAPY

Table 2 illustrates that some chemotherapy agents, especially if used at high doses, are considered capable of inducing nausea and vomiting in the majority of patients. Among these agents, CDDP is the symbol of highly emetogenic chemotherapy and the object of a large number of trials because it can cause nausea and vomiting in almost 100% of patients who have not received efficacious antiemetic therapy. Thus, when using CDDP, administration of the best antiemetic treatment available is mandatory. This is also the best way to avoid or reduce the unpleasant experience of anticipatory nausea and vomiting, more frequent when antiemetic protection at first cycle of chemotherapy is not complete.

In the late 1980s, clinical research made possible the development of an antiemetic regimen, and some variants of it, that was able to assure complete protection from nausea and vomiting in about 60–70% of CDDP-treated patients. This rather good result was the final step in a series of experiences that started with the intuition and the demonstration that very high doses of metoclopramide had good antiemetic potential (6). This effect was superior to that of the pharmacological doses (10–20 mg) considered capable of fulfilling the anti-dopaminergic capacity of the drug and was probably caused by its anti-serotoninergic activity when used at high doses. The antiemetic activity of metoclopramide was later confirmed to offer complete protection in about 20–40% of CDDP-treated patients; this figure substantially improved to 45–55% when steroids were added (3,7,8).

A further step toward even better antiemetic control was taken when diphenhydramine or lorazepam was added to the high-dose metoclopramide plus steroid combination. Neither of these compounds had a major antiemetic effect when used alone, but they were frequently used to treat the extrapyramidal effects of metoclopramide. When using them in prophylaxis, both the efficacy (over 60% complete protection from vomiting in untreated patients) and the tolerability of the combination regimen seemed to be improved in uncontrolled trials (9). This was confirmed in a double-blind trial in 367 patients showing that a combination of high-dose intravenous (IV) metoclopramide (3 mg/kg × 2 IV) plus dexamethasone (20 mg IV) plus diphenhydramide (50 mg IV) was significantly superior to the two-drug combination of metoclopramide (1 mg/kg × 4 IV) plus methylprednisolone (250 mg × 2 IV), in terms of both efficacy and tolerability (4). In fact, complete protection from vomiting was obtained in 72 and 56% of patients, respectively. Furthermore, the use of diphenhydramine, while increasing the rate of mild sedation, significantly decreased the incidence of extrapyramidal reactions, nervousness, and sweating. The reason for the increased efficacy of the three-drug combination regimens is probably the higher single dose of metoclopramide used (resulting in an antiserotoninergic effect, as shown in animal experiments), even if a diphenhydramide-related antiemetic action cannot be excluded.

Another trial in 120 patients compared the addition of diphenhydramine or lorazepam (1.5 mg/m^2 IV) to a combination of high-dose metoclopramide plus dexamethasone. Both these three-drug combinations offered similar complete protection from vomiting (56 and 63%, respectively), lorazepam decreasing the incidence of agitation and akathisia (10).

In conclusion, a three-drug antiemetic combination including metoclopramide plus dexamethasone plus diphenhydramine or lorazepam was shown to be the most efficacious and best tolerated regimen to prevent nausea and vomiting induced by CDDP. However, many problems remained to be solved with the use of metoclopramide:

1. Despite multidrug antiemetic treatment, 30–40% of patients still suffered from acute emesis. The response to therapy was even poorer in some subgroups of patients, such as females, young people, and patients with previous experience of nausea and vomiting induced by chemotherapy.
2. Complete protection from vomiting decreased significantly in the subsequent cycles of chemotherapy.
3. The tolerability of these combinations was not completely satisfactory because sedation, diarrhea, nervousness, and especially extrapyramidal reactions still affected about 3% of patients despite prophylactic treatment.

The introduction of the 5-HT_3 receptor antagonists in the late 1980s made possible new developments in antiemetic research. These drugs carry out their antiemetic activity by a selective antagonism of 5-HT_3 receptors; they have no activity on 5-HT1 or 5-HT2 receptors or on dopamine, histamine, muscarine, or opioid receptors. In animal experiments, antiserotoninergic drugs have proven to be potent and effective antagonists of emesis induced by CDDP, doxorubicin, and cyclophosphamide.

Table 3 lists the antiserotoninergic drugs currently being studied for prophylaxis against nausea and vomiting caused by chemotherapy. Many are still in phase I–II trials, and several years are needed before it can be verified whether they are suitable for therapeutic use.

Table 3 Antiserotoninergic Drugs

Drug	Producer	Dose and schedule
Ondansetron	Glaxo	0.15 mg/kg IV × 3 8 mg IV × 1 32 mg IV × 1
Granisetron	SmithKline Beecham	40 μg/kg IV × 1 3 mg IV × 1
Tropisetron	Sandoz	5 mg IV × 1
MDL 72222, MDL 73147	Merrell Dow	
Zacopride	Robins	
RG 12915	Rorer	
LAS 30451	Almirall	
Y-25130	Yoshitomi	

A. Ondansetron

Ondansetron (OND) is the most widely studied compound; it has recently been marketed in various countries in both oral and intravenous formulations. It possesses a relatively short-term half-life (about 3–3.5 h). OND was initially evaluated in patients submitted to high single-dose CDDP chemotherapy in several pilot studies using various schedules and doses. In these studies OND showed fairly good antiemetic activity, achieving complete protection from vomiting in 35–55% of patients, including some with emesis refractory to standard antiemetics. Tolerability was also fully satisfactory (11).

Subsequently, three controlled studies were published (12–14) that compared OND with high-dose metoclopramide. In all three studies, OND showed better antiemetic activity and lower toxicity than metoclopramide and, in the two crossover studies, was also preferred by the patients. Complete protection from vomiting was obtained in 40–45% of patients.

As already shown for metoclopramide, an increase in the antiemetic efficacy of OND when combined with dexamethasone was suggested by experiments conducted in ferrets and by pilot studies in humans.

The usefulness of such a combination was confirmed by a double-blind crossover study comparing OND alone (0.15 mg/kg IV every 2 h for three doses) versus OND (at the same dose and schedule) plus dexamethasone (20 mg IV) (15). This combination was significantly superior to the single drug (91 versus 64% complete protection from vomiting) and was preferred by the patients. Side effects were mild and not significantly different between the two antiemetic treatments. More recently, these results were confirmed by three other multicenter studies (16–18).

The next logical step in the search for the best treatment in the prevention of CDDP-induced acute emesis was to compare OND plus dexamethasone to a standard three-drug antiemetic combination containing metoclopramide.

The first of these studies was recently published (19). It is a multicenter randomized double-blind study including 289 patients submitted to ≥50 mg/m^2 of CDDP chemotherapy. OND plus dexamethasone was shown to be significantly more efficacious than metoclopramide plus dexamethasone plus diphenhydramine. In particular, complete protection from vomiting was obtained in 78.7 and 59.5% of patients, respectively, on day 1 after CDDP administration.

Furthermore, complete protection from vomiting was significantly superior with OND plus dexamethasone even on day 2 (83.9 versus 68.0%) and day 3 (86.3 versus 71.2%) after CDDP administration, while all patients were receiving the same antiemetics for prophylaxis of delayed emesis. The adverse events were also significantly less frequent with the OND plus dexamethasone regimen; in particular, slight sedation was reported by 2.1% of patients treated with OND with respect to 11.8% of those receiving high-dose metoclopramide, and extrapyramidal reactions were observed only with metoclopramide. Furthermore, in contrast to a metoclopramide-containing regimen, the persistence of the antiemetic activity of OND plus dexamethasone was demonstrated in subsequent cycles (20).

The side effects of OND are generally mild and infrequent. No extrapyramidal reactions have been published, except in two case reports, and in one of these the relationship between OND and the extrapyramidal reaction is questionable (21). The lack of CNS effects with OND is especially important for pediatric patients and for young adults, those most susceptible to experience extrapyramidal reactions. The most frequent side effects are headache (15–20% of patients) and constipation (5–10% of patients), easily controlled with adequate therapy. The transitory increase in transaminase levels shown in pilot studies was probably secondary to the CDDP chemotherapy itself.

In conclusion, OND plus dexamethasone seems to be the most efficacious and least toxic antiemetic therapy for prevention of CDDP-induced acute emesis (Table 4). The same is probably true for other highly emetogenic regimens, such as those utilizing high-dose cyclophosphamide (>750 mg), dacarbazine, and megadoses of alkylating agents in conditioning regimens for bone marrow transplantation, but a valid, specific demonstration in controlled studies is still lacking. Similar results have been obtained in the prevention of emesis induced by repeated low-doses of CDDP (20–40 mg/m^2 for 4–5 days). In this case, because the rate of extrapyramidal reactions is very high in patients submitted to repeated high doses of metoclopramide (over 20% of patients interrupted the antiemetic treatment), the OND plus dexamethasone combination should be considered the treatment of choice (22).

B. Granisetron

This drug is marketed in several countries in only an intravenous formulation, but an oral preparation is under development. It is characterized by a longer half-life (about 9–11 h) than ondansetron.

Table 4 Combination Antiemetic Regimens for High-Dose Cisplatin

Regimen with established antiemetics
Metoclopramide, 3 mg/kg IV every 2 h for two doses, plus
Dexamethasone, 20 mg IV, one dose, plus
Lorazepam, 1–2 mg IV × 1, or diphenhydramine, 50 mg IV
Regimen with 5-HT$_3$ receptor antagonists
Ondansetron (see Table 3 for dose and schedule) or other 5-HT$_3$ receptor antagonists, plus
Dexamethasone, 20 mg IV × 1

Source: Data from References 4, 10, 19, and 20.

In some pilot studies on patients submitted to high-dose CDDP chemotherapy, granisetron was shown to give complete protection from vomiting in 16–50% of patients. Its optimal dose seems to be 40 μg/kg in a single administration. In two studies relative to patients treated with high-dose CDDP, granisetron was equally efficacious and better tolerated than the metoclopramide plus dexamethasone (±diphenhydramine) combination (23,24). The evaluation of the additional efficacy of the combination of granisetron with steroids in moderately and highly emetogenic chemotherapy including CDDP is quite preliminary and needs further confirmation (25). The safety profile of granisetron appears very similar to that of OND.

C. Tropisetron

This drug also has a long half-life (8–15 h). In patients undergoing high single-dose CDDP, tropisetron has been evaluated in some pilot studies in doses varying from 5 to 48 mg/m^2 with complete protection from vomiting in 30–66% of patients. On the basis of phase I–II studies, a dose of 5 mg IV immediately before CDDP administration was chosen for phase III studies. Only one multicenter randomized study has so far been published regarding the prevention of acute emesis caused by CDDP (26). In 260 patients, tropisetron (5 mg IV) was compared to a combination of high-dose metoclopramide (3 mg/kg × 2 IV) plus dexamethasone (20 mg IV) with or without lorazepam (1 mg × 2 IV). The study showed the same percentage of complete protection from vomiting (63%) in the two treatments. Further studies are needed to define better the role of this drug and the potential usefulness of the addition of steroids.

D. Other 5-HT_3 Antagonists

The other 5-HT_3 antagonists reported in Table 3 are still in a preliminary stage of development, and their role must be better studied.

VI. THERAPY OF NAUSEA AND VOMITING IN MODERATELY EMETOGENIC CHEMOTHERAPY

Relatively few studies have been conducted on patients undergoing chemotherapy with drugs other than CDDP. Most of them are small, noncomparative trials in patients treated with various antiblastic drugs, usually lumped together under the heading of "moderately emetogenic drugs," although they may have very different emetic potentials. Often these studies claim the efficacy of one or the other antiemetic drug, without providing clear evidence of this in a specific antineoplastic regimen. Therefore, to provide sound information on this topic, we consider only the studies carried out in patients treated selectively with a single chemotherapic agent or a well-defined and widely used antineoplastic regimen.

Chemotherapeutic regimens containing doxorubicin, alone or in combination with cyclophosphamide and vincristine or with 5-fluorouracil and cyclophosphamide, are reported to produce acute vomiting in about 60% of patients. Although contrasting data have been published regarding the efficacy of metoclopramide in preventing emesis caused by doxorubicin, corticosteroids seem to be a better treatment. Furthermore, compared with metoclopramide, methylprednisolone (125 mg IV × 3 every 6 h) seems to have lower toxicity (27).

The IV combination of cyclophosphamide-methotrexate-5-fluorouracil (CMF), frequently used to treat breast cancer, induces acute emesis in 70–90% of patients. Again, contrasting results have been reported on the efficacy of metoclopramide. This compound at standard oral or high IV doses as administered in CDDP-treated patients has been shown to be no more efficacious than placebo, but with a 20 mg IV or intramuscular (IM) dose every 3 or 6 h contrasting results have been reported.

Again, methylprednisolone and dexamethasone seem to provide better control of emesis because they induce complete protection from vomiting in about 50–80% of patients according to different studies (28) and must be considered the optimal treatment for the prevention of vomiting caused by moderately emetogenic drugs.

The introduction of 5-HT_3 receptor antagonists also prompted research in this setting. In several pilot studies OND was shown to have good efficacy even in patients refractory to the usual antiemetic drugs, and recently two studies comparing different oral dosages of OND were published (29,30). From these studies it seems that an 8 mg twice per day oral dose of OND could be a good and convenient choice in the prevention of emesis in outpatients submitted to these chemotherapy regimens.

A recently published prospective, randomized double-blind study showed a significant advantage of oral OND (8 mg three times per day × 15 days) over placebo in CMF-treated patients (with cyclophosphamide given orally for 14 days), but the authors were cautious about considering this a first-line treatment (31).

Only one comparative double-blind trial has been published comparing OND with dexamethasone (32). In 112 patients, receiving IV anthracycline and/or cyclophosphamide and/or etoposide, dexamethasone (8 mg IV before chemotherapy and 4 mg orally four times per day on days 1 and 2, reduced to 2 mg four times per day on days 3 and 4 to 1 mg four times per day on day 5) was shown to have an efficacy similar to that of OND (4 mg IV and 4 mg orally every 6 h on days 1–5) in controlling acute and delayed emesis. Both antiemetic regimens were well tolerated.

Much less clinical experience has been accumulated with other 5-HT3 antagonists. Among these, granisetron is the most widely studied; it has been evaluated in some pilot studies and in three large controlled studies.

The first trial (33) was a double-blind study comparing two different doses of the drug (40 and 160 μg/kg). The complete protection from vomiting achieved was similar with the two dosages (76 and 81%, respectively). The other two comparative studies, one single blind (34) and the other double blind (35), showed that granisetron (40 or 80 μg/kg IV) had greater antiemetic activity than the combination of chlorpromazine or prochlorperazine plus dexamethasone (administered in a single dose before chemotherapy). Complete protection from vomiting was achieved in 70, 49, and 34% of patients, respectively, and tolerability was also better in granisetron-treated patients. At present, no studies have been published comparing granisetron with steroids used at repeated doses every 4–6 h. In conclusion, for the prevention of emesis induced by moderately emetogenic drugs, steroids are the treatment of choice. Orally administered 5-HT_3 antagonists, although as efficacious as dexamethasone, because of their higher acquisition cost, are indicated only in those patients refractory to corticosteroids or in those who cannot use them. More studies, some of which are in progress, are therefore necessary to define the role of 5-HT_3 antagonists in comparison to steroids and possibly to the combination of both.

VII. DELAYED EMESIS

Delayed emesis is defined as nausea or vomiting beginning 24 h or more after administration of chemotherapy. The pathophysiology of delayed emesis remains unclear. Its incidence varies from 20 to 93% in different studies. The symptoms are present with their maximal intensity on days 2 and 3 after chemotherapy and generally persist for 6–7 days and, more rarely, even until the next cycle of chemotherapy. Although delayed emesis is not generally as severe as acute emesis, it still represents a significant problem and may contribute to poor emetic control and possibly to the development of anticipatory nausea and vomiting in subsequent cycles of chemotherapy. Patients who had no emesis during the initial 24 h after CDDP, those who received lower doses of CDDP, and male patients are less likely to experience delayed emesis.

Despite its clinical relevance the phenomenon of delayed emesis has received much less attention than that of acute emesis. Only four randomized placebo-controlled studies with standard antiemetics have been published (36–39). In these, the activity of metoclopramide, dexamethasone, or adrenocorticotropic hormone used alone, although often superior to placebo in controlling delayed nausea or vomiting, is minimal and of limited clinical significance.

One study showed that the antiemetic activity of oral metoclopramide (0.5 mg/kg four times per day for 4 days) plus oral dexamethasone (8 mg twice per day on days 2 and 3 and 4 mg twice per day on days 4 and 5) was significantly superior to dexamethasone alone or to placebo. This combination was the most efficacious regimen for the prevention of delayed emesis (37), but despite this, over 40% of patients still suffer from it.

Only a limited amount of experience exists at present with 5-HT3 receptor antagonists. In a small phase II study of patients treated with more than 100 mg/mq of CDDP, treatment of delayed emesis with oral OND (16 mg orally three times per day × 4 days) achieved only 15% complete protection (40).

Only one small placebo-controlled study has been published on the use of the new 5-HT_3 antagonists in the prevention of delayed emesis (41). In this study, 48 patients receiving CDDP at doses ≥ 100 mg/m^2 were randomized to oral OND (16 mg three times per day, or placebo administered from day 2 to 5 after CDDP. OND showed superior efficacy in controlling delayed vomiting (statistically significant only on day 4) but not delayed nausea.

The poor control of delayed vomiting with OND may be because it is mediated by mechanisms not involving 5-HT_3 receptors. Data are not yet available on the efficacy and toxicity of a combination of oral OND (or other 5-HT_3 antagonists) with dexamethasone in the prevention of delayed emesis, nor are they available for the efficacy of granisetron or tropisetron. Until positive data are available, the routine use of oral 5-HT_3 receptor antagonists for delayed emesis outside clinical trials cannot be recommended (42). The combination of metoclopramide and steroids can be considered the best available treatment and the standard for clinical practice.

VIII. NAUSEA AND VOMITING CAUSED BY RADIOTHERAPY

In general, nausea and vomiting in radiotherapy practice is reported to be less severe than that seen with more aggressive chemotherapy treatments. This is one of the reasons the antiemetic treatment of such side effects of radiotherapy is today less studied than those caused by chemotherapy. Other reasons are the different radiotherapy techniques of treatment used in different centers, the empirical, personalized strategy, subject to change, for antiemetic treatment, and the paucity of well-planned controlled studies.

Typically, when nausea and vomiting occur, they first appear in the second hour after irradiation. The threshold for vomiting following irradiation of a large volume is approximately 1 Gy. The incidence of emesis is highest in the several hours following irradiation, and it increases with the dose of radiation.

The neurophysiopathological mechanism of radiation-induced nausea and vomiting can be compared to that already described for chemotherapy. In fact, it is today accepted that radiation induces the liberation of neurotransmitters, namely serotonin, especially if it is delivered to the gastrointestinal area, with the subsequent stimulation of 5-HT_3 receptors and their influence on the vomiting center.

There are variables that influence the incidence and severity of radiation-induced nausea and vomiting that should be considered. It is well known that the upper abdomen is the most sensitive site. Half-body radiation is a technique employed in some centers for the palliation of pain and the reduction of disseminated metastases. This technique requires high-dose (8 Gy) single-fraction irradiation of either the upper or lower half-body. Irradiation of the upper half-body results in about double the incidence of emesis.

In general terms, the greater the volume of tissue being irradiated the greater is the risk of sickness developing. The most obvious example is TBI for patients with leukemias and lymphomas. The dose and dose rate of radiation chosen for these therapies are usually the maximum that can be tolerated without evoking serious gastrointestinal symptoms, without incurring significant medium- or long-term morbidity and mortality from radiation-induced pneumonitis or morbidity from radiation enteritis. Vomiting in TBI patients has been particularly troublesome, because of both the coincident use of potent emetogenic chemotherapeutic agents and the high radiation dose (8–11 Gy). Among other factors, age seems important; in fact, children seem less susceptible to radiation-induced emesis than adults. Anxiety and apprehension also play a role; when present, the liklihood of sickness in radiotherapy patients may increase.

In the past, treatment of nausea and vomiting caused by radiotherapy was based mainly on the use of metoclopramide, phenothiazines, and domperidone. Unfortunately, as already stated, there are only a few controlled studies on the activity and safety of these drugs in such a setting. The introduction of 5-HT_3 receptor antagonists prompted a new wave of research in this area with an improvement in the methodological aspect of the clinical trials. Pilot studies with OND in radiotherapy-treated patients showed complete control of vomiting in about 60% of patients using an 8 mg three times per day schedule of treatment. The same dose of OND (for 5 days) was then used in a randomized trial in comparison with metoclopramide (10 mg three times per day) in patients who were to receive single doses of 8–10 Gy to the upper abdomen. In 105 evaluable patients complete control from vomiting was obtained in 92% of patients treated with OND and in 46% of those treated with metoclopramide. A similar advantage for OND was also evident for nausea even on subsequent treatment days. This study clearly shows that OND is superior to metoclopramide, although the dose of the latter could be considered too low in view of the experience accumulated with highly emetogenic chemotherapy (43).

Another controlled study examined patients undergoing fractionated irradiation to the upper abdomen who were to receive five or more daily treatments with fractions of 1.8 Gy or more. They were randomized to receive OND (8 mg three times per day) or prochlorperazine (10 mg three times per day). The recently published results showed a significant benefit for OND, with 58% complete protection from vomiting compared with 35% with prochlorperazine. In addition, OND provided significantly more emesis-free days (71 versus 56%) (44).

Granisetron has also been tested in radiotherapy-induced nausea and vomiting. In a small nonrandomized study, granisetron at two dose levels of 20 and 40 μg/kg was administered as an intravenous infusion 1 h before a radiotherapy regimen consisting of a single exposure of the lower half-body to a midline dose of 8 Gy. Complete response was observed in 15 of the 22 patients treated (45).

Nausea and vomiting are almost universal after TBI and equally prevalent whether treatment is given as a single dose or in a fractionated course with doses as low as 1.2 Gy daily, despite the use of conventional antiemetics, such as metoclopramide. Two nonrandomized studies have made initial assessments of 5-HT_3 antagonists in this situation (46, 47).

A very recent study compared granisetron (3 mg/day IV) versus the combination of metoclopramide (20 mg IV) plus dexamethasone (6 mg/m^2/day IV) and lorazepam (2 mg/day IV) before total-body irradiation (7.5 Gy in a single exposure) in 30 patients (48). It showed that after 24 h 53.3% of patients treated with granisetron had complete response (no vomiting and no moderate or severe nausea) compared with 13.3% in the other group. Time to first vomiting over the 7 day periods and the number of rescue doses of any antiemetic therapy were in favor of the granisetron group, but again, the low-dose metoclopramide-containing regimen cannot be considered the standard treatment.

The safety profile of the 5-HT_3 receptor antagonists in radiotherapy-treated patients is very similar to that already described for chemotherapy regimens. These drugs seem to have very good activity against emesis induced by radiotherapy, but further studies are necessary to define their value in comparison to the optimal antiemetic treatment using established antiemetics. Furthermore, it will be interesting to evaluate the possible additive role of steroids. Some trials are ongoing regarding this point, but it is too early to draw any definitive conclusion.

IX. NAUSEA AND VOMITING FROM OTHER CAUSES

Among the causes of nausea and vomiting other than chemo- and radiotherapy, two conditions are becoming increasingly important in oncology, namely narcotic analgesic and postoperative induced nausea and vomiting.

Nausea and vomiting are among the most common side effects of narcotic analgesics. Despite this, there is little evidence of studies aimed at quantifying the incidence of the phenomenon or comparing different antiemetic treatments. This can be explained by two considerations; first, the scarce interest in oncology for supportive therapy until the 1980s, and second, the difficulties in planning and performing controlled studies to evaluate the impact of therapy for such a side effect. In fact, it was only in 1991 that the first epidemiological study was conducted (49). A total of 260 patients treated with buprenorphine, codeine, morphine, and oxycodone were evaluated for 3 consecutive days. Of these, 32 patients (12%) presented with moderate to severe nausea and 69 (26%) with vomiting. Treatment with metoclopramide was unsuccessful in 56 patients, 22% of the total, who had to interrupt the analgesic treatment or go to an alternative treatment. Because of the limited number of patients, it is not possible to define the emetic potential of each analgesic drug. Studies are therefore necessary to establish the incidence of nausea and vomiting with the single drugs, timing of their appearance, duration of the symptom, appearance of tolerance with subsequent treatment, and importance of prognostic factors. These studies should be aimed at deciding whether a preventive treatment is necessary or if it is sufficient to treat nausea and vomiting once they appear (50).

At the present time, two prognostic factors for nausea and vomiting caused by narcotic analgesics have been identified: sex and in- or outpatient condition. Again, females vomit more frequently than males, as do outpatients in comparison with bedridden patients. Another important factor is the method of administration of the narcotic drug: IV morphine causes less nausea and vomiting than IM morphine, probably because a different receptor is involved in the vomiting center. The emetic effect of the opiates seems a result of an action on the chemoreceptor trigger zone because area postrema ablation prevents vomiting in animals. A peripheral action related to slow gastric emptying or to constipation induced by opiates cannot be excluded. In animals, the role of neurotransmitters, such as dopamine, histamine, endogenous opiates, and serotonin, has been documented, but it is not clear which of these mediators is the most important. Lacking this information, the use of antiemetic drugs has been based on personal experience more than on the results of controlled trials.

In Table 5 the antiemetic drugs that have been shown to be useful in preventing or treating narcotic analgesic-induced nausea and vomiting are reported. Some authors prefer to use haloperidol instead of prochlorperazine because the former induces less sedation and requires, because of its longer half-life, less frequent administration. If the sedation connected with the use of phenothiazines or butyrophenones is to be avoided, metoclopramide can be utilized, especially in the presence of gastric stasis or esophageal reflux. Recently a positive experience with the use of OND was published in a very small number of patients who were resistent to the established antiemetics. Five of the six patients obtained a marked improvement in their symptoms with OND used at the doses of 8–32 mg/day (51). This preliminary result must be confirmed by larger prospective studies.

X. FUTURE RESEARCH AND PERSPECTIVES

Control of chemotherapy and radiotherapy-induced emesis can today be obtained for a majority of patients. The responsibility of the clinician is to apply the best

Table 5 Antiemetics in Patients Treated with Narcotic Analgesics

Drug	Dose
Parenteral administration	
Haloperidol	1–2 mg SC
Chlorpromazine	25 mg IM
Prochlorperazine	10 mg IM
Metoclopramide	10 mg IM
Oral administration	
Prochlorperazine	5–10 mg every 4 h
Metoclopramide	10 mg every 4–6 h
Haloperidol	1–2 mg every 12 h
Dimenhydrinate	50–100 mg every 4 h
Ondansetron	8 mg every 12 h

available antiemetic treatment but also to pursue an always deeper understanding of the problem. This increases the probability of controlling emesis in all patients and permits a more appropriate and cost-effective approach to the specific emetic problem of each cancer patient. With this perspective, some points must be stressed.

The introduction of the 5-HT_3 antagonists meant a significant advantage because of their efficacy, safety, and ease of administration. On the basis of published literature, it appears clear that an OND-containing regimen should be the preferred choice of antiemetic for its greater efficacy in CDDP-treated patients but also for its efficacy over subsequent cycles. A consideration for any new drug is the greater acquisition cost with respect to the older drugs, and OND is no exception. Despite the higher acquisition cost, however, OND may be more cost effective than metoclopramide if one takes into consideration the dependence effect and/or its use in the group of patients at higher risk of vomiting (i.e., females and patients treated with high CDDP doses for multiple cycles) and superior side effect profile. In any case, even if OND plus dexamethasone must be considered the therapy of choice, they should be compared to the established antiemetic combination from a pharmacoeconomics point of view. Much research is being done with this very precise aim, and it is very important that it be conducted prospectively with a correct methodology based on proven assumptions.

In the continuous search for the ideal antiemetic, cost being very important, the definition of the optimal dose is therefore not irrelevant. This is particularly true for OND because of some contradictory results about the equivalence of a single low dose (8 mg) or a single high dose (32 mg), both showing a similar activity compared to the usual (0.15 mg/kg) regimen and, therefore, preferable from a practical point of view. The definition of this important problem requires further studies.

Another interesting point is the equivalence of the different 5-HT_3 receptor antagonists. Undoubtedly the most studied show similar levels of activity and the same toxicity profiles despite some structural and pharmacological differences. As a consequence, there is a trend in clinical practice toward considering them equivalent (42). If one must rely solely on the published evidence from well-conducted clinical trials, however, OND stands out as the best choice among the 5-HT_3 receptor antagonists for the reason that, among the available compounds, only OND has been studied with respect to three major issues in antiemetic therapy: (1) the efficacy potentiation by combination with corticosteroids (15–18); (2) the comparative efficacy with respect to the best standard antiemetic treatment (19); and (3) the persistence of efficacy in consecutive cycles of chemotherapy (20).

Therefore, although it may be possible that the other 5-HT_3 compounds already on the market have similar efficacy, data supporting such a possibility are still lacking. Randomized studies directly comparing the different agents are crucial for identifying the most efficacious compound, and these studies are being performed and their results are anxiously awaited.

Another area in which much remains to be done is that of delayed emesis, for which today's treatment cannot be considered satisfactory. A better understanding of the physiopathology of this problem and the recognition of the different prognostic factors that give rise to this side effect will, it is hoped, provide answers to the many questions still present.

An emerging problem facing the oncologist is the treatment of those patients who are, or become, resistant to the best available antiemetic therapy. They are very difficult to treat because of the lack of efficacious alternative treatments. This is another area that should be explored, but the difficulties in planning and executing such studies should be stressed. One possibility recently became evident with the use of propofol, an intravenous anesthesia-inducing agent associated with less post-operative nausea and vomiting than other anesthetics and, when used at subhypnotic doses, demonstrates direct antiemetic efficacy (52,53). In an open study, the addition of propofol to OND plus dexamethasone in patients who previously were not relieved of nausea and vomiting by this antiemetic regimen, 85–90% had complete protection from vomiting in the subsequent cycle of chemotherapy (54). This rather new approach should be evaluated in a double-blind study in patients exhibiting substantial emesis in previous CDDP chemotherapy courses.

The control of emesis is one of many important issues in the supportive care of patients with cancer. The considerable research efforts of the past decade in this area have resulted in improvements. The application of these findings continues to be the responsibility of all clinical oncologists and the recognition of the necessity of a continuous effort in basic and clinical research the basis for further improvements.

ANNOTATED BIBLIOGRAPHY

1. Aapro MS. 5-HT_3 receptor antagonists. An overview of their present status and future potential in cancer therapy-induced emesis. Drugs 1991; 42(4):551–568. This is a complete and up-to-date review of the 5-HT_3 receptor antagonists.
2. Andrews PLR, Sanger GJ, eds. Emesis in Anti-Cancer Therapy. Mechanisms and Treatment. London: Chapman & Hall Medical, 1993. This book provides a comprehensive review of the problems of emesis in a clinical context. Analysis of the neuropharmacology of emesis is particularly detailed, especially in relation to the 5-HT_3 receptor antagonists. It also covers practical aspects, such as measuring nausea and vomiting, as well as patient care from the specialist nurse's point of view.
3. European Journal of Cancer, Volume 29A, Supplement 1, 1993. Supportive Therapy in Cancer. Pergamon Press. This supplement, reporting the full papers presented at the Perugia International Cancer Conference III, presents a complete review of the 5-HT_3 antagonists. Particularly interesting is the full coverage of a roundtable discussion with the participation of the most experienced researchers in this field.
4. Gralla RJ. Antiemetic therapy. Adverse effects of treatment (Section 1). In: DeVita VT Jr, Hellman S, Rosenberg S, eds. Cancer Principles and Practice of Oncology, 4th ed. Philadelphia: JB Lippincott, 1993:2338–2348. The section on antiemetic therapy in this authoritative textbook provides a full picture of the treatment of chemotherapy-induced nausea and vomiting. The wide experience of the author and the results reported in the recent literature make this section a valuable updated reference for every oncologist. The section is divided into different parts that highlight specific problems.

REFERENCES

1. Tonato M, Roila F, Del Favero A. Methodology of antiemetic trials: a review. Ann Oncol 1991; 2:107–114.
2. Roila F, Tonato M, Basurto C, et al. Antiemetic activity of two different high doses of metoclopramide in cisplatin-treated cancer patients: a randomized double-blind trial of the Italian Oncology Group for Clinical Research. Cancer Treat Rep 1985; 69:1353–1357.
3. Roila F, Tonato M, Basurto C, et al. Antiemetic activity of high doses of metoclopramide combined with methylprednisolone vs metoclopramide alone in cisplatin-treated cancer patients: a randomized double-blind trial of the Italian Oncology Group for Clinical Research. J Clin Oncol 1987; 5:141–149.
4. Roila F, Tonato M, Basurto C, et al. Protection from nausea and vomiting in cisplatin-treated patients: high-dose metoclopramide combined with methylpredis-

olone vs metoclopramide combined with dexamethasone and diphenhydramine: a study of the Italian Oncology Group for Clinical Research. J Clin Oncol 1989; 7:1693–1700.
5. Kris MG, Tyson LB, Gralla RJ, et al. Extrapyramidal reactions with high-dose metoclopramide. N Engl J Med 1983; 309:433.
6. Gralla RJ, Itri LM, Pisko SE, et al. Antiemetic efficacy of high-dose metoclopramide: randomized trials with placebo and prochlorperazine in patients with chemotherapy-induced nausea and vomiting. N Engl J Med 1981; 305:905–909.
7. Allan SG, Cornbleet MA, Warrington PS, et al. Dexamethasone and high-dose metoclopramide: efficacy in controlling cisplatin induced nausea and vomiting. BMJ 1984; 289:878–879.
8. Strum SB, McDermed JE, Liponi DF. High-dose intravenous metoclopramide vs combination high-dose metoclopramide and intravenous dexamethasone in preventing cisplatin-induced nausea and emesis: a single-blind cross-over comparison of antiemetic efficacy. J Clin Oncol 1985; 3:245–251.
9. Kris MG, Gralla RJ, Clark RA, et al. Consecutive dose-finding trials adding lorazepam to the combination of metoclopramide plus dexamethasone: improved subjective effectiveness over the combination of diphenhydramine plus metoclopramide plus dexamethasone. Cancer Treat Rep 1985; 69:1257–1262.
10. Kris MJ, Gralla RJ, Clark RA, et al. Antiemetic control and prevention of side effects of anticancer therapy with lorazepam or diphenhydramine when used in combination with metoclopramide plus dexamethasone. A double-blind, randomized trial. Cancer 1987; 60:2816–2822.
11. Roila F, Tonato M, Basurto C, et al. Ondansetron. Eur J Cancer 1993; 29A(Suppl 1):S16–S21.
12. De Mulder PHM, Seynaeve C, Vermorken JB, et al. Ondansetron compared with high-dose metoclopramide in prophylaxis of acute and delayed cisplatin-induced nausea and vomiting. A multicenter, randomized, double-blind, crossover study. Ann Intern Med 1990; 113:834–840.
13. Hainsworth J, Harvey W, Pendergrass K, et al. A single-blind comparison of intravenous ondansetron, a selective serotonin antagonist, with intravenous metoclopramide in the prevention of nausea and vomiting associated with high-dose cisplatin chemotherapy. J Clin Oncol 1991; 9:721–728.
14. Marty M, Pouillart P, School S, et al. Comparison of the 5-hydroxytryptamine 3 (serotonin) antagonist ondansetron (GR 38032F) with high-dose metoclopramide in the control of cisplatin-induced emesis. N Engl J Med 1990; 322:816–821.
15. Roila F, Tonato M, Cognetti F, et al. Prevention of cisplatin-induced emesis: a double-blind multicenter randomized crossover study comparing ondansetron and ondansetron plus dexamethasone. J Clin Oncol 1991; 9:675–678.
16. Smith DB, Newlands ES, Rustin GJS, et al. Comparison of ondansetron and ondansetron plus dexamethasone as antiemetic prophylaxis during cisplatin-containing chemotherapy. Lancet 1991; 338:487–490.
17. Smyth JF, Coleman RE, Nicolson M, et al. Does dexamethasone enhance control of acute cisplatin induced emesis by ondansetron? BMJ 1991; 303:1423–1426.
18. Hesketh PJ, Harvey WH, Beck TM, et al. A randomized, double-blind comparison of intravenous ondansetron alone and in combination with intravenous dexametha-

sone in the prevention of nausea and vomiting associated with high dose cisplatin. (abstract). Am Soc Clin Oncol 1993; 12:1491.
19. Roila F, Tonato M, Ballatori E, et al. Ondansetron + dexamethasone vs metoclopramide + dexamethasone + diphenhydramine in prevention of cisplatin-induced emesis. Lancet 1992; 340:96–99.
20. Roila F, Tonato M, Favalli G, et al. Persistence of efficacy of ondansetron (OND) plus dexamethasone (DEX) vs metoclopramide (MTC) plus DEX and diphenhydramine (DIP) in acute emesis during three consecutive cycles of cisplatin (CDDP) chemotherapy (CT) (abstract). Proc Am Soc Clin Oncol 1993; 12:1490.
21. Kanarek BB, Curnow R, Palmer J, et al. Ondansetron: confusing documentation surrounding an extrapyramidal reaction. J Clin Oncol 1992; 10:506–507.
22. Weissbach L, Multi-day Cisplatin Emesis Study Group. Ondansetron. Lancet 1991; 338:753.
23. Chevallier B, Granisetron Study Group. Efficacy and safety of granisetron compared with high-dose metoclopramide plus dexamethasone in patients receiving high-dose cisplatin in a single-blind study. Eur J Cancer 1990; 26(Suppl. 1):33–36.
24. Venner P, Clinical Trials Group of the National Cancer Institute of Canada. Granisetron for high dose cisplatin (HDCP) induced emesis: a randomized double blind study (abstract). Proc Am Soc Clin Oncol 1990; 9:320.
25. Aapro M, Kirchner V, Terrey J-P, et al. Granisetron compared with granisetron plus dexamethasone. A placebo controlled double-blind randomised crossover study (abstract). Proc Am Soc Clin Oncol 1993; 12:1540.
26. Sorbe B, Frankendal B, Glimelius B, et al. A multicentre randomized study comparing the anti-emetic effects of the 5-HT3 antagonist ICS 205-930 with a metoclopramide-containing antiemetic cocktail in patients receiving cisplatin chemotherapy. Ann Oncol 1990; 1(Suppl. 1):113.
27. Basurto C, Roila F, Bracarda S, et al. A double-blind trial comparing antiemetic efficacy and toxicity of metoclopramide versus methylprednisolone versus domperidone in patients receiving doxorubicin chemotherapy alone or in combination with other antiblastic agents. Am J Clin Oncol 1988; 11:594–596.
28. Roila F, Basurto C, Minotti V, et al. Methylprednisolone versus metoclopramide for prevention of nausea and vomiting in breast cancer patients treated with intravenous cyclophosphamide, methotrexate, 5-fluorouracil: a double-blind randomized study. Oncology 1988; 45:346–349.
29. Fraschini G, Ciociola A, Esparza L, et al. Evaluation of three oral dosages of ondansetron in the prevention of nausea and emesis associated with cyclophosphamide-doxorubicin chemotherapy. J Clin Oncol 1991; 9:1268–1274.
30. Dicato M. Oral treatment with ondansetron in an outpatient setting. Eur J Cancer 1991; 27(Suppl. 1):518–519.
31. Buser KS, Joss RA, Piquet D, et al. Oral ondansetron in the prophylaxis of nausea and vomiting induced by cyclophosphamide, methotrexate and 5-fluorouracil (CMF) in women with breast cancer. Results of a prospective, randomized, double-blind placebo-controlled study. Ann Oncol 1993; 4:475–479.
32. Jones ALM, Hill AS, Soukop M, et al. Comparison of ondansetron vs dexamethasone in the prophylaxis of emesis induced by moderately emetogenic chemotherapy. Lancet 1991; 338:483–487.

33. Smith IE, Granisetron Study Group. A comparison of two dose levels of granisetron in patients receiving moderately emetogenic cytostatic chemotherapy. Eur J Cancer 1990; 26(Suppl. 1):19–23.
34. Marty M, Granisetron Study Group. A comparative study of the use of granisetron, a selective 5-HT3 antagonist, versus a standard anti-emetic regimen of chlorpromazine plus dexamethasone in the treatment of cytostatic-induced emesis. Eur J Cancer 1990; 26(Suppl. 1):28–32.
35. Warr D, Willan A, Fine S, et al. Superiority of granisetron to dexamethasone plus prochlorperazine in the prevention of chemotherapy-induced emesis. J Natl Cancer Inst 1991; 83:1169–1173.
36. Roila F, Boschetti E, Tonato M, et al. Prediction factors of delayed emesis in cisplatin treated patients and antiemetic activity and tolerability of metoclopramide or dexamethasone. A randomized single-blind study. Am J Clin Oncol 1991; 14:238–242.
37. Kris MG, Gralla RJ, Tyson LB, et al. Controlling delayed vomiting: double-blind, randomized trial comparing placebo, dexamethasone alone, and metoclopramide plus dexamethasone in patients receiving cisplatin. J Clin Oncol 1989; 7:108–114.
38. Passalacqua R, Cocconi G, Bella M, et al. Double-blind, randomized trial for the control of delayed emesis in patients receiving cisplatin: comparison of placebo vs adrenocorticotropic hormone (ACTH). Ann Oncol 1992; 3:481–485.
39. Shinkai T, Saijo N, Euguchi K, et al. Control of cisplatin-induced delayed emesis with metoclopramide and dexamethasone: a randomized controlled trial. Jpn Clin Oncol 1989; 19:40–44.
40. Kris MG, Tyson LB, Clark RA, et al. Oral ondansetron for the control of delayed emesis after cisplatin. Cancer 1992; 70:1012–1016.
41. Gandara DR. Progress in the control of acute and delayed emesis induced by cisplatin. Eur J Cancer 1991; 27(Suppl. 1):9–11.
42. Kaye SB. Antiemetic therapy—where do we go from here? (editorial). Ann Oncol 1993; 4:443–445.
43. Collis CH, Priestman TJ, Priestman S, et al. The final assessment of a randomized double-blind comparative study of ondansetron vs metoclopramide in the prevention of nausea and vomiting following high dose upper abdominal irradiation. Clin Oncol 1991; 3:241–242.
44. Priestman TJ, Roberts JT, Upadhyaya BK. Randomised, double-blind trial of ondansetron (OND) and prochlorperazine (PCP) in the prevention of fractionated radiotherapy (RT) induced emesis. Proc Am Soc Clin Oncol 1992; 11 (abstract 1370).
45. Logue JP, Magee B, Hunter RD, et al. The antiemetic effect of granisetron in lower hemibody radiotherapy. Clin Oncol 1991; 3:247–249.
46. Hewitt M, Cornish J, Pamphilon D, Oakhill A. Effective emetic control during conditioning of children for bone marrow transplantation using ondansetron, a 5-HT3 antagonist. Bone Marrow Transplant 1991; 7:431–433.
47. Hunter AE, Prentice HG, Pothecary K et al. Granisetron, a selective 5-HT3 receptor antagonist, for the prevention of radiation induced emesis during total body irradiation. Bone Marrow Transplant 1991; 7:439–441.
48. Prentice HG. Efficacy and safety of granisetron in the treatment of emesis induced

by total body irradiation: a comparison with standard antiemetic therapy (abstract). Proc Am Soc Clin Oncol 1993; 12:1574.

49. Campora E, Merlini L, Pace M, et al. The incidence of narcotic-induced emesis. J Pain Symptom Manage 1991; 6:428–430.
50. Hanks GW. Antiemetics for terminal cancer patients. Lancet 1982; 1:1410.
51. Gottlieb A, Luzzani M. Il problema della nausea e del vomito da oppiacei nel paziente neoplastico avanzato: nuovo approccio farmacologico con gli antagonisti dei recettori 5-HT3. Studio preliminare. In: International Congress on Nuove Acquisizioni sul Ruolo dei 5-HT3 Antagonisti, Verona, June 18, 1991, pp. 127–131.
52. McCollum JS, Milligan KR, Dundee JW. The antiemetic action of propofol. Anaesthesia 1988; 43:239–240.
53. Borgeat A, Wilder-Smith OHG, Saiah S, Rifat K. Subhypnotic doses of propofol possess direct antiemetic properties. Anesth Analg 1992; 74:539–541.
54. Borgeat A, Wilder-Smith OHG, Wilder-Smith CH, et al. Adjuvant propofol for refractory cisplatin-associated nausea and vomiting. Lancet 1992; 340:679–680.

5

Oral Care for the Cancer Patient

C. Daniel Overholser, Jr.
School of Dentistry and School of Medicine, University of Maryland at Baltimore, Baltimore, Maryland

I. INTRODUCTION

The first objective in the treatment of a patient with cancer is the eradication of the disease. Over the past two decades tremendous strides have been made in the diagnosis and treatment of these patients. However, intensive radiation and/or chemotherapy protocols disrupt the integrity and function of the tissues of the oral cavity. Such complications as mucosal ulceration, xerostomia, bleeding, and infections can cause significant morbidity and may compromise the systemic treatment of the patient. Fortunately, with proper oral evaluation before systemic treatment, many of the complications can be minimized or prevented.

II. RADIATION THERAPY

When upper mantle radiation therapy is indicated for the treatment of the cancer patient, consideration must be given to the numerous potential side effects of this form of cancer therapy. Most of these adverse sequelae can be prevented or at least diminished through a preoperative dental consultation (1). Dental evaluation should occur during the admission work-up of the patient to develop the most optimum treatment plan for that patient. The amount and portals of radiation, the urgency of the radiation therapy, prognosis of therapy, and oral health of the patient must all be considered when deciding on the most appropriate dental treatment plan for the patient. The oral health status that will be evaluated includes the severity of dental caries and periodontal disease, the estimated compliance of the patient in performing thorough oral hygiene procedures, and the need and extent of oral surgical procedures. Prevention of osteoradionecrosis is obviously of utmost importance. Secondarily, the reduction and/or elimination of other side effects, such as mucositis, radiation caries, and trismus, is attempted. The prevention of the side effects of radiation therapy is summarized in Table 1.

A. Mucositis

Mucositis, inflammation of the mucous membranes, is a very common reaction to radiation therapy. It is first seen 1–2 weeks after initiation of therapy and presents as an erythematous patch. The mucosa is thinned as a result of the killing of the rapidly dividing mucosal cells. Between 1000 and 3000 cGy, areas begin to desquamate and eventually develop into frank ulcerations. These ulcerations are extremely painful and often force interruption of the radiation therapy.

Normal oral mucosa acts as a barrier against chemicals that are ingested and, more importantly, against the ever present oral microorganisms. The disruption of the mucosal barrier thus leads to secondary infection, increased pain, delayed healing, and decreased nutritional intake.

Little can be done to prevent radiation mucositis. Occasionally stents can be constructed to prevent the irradiation of uninvolved tissues. Fractionation of the therapy into smaller doses over a longer period of time often reduces the severity. Recently, Kamillosan Liquidem (Asta Pharma, AG, Frankfurt, Germany) was reported to have diminished the severity of mucositis (2). Kamillosan Liquidem

Table 1 Prevention Protocol for Patients Receiving Radiation Therapy

Before radiation therapy	
Dental consultation: examination radiographs, treatment plan	3 weeks before
Oral surgery	3 weeks before
Dental care (restorative, endodontics, oral hygiene instructions, periodontics, fluoride treatment, diet counseling	Before radiation therapy
During radiation therapy	
Oral hygiene reinforcement	Weekly
Fluoride therapy	Daily
Dietary management	Weekly
After radiation therapy	
Oral evaluation	Monthly
Fluoride therapy	Daily for 6 months

is a solution prepared from the chamomile plant and contains chamazulene, levomenol, polyins, and flavonids. The study was uncontrolled and the drug therefore needs further evaluation. Teeth with sharp edges, fractures, restorations, and ill-fitting prostheses can damage the soft tissues and lead to further interruption of mucosal barriers. Correction of these problems before radiation therapy can diminish these complications.

Treatment of mucositis is symptomatic (3). Topical application of anesthetics, such as dyclonine hydrochloride or viscous 2% Xylocaine, helps to reduce the severity of the pain. A mouth rinse of Kaopectate and diphenhydramine often provides relief to many patients (4). If the patient is unable to eat a normal diet, food can be processed through a blender and diet supplements can be used. Occasionally a nasogastric tube must be placed to assist in proper nutrition. The patient should attempt to perform normal oral hygiene procedures to help prevent secondary infection. A mixture of salt and baking soda can be used to cleanse the hard and soft tissues of the mouth gently if normal oral hygiene becomes too difficult. When secondary infections occur, culture and sensitivity should be performed to determine the appropriate antibiotic to be used. An effective agent to treat superficial candidal infections is nystatin pastilles, 200,000 units four times a day. The tablet is held in the mouth until it dissolves, which allows sufficient contact time for the drug to be effective. Clotrimazole is also effective in managing these infections. Other secondary infections can be managed with the indicated systemic antibiotic.

B. Salivary Changes

Radiation to the salivary glands produces atrophy of the acini, fibrosis, and ultimately a decrease in the production of saliva. This decreased secretion is first seen 1–2 weeks after initiation of the radiotherapy. If all the major salivary glands are in the field, the decrease in saliva can be quite dramatic. Additionally, the saliva produced is increased in viscosity, which contributes to food retention and increased plaque formation. This increase in viscosity is likely caused by the more deleterious effects of the radiation on the serous portion of the salivary glands. Since saliva is necessary for bolus formation and deglutition, these xerostomic patients have difficulty in managing a normal diet. Normal saliva also has bacteriostatic properties that are compromised in these patients, which may help to account for the increase in plaque formation and bacterial colonization. Unless aggressive measures are taken, rampant dental caries results. Radiation-induced xerostomia is often irreversible, but partial return of salivary flow is seen, especially in younger patients (5).

Preventing salivary gland dysfunction is primarily dependent on shielding the major glands from the field of radiation. On occasion shields can be constructed to assist in this. Recent evidence indicates that the use of pilocarpine during radiation therapy may reduce the severity of the resulting dysfunction (6,7). The drug was previously cited as useful in the partial restoration of function of the glands. Others recommend the use of sugar-free chewing gum as a stimulant for saliva. Finally, a number of agents appear useful to ameliorate the symptoms. These include saliva substitutes (Xerolube or Oralube), proper hydration, and ice chips.

C. Radiation Caries

A rampant form of dental caries (dental decay) that sometimes follows radiation therapy is called radiation caries. It usually develops in the cervical region of the teeth adjacent to the gingiva. It often affects many teeth and proceeds to envelop the teeth very quickly. Originally thought to be a direct result of the radiation, it is now believed to be secondary to the damage done to the salivary glands. Radiation caries is initiated by dental plaque, but its rapid progress is caused by changes in saliva. In addition to the diminution in the amount of saliva, both the salivary pH and buffering capacity are diminished, which decreases the anticaries activity of saliva. The oral flora also changes with xerostomia, which may also lead to the increase in caries activity.

The prevention of radiation caries can be accomplished by improved oral hygiene, chlorhexidine rinses, daily applications of topical fluorides, and frequent dental recall visits (8). Part of the preradiation evaluation is an estimate of the patient's desire and ability to comply with the need for improved oral hygiene. In those patients who are not expected to be compliant, the extraction of many or all the remaining teeth is recommended to avoid extracting them after radiation therapy, thus decreasing the risk for the development of osteoradionecrosis. In patients who retain their dentition, custom-made mouth trays should be constructed to be utilized by the patient in applying the topical fluoride. A pH-neutral gel, such as Thera Flour N, can be used for 5 minutes each day, usually at bedtime. The patient should be advised not to eat or drink for 30 minutes after the application. This should be continued indefinitely. Dental evaluations should occur weekly during therapy and at least every 3 months upon completion of therapy. These recalls not only help to detect disease earlier but also serve to reinforce the importance of oral hygiene maintenance to the patient.

Treatment of radiation caries can be very problematical. In the early stages it can be treated by routine restorative therapy and increased use of topical fluorides. Later stages often result in irreversible pulpal pathology. Endodontic therapy is the treatment of choice because the extraction of such teeth should be avoided if at all possible to prevent osteoradionecrosis. When extractions must be performed, they must be done as atraumatically as possible.

D. Osteoradionecrosis

Osteoradionecrosis is the most severe complication of radiation therapy in the head and neck region. Radiation, trauma, and infection are the three major factors involved in this pathological process (9). Bone that has received heavy doses of radiation becomes hypovascular, hypocellular, and hypoxic. This results in permanent cellular and vascular damage. Trauma-induced spontaneous tissue breakdown occurs, which leads to a nonhealing wound. Teeth, gingiva, and damaged mucosa all can act as portals of entry for infectious agents. The resultant radionecrosis, if untreated, ultimately involves all dysplastic bone. The spread of this process is usually accompanied by intense pain, production of bony sequestra, purulence, and a marked fetor oris. In one series, 5% of the patients died from this complication with no evidence of their original neoplastic disease (10). The incidence of this lesion ranges from 4 to 35%, and the risk increases with increasing doses of radiation. Utilization of megavoltage instead of orthovoltage therapy has also decreased the risk of radionecrosis. With the advances in radiotherapy and proper dental management, the incidence should bc in thc 5–10% rangc.

1. Preradiation

The prevention of osteoradionecrosis begins during the admission process by obtaining a dental consultation. If the maxillary or mandibular arches will be exposed to significant amounts of radiation, consideration is given to several preventive measures. First, all compromised teeth should be extracted 21 days before radiation therapy begins to allow maximal healing. Alveolectomies and primary closure should be utilized to increase healing and decrease sharp bony spicules that later may damage the overlying soft tissues. Second, the remaining dentition should be treated to prevent the need for later extractions in areas to be irradiated. Third, the importance of preventive oral hygiene must be emphasized to the patient. Fourth, shielding of nontumor areas should be accomplished when possible. At one time it was recommended that all teeth in the path of the radiation be extracted before radiation therapy. However, a number of factors are taken into consideration when planning whether to retain or remove such teeth. Severe periodontal disease, irreversible pulpal pathology, and/or a high caries index are possible indications for the extraction of the involved teeth. Fewer extractions may be performed in patients who are thought to be motivated to maintain a high level of oral hygiene postoperatively. Because osteoradionecrosis occurs more often in the mandible, extraction of mandibular teeth is more frequently required. When irradiation of the major salivary glands cannot be avoided, indications for the removal of teeth increase. Decreased dosage of radiation and poor prognosis for tumor control are factors that decrease the necessity for dental extractions.

After the dental extractions, but before radiation therapy, it is most important that the remaining teeth and periodontium be brought to a maximal state of health. Routine dental care should be provided to prevent acute periodontal and pulpal exacerbation in the postradiation phase. Emphasis must be placed on the maintenance of a high level of oral hygiene, as well as daily applications of topical fluoride.

A number of prosthodontic stents can be constructed. Indications for stents include shielding structures from the radiation, fixation of movable structures (e.g., tongue), or assisting in the positioning of an external beam source. If at all possible, dental extractions should not be performed during radiation therapy. It has been shown that the trauma from the extraction and radiation is additive and therefore produces the highest risk for the development of osteoradionecrosis (9). When radiation therapy has begun, it is recommended that palliative measures be utilized until the mucositis or dermatitis signs and symptoms have subsided.

2. After Irradiation

The prevention of osteoradionecrosis after radiation therapy is accomplished by decreasing trauma to the bone. Therefore, both mechanical trauma (surgery) and microbiological trauma (periodontal disease, pulpal pathology and surgery) must be minimized. Maintenance of the optimal level of oral health established in the preradiation phase is the most effective way of preventing the development of osteoradionecrosis. During and immediately following radiation therapy, the patient should be evaluated weekly by the dental team. This allows detection of developing pathology and emphasis on the importance of good oral hygiene. Following this, the patient may be placed on a 2–3 month recall interval. Topical fluorides and a reemphasis of the importance of proper oral hygiene are used to reduce the incidence of periodontal disease and dental caries. Reducing the risk of caries also decreases the likelihood of subsequent pulpal pathology.

If the patient is edentulous, the prostheses must be evaluated routinely to assure that they fit properly and thus decrease the chance for soft tissue ulceration and secondary infectious involvement of underlying irradiated bone.

When possible, the use of endodontic therapy in teeth with irreversible pulpal pathology is preferred over dental extractions. When dental extractions or other surgery must be performed on the postradiation patient, the development of osteoradionecrosis is a distinct possibility. Hyberbaric oxygen treatment should be used both before and following surgical treatment. Hyperbaric oxygen has been shown to be more effective than prophylactic antibiotics in preventing osteoradionecrosis (11).

3. Therapy

In the past, the treatment of osteoradionecrosis was conservative. Topical application of zinc peroxide, antibiotics, and gentle wound irrigation were utilized. Systemic antibiotic therapy was administered when gross infection was found. Today, hyperbaric oxygen therapy has become a mainstay of treatment (12–14). Although loose, necrotic bone spicules should be judiciously removed, surgical interventions, such as partial or complete mandibulectomy, are indicated when conservative measures fail to control infections. It has been recommended by some that hyperbaric oxygen be combined with aggressive surgical techniques to reduce morbidity in severe cases of osteoradionecrosis (15).

4. Altered Nutrition

Several radiation-induced problems may compromise the nutritional status of these patients. If the muscles of mastication, especially the masseters, lie in the path of radiation, trismus may result. This form of trismus is thought to result from muscle fibrosis, producing a severely limited mandibular function. The diminished opening interferes with the patient's ability to masticate food and perform oral hygiene procedures. It is believed that trismus can be prevented by the use of a set of 20 maximal opening exercises three times daily during and following radiation therapy. These exercises are also used to treat postirradiation trismus but appear to be less successful when begun after therapy.

Dysgeusia is another side effect of therapy that may affect the nutritional status of the patient. The severity of these abnormal taste sensations ranges from loss of taste to altered perception of distinct flavors. Most patients are affected to some degree, and although apparently not preventable, taste sensations are reported to return gradually to near normal levels in the posttherapy period. Dysgeusia appears to contribute to the decrease in appetite that many patients experience.

III. CHEMOTHERAPY

Chemotherapy for neoplasia frequently results in oral complications. These may develop in more than 30% of patients being treated for malignancies other than of the head and neck (16). Infections and mucositis are the most common serious complications seen in patients receiving chemotherapy. By utilizing proper management, major hemorrhagic episodes are seldom encountered. Also occurring frequently are pain, altered nutrition, and xerostomia, which significantly affect the quality of life of the patient. With proper precautions, routine dental treatment, including periodontal therapy and the extraction of teeth, can be performed immediately preceding chemotherapy for leukemia with minimal risk of significant infectious or hemorrhagic complications. Neutropenic patients with counts less than 2000/mm^3 should receive prophylactic antibiotics before procedures that produce bacteremia. Likewise, patients with platelet counts less than 50,000/mm^3 should receive platelet transfusions before surgical procedures.

A major responsibility in oncology is the prevention and treatment of infectious complications. The prevention of these complications is summarized in Table 2. Infection is a leading cause of morbidity and mortality in patients with cancer. The patient's malignant disease and/or its treatment alter the host defenses and diminish the patient's ability to inhibit infectious agents. Two normally chronic oral infections, periodontal disease and pulpal pathosis, may

Table 2 Prevention Protocol for Patients Receiving Myelosuppressive Chemotherapy

Before chemotherapy	
Dental consultation: examination, radiographs, treatment plan	3–7 days before
Oral surgery	3 days before
Dental care: oral hygiene instruction, periodontics, endodontics, restorative	Before myelosuppression
During myelosuppression	
Oral hygiene	Daily
Peridex if indicated	Daily
After chemotherapy: routine care may be provided	

become acute during periods of granulocytopenia, leading to systemic sequelae. Viral and fungal infections are often seen in these patients. Their clinical presentation may be somewhat similar and resemble mucositis. A high index of suspicion and proper culturing techniques are obviously important in the diagnosis and management of these entities.

A. Mucositis and Ulceration

Mucositis is a frequent oral complication of cancer chemotherapy. The oral mucosa is susceptible to the toxic effects of these agents because of its high mitotic index. Certain chemotherapeutic agents, such as 5-fluorouracil, methotrexate, and doxorubicin, are more commonly associated with the development of oral mucositis. It is postulated that the basal cell activity of the mucosa is impaired, reducing the ability of the epithelium to regenerate. The mucosa is also probably less resistant to the trauma these tissues receive. The mucosal integrity is broken and then is secondarily infected by the normal oral flora. The resultant ulcerations can also act as a portal of entry for pathogenic organisms into the patient's bloodstream and may lead to systemic infections. Additionally, these oral ulcerations can lead to severe pain. This pain can lead to a decrease in nutritional intake and a reduction in chemotherapy dose. Obviously, this could alter the patient's prognosis. These lesions appear as oral ulcerations approximately 7–10 days after the initiation of chemotherapy and may be limited in range or involve upward of 50% of the mucosa of the oral cavity. The severity and extent of oral mucositis vary with the patient, the drugs used, and the severity of myelosuppression that is induced.

1. Prevention

It has been suggested that improved oral hygiene results in a decreased incidence of oral mucositis. However, conclusive evidence of this is not available at the present time. It seems reasonable that improved oral hygiene would at least result in the diminished severity of the secondary infections associated with these toxic reactions. As discussed later, reactivation of herpes simplex often cannot be clinically distinguished from mucositis. Prophylactic acyclovir effectively prevents much of the incidence of this form of mucositis today. A number of agents have been utilized to reduce the incidence, severity, and/or duration of chemotherapy-induced mucositis. Benzydamine hydrochloride, β-carotene, cryotherapy, oral sucralfate, and diphenhydramine syrup plus kaolin-pectin (3,4) have all shown some degree of efficacy in the management of mucositis. None have effectively prevented mucositis or the acute infections arising from mucositis. Further study in this area is obviously needed.

2. Management

Treatment of oral mucositis is mainly palliative, but steps should be taken to minimize secondary pathogenic infections. Culture and sensitivity data should be gathered to select the appropriate therapy for the bacterial, viral, or fungal organisms found. Numerous bacterial pathogens may be found, but the most common fungi isolated are *Candida* species, *Mucormycosis*, and *Aspergillus*. Herpes simplex and cytomegalovirus are the most frequent viral pathogens found in the oral cavity. They should be included in the differential diagnosis of any ulcerative lesions of the oral cavity.

A number of palliative treatments for mucositis are available. When the involved area is limited, topical application of Orabase with Benzocaine (Hoyt Laboratories, Norwood, MA) may be applied as necessary. Orabase is a solubilized adherent ointment base that serves to confine the anesthetic to the appropriate area, as well as lengthen the period of anesthesia. When the mucosal involvement is widespread, a variety of topical rinses may be employed. Such agents include lidocaine liquid, kaolin-pectin mixed equally with diphenhydramine elixir, dyclonine hydrochloride, and Tessalon perles (R. P. Scherer Laboratories, Detroit, MI), which provide varying degrees of symptomatic relief. All should be expectorated, not swallowed. If these are ineffective or cannot be tolerated by the patient, systemic analgesics may be necessary.

B. Infections

1. Periodontal Disease

It has been estimated that over 80% of patients aged 15–19 and over 90% of patients over age 35 are affected by periodontal disease. This disease represents the most common reason for the extraction of teeth in patients 35 years or older.

The periodontium is composed of four structures that maintain the teeth in the mouth. These are the gingiva, cementum, periodontal ligament, and alveolar bone. Periodontal disease includes gingivitis and periodontitis and is most commonly caused by poor oral hygiene that allows the accumulation of dental plaque and calculus. The microorganisms of the dental plaque that colonize the surface of the tooth adjacent to the gingiva induce a gingival inflammatory response. These microorganisms, chiefly bacteria, metabolize local nutrients and produce toxins that eventually lead to ulceration of the epithelium of the gingival sulcus. This process creates a gingival pocket or deepened gingival sulcus. The pockets next to the teeth deepen further, and additional accumulation of plaque is promoted. The patient's ability to perform proper oral hygiene (remove all dental plaque) is now impaired. The earliest clinical signs of gingivitis are inflammation and gingival bleeding resulting from minimal trauma. The gingival bleeding arises from the ulcerated sulcular epithelium. The pockets measured in gingivitis are generally less than 3 mm in depth when measured with a small calibrated probe.

Histologically, periodontitis begins with the loss of the connective tissue attachment that connects the gingiva to the crown of the tooth. The pocket epithelium is now able to migrate further along the root surface toward the apex of the tooth, creating a periodontal pocket. The inflammatory process now involves the underlying alveolar bone. This bone is resorbed in response to the inflammation, producing a net loss of bony support. Clinically this is characterized by mobility of the involved teeth and, unless treated, ultimately causes the loss of these teeth. Because the ulcerated epithelium lining the periodontal pockets can cover several square centimeters in advanced periodontal disease, it is easily understood why this can lead to infectious complications in myelosuppressed patients.

The extent of periodontal disease present in a cancer patient can best be determined by the dental staff using clinical and radiographic examinations. Pocket measurements in periodontitis can range from 4 to 10 mm or more. The deeper pockets are associated with more advanced disease. Many patients are unaware of the presence of the disease because it is usually asymptomatic. The incidence and severity of periodontal disease in cancer patients are comparable to those found in the general population. The ulcerative nature of the disease enables these tissues to act as a portal of entry for infectious agents into the systemic circulation. In one study, it was shown that up to 28% of all microbiologically and/or clinically documented infections in acute nonlymphocytic leukemia patients undergoing remission induction chemotherapy were periodontal in origin (17). These exacerbations are characterized by localized tenderness in the gingival area and temperature in excess of 38.3°C. These acute exacerbations of a normally chronic disease usually occurred during periods of profound granulocytopenia. Untreated periodontal disease therefore exposes a patient about to undergo myelosuppression to an increased risk of infectious complications.

Hospital-acquired organisms have been reported to cause 47% of all acute infections in myelosuppressed leukemia patients (18). In addition, it has been shown that the oral cavity acquires an enteric gram-negative flora in such patients. However, the surveillance cultures used to produce these data sample the flora of the gingiva and oral mucosa, not that of the ulcerated periodontal pocket. Because periodontal disease is an infectious process, the oncologist must be aware of potential shifts in the oral flora during hospitalization, producing systemic infectious episodes and requiring longer hospitalization and/or increased use of antibiotic therapy. *Staphylococcus epidermidis*, *Staphylococcus aureus*, and *Pseudomonas aeruginosa* have been found in the subgingival flora and are also associated with acute periodontal infections in these patients.

a. Prevention. When it was learned that the oral cavity could be a significant source of infection in chemotherapy-induced myelosuppressed patients, several recommendations were considered. In some centers it has been recommended to avoid manipulating the oral hard and soft tissues while patients are myelosuppressed. Included was the elimination of oral hygiene aids, such as brushing and flossing. This topic has been debated because oral hygiene measures, as well as the simple mastication of food, have been shown to produce transient bacteremias in noncancer patients with periodontal disease. However, it has been shown that oral hygiene measures do not result in an increase in systemic complications, including infections of the respiratory and upper alimentary tracts (19). Moreover, improved oral hygiene and other preventive measures have reduced the number of acute periodontal exacerbations in acute nonlymphocytic leukemia patients who undergo remission induction chemotherapy.

To prevent many of the oral complications, the dental evaluation must occur early in the admission work-up for any patient anticipated to receive myelosuppressive chemotherapy. Initial periodontal therapy, scaling and polishing the teeth, in combination with proper oral hygiene, effectively prevents most acute exacerbations of mild to moderate periodontal disease during periods of profound granulocytopenia. A major goal in periodontal therapy is to reduce pocket depths to the point that the patient can effectively perform oral hygiene measures on a daily basis. This objective is also sought for patients about to receive myelosuppressive chemotherapy, to reduce plaque accumulation and prevent this chronic infectious disease from becoming an acute infectious episode.

In patients with more severe periodontal disease, it has not been established whether initial periodontal therapy is the most efficacious method of preventing acute periodontal infections during periods of myelosuppression. Therefore, the extraction of such teeth is an alternative method of preventing acute infectious episodes (20). If extractions are contemplated several objectives should be met (see Table 3). First, the surgery must be accomplished quickly to allow approximately 10–14 days of healing before the onset of severe bone marrow suppression. Second, if the patient is already thrombocytopenic (<40,000/mm^3), platelet transfusion should be given to reach this level. Third, the surgeon should utilize alveolectomies to obtain primary closure with nonresorbable sutures. No packing materials should be placed in the extraction site to prevent secondary infection. Some patients, especially those with leukemia, may effectively present at admission with bone marrow suppression and thus not be candidates for dental extractions. They should therefore be managed more conservatively.

Emphasis on good oral hygiene techniques (brushing and flossing) must be continually reinforced to prevent the accumulation of dental plaque. Some patients are physically unable to accomplish this, and it may be necessary for the dental and/or nursing staff to provide this care for the patient. The only mouth rinse that has been shown to be effective as a chemical plaque-inhibiting agent in these patients is chlorhexidine (21). It can be most beneficial for patients who are unable to remove plaque properly by mechanical means and to reduce the overall oral microbial flora.

Powered water irrigation devices should not be used for these patients. In addition to producing bacteremias in patients with healthy periodontium, they have been shown to be ineffective in removing dental plaque. These devices do not seem indicated in patients receiving chemotherapy.

b. Treatment. When periodontal exacerbations occur, they should be treated conservatively. These usually occur during periods of profound granulocytopenia, and therefore the involved teeth should not be extracted. Acute periodontal infections are normally associated with mild gingival bleeding and some pain. The pain further diminishes the patient's ability to maintain proper oral hygiene. The staff can assist in the improvement of plaque removal. If the patient is not already utilizing chlorhexidine rinses, they should be instituted at this time.

Table 3 Guidelines for Dental Extractions in Patients Scheduled to Receive Myelosuppressive Cancer Therapy

10 days between extraction date and granulocyte count < 500 mm^2
Platelet transfusion if platelet count $< 40{,}000$ mm^3
Prophylactic antibiotics if granulocyte count < 2000 mm^3
Avoidance of intraalveolar hemostasis packing agents
Primary wound closure with multiple interrupted sutures

Source: From Overholser CD, et al. Dental extraction in patients with acute nonlymphocytic leukemia. Oral Maxillofac Surg 1982; 40:296–298.

Topical anesthetics, such as dyclonine hydrochloride or lidocaine, can be used to decrease the pain and allow the patient and/or staff to perform the oral hygiene procedures. All local irritants should be removed by gentle debridement.

Warm saline rinses and 3% hydrogen peroxide can be used as adjuncts to the regular brushing and flossing. If gingival bleeding occurs, topical thrombin (100–100,000 units/ml) can be applied. Generally no treatment is needed because the gingival bleeding is usually self-limiting. Appropriate systemic antibiotics should be administered for febrile patients.

2. Pulp and Periapical

Within the pulp chamber of each tooth is the dental pulp or dental nerve. This is connective tissue that has vascular, lymphatic, neural, and undifferentiated connective tissue cell components. Its chief function is to form dentin, which it does at varying rates throughout life. It responds to minor injuries, such as early caries, by mounting an inflammatory response and forming increased amounts of dentin as a protective measure. This often causes the tooth to be more sensitive to thermal stimuli. These teeth can be treated conservatively. If the injury received, most commonly caries or physical trauma, is too great, the inflammatory response becomes irreversible. Irreversible pulpal pathosis, including pulpitis and necrosis, cannot be treated conservatively and the tooth must be extracted or treated endodontically. Although these pulpal pathoses are invariably infectious in nature, they are not necessarily painful. The lack of discomfort in up to half of teeth with irreversible pulpal pathosis can mislead the clinician when the patient is facing significant myelosuppression. A thorough dental evaluation should identify most of these asymptomatic processes.

An established pulpal infection spreads toward the apex of the tooth. Ultimately the periapical region of alveolar bone can become involved and form a cyst, granuloma, or abscess. An abscess is usually painful, but the other two are often asymptomatic. These entities may lie dormant at the end of the tooth root for months or years before evolving further into an acute abscess and or osteomyelitis. It is not known why acute pathology develops in a previously quiescent lesion. Changes in the microflora may produce many of these exacerbations. The diminished host resistance of the myelosuppressed patient could conceivably contribute to this development. Pulpal pathosis accounts for up to 5–10% of all oral complications of chemotherapy. Periapical infections in myelosuppressed patients are serious infections that are difficult to manage when the patient is granulocytopenic (22).

a. Prevention. During the admission work-up, the dental consultant evaluates clinical and radiographic evidence of pulpal and/or periapical pathology. When reversible pulpal pathology is found, conservative dental restorative treatment is appropriate. If deep caries is found in a tooth but has not yet produced signs of irreversible pulpal pathosis, the dentist can remove the caries and insert a treatment restoration of zinc oxide and eugenol. These restorations stop the progress of the caries and have a palliative effect on the pulp. Any tooth that has turned dark, is crowned, has a history of acute trauma, or has deep caries or a deep restoration is a possible candidate for irreversible pulpal pathosis. If the evaluation indicates such pathology, endodontic therapy or extraction of the tooth is indicated before initiation of chemotherapy (see Table 4). If the infection is confined to within the pulp chamber, a one-appointment endodontic procedure appears to protect the patient adequately during subsequent chemotherapy. However, if radiographic or clinical evidence of asymptomatic periapical pathology exists, endodontic therapy or extraction is recommended. If symptomatic periapical pathology is found, extraction of the tooth is recommended when possible.

b. Management. Successful treatment of pulpal pathology found during or immediately after chemotherapy diminishes with increasing severity of the pulpal involvement. Shallow carious lesions and reversible pulpal pathology confined to the pulp chamber can usually be managed with conservative restorative treatment. Infection that has spread beyond the pulp into the surrounding alveolar bone presents a more difficult situation to manage. Routine endodontic therapy is less predictable for these infections in patients with normal host defenses. Leaving the tooth open for drainage exposes the patient to the risk of acquiring a nosocomial infection. Closing the tooth may lead to the formation of a sinus tract and again risk acquiring a hospital organism. Extraction of the tooth creates an even larger wound. Management with broad-spectrum antibiotics is successful until resistant organisms are encountered. Prevention of these adverse sequelae is therefore preferable to treatment during periods of myelosuppression.

3. Fungal

Fungal infections of the oral cavity are seldom primary events. They are seen in infants or are secondary to either systemic disease or systemic antibiotic therapy.

Table 4 Guidelines for Management of Patients with Pulpal Pathology Receiving Chemotherapy

Diagnosis	Prechemotherapy management	Postchemotherapy management
Reversible pulpitis	Caries control	Caries control
Irreversible pulpitis	Endodontics or extraction	Endodontics or extraction
Necrotic pulp with asymptomatic periapical pathology	Endodontics or extraction	Antibiotics if it becomes symptomatic
Necrotic pulp with acute periapical pathology	Extraction: endodontics only if extraction not possible	Antibiotics

It is not unusual for the patient receiving chemotherapy to develop oral fungal infections. The most common fungal infection is produced by *Candida albicans*, a normal inhabitant of the oral cavity (23). Infections caused by *Aspergillus* species and *Torulopsis glabrata* have also been reported with some frequency in recent years. Oral candidiasis may present as erythematous (diffuse mucosal erythema), pseudomembranous (white, creamy thrush with underlying ulceration), or hyperplastic (leukoplakialike) or as angular cheilitis. The erythematous and pseudomembranous types are usually accompanied by complaints of generalized oral pain. Smears and/or cultures can be used to confirm the diagnosis.

a. Prevention. Because oncologists already limit the utilization of systemic antibiotics when possible, little can be done to prevent fungal infections secondary to antibiotic therapy. Although many clinicians believe that improved oral hygiene will lead to decreased fungal infections, no clinical trial has confirmed this hypothesis.

b. Management. Superficial candidiasis can be treated with either topical nystatin or clotrimazole troches. Patients place them four times a day in the mouth and leave them until they completely dissolve. The increased contact time is necessary to control the organism. For deeper infections, fluconazole or amphotericin B can be used systemically. *C. albicans* can also complicate angular cheilitis. This usually can be controlled with Mycolog cream (Squibb and Sons, Inc., Princeton, NJ).

Fungal infections often occur in patients who wear removable dental prostheses. In addition to the patient regimen, the prosthesis must also be treated since the plastic can act as a reservoir to reinfect the treated mucosa. Prostheses may be placed in a denture cup with 100 ml nystatin suspension overnight for 6–8 h per day. Fungal infections caused by organisms other than *Candida* should be treated by the appropriate antifungal agent.

4. *Viral*

Viral infections in myelosuppressed patients can cause significant pain, interfere with function and nutrition, and be fatal under certain circumstances. Reactivation of latent herpes simplex virus infection is the most frequent viral complication, but primary herpes, varicella-zoster, and cytomegalovirus infections are also seen in these patients. They appear more commonly during therapy that produces intense and prolonged myelosuppression.

The clinical appearance of both recurrent herpes labialis and recurrent intraoral herpes in these patients presents in a much more severe form than in noncancer patients and may be overlooked in the differential diagnosis. Intraoral herpes simplex virus infection may present as a very difficult diagnostic challenge. Both forms of recurrent herpes labialis, intraoral herpes may begin as small vesicles. These vesicles quickly rupture, leaving small, shallow punctate ulcers. Usually these ulcers quickly coalesce to form larger ragged-shaped ulcerations that are quite painful. Apparently both forms of the infection are often not seen clinically until the latter stages. The lesions are then easily confused with chemotherapy-induced mucositis. The atypical presentations may account for the few descriptions of these lesions in the literature.

a. Prevention. Because almost all herpes infections in these patients are reactivation of the latent virus, identification of those patients at risk for reactivation during intensive myelosuppressive therapy is the best method of prevention. Identification of seropositive patients during the admission work-up enables the clinician to administer prophylactic acyclovir or have a high index of suspicion when unidentified mucocutaneous lesions are present. Early diagnosis of these lesions is important to institute effective therapy with acyclovir (24).

b. Treatment. Intravenous or oral acyclovir is effective in treating herpes simplex infections. The use of oral acyclovir in these patients is often limited because of the presence of nausea, vomiting, oral ulcerations, and other gastroenterological problems. Acyclovir therapy improves the quality of life, helps maintain nutrition, and helps prevent secondary bacterial and fungal infections in the ulcerated lesions.

5. Removable Dental Prosthesis

Approximately 20% of the population wears some type of removable dental prosthesis that serves functional and esthetic purposes. However, prosthetic devices can lead to complications during the treatment of patients receiving chemotherapy. Dentures that are worn constantly or fit improperly can produce mucosal ulcerations that readily become contaminated by the oral flora. The prostheses, their cleansers, and the containers in which they are soaked can be a source of reinfection for the patient, as well as cross-contamination among patients and staff. *C. albicans* is a common contaminant of dentures in the noncancer patient population. High concentrations of *P. aeruginosa*, *Klebsiella* species, *Enterobacter* species, *Escherichia coli*, other gram-negative bacilli, *S. aureus*, and *T. glabrata* are frequently found on the denture and denture-soaking containers of cancer patients. The potential for infection from such organisms in the myelosuppressed patient is readily apparent.

a. Prevention. To lessen the risk for oral infections during chemotherapy, patients with removable dental prosthetic devices should receive a dental evaluation preoperatively. Obviously, these prostheses assist in mastication and therefore are important in the maintenance of proper nutrition. In addition, these devices often promote the patient's self-image and loss of the prostheses can cause significant embarrassment. Therefore, the decision to remove the prosthesis during chemotherapy should not be made lightly. If time permits, improperly fitting prostheses should be modified to fit. However, the patient should not be allowed to use them if proper adaptation to the tissues cannot be established. Patients allowed to retain their dentures should not wear them more than 12 h in each 24 h period. When the prostheses are removed from the mouth they should be scrubbed clean with a denture brush, rinsed, and placed in an appropriate denture antiseptic solution. Denture-soaking agents with antiseptic properties include Efferdent (Warner-Lambert Co., Morris Plains, NJ), Polident (Block Drug Co., Jersey City, NJ), and Kleenite (Vicks Toiletry Products, Wilton, CT). These solutions must be changed on a daily basis. This prevents gross contamination, which may then allow growth of the pathogens described earlier. As mentioned, these containers and solutions represent not only a source of patient reinfection, but also a mechanism of cross-contamination via hospital staff members (25).

It must be kept in mind that the tissues beneath these prostheses continue to change slowly. Upon completion of chemotherapy, the adaptation of the dentures to the tissues must be periodically reevaluated by the dental staff to prevent subsequent complications.

b. Management. Appropriate antibiotic therapy should be instituted for infections arising from prosthetic contamination. It must be remembered that in the management of fungal infections, especially *C. albicans*, treatment of the prosthesis itself with the appropriate antifungal agent is important to prevent reinfection from the prosthesis. Additionally, the denture hygiene protocol and compliance should be reviewed to determine whether the infection was caused by an ill-fitting prosthesis, poor hygiene, or cross-contamination.

C. Hemorrhage

Bleeding complications occur commonly in patients receiving chemotherapy for cancer and are usually caused by the associated thrombocytopenia. Fortunately, most bleeding problems encountered are not seriously debilitating. Surgery, such as dental extraction, poses the greatest risk for bleeding diathesis. With proper evaluation before chemotherapy, there should seldom be a need for surgical procedures. Petechial hemorrhages are often seen in the gingiva, buccal mucosa, tongue, floor of the mouth, and hard and soft palate. Ecchymosis is more likely found in the tongue and floor of the mouth. Because gingival bleeding is one of the earliest clinical signs of gingivitis, this also commonly occurs in the thrombocytopenic patient. As in patients not receiving chemotherapy, gingivitis and gingival bleeding are a response to dental plaque. Effective oral hygiene usually prevents most such hemorrhages.

Physical trauma is a frequent cause of oral hemorrhagic events. Physical trauma includes improper oral hygiene (especially floss), mastication of soft tissues, and periodontal therapy. Traumatic episodes are often followed by local tissue necrosis. Such lesions often become secondarily infected.

1. Prevention

Dental evaluation of patients at admission should obviate the need for most surgical procedures during times of thrombocytopenia. The most common exception is the patient who presents as granulocytopenic and/or thrombocytopenic at admission. Hematoma formation in the floor of the mouth may slowly enlarge but seldom causes respiratory embarrassment. Serious hemorrhage is likely if surgery is performed in the presence of disseminated intravascular coagulation.

2. Treatment

Minor oral bleeding, commonly gingival in origin, can usually be controlled by pressure. Application of topical thrombin (100–100,000 units/ml) can be helpful if pressure is unsuccessful. Gingival bleeding is usually associated with the inflammation produced by dental plaque, and therefore improvement in the oral hygiene should be a primary goal. When estimating the amount of blood lost, the clinician and patient must be cognizant of presence of saliva, which dilutes the blood. This dilution significantly increases the apparent amount of bleeding observed.

Major oral bleeding most likely occurs when surgery is performed when platelet counts are below 40,000/mm^3. Ideally, such procedures as the extraction of teeth and periodontal surgery should have been accomplished before chemotherapy or be delayed until the patient's counts begin to return to normal. If necessary, however, teeth can be removed when appropriate platelet transfusions are given. Infection rather than hemorrhage is usually the greatest risk with surgery in the myelosuppressed patient. Bleeding from such wounds can be controlled by platelet transfusions and primary closure of the surgical site. No packing materials, such as oxidized cellulose or bone wax, should be placed in the extraction site (20).

D. Xerostomia

Xerostomia is occasionally a complication of chemotherapy that can interfere with nutrition, taste, and speech. Normal salivary output also provides some protection against shifts in the oropharyngeal microbial flora (26) that may help protect against mucosal infection. Although xerostomia as a result of chemotherapy cannot be prevented, it usually can be managed.

The primary goals in the management of xerostomia are restoration of moisture and alleviation of pain. Frequent rinses with sterile ice water or saline often provide sufficient relief to the patient. Some patients prefer saliva substitutes that replace many of the missing constituents of normal saliva. Chewing sugarless gum can be helpful in patients without oral mucositis. The patient must be advised to be careful not to damage the mucosa.

E. Graft-Versus-Host Disease

Except for graft-versus-host disease (GVHD), most oral complications in bone marrow transplant patients are similar to those found in patients receiving radiation and/or myelosuppressive chemotherapy (27–29). Acute GVHD (days 0–100 after transplant) and chronic GVHD (days 100–400 after transplant) are significant complications of allogeneic bone marrow transplant. They result when immunologically active T cells are transplanted into a recipient who is genetically different from the donor.

1. Acute GVHD

In the oral cavity it is difficult to distinguish the oral complications of GVHD from those toxic and infectious side effects of chemoradiotherapy. The lesions typically seen in acute GVHD are ulcers, which are usually painful. Biopsies that could differentiate GVHD from side effects of the conditioning regimen are usually contraindicated during this time period. Because viral and bacterial infections are often included in the differential diagnosis, appropriate culture and sensitivity should be performed. Prevention and treatment of oral GVHD is accomplished through the systemic management of GVHD. A number of drugs have found some usefulness in ameliorating the symptoms of the disease and include steroids, cyclosporine, and antithymocyte globulin. The response to these has been mixed.

2. Chronic GVHD

A number of oral manifestations of chronic GVHD have been described. These include mucosal erythema and atrophy, lichenoid reactions, pain, and xerostomia. In some cases the mucosal atrophy becomes frankly ulcerative and is often consistent with erosive lichen planus. As with acute GVHD, prevention and treatment are mainly accomplished through the systemic management of the disease. Topical steroids, appropriate antimicrobial agents, topical anesthetics, and systemic analgesics may be needed to treat the painful oral lesions. Management of the xerostomia is similar to that in the patient who has received radiation therapy and includes salivary stimulants, saliva substitutes, and fluoride treatments.

REFERENCES

1. Wright W. Pretreatment and oral care intervention for radiation patients. NCI Monogr 1990; 9:57–59.
2. Carl W, Emrich L. Management of oral mucositis during local radiation and systemic chemotherapy: a study of 98 patients. J Prosthet Dent 1991; 66(3):361–369.

3. Miaskowski C. Oral complications of cancer therapies. Management of mucositis during therapy. NCI Monogr 1990; 9:95–98.
4. Barker G, Loftus L, Cuddy P, Barker B. The effects of sucralfate suspension and diphenhydramine syrup plus kaolin-pectin on radiotherapy-induced mucositis. Oral Surg Oral Med Oral Pathol 1991; 71:288–293.
5. Liu R, Fleming T, Toth B. Salivary flow rates in patients with head and neck cancer 0.5 to 25 years after radiotherapy. Oral Surg Oral Med Oral Pathol 1990; 70:724–729.
6. Valdez I, Wolff A, Atkinson J, Macynski A, Fox P. Use of Pilocarpine during head and neck radiation therapy to reduce xerostomia and salivary dysfunction. Cancer 1993; 71:1848–1851.
7. Ferguson M. Pilocarpine and other cholinergic drugs in the management of salivary gland dysfunction. Oral Surg Oral Med Oral Pathol 1993; 75:186–191.
8. Epstein J, McBride B, Stevenson-Moore P, Merilees H, Spinelli J. The efficacy of chlorhexidine gel in reduction of *Streptococcus mutans* and *Lactobacillus* species in patients treated with radiation therapy. Oral Surg Oral Med Oral Pathol 1991; 71:172–178.
9. Marx, R, RP J. Studies in the radiobiology of osteoradionecrosis and their clinical significance. Oral Surg Oral Med Oral Pathol 1987; 64(4):379–390.
10. Watson WL, Scarborough JE. Osteoradionecrosis in intraoral cancer. Am J Roentgenol Radium Ther 1938; 40:524.
11. Marx R, Johnson R, Kline S. Prevention of osteoradionecrosis: a randomized prospective clinical trial of hyperbaric oxygen versus penicillin. J Am Dent Assoc 1985; 111:49–54.
12. Mainous E, Boyne P. Hyperbaric oxygen in total rehabilitation of patients with mandibular osteoradionecrosis. Int J Oral Surg 1974; 3(5):297–301.
13. Friedman R. Osteoradionecrosis: causes and prevention. NCI Monogr 1990; 9:145–149.
14. Myers R, Marx R. Use of hyperbaric oxygen in postradiation head and neck surgery. NCI Monogr 1990; 9:151.
15. Marx RE. Osteoradionecrosis: a new concept of its pathophysiology. J Oral Maxillofac Surg 1983; 41:283–288.
16. Sonis ST, Sonis AL, Lieberman A. Oral complications in patients receiving treatment for malignancies other than of the head and neck. J Am Dent Assoc 1978; 97:468–472.
17. Overholser CD, Peterson DE, Williams LT, Schimpff SC. Periodontal infection in patients with acute nonlymphocytic leukemia. Arch Intern Med 1982; 142:551–554.
18. Schimpff SC, Young VM, Greene WH, et al. Origin of infection in acute nonlymphocytic leukemia: significance of hospital acquisition of potential pathogens. Ann Intern Med 1972; 77:07–714.
19. Weikel DS, Peterson DE, Rubinstein LE, Samuels CM, Overholser CD. Incidence of fever following invasive oral interventions in the myelosuppressed cancer patient. Cancer Nurs 1989; 12:265–270.
20. Overholser CD, Bergman SA, Peterson DE. Dental extractions in acute and chronic myelogenous leukemia patients. Oral Surg 1982; 40:296–298.
21. Ferretti GA, Ash RC, Brown AT, et al. Chlorexidine for prophylaxis against oral

infections and associated complications in patients receiving bone marrow transplants. J Am Dent Assoc 1987; 114:461–467.
22. Peterson DE. Oral complications associated with hematologic neoplasms and their treatment. In: Peterson DE, Elias EG, Sonis ST, eds. Head and Neck Management of the Cancer Patient. Boston: Martinus Nihjoff, 1986:351–361.
23. Dreizen S, Brown LR. Oral microbial changes and infections during cancer chemotherapy. In: Peterson DE, Sonis ST, eds. Oral Complications of Cancer Chemotherapy, 1983:41–77.
24. Bustamante CI, Wade JC. Herpes simplex virus infection in the immunocompromised cancer patient. 1991; 9(10):1903–1915.
25. DePaola LG, Minah GE. Isolation of pathogenic microorganisms from dentures and denture soaking containers of myelosuppressed cancer patients. J Prosthet Dent 1983; 49:20–24.
26. Laforce FM, Hopkins J, Trow R, Wang WL. Human oral defenses against gram-negative rods. Am Rev Respir Dis 1976; 114:929–935.
27. Schubert MM, Sullivan KM, Truelove EL. Head and neck complications of bone marrow transplantation. In: Peterson DE, Elias EG, Sonis ST, eds. Head and Neck Management of the Cancer Patient. 1986:401–427.
28. Maxymiw WG, Wood RE. The role of dentistry in patients undergoing bone marrow transplantation. Br Dent J 1989; 167:229.
29. Brown AT, Shupe JA, Sims RE, et al. In vitro effect of chlorhexidine and amikacin on oral gram-negative bacilli from bone marrow transplant recipients. Oral Surg Oral Med Oral Pathol 1990; 70:715–719.

6

Mucositis

James G. Gallagher
Jefferson Medical College, Philadelphia, and Geisinger Clinic, Danville, Pennsylvania

I. INTRODUCTION

Toxicity to gastrointestinal mucous membranes is a frequent side effect of treatment for malignancy. Probably no other side effects so interfere with quality of life than mucositis and diarrhea. Both cause pain and hemorrhage and interfere with adequate hydration and nutrition. In addition, interruption of alimentary tract membranes may allow local invasion by bacteria, fungi, or viruses, singly or in combination. Some of these localized ulcerations may lead to systemic infections (bacteremia and fungemia). All such mucous membrane injuries require time to heal, during which intense supportive care must be given, frequently in the hospital, and at great expense.

Indeed, as newer chemotherapy and radiation therapy strategies are introduced, some of them result in unexpectedly severe mucositis or diarrhea. Sadly, each of these gastrointestinal toxicities can be fatal if not promptly recognized and treated. As long as aggressive treatment is done, mucositis and diarrhea will remain serious problems for oncologists. Recently, more attention has been paid to prevention and supportive care in this area. A number of international conferences on supportive care in cancer have been held in Europe and the United States. The practical applications of new knowledge in this area are presented in this volume and also in the new journal, *Supportive Care in Cancer*.

II. DEFINITION AND MAGNITUDE OF THE PROBLEM

Inflammation of the oral mucus membranes is a common toxicity of chemotherapy or irradiation with a wide spectrum of severity, from a few small patches of inflammation to widespread involvement causing severe pain and cessation of all oral intake. This process may extend down the esophagus, causing further dysphagia, odynophagia, and interrupted alimentation. Because this phenomenon is rarely seen outside cancer therapy or other acquired immunodeficiency states (e.g., acquired immunodeficiency syndrome and severe combined immunodeficiency), most general medicine and gastroenterology textbooks ignore mucositis. Because it is largely an iatrogenic phenomenon, stomatitis should be aggressively studied to minimize the suffering of those who must undergo systemic drug or oral irradiation treatment. Since mucous membranes are only one part of total oral care, dental prophylaxis (fluoride regimens for teeth before radiation therapy), endodontics, periodontics, and care of dental prostheses or intraoral or maxillofacial prostheses should be also considered at the outset of a treatment plan. These subjects are covered elsewhere (1–3). With increasing numbers of protocols delivering drugs on a "dose intensity" schedule, it should be expected that toxicity intensity will also result. Thus, the need for better supportive care to rescue surviving normal cells and ensure the survival of the individual should be apparent. Dose intensity makes sense only if it is both effective and results in less than fatal toxicity. Figure 1 shows the complex set of interactions that result in mucositis.

III. ETIOLOGY

Both irradiation and chemotherapy produce mucositis, and when both modalities and multiple agents are used to treat head and neck cancer, the toxicities are at least additive and result in a further cascade of morbidities: malnutrition, dehydration, bleeding, and infection. Many drugs have been observed to produce mucositis: 5-fluorouracil (5-FU), azathioprine, bleomycin, cyclophosphamide, dactinomycin, daunorubicin, doxorubicin, nitrogen mustard, melphalan, 6-mercaptopurine, methotrexate, mitomycin C, Novantrone (mitoxantrone), plicamycin (mithramycin), procarbazine, streptozotocin, 6-thioguanine, and Velban (vinblastine). Thus, about one-half of the most commonly used chemotherapy drugs have been reported to cause mucositis (4). Five drugs commonly cause severe mucositis: methotrexate, 5-FU, dactinomycin, doxorubicin, and daunorubicin. Combination chemotherapy with two or more of these drugs can be at least additive in toxicity to the mucous membranes. Other drugs that can occasionally produce clinically significant mucositis include nitrogen mustard, cyclophosphamide, ifosfamide, 6-thioguanine, idarubicin, mitoxantrone, vinblastine, bleomycin, mitomycin C, procarbazine, and malphalan. Methotrexate

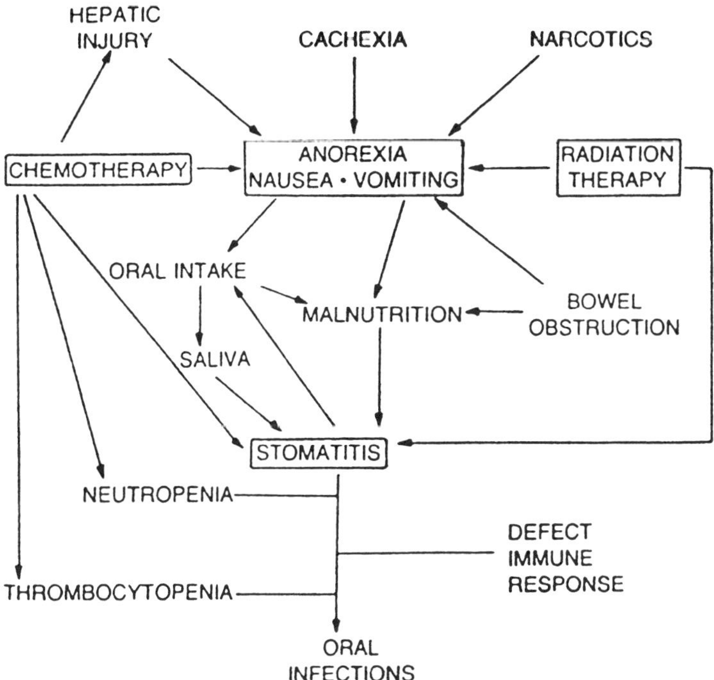

Figure 1 Interrelationships of common causal factors. (From Daeffer R. Oral hygiene measures for patients with cancer, part I. *Cancer Nurs* 1980; 3:347–355. Used by permission.)

can be particularly toxic when given to those with pleural effusions or ascites. The drug enters the effusion and then slowly reenters the circulation, causing severe mucositis and bone marrow suppression. Radiation therapy to head and neck sites produces inflammation acutely and decreased salivary function on a subacute and chronic basis. Concomitant chemotherapy and irradiation can produce very severe mucositis, and these treatments are often done sequentially to avoid the toxicity of simultaneous treatment. The most severe radiation mucositis occurs when 5-FU or methotrexate is given during a course of radiation to the head and neck region.

Besides direct toxicity to mucosal cells, immunosuppression and myelosuppression play a role in oral toxicity. Once the direct toxicity has occurred and is followed by immunosuppression or myelosuppression, infection is facilitated. This may be bacterial, fungal, or viral. In herpes simplex virus-seropositive bone marrow transplant patients (BMT), the majority reactivate within the first 5 weeks after transplant and have severe, deep, painful ulcers. Herpes simplex virus

(HSV) esophagitis occasionally follows the initial oral reactivation. None of these viral infections can be diagnosed on clinical grounds alone.

Candida albicans may present with any of several types of mucosal lesion: pseudomembranous candidiasis, chronic hyperplastic candidiasis, chronic erythematous candidiasis, and angular cheilitis (6).

Bacterial periodontal abscess, sialadenitis of major salivary glands, and gingivitis are seen and may be the portal of entry for bacteremia and sepsis (6). Empirical antibiotics are necessary while awaiting cultures and must include coverage for *Pseudomonas* species (6,7).

IV. PATHOPHYSIOLOGY

Cell death is the intended result of all cancer treatments. By whatever mechanism of injury to nucleic acid or protein synthesis, mitosis, or membrane integrity, it is hoped to kill more tumor than normal cells. This acknowledges the incidental killing of a fraction of normal cells, especially those with a rapid division rate and turnover time. Thus, mucosal and bone marrow cells sustain much of the incidental, unintended injury. This is particularly true when cell cycle-specific agents are used.

While sloughing of epithelial cells continues, replacement cells are slow to recover proliferative function. Histologically, dysplasia, hyperplasia, glandular degeneration, and collagen disruption are seen (8). Whereas intact oral mucosa serves as a chemical and microbiological barrier by surface sloughing and a regeneration time of 5–16 days, this protective function is disrupted when turnover time is prolonged. Bacteria that adhere and are normally carried away by surface sloughing maintain their position on the mucosa long enough to proliferate and invade. Similarly, *Candida albicans* may have more time to form germ tubes and penetrate mucosal epithelium, thus tipping the balance ordinarily present between mucosal clearance and pathogen (opportunist) virulence. Reduction in salivary gland and mucous gland function results in fewer humoral factors, such as antibody and antimicrobial proteins to degrade oral microorganisms.

Defenses against microorganisms are clearly multifactorial. The importance of mucosal barrier and clearance mechanisms, coupled with salivary flow, are most apparent when they are disrupted. Other host defenses are present in normal oral mucosa that are not as apparent but play an important role. Abundant lymphoid tissue is present in Waldeyer's ring and other oral mucosal sites. T cells, B cells, mast cells, and natural killer cells are all present. Secretory immunoglobulin (IgA) plays a role in preventing reinfection with previously recognized viruses and other microorganisms. Lymphoid tissue, with its important cellular and humoral defenses, is undoubtedly diminished by the same agents that injure mucosal epithelium directly. Thus, the final picture of inflamed, denuded epithelium, superficial or deep infection, and bleeding results from injury to all components of the oral defenses.

A. Bacterial Infections

Leukemic and other immunosuppressed cancer patients have a higher incidence of infection with gram-negative rods, such as *Escherichia coli*, *Klebsiella pneumonia*, and *Pseudomonas aeruginosa*. Frequently these occur as nosocomial infections when multiple-drug–resistant strains present in the hospital colonize the oropharynx and gastrointestinal tract or upper respiratory tract and then invade when mucosal barriers are disrupted. Since this usually coincides with a period of maximum neutropenia, systemic infections and endotoxic shock are very likely events. Antibiotic prophylaxis for this is controversial. It may decrease gram-negative rod infections at the cost of increased gram-positive coccal, fungal, and yeast infections. Empirical antibiotic therapy of the febrile neutropenic patient with many mucosal portals of entry is necessary and often lifesaving (9–11). Recently, gram-positive coccal organisms have become a more frequent cause of sepsis in granulocytopenic patients than gram-negative rods. These include *Staphylococcus epidermidis*, *Staphylococcus aureus*, *Streptococcus mitis*, and other strains. Multiple-drug–resistant *S. epidermidis* strains causing bacteremia in cancer patients have often been shown by DNA restriction endonuclease typing not to originate from contaminated intravenous catheters, as was thought, but to come from the gastrointestinal tract (12). These undoubtedly enter through disruptions of the mucosal barrier. Viridans streptococci from the mouth cause similar infections (4).

B. Fungal Infections

Candida species are the most commonly isolated yeast from oral lesions. Increased adherence time to mucosal cells and decreased phagocytic activity allow invasion of mucosa. Declining phagocytic activity against *Candida* can be demonstrated starting 30 minutes after exposure to alkylating agents. *Candida albicans* is most frequently encountered, but other species are seen in oral candidiasis: *Candida tropicalis*, *Candida krusei*, *Candida parapsilosis*, and *Candida glabrata*. The appearance of oral candidiasis ranges from discrete white "curds" to extensive white pseudomembranous lesions (4).

C. Viral Infections

Most oral viral lesions are caused by herpes simplex virus. In the normal host with reactivation of latent virus, the vesicles in the lips and oral mucosa have a characteristic appearance. In the compromised host, especially BMT patients, they are often far more extensive and their appearance is less characteristic or obscured altogether by concomitant mucosal inflammation and nonspecific ulceration, yeast infection (thrush), hemorrhage, and adherence of food particles and medicaments to the mucosa. Laboratory tests may be helpful in making a specific diagnosis (see later).

In the compromised host with painful ulcerated lesions who is already receiving antibiotics and does not have a fungal infection by clinical or laboratory criteria, the empirical use of acyclovir often produces clinical improvement. This may be the best test of whether HSV is part of a multiagent painful ulcerative process.

Graft-versus-host disease in BMT patients, either acute or chronic, affects both mucosal surfaces and salivary gland function.

V. CLINICAL PRESENTATION AND COURSE

Acute oral mucositis begins 7–10 days after cytoreductive therapy. Mucosal "burning" is often the first manifestation, accompanied by erythema. Erosion and ulceration next develop over a period of 3–5 days and then persist for days to weeks, depending on the dose and duration of the offending agent(s). This is accompanied by pain, bleeding, and infection. Brief pulses of chemotherapeutic drugs may produce short-duration patchy involvement of the mucosa, especially if the patient is practicing good oral hygiene. Continuous infusion of 5-FU or irradiation for head and neck tumors is often directly toxic to the entire mucosa, with very extensive involvement, which may occur despite the best oral hygiene.

VI. DIAGNOSTIC TESTS

Although nonspecific ulcerations occur secondary to leukemia or profound neutropenia, infection must always be ruled out. In BMT patients, graft-versus-host disease may also be present and confuse the diagnostic picture (6). During acute oral mucositis, cultures and stains for bacteria and fungi can be helpful in assessing the etiological role of these agents in the current episode. Viral cultures of ulcers may yield HSV because many patients who are serologically positive reactivate this virus. Swabs from ulcerated epithelium can be examined by immunofluorescence for HSV, but this is expensive and not always available.

There are tests for quantitating salivary flow and estimating the degree of xerostomia, but these are not of much benefit in managing acute toxicity.

When esophagitis is also present, endoscopy may be most helpful in differentiating between lesions caused by *Candida* and those caused by HSV.

VII. TREATMENT

Many topical oral preparations have been employed in the treatment of oral mucositis. A number were described as effective in the National Cancer Institute

Monograph (6): benzylamine hydrochloride in head and neck cancer patients; β-carotene in oral squamous cell carcinomas; allopurinol in gastrointestinal cancers; and sucralfate in acute nonlymphocytic leukemia in adults but not in children. It is sometimes effective to use a combination of therapies given sequentially through the day. Sucralfate given as a slurry to "swish and swallow" may protect both oropharynx and esophagus. Viscous 2% lidocaine (Xylocaine), 15 ml diluted with a small amount of water in a swish and spit treatment, reduces pain if used before meals. It is important that the lidocaine be expectorated to avoid cardiac toxicity from systemic absorption. Newer preparations that combine a long-lasting (6 h) barrier for denuded epithelium with an analgesic seem to be a worthwhile addition for those with discrete ulcers. A durable film of hydroxypropyl cellulose with 15% Benzocaine (Oratect gel) is formed after the application of the gel. Multiple discrete lesions of the tongue, gingiva, and buccal mucosa can be treated with this product, but it is impractical to treat very wide areas. For oral candidiasis, nystatin, clotrimazole, or oral ketoconazole can be used. Low-dose (3–5 mg) intravenous amphotericin B has been used for lack of response to the other agents.

Acyclovir should be given either as prevention for HSV in high-risk patients, such as leukemics and BMT patients, or for lower risk patients therapeutically as needed.

Radiation-induced decreased salivary flow often results in rampant caries. Increased flow can be stimulated with sialogogues, such as pilocarpine, or, more inexpensively, with sugarless chewing gum.

Additional recommendations can be found in comprehensive monographs (4,6). The pain from mucositis can be quite severe and should not be underestimated. Appropriate analgesics must be given, and this frequently includes parenteral morphine for adequate relief.

Parenteral nutritional support either as peripheral protein-sparing solution or total parenteral nutrition must often be administered to those with severe mucositis to rest inflamed mucosa and to promote healing. For those with less severe mucositis, a full liquid diet (e.g., Ensure, Sustacal, or surgical liquid diet) may suffice. Consultation with the nutritional support service may be helpful for calculation of caloric requirements in a catabolic, malnourished patient and counting the actual number of calories delivered orally and intravenously, for example.

VIII. PREVENTION

Preexisting oral disease unrelated to the cancer or its therapy increases the complication rate after therapy. The mouth is a "trauma-intense" environment. Rough teeth, dental plates, bridges, and hard food particles frequently abrade the mucosa. If possible, a dental evaluation and corrective plan should be initiated before the onset of chemotherapy or radiation therapy. In this way, plaque can be removed and roughened or ill-fitting teeth and appliances can be repaired. Carious teeth should be repaired or removed. Gingivitis should be controlled before treatment because it can easily exacerbate and be a source for systemic infection.

While on therapy for cancer, consistent oral hygiene with a fluoride toothpaste and a soft toothbrush should be done after meals and at bedtime. For those in whom use of a toothbrush causes hemorrhage because of friability of thrombocytopenia, topical rinses, such as chlorhexidine, are available. Chlorhexidine with an aminoglycoside prevents the emergence of gram-negative rods. Oral nonabsorbable antibiotic mixtures, such as gentamicin, vancomycin, and nystatin, are falling from favor because their foul taste markedly reduces patient compliance. Less compromised hosts are often advised to rinse with normal saline solution, 3% hydrogen peroxide solution, or sodium bicarbonate solution. Other strategies include a soft diet to reduce mechanical trauma and avoidance of thermal trauma. A cooked food diet and avoidance of fresh fruit and vegetables reduce the acquisition of new gram-negative rods. For leukemics or BMT patients, antifungal prophylaxis and antiviral prophylaxis with acyclovir have been shown to be helpful (11). Not all preventive measures are effective. Citrovorum mouthwash during methotrexate infusion has failed to prevent mucositis. Recently, a controlled trial of oral cryotherapy for preventing stomatitis from 5-FU modulated with leucovorin was found to be effective (13). Patients used ice chips to cool the mouth for 30 minutes while a bolus of 5-FU was given. Since the drug has a half-life of 10–20 minutes, it was hoped that decreasing blood flow by cooling would limit exposure of mucosal cells. This is an inexpensive prophylactic against an expensive toxicity.

Synthetic saliva (Salivart) is often used to prevent dryness (xerostomia) when salivary flow is decreased. The duration of such an effect is usually very brief. Longer acting saliva substitutes with mucopolysaccharides are becoming available (MouthKote). Some add diphenhydramine or benzyl alcohol for anesthetic purposes.

An exciting recent finding is that granulocyte colony-stimulating factor not only reduces the duration of neutropenia but decreases the severity of mucositis (6). If confirmed, this would be a major, although expensive, advance in preventing chemotherapy-related mucositis.

IX. FUTURE RESEARCH

Future cooperative group protocols should incorporate data collection on the incidence and prevalence of oral complications related to different types of anticancer therapies. These trials should also incorporate state-of-the-art treatment for oral toxicity. It would be useful to have radioprotective and chemoprotective agents. Further investigation of the role of biologic response modifiers, such as the colony-stimulating factors, in the prevention of myelosuppression and mucositis is needed. Further definition of the patient populations that benefit from prophylactic antiviral therapy should be done. More information is needed about the optimal antifungal prophylaxis and therapy of overt infection. Controlled studies of chlorhexidine and other oral antimicrobials for the prevention of infection and control of mucositis are needed in defined patient populations. It will be useful to know the cost of oral toxicity to determine the cost effectiveness of strategies for dealing with these toxicities.

ANNOTATED BIBLIOGRAPHY

Fisher DS, Knobf MT. The Cancer Chemotherapy Handbook, 3rd ed. St. Louis: Mosby-Year Book, 1989. The stomatitis section is a useful guide to management. The figure illustrating the multifactorial etiology of mucositis is helpful. The treatment of diarrhea is less adequate. Overall, this is an excellent example of the many such handbooks available.

National Cancer Institute. Consensus Development Conference on Oral Complications of Cancer Therapies: Diagnosis, Prevention, and Treatment. NCI Monograph Vol. 9, 1990. This is the most extensive reference ever produced on oral toxicities and their management. A total of 30 presentations on pretreatment assessment, pretreatment strategies, management of acute problems, and management of chronic toxicities are followed by a consensus statement. There is more information about tooth and bone problems in irradiated and BMT patients than in most other reviews. The pediatric population is well covered.

National Institutes of Health. Oral Complications of Cancer Therapies: Diagnosis, Prevention and Treatment. NIH Consensus Development Conference Statement. 1989, Vol. 7, No. 7. This is the consensus statement alone and should not be confused with the much larger conference proceedings. This brief consensus statement, however, is a remarkable summary of current recommendations for the management of oral toxicities and directions for future research.

Peterson DE. Oral toxicity of chemotherapeutic agents. Semin Oncol 1992; 19:478–491. This is a thorough treatment of oral toxicities emphasizing dental problems. Mucositis and salivary gland dysfunction are well covered, and the reference list is excellent: a recent and highly recommended reference.

REFERENCES

1. McElroy TH. Oral care of the cancer patient. In: Schein PS, ed. Decision Making in Oncology. Philadelphia: B.C. Decker, 1989:230–231.
2. Toth BB, Frame RT. The management of disease and treatment-related oral dental complications associated with chemotherapy. Curr Prob Cancer 1983; 7:7–35.
3. McElroy TH. Infection in the patient receiving chemotherapy for cancer: oral considerations. J Am Dent Assoc 1984; 109:454–456.

4. Peterson DE. Oral toxicity of chemotherapeutic agents. Semin Oncol 1992; 19:478–491.
5. Perry MC. Toxicity: ten years later. Semin Oncol 1992; 19:453–457.
6. National Cancer Institute. Consensus Development Conference on Oral Complications of Cancer Therapies: Diagnosis, Prevention, and Treatment. NCI Monograph Vol. 9, 1990.
7. Gallagher JG. Empiric antimicrobial therapy in the community hospital setting for the cancer patient with fever and neutropenia: the need for vigilance and attention to detail. Recent Results Cancer Res 1993; 132:89–96.
8. Lockhart PD, Sonis ST. Alterations in the oral mucosa caused by chemotherapeutic agents. J Dermatol Surg Oncol 1981; 7:1019–1025.
9. Klastersky J, Zinner SH, Calandra T, et al. Empiric antimicrobial therapy for febrile granulocytopenic cancer patients: lessons from four EORTC trials. Eur J Cancer Clin Oncol 1988; 24(Suppl 1):S35–S45.
10. Hughes WT, Armstrong D, Bodey GP, et al. Guidelines for the use of antimicrobial agents in neutropenic patients with unexplained fever. J Infect Dis 1990; 161:381–396.
11. Schimpff SC. Prevention of and therapy for infections in cancer patients. Curr Opin Oncol 1990; 2:919–923.
12. Wade J. Controversies in new anti-infectious therapies. Fourth International Symposium on Supportive Care in Cancer. St. Gall, Switzerland, February, 24–27, 1993.
13. Mahood DJ, Dose AM, Loprinzi CL, et al. Inhibition of fluorouracil-induced stomatitis by oral cryotherapy. J Clin Oncol 1991; 9:449–452.

7

Diarrhea

James G. Gallagher
Jefferson Medical College, Philadelphia, and Geisinger Clinic, Danville, Pennsylvania

I. INTRODUCTION

Toxicity to gastrointestinal mucous membranes is a frequent side effect of treatment for malignancy. Probably no other side effects so interfere with quality of life as mucositis and diarrhea. Mucositis is covered in the previous chapter; diarrhea is the subject of this chapter. Both cause pain and hemorrhage and interfere with adequate hydration and nutrition. In addition, interruption of alimentary tract membranes may allow local invasion by bacteria, fungi, or viruses singly or in combination. Some of these localized ulcerations may lead to systemic infections (bacteremia and fungemia). All such mucous membrane injuries require time to heal, during which intense supportive care must be given, frequently in the hospital and at great expense.

Indeed, as newer chemotherapy and radiation therapy strategies are introduced, some of them result in unexpectedly severe mucositis or diarrhea. Sadly, each of these gastrointestinal toxicities can be fatal if not promptly recognized and treated. As long as aggressive treatment is done, mucositis and diarrhea will remain serious problems for oncologists. Recently, more attention has been paid to prevention and supportive care in this area. A number of international conferences on supportive care in cancer have been held in Europe and the United States. The practical applications of new knowledge in this area are presented in this volume and also in the new journal, *Supportive Care in Cancer*.

II. DEFINITION AND MAGNITUDE OF THE PROBLEM

Many cancer patients are troubled by diarrhea at some time during therapy for malignancy. Usually this is simply an excess number of loose stools for a limited time and is easily managed. Life-threatening diarrhea is seen infrequently and is observed mostly for those on continuous chemotherapy infusions, those receiving radiation to the abdomen or pelvis, and those with pseudomembranous enterocolitis or secretory diarrheas. The Cancer Clinical Trials common toxicity criteria for grading diarrhea are found in Table 1.

III. ETIOLOGY AND PATHOPHYSIOLOGY

Normal bowel function has considerable variation in the healthy adult human, but average values for frequency, weight, water content, and solids are available (1). Normal frequency is defined as up to two stools per day. Diarrhea is defined by one or more of the following: (1) abnormal increase in stool frequency, (2) abnormal increase in stool liquidity, and (3) abnormal increase in stool weight (2,3). These are often accompanied by urgency, incontinence, and abdominal pain and cramps. In a normally nourished adult, approximately 9 liters fluid per day is delivered to the duodenum. Of this, the small bowel absorbs approximately 8 liters per day, the colon absorbs approximately 0.9 liter, and approximately 0.1 liter is excreted as stool liquid. This is an enormous capacity for absorption of fluid while maintaining osmolality and ion concentrations, and there is little reserved capacity; therefore, normal bowel function is easily tipped toward constipation or diarrhea (2).

There are multiple etiologies of diarrhea: (1) unusual amounts of poorly absorbed osmotically active solutes; (2) intestinal ion secretion; (3) inhibition of normal ion absorption and stimulation of ion secretion (secretory diarrhea); (4) abnormal intestinal motility; and (5) inflammatory exudation of mucus, blood, and protein (1–3).

Osmotic diarrheas result from disaccharidase deficiency or mannitol, sorbitol, or lactulose ingestion or poorly absorbed salts and mineral ions in cathartics and antacids, such as magnesium citrate and magnesium hydroxide.

Secretory diarrhea results when enterotoxins or endocrine tumors elaborate secretagogues, such as vasoactive intestinal peptide (VIP) or serotonin, that cause net increases in luminal ions and water. This is often a combination of abnormal ion secretion and inhibition of normal ion absorption.

Deranged motility hurries fluid through the small intestine, with consequent reduced contact time between bowel mucosa and contents. The result is delivery of abnormally large and qualitatively abnormal boluses of fluid to the colon. Overwhelming of colonic absorption or reduced time in transit results in increased

Table 1 Toxicity Criteria

	Grade				
Toxicity	0	1	2	3	4
Diarrhea	None	Increase of 2–3 stools/day over pretherapy	Increase of 4–6 stools/day, or nocturnal stools, or moderate cramping	Increase of 7–9 stools/day, or incontinence, or severe cramping	Increase of ≥10 stools/day or grossly bloody diarrhea, or need for parenteral support
Diarrhea + colostomy	None	Mild increase in loose watery colostomy output compared with pretreatment	Moderate increase in loose watery colostomy output compared with pretreatment	Severe increase in loose watery colostomy output compared with pretreatment	Grossly bloody diarrhea or loose water colostomy output requiring parenteral support

volume and liquidity of stools. The mildest example might be irritable bowel syndrome and a severe example the diarrhea of carcinoid syndrome.

Exudation of fluid, mucus, and blood in variable quantities follows disruption of mucosal integrity by inflammation, infection, or cytotoxic drugs. Arrest of rapidly dividing mucosal cells in the crypts results in atrophy of villus formation and patches of inflamed and infected mucosa.

Most diarrheas are not the result of a single operant mechanism. Most are a combination of mechanisms and, in addition, may be exacerbated by diabetic autonomic neuropathy, thyroid dysfunction, previous bowel surgery, radiation, or advanced age.

Clues to the etiology of an episode of diarrhea are provided in most patients with an established diagnosis of malignancy by their immediate previous therapies: 5-fluorouracil (5-FU) ± leucovorin, 5-FU by continuous infusion, abdominal or pelvic radiation, or antibiotic therapy predisposing to pseudomembranous enterocolitis. In a summary of the toxicity of the 33 most commonly used chemotherapy drugs, only 9 of 33 were noted occasionally to cause diarrhea (4). Only 5-FU was noted as a frequent cause of clinical diarrhea. When 5-FU is given over multiple days or as modulated by folinic acid (leucovorin), diarrhea is a major problem. In a study of 5-FU + high-dose folinic acid for metastatic colon cancer, Asbury et al. reported that 58% had enteritis, severe enough for admission in 30% and fatal in 9% (5). Numerous other reports note that aggressive 5-FU therapy protocols, especially those with folate modulation, can result in death from either diarrhea and dehydration alone or combined with neutropenia and sepsis (6).

Radiation-induced enteritis is most frequently observed after pelvic irradiation for prostate, bladder, or gynecological malignancies (3). Total dose, fractionation, vascular disease, and previous surgery that may have fixed bowel in the pelvis are important variables in the etiology of enteritis. Most patients undergong pelvic irradiation have signs or symptoms of proctitis. Those with a history of ulcerative colitis or diverticular disease have less tolerance to radiation therapy. As with chemotherapy toxicity to the mucosa, there are acute reversible mucosal changes: reduction in the mitotic figures and progressive flattening of columnar cells. This results in villus flattening after 1 week. Late effects include ulceration, stricture, and even perforation. Connective tissue shows amorphous hyalne change and atypical fibroblasts. Smooth muscle atrophy is often present. Radiation vasculitis results in ischemic lesions (3). The bowel may ultimately become narrow, straight, and tubular and lose its haustra; it may resemble ulcerative colitis in gross appearance. The small bowel may histologically resemble Crohn's disease (3). Acutely, there is diarrhea ± tenesmus and rectal bleeding. Malabsorption of B_{12}, bile salts, lactose, and water are noted (7,8). Excess bile acids induce water and electrolyte secretion, increase motility, and decrease transit time (9–11).

The diarrheas caused by endocrine neoplasms are secondary to the circulating hormones produced by these tumors. Their characteristics, diagnosis, and treatment are adequately reviewed in the standard texts (2,12,13). The infectious diarrheas are covered in Chapter 1 and are not covered here, except for pseudomembranous enterocolitis caused by *Clostridium difficile* toxin. This is an often serious and sometimes lethal diarrhea that follows antibiotic therapy, especially with clindamycin, ampicillin, and cephalosporines (2). Some patients seem to develop pseudomembranous enterocolitis after combination chemotherapy, without recent exposure to antibiotics or gastrointestinal surgery. Pseudomembranes composed of fibrin, mucin, inflammatory cells, and sloughed mucosa are noted on examination of the colon. A more advanced stage shows gland disruption. The most advanced form shows necrosis down to the lamina propria, with a correspondingly thicker pseudomembrane (14). Infectious diarrheas were recently reviewed in the literature (15).

IV. CLINICAL PRESENTATION AND COURSE

Many patients with mild to moderate diarrhea delay seeking help until they have tried an over-the-counter preparation that helped in the past. Because these have been intensely promoted in recent years, most patients have ready access to Kaopectate, antispasmodics, and anticholinergics.

Most diarrhea episodes are either self-limited or self-treated to resolution. Those that resist self-medication, are accompanied by considerable spasm and pain, awaken the patient from sleep, or are accompanied by blood trigger medical consultation. Unfortunately, volume loss and dehydration do not, of themselves, seem to trigger appropriate concern in the sufferer. This is especially true in the elderly and very young. Fatalities have been observed in the elderly from excessive volume loss and failure of early recognition and correction of volume and electrolyte depletion (6). Most patients have some degree of crampy abdominal pain with the diarrhea. Varying amounts of mucus and blood may be present. Clinical symptoms at presentation may give some clues to the etiology, as may the history of drug treatment, but diagnostic tests are necessary for definiive diagnosis because diverse etiologies may have similar clinical presentations.

V. DIAGNOSTIC TESTS

Diarrhea in a patient receiving chemotherapy or radiation therapy is usually attributed to the treatment modality involved. This is often the correct assessment, but it remains important to rule out other causes, such as infectious or toxin-mediated enterocolitis, because these may require very specific therapies. A relatively simple and inexpensive diagnostic approach should narrow the

Table 2 Differential Diagnosis of Diarrhea in Cancer Patients[a]

Excessive volume

- I. Impaired absorption
  - A. Malabsorption secondary to loss of normal mucosal integrity
    - 1. Inflammatory diseases
      - a. Radiation enteritis
      - b. Regional enteritis
      - c. Ischemic colitis
      - d. Ulcerative colitis
      - e. Stevens-Johnson syndrome
      - f. Celiac sprue
      - g. Pseudomembranous enterocolitis
    - 2. Invasive infectious diseases
      - a. Bacteria: *Shigella*, *Salmonella*, enteropathogenic *Escherichia coli*
      - b. Viruses
      - c. Protozoa: giardiasis, amebiasis
      - d. Helminths: *Ascaris lumbricoides*, *Necator americanus*, and *Strongyloides stercoralis*
    - 3. Infiltrative diseases
      - a. Intestinal lymphoma
      - b. Intestinal amyloidosis
      - c. Intestinal scleroderma
    - 4. Miscellaneous
      - a. Massive small bowel resection
      - b. Postgastrectomy diarrhea
      - c. Bile salt diarrhea
      - d. Steatorrhea
  - B. Maldigestion
    - 1. Pancreatic insufficiency
    - 2. Lactase deficiency
    - 3. Disaccharidase deficiency
    - 4. Other enzyme deficiencies
- II. Increased secretion
  - A. Bacterial toxins
    - 1. *Clostridium difficile*
    - 2. Enterotoxigenic *E. coli*
    - 3. Food poisoning with *Staphylococcus*, *Bacillus*, or *Clostridium* species
  - B. Humoral factors
    - 1. Non-β islet cell tumors of the pancreas
      - a. Zollinger-Ellison syndrome (gastrin)
      - b. Vasoactive intestinal peptide (VIP-producing tumors)
      - c. Other vasoactive substances
    - 2. Medullary carcinoma of the thyroid
  - C. Miscellaneous: villous adenoma

Table 2 *(Continued)*

Abnormal gastrointestinal motility
- I. Hypermotility with decreased transit time
  - A. Gastrointestinal hemorrhage
  - B. Postgastrectomy with "dumping syndrome"
  - C. Cathartics
  - D. Carcinoid tumors
- II. Hypomotility with intestinal stasis, bacterial overgrowth, secondary malabsorption, and maldigestion
  - A. Stricture
  - B. Diverticula
  - C. Blind loops
  - D. Neuromuscular disease
- III. Miscellaneous
  - A. Diabetic diarrhea
  - B. Postvagotomy
  - C. Irritable bowel syndrome

[a]Diarrhea is categorized according to pathophysiological mechanisms as described in the text. Any one episode may be mediated by several mechanisms. All patients are presumed to have received chemotherapy drugs and/or radiation therapy.
Source: Adapted from Ref. 17.

differential diagnosis. White cells ± blood in the stool denote inflammation and help to distinguish bacterial from nonbacterial causes of diarrhea. Blood without white cells indicates either tumor invasion of the bowel or recent bowel surgery. Cultures should be done to rule out *Salmonella*, *Shigella*, *Campylobacter*, and enterotoxigenic *Escherichia coli*. Smears for *Cryptosporidium* are occasionally indicated, especially in those with acquired immunodeficiency syndrome (AIDS). Toxin assay for *C. difficile* should not be overlooked. A problem-oriented approach to differential diagnosis is found in Table 2. This is intended as a first approach to diagnosis in an adult with an established diagnosis of malignancy undergoing treatment. It should be emphasized that for patients without a previous history of gastrointestinal illness and whose diagnosis does not appear in Table 2, consultation with a gastroenterologist or reference to a more comprehensive differential diagnosis is imperative (2,3,16–18).

Most acute diarrhea episodes resolve with a week or less of supportive care if the chemotherapy agents are discontinued and no other etiology is identified. Those that persist beyond this time must be evaluated for other etiologies besides chemotherapy associated, for example infectious agents, toxins, or ischemia. Most acute episodes of diarrhea following chemotherapy respond well to simple supportive measures, but those with grade III or IV toxicity (Table 1) require considerably more attention and support to avoid catastrophic outcome.

VI. THERAPY OF DIARRHEA

It is difficult to assess over the telephone the severity of diarrhea and the need for intervention. Many patients seem to underestimate the number of stools per day, duration of diarrhea, and extent of volume loss. Often when such patients present to the clinic, they are significantly volume depleted, as manifested by postural hypotension, decreased skin turgor, and oliguria. Such acute fluid and electrolyte losses can be life threatening unless replaced in a timely fashion. Standard texts contain recommendations for estimating extracellular fluid and electrolyte deficits and acid-base imbalance (2,3,18). These recommendations should be followed to determine the volume and electrolyte composition of replacement fluids. Water deficit can be estimated by the following equation, in which body weight is estimated weight in kg when fully hydrated; Na^+ is serum or plasma sodium.

$$\text{Water deficit} = 0.6 \times \text{body weight} \times \left[1 - \left(\frac{140}{Na^+}\right)\right]$$

Corrected sodium is necessary if blood glucose is greater than 150, and for each kg water deficit, 1 liter appropriate crystalloid is given as replacement (15,19).

Normal saline solutions can be given rapidly (300–500 ml/h) until 2–3 liters is delivered, as long as the patient is closely observed for pulmonary edema and the solution does not result in the delivery of more than 10 mEq/h of potassium. Potassium deficit should be estimated based on the serum potassium concentration. A serum potassium of 3.0–3.5 corresponds to a 150–300 mEq deficit, a serum potassium of 2.5–3.0 is equivalent to a 300–500 mEq deficiency, and for each additional decrease in serum potassium by 1.0 mEq/liter, there is approximately a 200–400 mEq additional deficit. Correction of hypokalemia is most important in patients with cardiac disease and those on digitalis to decrease conduction disturbances and dysrhythmias. For serum potassium levels greater than 2.5 mEq/liter, potassium can be given at a rate of up to 10 mEq/h and in concentrations of up to 30 mEq/liter. If estimated potassium deficit is large, a portion can be given orally to limit the intravenous (IV) amount so that rapid infusion rates and larger volumes can be delivered when necessary. It is inefficient to rehydrate at 100–200 ml/h when most adults without a history of congestive heart failure can tolerate 500 ml/h of crystalloid for long enough to replace a multiliter volume deficit. This type of rehydration is best done in a hospital setting, especially if diarrhea remains an ongoing process. Strict measurements of input and output and electrolyte changes are required. A measure of successful hydration is a urine output $\geq$30 ml/h, urine specific gravity

≥1.010, and resolution of postural hypotension. For those with lesser volume deficits and some oral intake, daily IV hydration of 1–2 liters may be sufficient. Some patients can use oral home hydration with isotonic fluids, such as Gatorade. Because chemotherapy-related acute diarrhea is often self-limited, rehydration and maintenance fluids for several days should be adequate therapy.

Patients often self-medicate or seek prescriptions for symptoms associated with diarrhea. Such adsorbents as Kaopectate do not affect the course of disease but, in milder cases, may help solidify stools and allow more voluntary control of defecation. They usually fail to help those diarrheas that need medical attention. Opiates diminish peristalsis and slow gut transit time but are contraindicated in toxin-mediated or infectious diarrheas because they allow the toxic gut contents to remain in mucosal contact in pooled secretions in hypoactive loops of bowel.

Anticholinergics, such as dicyclomine (Bentyl Hydrochloride), are not useful. Antisecretory agents, such as octreotide, may help in secretory diarrheas and are occasionally used empirically in other refractory diarrheas for which toxin and infectious etiologies have been excluded. For those who are febrile and neutropenic as well, empirical antibiotics are given. Specific antimicrobial therapies of infectious diarrheas are available from many references (e.g., Refs. 15 and 18).

An excellent guide to the assessment and treatment of diarrhea in children was published recently (19). It contains useful information regarding at-home oral rehydration fluids, as well as intravenous rehydration and nutritional support.

VII. PREVENTION OF DIARRHEA

Unfortunately, there is no a priori method of determining who will have severe gastrointestinal toxicity from chemotherapy regimens. However, experience has identified those drugs and delivery strategies that place the patient at most risk (see Secs. III and IV). Thus, patients receiving 5-FU modulated with leucovorin, 5-FU by continuous infusion, or by multiple daily bolus doses to saturate degradation enzymes are at high risk. They should be cautioned that this treatment can induce life-threatening diarrhea so that early evaluation and therapy are possible. Most protocols require significant reductions in drug doses following an initial episode of severe diarrhea. The Cancer Clinical Trials Common Toxicity Criteria for diarrhea are reproduced in Table 1. A grade II toxicity requires a 20% reduction in 5-FU in many colon cancer protocols, and grade III or IV toxicity requires a 30% reduction in drug dose. This strategy helps prevent subsequent episodes. For those patients for whom dose reduction does not prevent grade II or III recurrent episodes of diarrhea, daily outpatient hydration of 1–2 liters saline solution often reduces the worst of the volume, electrolyte, and acid-base disturbances so that the chemotherapy regimen need not be abandoned.

Prevention of irradiation-induced bowel spasm and diarrhea has long been a desirable goal of research. Steroid enemas and bile acid sequestering resins have only provided brief palliation and may have a considerable number of side effects. A more effective therapy may be sucralfate, a sulfated sucrose compound used for healing gastric ulcers. In a prospective, randomized, double-blind placebo-controlled trial in pelvic malignancies treated with curative intent, to doses of 62–66 Gy, it was shown that sucralfate decreased stool frequency and increased stool consistency compared with placebo (20). Diminished bowel discomfort was also reported in the treated group. The authors speculate that sucralfate served as a protective barrier from acids, enzymes, and bacteria for denuded mucosa. The increased concentrations of bile acids as a result of malabsorption are controlled by binding with sucralfate, reducing their activity on the mucosa. This study suggests real benefit from a simple oral therapy for the many patients who undergo definitive radiation therapy for bladder, prostate, and cervix cancers.

The role of nutritional support in limiting gastrointestinal toxicity and maintaining weight is an important area for research. It has been shown that maintaining normal protein intake during 5-FU chemotherapy of tumor-bearing animals resulted in decreased incidence and duration of diarrhea and increased body weight compared with similarly treated tumor-bearing animals fed a protein-depleted but isocaloric diet (21). Perhaps in the human, earlier therapy with intravenous protein-sparing solutions would similarly decrease the severity of mucositis and diarrhea compared with therapy when these toxicities are already well established. As with burns, mucosal injury is better prevented than treated.

VIII. FUTURE RESEARCH ON DIARRHEA

There is much research and progress on the roles of bile salts and disaccharides in chemotherapy-induced diarrhea. In addition, data are being gathered from cooperative group clinical trials on the grade and duration of diarrhea experienced, as well as the type and duration of supportive care required. Retrospective analysis of these data will better define risk of diarrhea by regimen, patient age, functional status at enrollment, and numerous other parameters. Thus, high-risk situations can be better defined, allowing the oncologist to closely watch the patients at highest risk. Further attention should be directed toward oral rehydration solutions for inexpensive therapy of less severe grades of diarrhea. Most patients can take oral fluid but often are not sure what to take. Coca or ginger ale (after decarbonation) is often recommended, but in my experience, Gatorade and similar dilute salt solutions with less carbohydrate are more tolerable and more effective as oral rehydration. A prospective randomized trial of Gatorade versus some more traditional rehydration fluid would be useful in advancing outpatient therapeutic options.

Some oncologists recommend empirical use of octreotide in secretory diarrheas for which toxins or infectious agents have been ruled out. Further definition of the role of octreotide in noncarcinoid diarrheal syndromes is needed. Further work on the role of cost-effective nutritional support in limiting gastrointestinal toxicity would be most helpful.

ANNOTATED BIBLIOGRAPHY

Davenport HW. Physiology of the Digestive Tract, 4th ed. Chicago: Yearbook Medical, 1977. An excellent compendium of human gastrointestinal motility secretion, digestion, and absorption.

Mitchell EP. GI toxicity of chemotherapeutic agents. Semin Oncol 1992; 19:572–579. This is the most recent and comprehensive review of the subject. The table on pages 454–455 summarizes a great deal of reference material in a concise manner. Highly recommended reading.

U.S. Public Health Service. The management of acute diarrhea in children: oral rehydration, maintenance, and nutritional therapy. 1992; MMWR 41:RR–16. This "recommendation and report" discusses home as well as hospital rehydration solutions. It is an excellent guide to assessment and treatment.

Slesinger MH, Fordtran JS. Gastrointestinal Diseases, 4th ed. Philadelphia: W. B. Saunders, 1989. A comprehensive two-volume work. Of interest are chapters on neoplasms causing secretory diarrhea, lymphoma of the gastrointestinal tract, and AIDS enteropathy.

Spiro HM. Gastroenterology, 3rd ed. New York: Macmillan, 1983. A classic reference, slightly dated. Radiation enteritis is well considered here.

REFERENCES

1. Davenport HW. Physiology of the Digestive Tract, 4th ed. Chicago: Yearbook Medical, 1977.
2. Slesinger MH, Fordtran JS. Gastrointestinal Diseases, 4th ed. Philadelphia: W. B. Saunders, 1989.
3. Spiro HM. Gastroenterology, 3rd ed. New York: Macmillan, 1983.
4. Mitchell EP. GI toxicity of chemotherapeutic agents. Semin Oncol 1992; 19:572–579.
5. Asbury RF, Boros L, Brower M, et al. 5-FU and high dose folic acid treatment for metastatic colon cancer. Am J Clin Oncol 1987; 10:47–49.
6. Grem JL, Shoemaker DD, Petrelli NJ, Douglass HO Jr. Severe and fatal toxic effects observed in treatment with high- and low-dose leucovorin plus 5-fluorouracil for colorectal carcinoma. Cancer Treat Rep 1987; 71:1122.
7. Thomas PRM, Lindblad AS, Stablein DM. Toxicity associated with adjuvant postoperative therapy for adenocarcinoma of the rectum. Cancer 1986; 57:1130–1134.
8. Kelvin FM, Gramm HF, Gluck WL, et al. Radiologic manifestations of small bowel toxicity due to floxuridine therapy. Am J Radiol 1986; 146:39–43.

9. Arlow FL, Dekovich AA, Priest RJ, et al. Bile acids in radiation-induced diarrhea. South Med J 1987; 80:1259–1261.
10. Yeoh EK, Lui D, Lee NY. The mechanism of diarrhea resulting from pelvic and abdominal radiotherapy; a prospective study using selenium-75 labeled conjugated bile acid and cobalt-58 labeled cyanocobalamin. Br J Radiol 1984; 57:1131–1136.
11. Fernandez-Banares F, Villa S, Esteve M, et al. Acute effects of abdominal pelvic irradiation on the orocecal transit time: its relation to clinical symptoms, and bile salt and lactose malabsorption. J Gastroenterol 1991; 86:1771–1776.
12. Moossa AR, Schimpff SC, Robson MC. Comprehensive Textbook of Oncology. Baltimore: Williams & Wilkins, 1991.
13. Krejs GJ, ed. Diarrhea. Clin Gastroenterol 1986; 15:603–629.
14. Bartlett JG. The pseudomembranous enterocolitides. In: Slesinger MH, Fordtran JS, eds. Gastrointestinal Diseases, 4th ed. Philadelphia: W. B. Saunders, 1989.
15. Woodley M, Whelan A., eds. Manual of Medical Therapeutic. Boston: Little, Brown, 1992:261–264.
16. Friedman HH, ed. Problem-Oriented Medical Diagnosis, 5th ed. Boston: Little, Brown, 1991.
17. Gottlieb AJ, Zamkoff KW, Jastremski MS, Scalzo A, Imboden KJ. The Whole Internist Catalog. Philadelphia: W. B. Saunders, 1980.
18. Eastwood GL, Avunduk C, eds. Manual of Gastroenterology, Diagnosis, and Therapy. Boston: Little, Brown, 1988.
19. U.S. Public Health Service. The management of acute diarrhea in children. MMWR 1992; 41:RR–16.
20. Henriksson R, Franzen L, Littbrand B. Prevention of irradiation-induced bowel discomfort by sucralfate: a double-blind placebo-controlled study when treating localized pelvic cancer. Am J Med 1991; 91(suppl. 2A):151S–156S.
21. Torosian MH, Jaloli S, Nguyaen HQ. Protein intake and 5-fluorouracil toxicity in tumor bearing animals. J Surg Res 1990; 49:298–301.

8

Nutritional Support

Anders Hyltander, Rolf Sandström, and Kent Lundholm
Sahlgrenska University Hospital, Göteborg, Sweden

I. INTRODUCTION

Malnutrition is a common feature of cancer patients and constitutes an ominous sign to clinicians and family members because weight loss is often the first symptom of a serious and potentially life-threatening illness. Unless the patient is cured or in a stable state of remission, the continuous breakdown of lean tissues ensues, eventually leading to cachexia with a reduced quality of life, and in the long run it is inconsistent with survival. Clinicians have since long experienced that malnutrition may jeopardize successful surgical treatment (1,2). Such risks also occur in undernourished patients who receive treatment with chemotherapy, radiation, and biological response modifiers (3,4). The development and refinement of enteral and parenteral nutrition introduced some 30 years ago was expected to be a significant adjunct to cancer therapy. However, despite numerous efforts and attempts to prove its benefit in malnourished patients as adjunct to surgery and other therapies, very few reports demonstrating such improvements have been published. Several explanations may exist. Most studies have been inappropriately designed (5). Artificial nutrition is only one of several treatments in a multifactorial scenario. To demonstrate the effect of nutrition on outcome and mortality, numerous patients are required, exceeding the patient population by severalfold the number generally presented in most studies. However, investigations aimed to evaluate biochemical alterations and reversal of signs of undernutrition have been more rewarding (6,7). Thus, it can be safely concluded that artificial nutrition, either parenteral or enteral, impacts on the nutritional state in most cancer patients irrespective of type of tumor or concomitant therapy. If so, has nutritional therapy proved its efficacy as a meaningful adjunct to interventional therapy and palliative procedures? We require evidence to justify the medical feasibility of artificial nutrition economically, functionally, and ethically. Nutritionists are not alone in this regard: for example, very few well-recognized surgical procedures have actually been evaluated for their economical and therapeutic effectiveness. There is now a trend from authorities to request confirmation of superior results compared to current methods before new strategies and concepts are formally accepted, which is sound. This trend has not left the field of nutrition research uninfluenced. However, before we can start to adopt such requirements on nutrition, we must define and determine the purpose of nutrition in medicine. After all, provision of substrates and nutrients to patients under medical treatment may be compared with food supply only. It is therefore not equal to drug administration in most aspects, although future development of the concept of "nutritional pharmacology" opens up exciting possibilities (8). However, even in its present and more conservative setting, the optimal use and indications for nutrition must be defined.

II. PATHOPHYSIOLOGY

A. Anorexia

The importance of anorexia as a contributing factor to cancer cachexia is sometime underestimated (9). Anorexia in cancer disease may be such a potent factor that it is not possible to overcome with encouragement of patients to consume extra meals or energy-enriched food. Nausea and vomiting may develop in association with progression of the disease and are extremely common in patients undergoing chemotherapy. It is generally not possible to support such patients by the enteral route, leaving the clinician with partial or total parental nutrition as the only alternative. In cancer disease, anorexia may be an appropriate adaptation, at least in the short term: it has been demonstrated that starvation in the experimental setting retards tumor growth and partially inhibits tumor proliferation in the G_0–G_1 phase (10).

The role of cytokines as promoters of anorexia has been proposed in recent years. Administration of interleukin-1 (IL-1) and tumor necrosis factor (TNF) to experimental animals induces wasting comparable to clinical conditions associated with inflammation and cancer and reduction of food intake in a dose-dependent manner (11). Administration of antibodies against the TNF molecule and the IL-1 receptor improved food intake in experimental tumor systems, with a simultaneous reduction in tumor growth (12).

B. Elevated Energy Expenditure

Although anorexia has been identified as a common phenomenon, the role of increased energy expenditure has been controversial, and there are conflicting reports in the literature about whether cancer patients exhibit elevated resting energy expenditure. We investigated a large cohort of surgical patients with various types of solid tumors in patients with or without weight loss (13). Resting energy expenditure (REE) was compared with resting metabolism in matched patients without cancer. The large number of investigated patients allowed extended statistical and mathematical evaluation. Elevated energy metabolism was a consistent finding, not only in weight-losing but also in weight-stable cancer patients irrespective of whether REE was normalized to body weight or to body surface area (Fig. 1) (13). Fat oxidation was increased in both weight-losing and weight-stable cancer patients. Therefore, increased resting energy expenditure seems to be a metabolic event that may occur early in the clinical course of cancer. Although small in absolute magnitude, increased REE in cancer patients may explain the loss of several kilograms body weight over a period of 4–6 months. Evaluation of covarying factors suggested heart rate as a factor with significant predictive value, explaining in part elevated REE in cancer patients. This finding supports the contention that cancer patients have increased adrenergic activity compared with malnourished patients without cancer disease, who generally show a decreased adrenergic tone and catecholamine turnover (14). Investigations from our laboratory also indicated the appearance of a myocardial β receptor with high affinity for adrenergic agonists in malnourished tumor-bearing rats (15). This finding was suggested as a compensatory mechanism to maintain pumping capacity during progressive depletion because heart

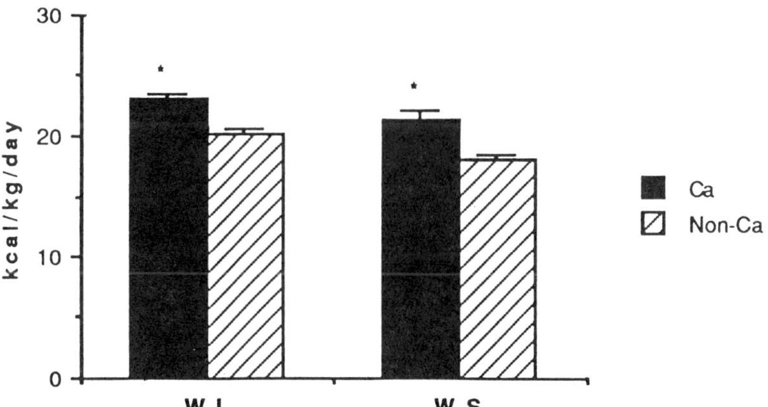

Figure 1 Differences in resting energy expenditure in 204 patients with (solid bars) and without (hatched bars) cancer. The patients were classified as either weight losing (WL) if they had experienced a loss of more than 4% body weight within the last 3 months or weight stable (WS). Cancer patients had a significantly increased energy expenditure compared with noncancer controls irrespective of weight loss.

muscle mass is reduced to a similar extent as in skeletal muscles in weight-losing cancer-bearing hosts. The heart may thus be one organ that consumes disproportionally more oxygen than normally, accounting for the degree of malnutrition. An increased cardiac sensitivity to adrenergic agonists may then increase the risk for arrythmias in situations with increased stress, such as induction of anesthesia and surgery.

In agreement with high adrenergic activity in cancer patients, we found a reduction in REE by propranolol treatment in cancer patients corresponding to approximately 10% (Fig. 2) (16). Propranolol also reduced REE in a group of healthy volunteers, but to a lower extent. Treatment with antiinflammatory drugs, such as indomethacin, seemed not to have significant effects on REE compared with placebo treatment. Therefore, it is likely that adrenergic factors are significant in increased energy expenditure in cachectic cancer patients, and inflammation may be less important in this respect (16).

C. Additional Changes in Metabolism

The metabolic adaption in progressive cancer disease differs in some respects from that in pure starvation (17). The turnover of body proteins is usually increased in cachectic cancer patients. In experimental cancer-bearing animals, the site of increased protein turnover was mainly in visceral and immune tissues. However, the expectation that cancer patients have increased skeletal muscle breakdown activity has not been confirmed in a majority of investigations. It is

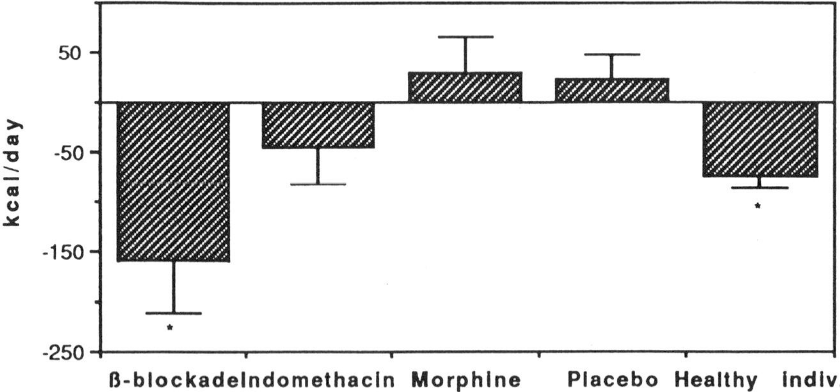

Figure 2 Changes in resting energy expenditure after drug treatment for 5 days in weight-losing cancer patients. Only β blockade (propranolol) reduced resting energy expenditure significantly in cancer patients as in healthy control patients. (Reproduced from Ref. 16.)

thus more likely that the loss of muscle tissues in cancer patients is generally explained by reduced synthesis rather than increased breakdown (18).

Early studies of substrate metabolism in cancer disease demonstrated an increased recycling of glucose through lactate, although studies have shown that this "futile cycling" can account for only a minor fraction of the increased energy expenditure. The most simple explanation for this increased reutilization of glucose carbons is the finding of elevated gluconeogenesis, with alanine, lactate, and glycerol as important precursors (19).

Studies of lipid metabolism in cancer patients have shown increased plasma concentrations of free fatty acids and glycerol without evidence of increased reesterification of free fatty acids. Measurements of glycerol dynamics confirmed an increased plasma turnover of glycerol in weight-losing cancer patients, explained in part by increased whole-body lipolysis (20). Such alterations in lipid metabolism may be explained by insulin resistance as the causal factor, perhaps as a result of elevated adrenergic activity promoting lipolysis.

III. EFFECTS OF ARTIFICIAL NUTRITION ON MALNOURISHED SUBJECTS

A. Nutrition in Cancer Surgery

Two controlled studies have shown that perioperative, particularly preoperative nutrition, is efficient in improving outcome by reducing postoperative morbidity and mortality (21, 22).

We recently reported the effect of total parenteral nutrition (TPN) on outcome following surgery: 300 unselected patients undergoing major surgical procedures (mainly cancer surgery) were randomized to receive either total parenteral nutrition or glucose alone with electrolytes from the first postoperative day until they could start eating freely (23). The parenteral regimen was defined to provide patients with an individual daily support of nonprotein energy corresponding to 120% of their daily measured resting energy expenditure, which was regarded as a standard therapy (24). Nonprotein energy was provided as 60% glucose and 40% fat in the form of long-chain triglycerides (LCT). Nitrogen was supplied in the form of crystalline amino acid solutions to cover the total nitrogen loss determined individually on a daily basis for all patients. Our results showed an overall mortality rate of 6–7% in all patients. No significant differences were found between TPN and glucose-treated patients when statistical evaluation was performed according to *intention to treat*. This unexpected finding was certainly explained by the fact that around 60% of all patients succeeded in eating within 8–9 days postoperatively, and this length of time was obviously not long enough to allow insufficient intake to be translated into a limiting factor. However, in the remaining 40% of our patients other results were found. Subgroup analyses revealed a very high mortality and complication rate in some patients. Thus, around 20% of all patients were not able to start eating within 14 days postoperatively, and they were therefore by definition treated by TPN for the remaining and following days until they were able to eat. The mortality rate was 21% in this group, which was significantly higher than in those patients who were able to start eating early (mortality 6–7%). However, in additional TPN-treated patients, representing 20% of all randomized patients, TPN according to the protocol had a very low treatment compliance because of numerous early side effects, mainly of a cardiopulmonary nature. This group of patients had a mortality rate of around 36%. We concluded from our study that around 40% of patients scheduled for major cancer surgery may represent high-risk patients in whom inappropriate nutrition may be detrimental. In this sense, inappropriate nutrition may be both under- and overfeeding. Thus, depending on the degree of preceding malnutrition, it can be concluded that artificial nutrition becomes a life-supporting modality beyond 12–14 days in postoperative patients following major surgery in patients who have not started with sufficient spontaneous oral intake around 10 days postoperatively.

B. Nutrition and Quality of Life

Most studies evaluating the role of nutrition in oncology service have focused on tumor treatment outcome without impressive benefit to the patient. This negative situation was certainly in part dependent on the fact that most tumor treatment modalities under test were less than effective in themselves. Therefore, it is not unexpected to find that the role of an adjunct therapy was difficult to delineate. A principally different condition is the role of nutrition in bone marrow transplantation following chemotherapy (25). However, artificial nutrition in such randomized controlled studies has not appeared to be rewarding, which again may be explained by the fact that bone marrow cellular recoveries were more dependent on growth factor regulation than substrate availability, although it has been emphasized that for these factors to exert their optimal effects—appropriate cell growth—nutritional requirements must be present (26).

Available information on the role of nutrition in oncology suggests that more focus should be related to those aspects that are primarily dependent on organ function and quality of life aspects (27). Few attempts have been made to study the role of nutrition for quality of life improvement. This may be because few clinical test models can evaluate integrated function and quality of life in patients suffering from severe disease. Some attempts have been made to correlate involuntary muscular strength to the degree of undernutrition and to correlate the subjective feeling of fatigue to abnormalities in nutritional state, particularly in the postoperative period (28). It is our clinical impression that the sensation of fatigue may be a more initial and sensitive marker for abnormality than involuntary muscle function. Therefore, such approaches should be encouraged in the future.

C. Nutrition and Chemotherapy

Chemotherapy usually induces undernutrition. This can be explained either by the induction of anorexia or by a direct toxic effect at the cellular level with inhibition of DNA and RNA synthesis.The next result is progressive malnutrition associated with increased morbidity and decreased quality of life. Thus, it was assumed that patients undergoing chemotherapy should benefit from nutritional support, especially with respect to the patient's ability to fullfill the planned treatment. It was also expected that serious side effects, such as bone marrow depression with granulocytopenia and anemia followed by intercurrent infections, should be reduced (3,4). These assumptions were based on the finding of an association between severe malnutrition and increased morbidity in infectious diseases. However, despite numerous studies, no controlled prospective study has demonstrated a major beneficial effect of parenteral nutrition as adjunct to patients undergoing chemotherapy. On the contrary, meta analyses of such studies suggested increased morbidity and mortality in infectious complications even when catheter-related septicemia was excluded in patients receiving nutritional support (3). On the basis of our present knowledge, this may not be surprising because chemotherapeutic agents exert direct toxic effects on gastrointestinal mucosal cells and bone marrow stem cells. These effects are thus not the alterations usually associated with pure substrate deficiency, although it has been reported that a reduced oral intake may lead to atrophy of the intestinal mucosa in experimental animals (29).

In our own attempts to evaluate the role of artificial nutrition during chemotherapy, young men with testicular carcinoma were studied (30). Such patients generally do not suffer from overt malnutrition at the beginning of the treatment, which was a combination of surgery and heavy combination chemotherapy with iterated courses of cisplatin (Platinol), vincristine, and bleomycin (PVB treatment). This treatment is superior to many other chemotherapeutic regimens for solid tumors because it is effective and dramatically influences the natural course of the disease in terms of disease-free survival and probably also survival. The severe state of undernutrition that patients develop during PVB treatment was thus entirely caused by the drugs and less by a progressive component of the underlying disease. This model therefore had several advantages in clarification of the effect of nutritional support to cancer patients on chemotherapy.

One question to address in patients with testicular carcinoma was whether vigorous nutritional support could protect body composition. This should be so, since a part of patients' weight loss could be explained by insufficient spontaneous intake because of anorexia and drug toxicity. Hospital intravenous nutrition covering more than the basal expenditure, however, did not improve the protein status compared with control patients, who were allowed to rely on spontaneous oral intake only (30). This was an unexpected observation, because provision of nitrogen and calories could be utilized according to additional experiments. Additional measurements revealed that the hospital TPN-treated patients had such a low oral intake at home between courses of chemotherapy that the cumulative intake of nonprotein energy and proteins was insufficient to cover the maintenance of normal body composition over several months. Food intake at home in the TPN group was as low as the intake by the spontaneously eating control group. Thus, hospital nutrition did not overcome the undernutrition in outpatients with prolonged anorexia and drug toxicity when time was considered (30). The next question was to evaluate whether continuous intravenous nutrition, with combined hospital and home parenteral nutrition, could improve the situation. Study patients were randomized to receive continuous intravenous nutrition from the first day of chemotherapy treatment (PVB) until they finished all courses (31). Again, the control group had spontaneous oral intake only. This study revealed that continuous nutrition was effective to prevent loss in body weight, and several patients even increased their body weight; the control group lost weight, as expected. Measurement of body composition revealed that weight maintenance was mainly a result of fat accumulation without protection of whole-body protein status. Evaluation of exercise capacity revealed that chemotherapy decreased the maximum working capacity from around 185 W before treatment to 135 W after treatment (Fig. 3). This decline in exercise capacity, which represents a substantial decrease in function, was not improved by home parenteral nutrition.

There is no evidence that cancer patients not receiving chemotherapy should be unable to utilize nutrition to the same extent as patients without cancer irrespective of being malnourished (32). However, standard TPN support did not allow protection of normal body composition and thereby preservation of body function in conjunction with chemotherapy. The question of whether toxic drugs have anything to do with this finding is not yet definitely clarified, although our initial investigation gave support to the suggestion that the patients were able to utilize nitrogen provision.

D. Nutrition and Tumor Growth

The ultimate goal for nutritional therapy in cancer patients is an efficient repletion of lean body mass and fat stores without stimulation of tumor growth. Stimulation of tumor growth by intravenous nutrition has repeatedly been demonstrated in experimental cancer, with increases in tumor weight and mitotic activity (10). Conversely, food restriction has resulted in inhibition of tumor growth (10).

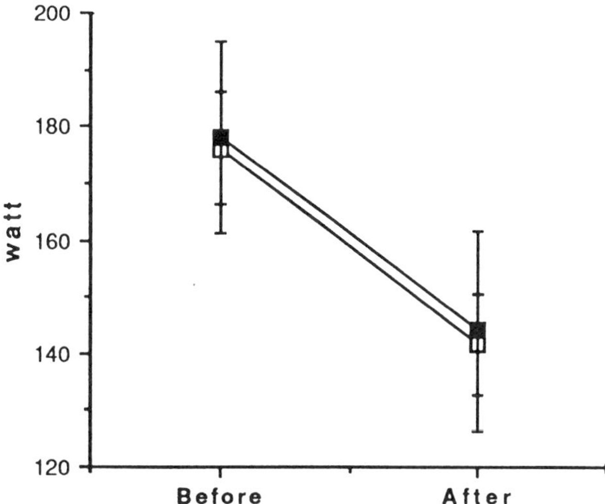

Figure 3 Changes in maximal exercise capacity in young men with testicular carcinoma before and after chemotherapy. The decline in exercise capacity both in patients receiving TPN (open symbols) and in patients confined to spontaneous oral intake (control patients, closed symbols) during the entire course of chemotherapy was statistically significant. (Reproduced from Ref. 31.)

Measurements of tumor response to feeding with flow cytometry for analysis of cell cycle distribution and the proportion of aneuploid cells have demonstrated that tumor growth in response to starvation and refeeding was rapid and highly reproducible (33). Analyses of substrate utilization in experimental cancer have demonstrated that the carbohydrate component in food had the most pronounced effect in stimulating tumor growth (34). However, whether these effects are transferable to human cancer is unclear because there may be differences in tumor sensitivity between experimental and clinical cancer. In animal experiments the tumors are often bulky, constituting 20–25% of carcass weight, and they grow very quickly and kill the animal within weeks.

Studies of substrate utilization in vivo across human malignant gastric and colon cancers have revealed that glucose is preferentially extracted by tumor tissue, supporting data from animal studies (35,36). Moreover, studies with repeated biopsies of human colon cancer have demonstrated a powerful stimulation of protein synthesis, measured as leucine incorporation, in tumor in response to short-term nutritional provision (37). These data suggest that tumor cell kinetics may be influenced by intravenous nutrition. This area of research is important, because the frequency of nutritional support to cancer patients is steadily increasing. Present knowledge about the role of nutrition stimulation of tumor growth is restricted, however, and does not yet allow recommendations for a specially designed nutritional therapy for cancer patients.

E. Nutrition Kinetics

Based on studies in our laboratory, we suspect that inefficient protection of body composition in cancer patients on either TPN or enteral nutrition may be less efficient than generally expected. We have repeatedly observed that patients on artificial nutrition do not switch amino acid kinetics to clear-cut anabolism, which was evident for other substrates as glucose, glycerol, free fatty acids when measured across peripheral tissues (38). It has also been pointed out by many authors that it is usually difficult to reverse undernutrition in patients suffering from stress. It may be easier to replenish protein status in patients with overt protein depletion, however, than in those suffering from only mild or no protein deficiency. Thus, Hill and coworkers recently emphasized that pronounced protein depletion must be present in patients before they can accrete proteins following intravenous nutrition (39). These results make sense, because nitrogen provision should not expand protein compartments beyond their individual normal size; that is, it is not possible to expand normal muscle mass merely by eating. Protein mass in a subject is genetically determined and is significantly expanded beyond normality, mainly by physical training. However, one of the most significant observations in the report by Hill and colleagues was that intravenous nutrition did not *protect* from further protein loss in those patients suffering from no or mild protein undernutrition. These results obtained with long-term (14 days) nutritional intervention agree with our results obtained in both acute investigations evaluating amino acid kinetics (38) and long-term nutritional interventions (3 months) (31). Thus, artifical nutrition was surprisingly often accompanied by amino acid flux that did not confirm anabolism in peripheral tissues. This was particularly so in the skeletal muscles, which represent a functional reservoir of proteins that can be rapidly degraded for support of both amino acids and the generation of putative carbon 3 fragments for intermediary metabolism in other cells. Similar results were available from numerous studies of both cancer and noncancer patients on nutritional support irrespective of being on active cancer treatment (40,41).

F. New Substrates

Among other important issues to be addressed to improve effectiveness of TPN is the composition of nutrient solutions, that is, lipid and amino acid solutions. Based on animal experiments, it has been proposed that emulsions with medium-chain triglycerides (MCT) may have advantages to the traditional long-chain triglyceride emulsions, such as higher plasma clearance and more rapid oxidation rate (42). MCT-containing lipid solutions may also accumulate to a lower extent in the reticuloendothelial system (RES) during long-term treatment (43). The clinical significance of less pronounced effects on RES function is still unclear, however. Pure MCT emulsions may be toxic in high doses, and they do not contain essential polyunsaturated fatty acids, as do LCT emulsions. A possible method of combining the advantageous effects of LCT and MCT emulsions would be to esterify LCTs and MCTs in a random fashion on the carbon skeleton of glycerol, which would result in "structured triglycerides." Preliminary clinical studies in our laboratory have demonstrated that structured triglycerides are comparable to LCT-containing emulsions with regard to tolerance and safety (44). Evaluations of the oxidation rate of structured triglycerides compared to oxidation of LCT emulsions are now under investigation. It is possible that lipid emulsions consisting of structured triglycerides may provide an energy-rich substrate that is rapidly oxidized, offering advantages in patients in whom a reduced carbohydrate supply is necessary.

Amino acids constitute precursors essential for protein synthesis. Glutamine is one of the most abundant amino acids in the body and is an important substrate and regulator in a wide variety of metabolic reactions. Glutamine has also been suggested as an essential nutrient for enterocytes, although it is not present in commercially available parenteral nutrient solutions. There are several examples in which adding glutamine to the diet can alter outcome in laboratory animals. Glutamine has been reported to reduce endotoxinemia in a lethal model of methotrexate-induced enterocolitis, and bacteremia caused by translocation from the gut could be reduced from 51 to 7% after severe burn injury in rats by the administration of bombesin, which prevents mucosal atrophy (29). Glutamine has also been reported to prevent pancreatic atrophy and fatty liver during elemental feeding following extensive jejunoileal resection in rats (45), and it protected the intestinal mucosa from radiation injury by supporting crypt cell proliferation (46). However, although both glutamine and fiber supplementation of a defined formula diet prevented loss of bowel mass, neither substances resulted in effective protection against spontaneous bacterial gut translocation, endotoxin-induced bacterial translocation, or mortality when animals were challenged with exogenous endotoxin (47). Although interesting, the role of glutamine in supporting enterocyte proliferation and gut barrier function in humans remains to be determined. However, glutamine can be provided without clinical evidence of toxicity or appearance of toxic metabolites (ammonia and glutamate) when infused intravenously in normal subjects during 4 h at doses of 0.0125 and 0.025 g/kg/h (48).

Glutamine supplementation of amino acid solutions may thus represent a significant modification of today's TPN treatment. Our own studies of amino acid fluxes across peripheral muscle tissues in TPN-treated patients have repeatedly demonstrated a negative balance of tyrosine and phenylalanine (38). These amino acids are not metabolized in skeletal muscle tissue and may therefore represent suitable indicators for protein balance in peripheral tissues. The negative balance of these amino acids across peripheral muscle tissues during TPN infusion indicates a subnormal supply, particularly of tyrosine. Whether increased amounts of tyrosine in amino acid solutions have any positive effect on protein accretion in peripheral skeletal muscle remains to be evaluated. Interest has also been focused on arginine because of its effects as an immune stimulator (49). L-arginine is also the substrate for nitrous oxide synthesis, which is an important modulator of vasoactivity (50). The role of arginine supply is unclear.

G. Pharmacological and Hormonal Manipulation

In most textbooks insulin is described as a potent stimulator of protein synthesis. However, the role of insulin in regulating protein balance is not clear. Studies on the cellular level with either perfused organs or fortified cellular systems have generally demonstrated that insulin stimulates protein synthesis (51), but results obtained from intact animals and humans have been less convincing (52). The lack of insulin in a diabetic subject induces loss of body nitrogen. However, this is not equivalent to the effect of insulin in stimulating protein synthesis (53). Recent investigations in humans have confirmed that insulin attenuated protein breakdown selectively without effects on protein synthesis (54). These results have also been observed in our own studies on healthy volunteers with simultaneous infusion of amino acids to elevate plasma concentrations of amino acids (55). In this study a postabsorptive increase in plasma insulin improved protein balance by decreasing protein breakdown, however, without inhibition of breakdown of the major myofibrillar protein pool as measured with 3-methylhistidine release from skeletal muscle. Therefore, it seems likely that insulin selectively attenuates breakdown of nonmyofibrillar proteins in human without stimulation of protein synthesis.

Administration of growth hormone to patients identified as candidates for parenteral nutrition has demonstrated an improved protein metabolism (56). The anabolic effect of growth hormone is believed to be mediated via insulin-like growth factor I (IGF-I). This hypothesis has support in experimental studies in which IGF-I administration significantly improved protein status, mainly by reducing protein catabolism (57). Studies on healthy human subjects receiving IGF-I have shown a decreased plasma urea concentration, further supporting this hypothesis (58). The effect of IGF-I on nitrogen metabolism in postoperative patients is now under investigation in several laboratories, including our own.

Studies of selective β_2 agonists have repeatedly confirmed a rapid and potent anabolic effect on skeletal muscle in a number of species during food restriction. Among various agonists, clenbuterol has proven to be one of the most potent (59). The exact mechanisms of clenbuterol action remain unclear, but its dependence on changes in major anabolic hormones, such as insulin, growth hormone, and gonadal hormones, has been excluded. The anabolic effect seems to be dependent on interaction with the β_2 receptor (60). A combination of TPN and clenbuterol treatment during experimental conditions with tumor-bearing animals demonstrated increased muscle mass and muscle protein content, but treatment with either of the two regimens had no such anabolic effects (61). The effect on muscle protein content of the combined therapy with nutrition and β_2 agonists opens interesting perspectives for the future.

IV. CONCLUSIONS

Considering available information about the lack of protein accretion in response to artificial nutrition, it may be possible that a therapeutical deficiency exists with respect to the nutrition therapy itself. When eating normal food, the substrate/calorie load is delivered as a very condensed bolus with high concentration of nutrients. This load elicits the well-recognized metabolic and hormonal response to feeding, which includes high plasma concentrations of various components, for example amino acids. Such high concentrations may not be obtained when infusing artificial diets either intravenously or gastrointestinally. Our own studies have indicated that the arterial concentration of amino acids is a strong predictor for uptake of amino acids into peripheral tissues—actually a more powerful predictor than plasma insulin concentration when determined in amino acid infusion experiments on normal volunteers (62). Therefore, a simple explanation for inefficient therapy by infusion-delivered nutrition is that plasma concentrations are too low to achieve an appropriate combination of circulating hormones and substrates. If so, it should be more rewarding to infuse liquid meals in a bolus-fashioned delivery. In line with this theory, investigations in our laboratory have confirmed that intermittent infusions of TPN improved further nitrogen balance in patients after elective cholecystectomies compared with constant infusion at low rate (Fig. 4) (63). Another factor that must be considered is the composition of the nutrition formulas, particularly that of the amino acid solutions. It has become evident that present formulas, as defined in growing animals and infants, may not be appropriate in adults. The most spectacular suggestion in this respect may be increased need for glutamine in stressed patients (64), but similar concepts can also be developed for other amino acids, such as arginine (65), tyrosine, cysteine, and methionine and, possibly, tryptophan (unpublished). Pharmacological treatment with IGF-I, clenbuterol, and insulin as adjunct to nutritional therapy may also be rewarding, at least from a theoretical view. We can certainly anticipate that artificial nutrition will be further developed in the near future. An improved metabolic efficiency of intravenous nutrition will provide physicians with a powerful tool to treat malnourished patients. Death in cancer disease and progressive malnutrition are closely related. Hence, an

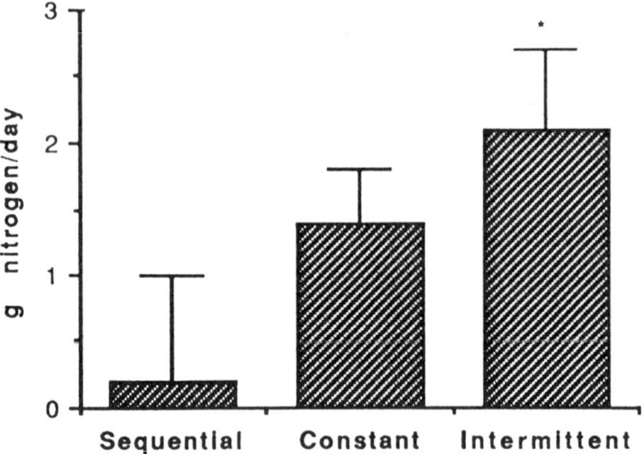

Figure 4 Nitrogen balance in patients randomized to receive one of three TPN regimens postoperatively. *Sequential*: crystalline amino acids and lipid emulsion given for 12 h in the daytime and glucose infusion infused for 12 h during the night. *Constant*: all substrates infused simultaneously during 24 h. *Intermittent*: all substrates infused simultaneously during 1 h, six times/24h. All regimens with the same energy and nitrogen content. Nitrogen balance was significantly improved in patients receiving intermittent infusions. (Reproduced from Ref. 63.)

efficient nutrition therapy to cancer patients would most certainly offer an important and valuable palliation with increased quality of life.

V. SUMMARY

The role of artificial nutritional support, that is, both intravenous and enteral nutrition by infusion of chemically defined nutrients, is considered an adjunct to cancer treatment. Despite a vast literature reflecting numerous attempts to demonstrate a supportive role for nutrition, little benefit has actually been confirmed in controlled investigations regarding outcome and objective remission in progressive cachexia. The impact of nutritional support on quality of life has only been considered in preliminary studies, however, and few attempts have been made in cancer patients. We suggest that the lack of evidence in cancer treatment for a significant role of nutritional support in a general sense is probably explained by both inappropriately designed investigations and by the unrecognized fact that standard clinical nutrition is hampered by nutrition-related inefficiencies that have not yet been well described. Improved understanding of such deficiencies and the development of more sophisticated regimens in line with "nutrition pharmacology" instead of plain feeding with calories and protein may change this situation in the near future.

ACKNOWLEDGMENTS

Supported in part by Grant Nos. 93-B89-22XA, 2014-B88-01XA, and 2147-B89-04XA from the Swedish Cancer Society, and B89-17X-00536-25A and B89-17K-08712-01A from the Medical Research Council and by the Tore Nilson Foundation, the Assar Gabrielsson Foundation (AB Volvo, Sweden), the Jubileumskliniken Foundation, the Ingabritt and Arne Lundbergs Research Foundation, the Swedish and Göteborg Medical Societies, and the Medical Faculty, University of Göteborg, Sweden.

SELECTED READINGS

Apovian CM, McMahon MM, Bistrian BR. Guidelines for refeeding the marasmic patient. Crit Care Med 1990; 18:1030–1033. The authors discuss practical aspects of importance in nutritional treatment of severely undernourished individuals.

Hill GH, Witney GB, Christie PM, Church JM. Protein status and metabolic expenditure determine response to intravenous nutrition—a new classification of surgical malnutrition. Br J Surg 1991; 78:109–113. This is an additional example of standard TPN failing to protect body stores of proteins when given to hospitalized patients.

Lowell JA, Parnes HL, Blackburn GL. Dietary immunomodulation: beneficial effects on oncogenesis and tumor growth. Crit Care Med 1990;18:S145–S148. The authors discuss and suggest several fields in medicine in which modified nutrition may be regarded as an organ- or a condition-oriented therapy in the near future. Of particular interest are the aspects of the possible role of fish oils to modify tumor progression and transplantation reactions.

Lowell JA, Schifferdecker C, Driscoll DF, Benotti PN, Bistrian BR. Postoperative fluid overload: not a benign problem. Crit Care Med 1990; 18:728–733. The authors raise an extremely important issue in the handling of severely ill patients, namely the risk for fluid accumulation, which is probably tremendously underestimated worldwide.

McGeer AJ, Detsky AS, O'Rourke K. Parenteral nutrition in cancer patients undergoing chemotherapy: a meta-analysis. Nutrition 1990; 6:233–240. The results from meta analysis of chemotherapy-treated cancer patients are described. The results show no benefit from intravenous nutrition. In contrast, the results suggest net harm to TPN-treated patients, with increased susceptibility to infection even when catheter-related sepsis is omitted from the calculations.

Otto DA, Kahn DR, Hamm MW, Forrest DE, Wooten JT. Improved survival of heterotopic cardiac allografts in rats with dietary *n*-3 polyunsaturated fatty acids. Transplantation 1990; 50:193–198. The data indicate that providing dietary n-3 polyunsaturated fatty acids before and after cardiac transplant to recipient animals provides a significant protection against acute rejection.

REFERENCES

1. Holmes S, Dickerson JW. Malignant disease: nutritional implications of disease and treatment. Cancer Metastasis Rev 1987; 6:357–381.

2. Mullen JL, Buzby GP, Matthews DC, Smale BF, Rosato EF. Reduction of operative mortality by combined preoperative and postoperative nutritional support. Ann Surg 1980; 192:604–613.
3. McGeer AJ, Detsky AS, O'Rourke K. Parenteral nutrition in cancer patients undergoing chemotherapy: a meta-analysis. Nutrition 1990; 6:233–240.
4. Nixon DW. The value of parenteral nutrition support. Chemotherapy and radiation treatment. Cancer 1986; 58:1902–1903.
5. Brennan MF. Total parenteral nutrition in the cancer patient. N Engl J Med 1981; 217:375–382.
6. Edén E, Bennegård K, Bylund-Fellenius A-C, Scherstén T, Lundholm K. Whole body energy metabolism and metabolic capacity of skeletal muscles in malnourished patients before and after total parenteral nutrition. Hum Nutr Clin Nutr 1983; 37C:185–196.
7. Bennegård K, Edén E, Ekman L, Scherstén T, Lundholm K. Metabolic response of whole body and peripheral tissues to enteral nutrition in weight-losing cancer and non-cancer patients. Gastroenterology 1983; 85:92–99.
8. Alexander JW, Peck MD. Future prospects for adjunctive therapy: pharmacologic and nutritional approaches to immune system modulation. Crit Care Med 1990; 18:S159–S164.
9. Lundholm, K, Karlberg I, Ekman L, Edström S, Scherstén T. Evaluation of anorexia as the cause of altered protein synthesis in skeletal muscles from non-growing mice with sarcoma. Cancer Res 1981; 41:1989–1996.
10. Westin T, Edström S, Lundholm K. Tumour cell proliferation and nutrition. Am J Clin Nutr 1991; 53:764–768.
11. Moldawer LL, Georgieff M, Lundholm K. Interleukin-1, tumour necrosis factor-alpha (cachectin) and the pathogenesis of cancer cachexia. Clin Physiol 1987; 7:263–274.
12. Gelin J, Moldawer LL, Lönnroth C, Sherry B, Chizzonite R, Lundholm K. The role of endogenous TNF-α and interleukin-1 for experimental tumor growth and the development of cancer cachexia. Cancer Res 1991; 51:415–421.
13. Hyltander A, Drott C, Körner U, Sandström R, Lundholm K. Elevated energy expenditure in cancer patients with solid tumours. Eur J Cancer 1991; 27:9–15.
14. Jayarajan MP, Shetty PS. Cardiovascular β-adrenoceptor sensitivity of undernourished subjects. Br J Nutr 1987; 58:5–11.
15. Ransnäs L, Drott C, Lundholm K, Hjalmarson Å, Jacobson B. Effcts of malnutrition on rat myocardial β-adrenergic and muscarinic receptors. Circ Res 1989; 64:949–956.
16. Hyltander A, Körner U, Lundholm K. Evaluation of mechanisms behind elevated energy expenditure in cancer patients with solid tumours. Eur J Clin Invest 1993; 23:46–52.
17. Lundholm K. Origins of emaciation in cancer patients. Med Oncol Tumor Pharmacother 1985; 2:183–187.
18. Svaninger G, Bennegård K, Ekman L, Ternell M, Lundholm K. Lack of evidence for elevated breakdown rate of skeletal muscles in weight-losing tumor-bearing mice. J Natl Cancer Inst 1983; 71:341–346.
19. Holroyde CP, Skutches CL, Boden G, Reichard GA. Glucose metabolism in cachectic patients with colorectal cancer. Cancer Res 1984; 44:5910–5913.

20. Edén E, Edström S, Bennegård K, Lindmark L, Lundholm K. Glycerol dynamics in weight-losing cancer patients. Surgery 1985; 97:176–184.
21. Müller JM, Brenner U, Dienst C, Pichlmaier H. Preoperative parenteral feeding in patients with gastrointestinal carcinoma. Lancet 1982; 1:68–71.
22. Meijerink WJ, von Meyenfeldt MF, Rouflart, MM, Soeters PB. Efficacy of perioperative nutritional support (letter). Lancet 1992; 18; 340:187–188.
23. Sandström R, Drott C, Hyltander A, et al. The effect of postoperative intravenous feeding (TPN) on outcome following major surgery evaluated in a randomized study. Ann Surg 1993; 217:185–195.
24. McClave SA, Short AF, Mattingly DB, Fitzgerald PD. Total parenteral nutrition. Conquering the complexities. Postgrad Med 1990; 88:235–248.
25. Lough M, Watkins R, Campbell M, Carr K, Burnett A, Shenkin A. Parenteral nutrition in bone marrow transplantation. Clin Nutr 1990; 9:97–101.
26. Wilmore DW. The practice of clinical nutrition: how to prepare for the future. J Parenter Enter Nutr 1989; 13:337–343.
27. Windsor JA, Hill GL. Weight loss with physiological impairment. Ann Surg 1988; 207:290–296.
28. Russell DM, Leiter LA, Whitwell J, Marliss EB, Jeejeebhoy KN. Skeletal muscle function during hypocaloric diets and fasting: a comparison with standard nutritional assessment parameters. Am J Clin Nutr 1983; 37:133–138.
29. Rombeau JL. A review of the effects of glutamine-enriched diets on experimentally induced enterocolitis. J. Parenter Enter Nutr 1990; 14:100S-105S.
30. Drott C, Unsgaard B, Scherstén T, Lundholm K. Total parenteral nutrition as an adjuvant to patients undergoing chemotherapy for testicular carcinoma: protection of body composition—a randomized prospective study. Surgery 1988; 103:499–506.
31. Hyltander A, Drott C, Unsgaard B, et al. The effect on body composition and exercise performance of home parenteral nutrition when given as adjunct to chemotherapy of testicular carcinoma. A randomized and prospective study. Eur J Clin Invest 1991; 21:413–420.
32. Hyltander A, Warnold I, Edén E, Lundholm K. Effect on whole-body protein synthesis after institution of intravenous nutrition in cancer and non-cancer patients who lose weight. Eur J Cancer 1991; 27:16–21.
33. Westin T, Gustavsson B, Edström S, et al. Tumor cytokinetic effects of acute starvation versus polyamine depletion in tumor-bearing mice. Cytometry 1991; 12:628–635.
34. Westin T, Edström S, Lundholm K. Ornithine decarboxylase activity in tumor tissue in response to refeeding and its dependancy on diet components. Eur J Cancer 1991; 27:1282–1288.
35. Greschner M, Saeger HD, Barth H, Leweling H, Holm E. Balances of energy-yielding substrates across malignant gastric tumors in man. Clin Nutr (Suppl) 1991; 10:12.
36. Günther HJ, Hagmüller E, Kollmar H, Saeger HD, Holm E. In-vivo investigation of substrate exchange concerning energy-metabolism by human colon carcinomas. Clin Nutr (Suppl) 1992; 11:17–18.
37. Heys SD, Park KGM, McNurlan MA, et al. Stimulation of protein synthesis in

human tumours by parenteral nutrition: evidence for modulation of tumour growth. Br J Surg 1991; 78:483–487.
38. Warnold I, Edén E, Lundholm K. The inefficiency of total parenteral nutrition to stimulate protein synthesis in moderately malnourished patients. Ann Surg 1988; 208:143–149.
39. Hill GH, Witney GB, Christie PM, Church JM. Protein status and metabolic expenditure determine response to intravenous nutrition—a new classification of surgical malnutrition. Br J Surg 1991; 78:109–113.
40. Bozzetti F. Effects of artificial nutrition on the nutritional status of cancer patients. J Parenter Enter Nutr 1989; 13:406–420.
41. Shike M, Russel DMcR, Detsky A, et al. Changes in body composition in patients with small-cell lung cancer. The effect of total parenteral nutrition as an adjunct to chemotherapy. Ann Intern Med 1984; 101:303-309.
42. Bach AC, Babayan VK. Medium-chain triglycerides: an update. Am J Clin Nutr 1982; 36:950–962.
43. Sobrado J, Moldawer LL, Pomposelli JJ, Mascioli EA. Lipid emulsions and reticuloendothelial system function in healthy and burned guinea pigs. Am J Clin Nutr 1985; 42:855–863.
44. Sandström R, Hyltander A, Körner U, Lundholm K. Structured triglycerides to postoperative patients: a safety and tolerance study. J Parenter Enter Nutr 1993; 17:153–157.
45. Helton WS, Smith RJ, Rounds J, Wilmore DW. Glutamine prevents pancreatic atrophy and fatty liver during elemental feeding. J Surg Res 1990; 48:297–303.
46. Klimberg SV, Souba WW, Dolson DJ, et al. Prophylactic glutamine protects the intestinal mucosa from radiation injury. Cancer 1990; 66:62–68.
47. Barber AE, Jones WG II, Minei JP, et al. Harry M. Vars Award. Glutamine or fiber supplementation of a defined formula diet: impact on bacterial translocation, tissue composition, and response to endotoxin. J Parenter Enter Nutr 1990; 14:335–343.
48. Smith RJ, Wilmore DW. Glutamine nutrition and requirements. J Parenter Enter Nutr 1990; 14:94S–99S.
49. Daly MJ, Reynolds J, Thom A, et al. Immune and metabolic effects of arginine in the surgical patient. Ann Surg 1988; 208:512–523.
50. Palmer RMJ, Ashton DS, Moncada S. Vascular endothelial cells synthesize nitric oxide from L-arginine. Nature 1988; 333:664–666.
51. Lundholm K, Edström S, Ekman L, Karlberg I, Walker P, Scherstén T. Protein degradation in human skeletal muscle, the effect of insulin, leucin, amino acids and ions. Clin Sci 1981; 60:319–326.
52. Inculet RI, Finley RJ, Duff JH, et al. Insulin decreases muscle protein loss after operative treauma in man. Surgery 1986; 99:752–758.
53. Bennet WM, Connacher A, Smith K, Jung RT, Rennie MJ. Inability to stimulate skeletal muscle or whole body protein synthesis in type I diabetic patients by insulin-glucose during amino acid infusion: studies of incorporation and turnover of tracer L-[1-^{13}C] leucine. Diabetologica 1990; 33:43–51.
54. Gelfand RA, Barrett EJ. Effect of physiologic hyperinsulinemia on skeletal muscle protein synthesis and breakdown in man. J Clin Invest 1987; 80:1–6.

55. Möller-Loswick AC, Zachrisson H, Hyltander A, Körner U, Matthews DE, Lundholm K. Insulin attenuates selectively the breakdown of nonmyofibrillar proteins in peripheral tissues in normal man. Submitted for publication, 1992.
56. Jiang ZM, He GZ, Zhang SY. Low-dose growth hormone and hypocaloric nutrition attenuate the protein-catabolic response after major operation. Ann Surg 1989; 210:513–524.
57. Gluckman PD, Douglas RG, Ambler GR, Breier BH. The endocrine role of insulin-like growth factor I. Acta Paediatr Scand 1991; 372:97–105.
58. Guler HP, Schmid C, Zapf J, Froesch ER. Effect of recombinant insulin-like growth factor I on insulin secretion and renal function in normal human subjects. Proc Natl Acad Sci USA 1989; 86:2868-2872.
59. Choo JJ, Horan MA, Little RA, Rothwell NJ. Effects of the β_2-agonist clenbuterol on muscle atrophy due to food deprivation in the rat. Metabolism 1990; 39:647–650.
60. Choo JJ, Horan MA, Little RA, Rothwell NJ. Anabolic effects of clenbuterol on skeletal muscle are mediated by β_2-adrenoceptor blockade. Am J Physiol 1992; 263:E50–E56.
61. Chance W, Cao L, Zhang FS, Foley-Nelson T, Fisher J. Clenbuterol treatment increases muscle mass and protein content of tumor-bearing rats maintained on total parenteral nutrition. J Parenter Enter Nutr 1991; 15:530–535.
62. Lundholm K, Bennegård K, Zachrisson H, Lundgren F, Edén E, Möller-Loswick AC. Transport kinetics of amino acids across the resting human leg. J Clin Invest 1987; 80:763–771.
63. Hyltander A, Arfvidsson B, Körner U, Sandström R, Lundholm K. Metabolic rate and nitrogen balance in patients on bolus intermittent TPN infusion. Submitted for publication, 1992.
64. Stehle P, Mertes N, Puchstein CH, et al. Effect of parenteral glutamine peptide supplements on muscle glutamine loss and nitrogen balance after major surgery. Lancet 1989; 1:231–233.
65. Lowell JA, Parnes HL, Blackburn GL. Dietary immunomodulation: beneficial effects on oncogenesis and tumor growth. Crit Care Med 1990; 18:S145–S148.

9

Sexual Dysfunction

Ursula S. Ofman
Memorial Sloan-Kettering Cancer Center, New York, New York

I. INTRODUCTION

Sexual quality of life of the cancer survivor is a topic that has received increasing attention with the advent of more effective cancer therapies. The focus of the concerned literature is on prevalence of sexual dysfunction after cancer treatment, and most reports in the literature confirm that cancer treatment has a deleterious effect on sexual functioning. Derogatis and Kourlesis (1) found in a review of the literature incidences of sexual dysfunction ranging from 40 to 100% after treatment. This chapter briefly reviews the prevalence and nature of sexual dysfunction after cancer treatment by disease site, followed by a discussion of preventative measures the medical team can provide, as well as evaluation and treatment issues in this population.

II. PREVALENCE OF SEXUAL DYSFUNCTION IN PATIENTS AFTER CANCER THERAPY BY SITE OF DISEASE AND TREATMENT MODALITY

A. Breast Cancer

As a diagnostic category, breast cancer patients may very well be the best researched group in terms of sexual impact of treatment on sexual functioning. In recent years it has been widely accepted that comparative survival rates may be obtained in early breast cancer patients treated either with traditional surgical procedures (modified radical mastectomy) or with breast-conserving techniques combined with radiation and, increasingly, chemotherapy. The psychological and psychosexual outcomes of these two approaches have been compared in a number of studies. Some studies found a tendency toward better preservation of body image and sexual functioning in patients who elected breast-conserving treatment (2–4), but there is no conclusive evidence that these women also have better overall adjustment. Schover (5) questioned the frequently assumed connection between mutilating breast surgery and poor sexual adjustment following treatment. She suggested rather that a woman's overall psychological health, relationship satisfaction, and premorbid sexual life appear to be far stronger predictors of postcancer sexual satisfaction than the extent of the damage to the breast, and that even a less damaged sense of desirability and better preserved body image may have only a subtle impact on actual sexual functioning after surgery.

In an effort to clarify the nature of women's response to lumpectomy, McCormick and coworkers (6) studied how 74 women treated with lumpectomy and radiation perceived their breasts and reported that 39% of the sexually active patients in their study avoided the treated breast, 20% stated that their partner avoided it, and 48% noted breast discomfort during sexual activity; still, 90% indicated a high level of satisfaction with the results of treatment. The implications of reconstruction for the psychological adjustment of the mastectomy population is also beginning to receive attention; Rowland et al. (7) studied 83 women who had undergone reconstruction after modified radical mastectomy for early stage breast cancer and reported that patients generally returned to premorbid levels of sexual satisfaction and comfort.

There is now a growing body of research dealing with the emotional and sexual consequences of surgery for early stage breast cancer, but little is known about the effects of systemic regimens for breast cancer on sexual functioning. With large cohorts of women now receiving hormonal treatment, especially tamoxifen, for long periods of time, such questions become more pressing. Research to date suggests that tamoxifen may actually produce estrogenic changes in the vaginal mucosa of postmenopausal women (8,9). However, its impact on symptomatic vaginal atrophy in these women is unknown (10).

B. Cancer of the Male Reproductive Organs

1. Prostate Cancer

Prostate cancer is the most commonly diagnosed cancer in men. It affects mostly older men: 80% of all diagnoses are made in men of 65 years and older. Men and their partners in this age group are often at a developmental stage dominated by loss: retirement, death of peers, and separation from adult children who move away. Part of these losses may also be loss of sexual activity secondary to sexual dysfunction that precedes the cancer diagnosis. Changes in sexual functioning as a result of normal aging are often compounded by age-related chronic diseases, such as hypertension, and their treatment. Schover and von Eschenbach (11) found in a prospective study of 22 men with stage B or C prostate cancer that 23% reported painful ejaculation before therapy and 40% reported erectile difficulties. More recently, Zinreich et al. (12) reported in a sample of 43 patients with adenocarcinoma of the prostate at varying stages (mean age 67.7 years) and their partners, that 63% of the patients had erectile dysfunction before cancer treatment. Of these, 44% were never able to obtain an erection and 56% reported difficulty maintaining erections during intercourse. For many elderly couples the man's erectile difficulty results in a complete cessation of sexual activity.

Treatment for early-stage disease commonly consists of surgery or radiation therapy. In early-stage prostate cancer, the advances in medical technology have meant gains for sexual functioning after treatment. Quinlan et al. (13), in a case series of 500 men, reported an incidence of erectile dysfunction of 32% with nerve-sparing surgery techniques, compared with 85% after traditional radical prostatectomy. In any case, recovery of erectile functioning is often slow and may exceed 6 months in some individuals (14). Traditional radiation regimens for prostate cancer may also produce erectile dysfunction as a long-term side effect. Schover (15) found in a review of the literature that the generally estimated 50% of erectile dysfunction after definitive radiotherapy may be inflated and may actually be between 14 and 46% of all cases. The mechanism believed to be responsible for the development of erectile dysfunction in radiation patients is vascular scarring, which may develop 6 months after treatment or later.

Advanced stage prostate cancer is commonly treated with testosterone deprivation, accomplished by bilateral orchiectomy, or the administration of estrogen, flutamide, or luteinizing hormone releasing hormone analogs. All these interventions produce sexual side effects, including loss of desire for sexual activity and impaired erectile functioning. Men undergoing hormone treatments are also confronted with body image issues, reduced energy levels, and hot flashes, which may contribute to the development of sexual problems.

2. Testicular Cancer

Unlike prostate cancer, testicular cancer typically affects young men. It is the most common cancer in men aged 17–34 in the United States. They are confronted with a life-threatening disease at a life stage in which they are supposed to separate from their families of origin and find their own identities as an adult. The demands of the illness interfere with the developmental goal of this population, interfering with the young man's concept of himself as an independent, strong, and virile person.

Treatment in the past routinely included unilateral orchiectomy, retroperitoneal lymphadenectomy (RLND), and either chemotherapy for nonseminomatous tumors or radiation for seminomas. Men with metastatic seminomas may receive chemotherapy in addition to radiation. Fertility issues as a result of retrograde ejaculation caused by surgical damage to paraaortic sympathetic nervous system pathways are a prominent concern for men after RLND (16). Antegrade ejaculation may return with time and in some men. Sympathomimetic drugs (ephedrine) or anticholinergic drugs, such as diphenhydramine or imipramine, may help facilitate normal ejaculation. Recently there has been more of an effort to preserve ejaculatory function and avoid other treatment side effects in men with nonseminomatous tumors who do not evidence of metastatic spread. In these cases unilateral orchiectomy may now be followed by careful observation. New nerve-sparing surgery techniques may also contribute to the preservation of ejaculatory functioning by sparing the superior hypogastric plexus (17).

Fertility concerns relating to this problem and to chemotherapy appear to be the most common sexual side effects of testicular cancer, but a number of reports document further sexual difficulties after treatment (18). Rieker et al. (19) found in a retrospective study of 223 testis cancer survivors who were more than 1 year after diagnosis that 30% experienced overall performance distress, 10% had erectile difficulties, and 6% were anorgasmic. These findings point to the continued need for help in patients who appear to be disease free and whose sexual functioning has at least to a significant degree returned; these patients often remain troubled in their relationships because of persisting low-grade sexual dysfunction that is treatable (20).

C. Cancer of the Female Reproductive Organs

The incidence of sexual problems in women after gynecological cancer treatment ranges in various reports from 0 to virtually 100% (21). This reflects both the many methodological difficulties of assessment in this field and the wide range of treatments for gynecological malignancies, from laser surgery for cervical carcinoma in situ, to total pelvic exenteration and vigorous chemotherapies for advanced gynecological tumors. The gynecological malignancies, with their obvious significance for sexual function, deserve comprehensive study to help women recover sexually as fully as possible. As van de Wiel et al. (22) point out in their review of the literature on sexual function after cervical cancer treatment, many studies use frequency of intercourse as the sole indicator of the quality of sexual relations; this sheds little light on the true sexual status of the gynecological cancer survivor. Further refinements in research instruments and methodology should benefit this population. A review of the research in this area is also available in Berek and Andersen (23).

1. Cervical Cancer

Cervical cancer is the fourth most common neoplasm in women, with 13,000 new cases of invasive disease diagnosed annually in the United States. Excluding in situ lesions, treatment consists of radical hysterectomy, radiation therapy, or a combination of both approaches. For almost two decades researchers have explored and compared the relative incidence of sexual dysfunction in women with cervix cancer after surgery versus after radiation treatment (24,25). It appears that although 6 months after treatment both surgery and radiation patients report no significant changes in sexual functioning, 1 year after treatment both populations report decreased sexual interest, radiation patients reporting significantly diminished sexual functioning with severe dyspareunia, postcoital bleeding, and pain on penetration. These studies highlight the dilemmas posed for sexual recovery by pelvic irradiation for gynecological cancer. The sequelae of fibrosis, vaginal stenosis, and decreased lubrication (26) are likely to interfere with sexual function unless treated appropriately, promptly, and continuously with vaginal dilators, effective vaginal lubricants (AstroGlide® and others), and, in some cases a hormone-free vaginal moisturizer (Replens®).

Total pelvic exenteration is a major surgical procedure occasionally performed to excise advanced pelvic tumors en bloc in the absence of distant metastases. The surgery entails removal of the bladder, urethra, vagina, uterus, ovaries, and rectum; two ostomies are created. The treatment comprises such a serious challenge to both physical and emotional recovery that early clinical reports explored whether postoperative quality of life justified the continued use of so radical an approach (27,28). Some researchers have reported that construction of a neovagina combined with special support and counseling efforts offers an improved chance for sexual rehabilitation after surgery (29–31).

At present, however, many questions remain regarding vaginal reconstruction. The long-term advantage to patient adjustment and satisfaction must be weighed against the risk of these procedures. The psychological and practical adjustments required by exenteration, which include body image, ostomy, and mortality concerns, also merit further study.

The impact of gynecological cancer on a woman's sexual self-esteem or sense of worth as a sexual partner remains an intuitively powerful yet little studied factor in postcancer distress. Van de Wiehl et al. (32) compared 11 women treated for cervical carcinoma with a group of nonpatient controls and found that although the frequency of sexual activity did not differ between the groups, the cervix cancer patients valued sexual interactions significantly less, and had a lower appraisal of themselves as sexual partners. The small population studied, and retrospective nature of the work curtail conclusions, but this report marks a valuable effort to illuminate the subtler, but far-reaching consequences of gynecological cancer for sexual well-being.

2. Endometrial and Ovarian Cancer

Endometrial cancer presents most commonly in postmenopausal women. Treatment consists of surgery, radiation therapy, or a combination of both modalities.

Ovarian cancer presents in pre- and postmenopausal women; surgical evaluation and debulking is ordinarily the first step in treatment, followed by a chemotherapy regimen with a combination of agents. Only with the relatively recent advent of chemotherapy for ovarian cancer in the last several years has the previously dismal prognosis for this tumor improved markedly. Partly for this reason, studies of the long-term implications of this illness for the survivor's sexual function have begun to appear (33–35). Compared with healthy controls, women with these cancers report lower frequency of sexual behaviors, lower levels of arousal, increased incidence of dyspareunia, and problems with body image.

The ovarian cancer patient faces the serial traumata of a serious cancer diagnosis, major pelvic surgery with resultant changes to the vagina, a demanding chemotherapy regimen, and treatment-related onset of menopause in the premenopausal patient with complete loss of fertility. The psychological, physical, and hormonal impact on sexual function in this population merits futher careful study.

The endometrial cancer patient must often contend with radiation changes to the vagina and pelvis (36). Vaginal changes include fibrosis with resultant shortening and narrowing, reduced elasticity of the vaginal wall, and diminished lubrication, creating a high risk of dyspareunia. As mentioned earlier, the consequences of radiation to the vagina may be avoided or alleviated by the regular use of vaginal dilators and sexual comfort improved by use of appropriate lubricants, vaginal moisturizers, and intercourse positions. Therefore, an important area for future inquiry is the implementation of patient support and education plans for women facing pelvic radiation, to maintain contact and encourage crucial patient compliance with these strategies during the demanding months of treatment and especially during the first year after treatment, as radiation changes evolve and produce physical and relationship distress.

3. Vulvar Cancer

Vulvar carcinoma is a rare tumor, arising primarily in older women. In early-stage disease treatment may consist of wide local excision. In more advanced disease with its often multicentric lesions, radical vulvectomy is performed, which entails removal of clitoris and labia minora, and majora and bilateral inguinal lymph node dissection. Postoperatively patients may experience a high degree of complications, including wound infections and lymphedema of the lower extremities, as well as introital stricture. Research attention has begun to focus on this population in recent years (37–39), and reports document that sexual dysfunction after treatment for vulvar cancer is common and affects all phases of the sexual response cycle.

Gynecological cancer patients as a group merit further inquiry not only as treatment advances create a growing population of survivors but because many factors often converge to place these patients at high risk for sexual and relationship dysfunction after treatment. These factors are cancer site, gravity of diagnosis, magnitude of therapy, impact on hormonal status, impact on fertility and impact of all these factors on partners. The psychosocial aspects of treatment and recovery from gynecological cancer are covered in detail by McCartney and Auchincloss (40).

D. Cancer Sites in Both Sexes

1. Bladder Cancer

Bladder cancer arises primarily in older men and women, who may already have experienced age-related changes in sexuality. In the United States treatment previously consisted of cystectomy for lesions of any stage, but early bladder carcinoma in situ without infiltration may now be treated with local excision and bacillus Calmette-Guérin.

In patients with invasive bladder cancer, cystectomy is the treatment of choice in the United States. A common sexual side effect for men after radical cystectomy is erectile dysfunction, with difficulty attaining or maintaining erections because of transection of the nerves governing erection (41), and loss of ejaculation secondary to excision of the prostate at the time of surgery. Changes in sensations of orgasm may ensue. The patient's response to this additional loss occasioned by cancer is little studied in this population.

In women, cystectomy may result in a narrowed or shortened vagina, scarring, and numbness or loss of sensation, all of which may impair the excitement response. Furthermore, since both ovaries are also removed during surgery, premature menopause occurs in premenopausal patients, which may lead to reduced vaginal lubrication and desire. The simultaneous creation of a stoma and external diversion of urine generate concern about body image, odor, leakage, and spills and thus may contribute to sexual avoidance and other difficulties (42).

2. Colorectal Cancer

Cancer of the colon and rectum is the second most common cancer in the United States: approximately 140,000 new cases are diagnosed annually, primarily in older men and women. Surgery remains the mainstay of treatment; resection of the tumor with pelvic lymphadenectomy may be followed by radiation and/or chemotherapy. Pelvic lymphadenectomy may result in damage to the parasympathetic nervous system, causing erectile dysfunction, and to the sympathetic nervous system, causing retrograde or diminished ejaculation. Past clinical studies have reported varying incidence of these side effects after treatment (43–45). More recently, Havenga and Welvaart (46) studied 26 men with rectosigmoid carcinoma, 9 treated with abdominoperineal resection and 17 treated with low anterior resection. They found that of patients with abdominoperineal resection only 2 returned to sexual activity; 5 had erectile dysfunction and 7 were anorgasmic. Patients who had low anterior resection reported fewer sexual dysfunctions after surgery; 12 maintained sexual activity, and 4 reported either erectile dysfunction or anorgasmia. Further evidence that abdominoperineal resection produces significant sexual dysfunction comes from Koukouras et al. (47), who studied 60 sexually active male patients with colorectal cancer who were treated with higher anterior resection, low anterior resection, or abdominoperineal resection. They found that patients with the abdominoperineal resection had the highest incidence of sexual dysfunction: 65% became sexually inactive, 45% lost all erectile ability, and 50% reported absence of ejaculation. Hojo et al. (48) described the use of a nerve-sparing approach to pelvic lymphadenectomy in 134 patients with advanced disease. They found that although bladder dysfunction was best prevented with a nerve-sparing procedure, preservation of sexual function in men is more difficult, requires a high degree of nerve preservation, and therefore is not advisable for patients with extended disease.

In patients with early-stage disease who are treated with the amputation of the rectum alone, erectile dysfunction appears to be less prevalent but orgasm-phase problems persist (49). There is a glaring shortage of studies focusing on the sexual side effects of treatment for colorectal neooplasms in women.

After the creation of a colostomy, both men and women must contend with issues of changed body image and sensitivity about cleanliness, odor, and fear of accidents. The early studies of Sutherland et al. (50) have remained clinically on target; this researcher found that the sexual impact of the ostomy far exceeds the extent of physical handicap. Depression, anger, and fear of being repugnant are common emotional reactions postoperatively and may contribute to a pattern of sexual avoidance. The medical staff must anticipate these issues and offer support to the patient, whose challenges include self-care of the ostomy, overcoming fears concerning changed appearance, and regaining physical self-esteem. Other patients who are further along in this process may provide invaluable help to the recovering colorectal patient in this regard. Overall adjustment to the colostomy may take more than a year, as documented by Hurny and Holland (51).

Sexual response after colorectal surgery remains an insufficiently understood area, which is particularly disturbing in view of the current high prevalence of this tumor in the population. Issues of sexual recovery of women in particular after colorectal and bladder cancer remain too little explored, although the impact of these pelvic surgeries on the female excitement and orgasm responses, as well as the impact of the ostomy issues on desire, may be surmised to be very significant. The value of treatment interventions for sexual dysfunction in this population, including both penile prosthesis implantation and sexual counseling for the patient or couple, is also an appropriate area of study. Currently research endeavors are being undertaken in this area at our institution, which we hope will further illuminate these concerns for both oncology professionals and the patients facing these dilemmas.

E. Other Cancers

Patients with less common tumors, or with commonly occurring tumors that do not appear directly to affect the organs of sexual response, have received little or no research attention with regard to the sexual sequelae of treatment. Diagnosis and treatment of any cancer have far-reaching psychological implications for the patient and family, beyond the scope of this chapter. These matters are covered comprehensively elsewhere (52). Some cancer treatments pose a particularly severe challenge to the recovery of normal self-esteem and restored body image; tumor treatments involving limb amputation, marked facial and other appearance changes, or loss of normal phonation are examples.

The simple passage of time does not heal all wounds; in the area of sexuality it is not uncommon for problems to become more severe with time (53). The adjustment to cancer and its elements of disfigurement is by nature a slow process, but problems with adjustment and recovery, including those in the sexual and relationship arena, may often be more accessible to counseling by oncology mental health professionals during the first and second posttreatment years than at a later stage in cancer survivorship.

Cancers that require systemic treatment with chemotherapy, whole-body irradiation, or bone marrow transplantation challenge the patient physically and emotionally more than most surgeries or radiation regimens. Treatments may be lengthy and arduous, depleting the patient of energy and causing severe side effects. Sexual functioning is clearly affected by many of these regimens. In recent years the sexual concerns of female bone marrow transplant patients have received some research attention. It was found that ovarian failure secondary to conditioning treatment with melphalan or cyclophosphamide and with total-body irradiation is associated with profound effects on sexual functioning, most commonly vaginal dryness, loss of desire for sexual activity, and difficulties with sexual intercourse (54). Ostroff et al. (55) found that standard regimens of hormone replacement therapy did not alleviate all sexual impairment experienced by women with treatment-related ovarian failure. In a study comparing bone marrow transplant survivors and a matched sample undergoing maintenance chemotherapy, Altmeier et al. (56) found, that although overall the two groups showed few significant differences, bone marrow transplant patients reported a higher incidence of sexual difficulties. Ostroff and Lesko (57) confirmed the prevalence of sexual dysfunction in bone marrow transplant survivors. Clearly, this population is at increased risk for sexual dysfunction and would benefit from further research attention.

Patients with Hodgkin's disease are now often successfully treated with aggressive chemotherapy. However, treatment is associated with a high degree of infertility in both men (80–90%) and women (50%) (58). The interrelationship in young cancer survivors between cancer treatment, loss of desire and sexual dysfunction, lost or impaired fertility, and relationship distress remains clinically inescapable but very little studied.

III. PREVENTION AND MANAGEMENT OF SEXUAL DYSFUNCTION IN CANCER PATIENTS

Currently efforts are made in several areas to refine surgical and radiation therapies to reduce sexual morbidity while retaining medical efficacy. Examples of efforts to preserve sexual quality of life include the development of nerve-sparing surgery techniques for prostate cancer (59) and wide local excision for vulvar cancer (37). A further example of the attempt to preserve quality of life is the strategy of offering observation as a treatment for nonmetastatic seminomatous testicular cancer instead of immediately proceeding with chemotherapy after retroperitoneal lymph node dissection. These developments reflect the growing willingness of the oncology world to try to preserve and maintain sexual function while providing appropriately aggressive cancer therapy.

However, impaired sexual functioning during and/or after cancer treatment can occur regardless of the specific physiological changes that may have taken place. Even patients whose treatments did not affect sexual end organs report being impaired in sexual enjoyment after cancer treatment. Sexual functioning is a complex process that may be disrupted by a wide range of factors, both physiological and psychological. Sexual response during and after cancer treatment is vulnerable to the impact of the cancer itself, medical treatment side effects, other medical problems, medications, pain, depression, anxiety, partner response, and subtler psychological effects, such as changed body image and belief in cancer myths. Cancer patients must face their own mortality, undergo uncomfortable, sometimes lengthy, and/or disfiguring treatments, and deal with the effect of the illness on spouse, family, and work. An understandable consequence of this process can be loss of sexual desire and impaired sexual response. Von Eschenbach and Schover (60) found that the most frequent sexual side effect of men with cancer is erectile dysfunction, but women are more likely to lose interest in sex altogether. Loss or impairment of sexual desire may be triggered by the trauma of diagnosis and treatment, which interferes with the patient's perception of self as a sexual person. There may be concerns about one's attractiveness and the partner's reaction that contribute to an overall withdrawal from sexual activity. Concerns about sexual functioning may contribute to sexual avoidance even if sexual desire per se is not impaired. Although inhibited sexual desire, sexual avoidance, and erectile dysfunction may be the most frequently observed sexual difficulties in this context, any sexual dysfunction may be caused by the patient's and/or partner's reaction to the trauma of the experience.

The medical team often fails to help prevent the development of sexual dysfunction by not addressing the topic with the patient. This may be because of a number of factors, such as discomfort with the topic or a concern not to appear intrusive or presumptuous. When the patients are elderly, young, single, widowed, or gay, sexual concerns appear to be particularly difficult to address (20). All too often, sexuality is viewed as a concern only for men and women who are sexually active within a committed relationship. Every patient, however, regardless of current level of sexual activity, has a perception of self as a sexual being and is invested in knowing that he or she can function sexually, even if they choose not to pursue sexual relationships at the moment. Often the medical staff waits for the patient to open the topic and concludes that there is no interest in sexual issues if the patient remains silent. Vincent et al. (24) found that 80% of patients receiving cancer treatment were interested in more information about sex, although 75% said they would not initiate conversation about it with their doctor. Cancer patients often feel that they should be glad to be alive. Asking about sexual concerns may seem ungrateful and frivolous. If physicians and nurses initiate communication about the sexual side effects of proposed treatments at the time of treatment decisions, they signal to the patient that sexual functioning is a legitimate concern that can be addressed with them.

Privacy and confidentiality are crucial prerequisites for discussing sexual concerns with patients. Sexual matters cannot be productively discussed during rounds, when several staff members are present, or when a roommate is within earshot. Under such conditions the clinician is likely to encounter vague responses and little enthusiasm about the topic. Assessment of the patient's sexual status and history at the time of treatment decision provides the crucial basis for members of the medical team to give appropriate support and information about the possible impact of treatment options on sexual functioning. It also signals to the patient that sexual concerns are understood to be an integral component of quality of life. The time of diagnosis and treatment decision is very stressful for the patient and his or her partner, and sexual concerns are not likely to be in the forefront of their minds. However, sexual functioning must be addressed from the start to support the patient optimally in his or her struggle to adjust to the impact of cancer treatment on his or her self-image and functioning.

Clear and detailed information enables patients and their partners to anticipate problems and prepare for them. The nursing staff in particular can be instrumental in helping patients and their partners deal with both emotional and physical side effects by explaining the physiology involved, normalizing the experience, and giving pragmatic advice and coping strategies. The timing of these interventions is determined by the situation the patient presents. Certainly in emotional or medical crisis situations, as when a relapse of the cancer is discovered, it is not helpful for the patient to be asked about sexual matters. Sexual advice is best received when it specifically addresses the problems with which patient and partner are currently struggling.

At the time of treatment decision, the patient needs to know the sexual issues that may arise from the treatment he or she is about to receive, and that help is available if sexual difficulties should occur. As treatment proceeds and patients are seen for follow-up visits, the sexual status should be assessed by asking open-ended questions: How are things going in your relationship? How are things sexually? As patients express difficulty, it is easy for the caregiver to normalize the experience of the patient, and to offer specific advice on how to improve matters sexually. Table 1 provides an example of the kind of specific coping strategies that may be helpful to patients, in this case individuals with ostomy appliances who have difficulty with resuming sexual activity.

Because any kind of change in appearance and functioning may have sexual consequences, the medical staff must consider the potential sexual implications of all treatments that are offered to the patient and must address them with all patients. A good resource for both staff and patients is a pair of booklets published by the American Cancer Society that address the sexual concerns of male and female patients after cancer treatment and are lucid, practical, and informative about both sexual side effects and strategies to deal with them (61). If patients

Table 1 Strategies for Patients with Ostomy Appliances to Ease Resumption of Sexual Activity

1. Odor can be prevented by having a well-fitting seal and by avoiding foods that produce smelly urine, such as asparagus.
2. Use the smallest pouch available, which will suffice for the duration of sexual activity and be less distracting than the size used ordinarily.
3. Empty the ostomy pouch before sexual activity.
4. Experiment with cloth pouch covers that can be sewn from patterns available from the enterostomal therapist.
5. Try taping the pouch sideways to the body. This keeps the appliance out of the way and prevents distracting flapping.
6. Crotchless panties for women and boxer shorts for men completely cover the pouch.
7. Use a position for intercourse that minimizes friction on the ostomy appliance. A small cushion placed over the ostomy appliance when in the missionary position also helps deflect friction.
9. A rubber undersheet or an absorbing towel in the bed may add to the level of comfort and may reduce concerns about what to do when leakage occurs.
10. Discuss with the partner beforehand what to do if the pouch seal should leak. This helps both partners relax during sexual activity.

continue to experience sexual difficulty after cancer treatment, referral to a sex therapist for careful evaluation and treatment is indicated.

Often a short course of sexual counseling suffices to facilitate better adaptation and functioning. This is particularly true for patients who had a satisfactory sex life before the cancer diagnosis. Sex therapy with cancer patients is geared to address the specific difficulty that patients and/or partners experience. Sexual attitudes and fears are explored, and frequently physical exercises are prescribed for the patient (and his or her partner) to do at home. These exercises are designed to reintroduce sexual activity slowly. Usually these exercises follow a graded approach, beginning with general physical pleasuring and gradually becoming more sexually focused. This approach is particularly helpful to patients who have a great deal of performance anxiety; who may avoid sexual activity for fear they might not be able to complete it; whose confidence in their ability to function is shaken; or who feel unattractive and shy about how their bodies were affected by cancer treatment. Partners similarly can be traumatized by the experiences they had in the course of the treatment and may feel similarly uncomfortable. Recently there have also been some encouraging medical developments to help patients overcome sexual difficulties. Particularly notable in this context is pharmacological injection therapy for erectile dysfunction and ongoing research exploring the use of topical agents to promote erections in men with organic impotence.

IV. SUMMARY

The focus of the available literature is primarily on incidence of sexual dysfunction after cancer treatment. The effect of different sexual treatment interventions on incidence, severity, and duration of sexual dysfunction after cancer treatment is unknown. However, oncologists and nurses can play an important role in helping patients and their partners adjust to physical changes after cancer treatment. A range of possibilities exist: general mention of sexual side effects of treatment at the point of diagnosis and treatment decision; discussion of any sexual concerns during treatment by oncology staff, at times with specific recommendations for particular problems, such as the use of a vaginal lubricant in the woman with treatment-related atrophic vaginitis; follow-up by oncology staff; referral as needed for more comprehensive evaluation by colleagues, including competent specialists in sexual medicine or sex therapy; and self-help measures proposed by cancer patient groups or organizations.

Research on sexual dysfunction in cancer patients is a relatively young discipline, but the increasing attention of the oncology world to this topic is most encouraging. For the clinical oncologist and nurse it is important to be aware that any cancer patient can experience sexual side effects. The process of providing information, education, and help for sexual dysfunction related to cancer starts at the point of diagnosis; patients and partners who are prepared this way are spared the dreary experience of encountering sexual problems as an unexpected and unwanted new burden during or after treatment and then being at a loss about where to turn. Patients are often grateful for direct discussion of sexual concerns; with permission to ask questions without embarrassment many problems may be obviated altogether, and those requiring further attention may be evaluated or referred before long-term consequences, including relationship dysfunction, have been incurred. Common sexual concerns of cancer patients are as follows:

1. Will sexual activity worsen my condition?
2. Will I infect my partner?
3. Will I be attractive to my partner?
4. Will I be able to function and to satisfy my partner?

When sexual problems persist, a brief course of counseling by a professional with training in sexual medicine and sex therapy may be effective in fostering recovery.

REFERENCES

1. Derogatis LR, Kourlesis SM. An approach to evaluation of sexual problems in the cancer patient. CA 1981; 31:46–50.
2. Kiebert GM, De Haes JCJM, Van de Velde CJH. The impact of breast-conserving treatment and mastectomy on the quality of life of early-stage breast cancer patients: a review. J Clin Oncol 1991; 9(6):1059–1070.
3. Wolberg WH, Tanner MA, Romsaas EP, Trump DL, Malec JF. Factors influencing options in primary breast cancer treatment. J Clin Oncol 1987; 5(1):68–74.
4. Fallowfield LJ, Hall A. Psychosocial and sexual impact of diagnosis and treatment of breast cancer. Br Med Bull 1991; 47(2):388–399.
5. Schover LR. The impact of breast cancer on sexuality, body image, and intimate relationships. CA 1991; 41(2):112–120.
6. McCormick B, Yahalom J, Cox L, Shank B, Massie MJ. The patient's perception of her breast following radiation and limited surgery. Int J Radiat Oncol Biol Phys 1989; 17(6):1299–1302.
7. Rowland J, Holland JC, Chaglassian T, Kinne D. Psychological response to breast reconstruction; expectations for and impact on postmastectomy functioning. Psychosomatics 1991; 34(3):241–250.
8. Jordan VC. Long-term adjuvant tamoxifen therapy for breast cancer: the prelude to prevention. Cancer Treat Rev 1990; 17:15–36.
9. Love RR. Antiestrogen chemoprevention of breast cancer: critical issues and research. Prev Med 1991; 20:64–78.
10. Schover LR, Montague DK, Schain WS. Sexual problems. VT DeVita, S Hellman,

Rosenberg S, eds. In: Cancer. Principles and Practice of Oncology, Vol. 2. 1993:2464–2480.
11. Schover LR, von Eschenbach AC. Erectile function in bladder and prostate cancer patients before treatment. Presented at meeting of the American Urologic Association, Las Vegas, 1983, Abstract 17.
12. Zinreich ES, Derogatis LR, Herpst J, Auvil G, Piantadosi S, Order SE. Pretreatment evaluation of sexual function in patients with adenocarcinoma of the prostate. Int J Radiat Oncol Biol Phys 1990; 19(4):1001–1004.
13. Quinlan DM, Epstein JI, Carter BS, Walsh PC. Sexual function following radical prostatectomy: influence of preservation of neurovascular bundles. J Urol 1991; 145(3):998–1002.
14. Schover LR, Von Eschenbach AC, Smith DB, Gonzalez J. Sexual rehabilitation of urologic cancer patients: a practical approach. CA 1984; 34(2):66–74.
15. Schover LR. Sexual rehabilitation after treatment for prostate cancer. Cancer 1993; 71(3 Suppl):1024–1030.
16. Bracken RB, Johnson DE. Sexual function and fecundity after treatment for testicular tumors. Urology 1976; 7:35–38.
17. Takasaki N, Okada S, Kawasaki T, et al. Studies on retroperitoneal lymph node dissection concerning postoperative ejaculatory function in patients with testicular cancer. [Hinyokika Kiyo] Acta Urol Jpn 1991; 37(3):213–219.
18. Schover LR, Von Eschenbach AC. Sexual and martial relationships after treatment for nonseminomatous testicular cancer. Urology 1985; 25(3):251–255.
19. Rieker PP, Fitzgerald EM, Kalish LA, et al. Psychosocial factors, curative therapies, and behavioral outcomes. A comparison of testis cancer survivors and a control group of healthy men. Cancer 1989; 64(11):2399–2407.
20. Auchincloss SS. Sexual dysfunction in cancer patients: issues in evaluation and treatment. In: Holland JC, Rowland JH, eds. Handbook of Psychooncology. New York: Oxford University Press, 1989:383–413.
21. Andersen BL, Jochimsen PR. Sexual functioning among breast cancer, gynecologic cancer, and healthy women. J Counseling Clin Psychol 1985; 53(1):25–32.
22. Van de Wiehl HBM, Weijmar Schultz WCM, Hallensleben A, Thurkow FG, Bouma J. Sexual functioning following treatment of cervical carcinoma. J Gynaecol Oncol 1988; 9:275–281.
23. Berek JS, Andersen BL. Sexual rehabilitation: surgical and psychological approaches. In: Hoskins WJ, Perez CA, Young RC, eds. Principles and Practice of Gynecologic Oncology. Philadelphia: J. B. Lippincott, 1992:401–416.
24. Vincent CE, Vincent B, Greiss FC, Linton EB. Some marital-sexual concomitants of carcinoma of the cervix. South Med J 1975; 68:52–58.
25. Schover LR, Fife M, Gershenson DM. Sexual dysfunction and treatment for early stage cervical cancer. Cancer 1989; 63:204–212.
26. Seibel MM, Freeman MG, Graves WL. Carcinoma of the cervix and sexual function. Obstet Gynecol 1980; 55:484–487.
27. Knorr NJ. A depressive syndrome following pelvic exenteration and ileostomy. Arch Surg 1967; 94:258–260.
28. Andersen BL, Hacker NF. Psychosexual adjustment following pelvic exenteration. Obstet Gynecol 1983; 61(3):331–338.

29. Morley GW, Lindenauer SM, Youngs D. Vaginal reconstruction following pelvic exenteration: surgical and psychological considerations. Am J Obstet Gynecol 1973; 116:996–1002.
30. Lamont JA, DePetrillo AD, Sargent ES. Psychosexual rehabilitation and exenterative surgery. Gynecol Oncol 1978; 6:236–242.
31. Lacey CG, Stern JL, Feigenbaum S, Hill EC, Braga CA. Vaginal reconstruction after exenteration with use of gracilis myocutaneous flaps: the University of California, San Francisco experience. Am J Obstet Gynecol 1988; 158:1278–1284.
32. Van de Wiehl HBM, Weijmar Schultz WCM, Hallensleben A, Thurkow FG, Bouma J. Sexual functioning following treatment of cervical carcinoma. J Gynaecol Oncol 1988; 9:275–281.
33. Andersen BL, Jochimsen PR. Sexual functioning among breast cancer, gynecologic cancer, and healthy women. J Counseling Clin Psychol 1985; 53(1):25–32.
34. Andersen BL, Lachenbruch PA, Anderson B, DeProsse C. Sexual dysfunction and signs of gynecologic cancer. Cancer 1986; 57(9):1880–1886.
35. Mitchell MF, Gershenson DM, Soeters RP, Eifel PJ, Delclos L, Wharton JT. The long-term effects of radiation therapy on patients with ovarian dysgerminoma. Cancer 1991; 67(4):1084–1090.
36. Jenkins B. Sexual healing after pelvic irradiation. Am J Nurs 1986; 86(8):920–922.
37. Stehman FB, Bundy BN, Dvoretsky PM, Creasman WT. Early stage I carcinoma of the vulva treated with ipsilateral superficial inguinal lymphadenectomy and modified radical hemivulvectomy: a prospective study of the gynecologic oncology group. Obstet Gynecol 1992; 79(4):490–497.
38. Andersen BL, Hacker NF. Psychosexual adjustment following pelvic exenteration. Obstet Gynecol 1983; 61(3):331–338.
39. Andreasson B, Moth I, Jensen SB, Bock JE. Sexual function and somatopsychic reactions in vulvectomy-operated women and their partners. Acta Obstet Gynecol Scand 1986; 65:7–10.
40. McCartney CF, Auchincloss SS. Psychosocial aspects of gynecologic cancer care. In: Hoskins WJ, Perez CA, Young RC, eds. Principles and Practice of Gynecologic Oncology. Philadelphia: J. B. Lippincott, 1992: 387–400.
41. Schover LR, Evans R, Von Eschenbach AC. Sexual rehabilitation and male radical cystectomy. J Urol 1986; 136(11):1015–1017.
42. Schover LR, Von Eschenbach AC. Sexual function and female radical cystectomy: a case series. J Urol 1985; 134(9):465–468.
43. Bernstein WC, Bernstein EF. Sexual dysfunction following radical surgery for cancer of the rectum. Dis Colon Rectum 1966; 9:328–332.
44. Bernstein WC. Sexual dysfunction following radical surgery for cancer of rectum and sigmoid colon. Med Aspects Hum Sexuality 1972; 6(3):156–163.
45. Yeager ES, Van Heerden JA. Sexual dysfunction following proctocolectomy and abdominoperineal resection. Ann Surg 1980; 191:169–170.
46. Havenga K, Welvaart K. Sexual dysfunction in men following surgical treatment for rectosigmoid carcinoma. Ned Tijdschr Geneeskd 1991; 135(16):710–713.
47. Koukouras D, Spiliotis J, Scopa CD, Kalfarentzos F, Tzoracoleftherakis E, Androulakis J. Radical consequence in the sexuality of male patients operated for colorectal carcinoma. Eur J Surg Oncol 1991; 17(3):285–288.

48. Hojo K, Vernava AM III, Sugihara K, Katumata K. Preservation of urine voiding and sexual function after rectal cancer surgery. Dis Colon Rectum 1991; 34(7):532–539.
49. Zenico T, Neri W, Zoli M, Tamburini C, Fabri F, Maltoni G. Sexual dysfunction after excision of the rectum. Acta Urol Belg 1989; 57(1):213–216.
50. Sutherland AM, Orbach CE, Dyk RB, Bard M. The psychological impact of cancer and cancer surgery. I. Adaptation to the dry colostomy: preliminary report and summary of findings. Cancer 1952; 5:857–872.
51. Hurny C, Holland JC. Psychosocial sequelae of ostomies in cancer patients. CA 1985; 36:170–183.
52. Holland JC, Rowland JH, eds. Handbook of Psychooncology. Psychological Care of the Patient with Cancer. New York: Oxford University Press, 1989.
53. Chang AE, Steinberg SM, Culnane M, et al. Functional and psychosocial effects of multimodality limb-sparing therapy in patients with soft tissue sarcomas. J Clin Oncol 1989; 7(9):1217–1228.
54. Cust MP, Whitehead MI, Powles R, Hunter M, Milliken S. Consequences and treatment of ovarian failure after total body irradiation for leukaemia. BMJ 1989; 299:1494–1497.
55. Ostroff J, Stern V, Dukoff R, Bajournas D, Lesko LM. The psychosocial adjustment of prematurely menopausal cancer survivors treated with hormone replacement therapy. American Psychosomatic Society Meeting, 1991.
56. Altmaier EM, Gingrich RD, Fyfe MA. Two-year adjustment of bone marrow transplant survivors. Bone Marrow Transplant 1991; 7(4):311–316.
57. Ostroff J, Lesko LM. Psychosexual adjustment of patients undergoing bone marrow transplanation: clinical/research issues and intervention programs. In: Whedon M, ed. Bone Marrow Transplantation: Principles, Practice and Nursing Care. Monterey, CA: Jones and Bartlett, 1991:312–333.
58. Cella DF. Cancer survival: psychosocial and public issues. Cancer Invest 1987; 5(1):59–67.
59. Walsh PC, Lepor H, Eggelston JC. Radical prostatectomy with preservation of sexual function. Prostate 1983; 4:473.
60. Von Eschenbach AC, Schover LR. The role of sexual rehabilitation in the treatment of patients with cancer. Cancer 1984; 54:2662–2667.
61. Schover LR, Randers-Pehrson M. Sexuality and Cancer for the Woman Who Has Cancer, and Her Partner; Sexuality and Cancer for the Man Who Has Cancer, and His Partner. New York: American Cancer Society, 1988.

10

Pain Control in Patients with Cancer

Stuart A. Grossman
Johns Hopkins Oncology Center, Baltimore, Maryland

I. IMPORTANCE OF CANCER PAIN

Pain is one of the most common and feared symptoms associated with cancer. Approximately 20–50% of patients with cancer present with pain, 33% have pain during the treatment of their disease, and 75–90% in the advanced stages of their disease experience moderate to severe pain requiring treatment with opioids (1–3). Unrelieved pain has a substantial effect on patients' activities, affect, motivation, interactions with family and friends, and overall quality of life.

The importance of this symptom and the excellent therapies available make it imperative that physicians and nurses caring for cancer patients be adept at the assessment and treatment of cancer pain. This requires familiarity with the pathogenesis of cancer pain, pain assessment techniques, the common barriers to the delivery of appropriate analgesia, and the pertinent pharmacological, anesthetic, neurosurgical, and behavioral approaches to the treatment of cancer pain.

II. ETIOLOGY OF CANCER PAIN AND IMPLICATIONS FOR THERAPY

Approximately 70% of all pain in cancer patients results from tumor invading or compressing soft tissue, bone, or neural structures (3). Common cancer pain syndromes are listed in Table 1. Failure to define the etiology of pain is a common

Table 1 Etiology of Pain in Cancer Patients

Etiology
Direct tumor involvement (70%)
1. Invasion of bone
2. Invasion or compression of neural structures
3. Obstruction of hollow viscus or ductal system of solid viscus
4. Vascular obstruction or invasion
5. Mucous membrane ulceration or involvement
Associated with antineoplastic therapy (20%)
1. Diagnostic and staging procedures
2. Postoperative (acute postoperative pain or postsurgical syndromes: postmastectomy, postthoracotomy, postamputation)
3. Postradiation (injury to plexus or spinal cord, mucositis, enteritis)
4. Postchemotherapy (mucositis, peripheral neuropathy, aseptic necrosis)
Cancer-induced syndromes (<10%)
1. Paraneoplastic syndromes
2. Pain associated with debility (bedsores, constipation, rectal or bladder spasm)
3. Other (postherpetic neuralgia)
Pain unrelated to the malignancy or its treatment (<10%)

reason for inadequate pain relief and for poor patient outcome. This is exemplified by the following case history.

A 65-year-old woman with lung cancer presented with a 3 week history of worsening pain in the midthoracic region. She had no other symptoms on a complete review of systems, and careful neurological examination was entirely normal. Her chest roentgenograph revealed a posterior mediastinal mass that had not changed since her last evaluation. Oral opioids were initiated, and the doses were rapidly increased in an unsuccessful attempt to control her pain. She developed sudden bilateral lower extremity weakness 2 weeks later, with loss of bowel and bladder continence. On examination she had a T6 sensory level and myelography revealed a T6–9 epidural cord compression. Despite aggressive treatment with surgery, radiation therapy, and glucocorticoids, she failed to regain strength in her lower extremities or sphincter function.

Impending epidural cord compressions are an important cause of unrelieved pain in patients with cancer (4). These patients usually present with weeks to months of back pain, which may have a radicular component. Tumor can reach the epidural space from a metastatic site in the vertebrae or from a posterior mediastinal or retroperitoneal mass that extends through the intervertebral foramina. Over 70% of patients with cancer, back pain, a normal neurological examination, and an abnormal roentgenogram of the spine have epidural tumor evident on myelography or magnetic resonance imaging (MRI) (5). These patients often remain in substantial pain on opioids before they develop an acute and usually irreversible loss of neurological function. A high index of suspicion and early evaluation allow the diagnosis to be made before neurological function is compromised. Pain relief with the administration of glucocorticoids can be dramatic, and radiation usually provides excellent local control. Thus, this patient could have received excellent pain relief and preservation of neurological function with a prompt evaluation and appropriate therapy.

Other common clinical scenarios also highlight the need for a proper pain diagnosis rather than the "empirical" use of opioids in this patient population. Headaches in cancer patients may result from many causes, and opioid analgesics are often not the treatment of choice. Herniation and death may result from untreated brain metastases. Progressive pain and irreversible cranial nerve palsies occur when metastases to the base of the skull are not suspected and treated with radiation therapy. Multifocal neurological signs and symptoms and a rapid demise are likely in patients with untreated leptomeningeal metastases. Likewise, pain in the hip can result from extensive bone metastases and an impending pathological fracture or from referred pain secondary to a spinal lesion. Proper treatment of the pain in these and other situations requires an accurate diagnosis.

Pain also occurs from causes other than the cancer itself. Nearly 20% of all cancer pain results from diagnostic tests, staging procedures, or antineoplastic therapy (3). Surgery can result in significant pain. Of women who undergo a mastectomy for breast cancer, 10% develop a tight, burning pain in the posterior arm, axilla, or anterior chest following surgery. This postmastectomy syndrome must be differentiated from brachial plexus involvement by tumor, a transient inflammatory plexopathy, radiation fibrosis, or an injury related to surgical positioning. Post-thoracotomy syndromes are also common. Radiation and chemotherapy can also cause significant discomfort. Severe oral mucositis is common with these treatment modalities. Cisplatin, vincristine, and taxol can produce painful peripheral neuropathies, and other agents, such as cyclophosphamide, can cause a painful hemorrhagic cystitis. In addition, many patients have pain from illness unrelated to the neoplasm. Migraine headaches, osteoarthritis, gout, and degenerative disk disease are examples of painful illnesses frequently seen in patients with cancer.

Pain is often classified as nociceptive, neuropathic, or sympathetically maintained to guide the evaluation and therapy in cancer patients. Nociceptive pain occurs with the activation of somatic or visceral nociceptors. Painful bone metastases are a common example of somatic nociceptive pain, and visceral nociceptive pain occurs with organ distension. The referral of visceral pain to cutaneous sites can be confusing to the examiner. Neuropathic pain results from direct injury to peripheral or central nervous system structures. It is typified by the burning discomfort or shock-like paroxysms seen in brachial plexopathies. This pain may not respond to opioids but sometimes improves with agents that affect spontaneous discharges in nerves, such as anticonvulsants or antidepressants. Sympathetically maintained pain is much less prevalent than nociceptive or neuropathic pain in cancer patients. It is characterized by a burning discomfort, allodynia, hyperpathia, brawny edema, and osteoporosis. Prompt sympathetic blockade and physical therapy are important in the management of this type of cancer pain.

III. ASSESSMENT OF CANCER PAIN

The goals of a comprehensive cancer pain assessment are to estimate the severity of pain, formulate a differential diagnosis of the etiology of the pain, determine the need for further diagnostic studies, and plan therapy that considers the patient's overall medical and psychosocial status. The assessment of cancer pain, not unlike the assessment of any other serious medical problem, is comprised of a detailed history, physical examination, and review of available records, laboratory data, and imaging studies. Aggressive treatment with analgesics should be initiated while the etiology of the pain is being evaluated. This facilitates the evaluation and reassures patients that their discomfort is being taken seriously. The entirely subjective nature of pain, the complex multisystem involvement in patients with advanced malignancies, and the ever-changing clinical situation in this patient population pose special challenges in the assessment of cancer pain.

A detailed pain history is the cornerstone of the assessment. This may be complex because most patients with advanced cancer have several painful sites and almost one-third have four or more separate pains (1,6). Each pain must be identified and characterized as to its intensity, location, radiation, how and when it began, how it has changed over time, and what makes it better or worse. The quality of each pain (burning and stabbing, for example), its temporal pattern (constant or intermittent), whether it is associated with neurological or vasomotor abnormalities, how it interferes with the patient's life, and an account of the successes and failures of current and prior therapies can provide valuable insight.

Patients with severe, chronic pain often do not "appear" to be in pain (7). Thus, it is imperative that health care providers believe the patient's report of pain and use pain intensity ratings to assess the efficacy of therapeutic interventions. The most useful measure of a patient's pain in his or her subjective pain rating. A formal assessment of pain intensity should be performed using a validated pain intensity scale, such as the visual analog or visual descriptor scale. Many instruments have been developed to aid in pain assessment (Table 2) (8,9). These attempt to characterize and quantify the quality and/or intensity of a patient's pain and represent the best available means to document the discomfort and to follow serially the results of therapy. Several of these instruments have been validated in patients with cancer pain and can be practically incorporated into clinical practice. Most contain a variant of the unidimensional visual analog

Table 2 Valid and Practical Cancer Pain Assessment and Staging Tools

Wisconsin brief pain inventory
Memorial pain assessment card
Hopkins pain rating instrument
Edmonton staging system

scale (VAS) and a schematic representation of the body for the patient to indicate where the pain is located. The Wisconsin brief pain inventory provides information on the characteristics, severity, and location of the pain, its interference with normal life functions, and the efficacy of prior therapy (10). The Memorial pain assessment card is a simple instrument that can be completed in under a minute and features scales for the measurement of pain intensity and pain relief (11). It is also designed to provide some insight into global suffering or psychological distress. The Hopkins pain rating instrument is a validated plastic version of the VAS that obviates the need for the paper, pencil, ruler, and measurements associated with the standard VAS (12). This simplifies repeated pain intensity measurements, making it easier to reassess frequently the efficacy of therapeutic endeavors. The Edmonton staging system for cancer pain provides information on how likely a specific patient is to respond to therapy (13). This staging system relies on the underlying reason for the pain, prior treatment with opioids, and presence of incident pain, impaired cognitive function, psychological distress, tolerance to opioids, and history of alcoholism or drug abuse.

A complete oncological history is essential: 70% of the pain in cancer patients results from tumor invading or compressing normal tissues, and 20% stems from surgery, radiation, chemotherapy, or diagnostic studies performed to evaluate the extent of the tumor. As a result, information about the tumor's histology, presentation, stage, sites of involvement, and natural history is indispensable. All surgery, radiation, chemotherapy, and hormonal treatments should be noted, as should the dates, doses, toxicities, and responses to each. In addition, it is important to determine if the malignancy is responding to therapy, stable, or progressing.

Pain treatments can affect coexisting medical problems, exacerbate constitutional symptoms, or interact with other medications. As a result, a general medical history is critical. A history of severe peptic ulcer disease, benign prostatic hypertrophy, or obstructive pulmonary disease with CO_2 retention is a significant factor in decisions to prescribe potent antiinflammatory drugs or opioids. The route of drug administration is also influenced by a patient's ability to take food or fluids by mouth, the presence of an indwelling venous access device, or a history of substance abuse. The patient's age, functional status, social support, education, residence, health insurance, finances, and religious and cultural background may also figure prominently in planning therapy.

A thorough physical examination with emphasis on the neurological system can also provide important clues to the etiology of the pain. Added insight may come from a review of available laboratory and imaging data, medical records, and discussions with family members and physicians familiar with the patient and his or her illness. Appropriate diagnostic studies may include blood tests, bone scans, plain roentgenograms, myelography, lumbar puncture, electromyography, nerve conduction studies, or computed tomographic or MRI scans of the head, brachial plexus, chest, abdomen, pelvis, or spine.

The history, physical examination, and laboratory and other data should provide the clinician with sufficient information to formulate a differential diagnosis for each of the patient's distinct pains and to make recommendations regarding the work-up and therapy. However, frequent reassessment of cancer pain relief is key to providing optimal care. Excellent pain relief suggests an accurate initial diagnosis and appropriate therapy; suboptimal control or new symptoms may prompt a new treatment approach or a search for a different etiology to the pain. The toxicities of the analgesic therapies must also be periodically reevaluated. Many of the agents used to treat cancer pain can substantially affect quality of life and can be replaced by alternative approaches is they are associated with excessive toxicity. One of the most difficult aspects of cancer pain management is that the patient's clinical situation is rarely static. The underlying malignancy, antineoplastic therapy, tolerance to opioids, and psychosocial status change continually during the course of the illness. As a result, the etiology and intensity of each new or worsening pain must be reassessed.

IV. TREATMENT OF CANCER PAIN

Over 80% of patients with cancer pain can receive excellent analgesia with conventional oral medications (14). More aggressive or invasive therapies should provide pain relief in an additional 10% of patients, leaving only a small portion of cancer patients with inadequate pain relief. However, current data suggest that only a minority of patients with cancer pain receive adequate analgesia (15,16). Many reasons have been proposed to explain these therapeutic inadequacies. Some of these have directly to do with patient concerns or misconceptions. Many patients are reluctant to take opioids, fearing addiction, tolerance, and the potential side effects of these agents. Others fail to communicate the intensity of the discomfort to the health care provider. Some patients elect not to discuss pain with caregivers, believing that cancer pain is unavoidable or fearing that it signifies progressive cancer or that they may divert physician attention from treating the tumor.

Health care providers also contribute to inadequate pain treatment for these patients. Physicians and nurses receive little formal cancer pain instruction during training. As a result, studies demonstrate that physicians and nurses neglect pain control issues, fail to evaluate the underlying etiology of cancer pain, are overly concerned about addiction, tolerance, and opioid toxicities, lack essential opioid-prescribing skills (17), and have little understanding of the intensity of cancer pain in patients (18). In addition, they are frequently confused by the differences between opioid tolerance, dependence, and addiction (Table 3) and intimidated by the special problems of pediatric patients and those with cognitive or communication handicaps or a history of substance abuse. Regulatory efforts to control opioid diversion also result in physicians being overly cautious in prescribing these important drugs (19,20).

Pharmacological approaches are the most commonly used treatments for cancer pain because they are effective, safe, and inexpensive (21,22). Aspirin, acetaminophen, or nonsteroidal antiinflammatory agents (NSAID) are preferred for mild to moderate pain. If these do not provide adequate analgesia, codeine, oxycodone, or hydrocodone frequently provide excellent relief (Table 4). For persistent or severe pain, codeine (or its congener) can be replaced by a potent opioid, such as morphine (Table 5). Drug substitution should be considered before an entire class of agents is abandoned, because patients frequently tolerate one NSAID or opioid better than another.

Table 3 Important Definitions in the Treatment of Cancer Pain

Physical Dependence
Normal physiological response to chronic opioid administration characterized by development of the abstinence syndrome on abrupt withdrawal of opioids
Potential problem in virtually all patients receiving moderate to high doses of opiates
Tolerance
Normal pharmacological response to chronic opioid therapy characterized by the development of a relative resistance to analgesic and other effects of the drug
Overcome by increasing the dose administered
Psychological dependence (addiction)
Abnormal behavior pattern characterized by an all-consuming desire to obtain opioids for reasons other than pain relief, often at the expense of the patient's physical, social, and environmental well-being
Extraordinarily rare in patients with cancer pain
Not to be confused with "pseudoaddiction," which is behavior commonly seen in patients who are undertreated and in pain and are attempting to obtain appropriate analgesia

Table 4 Weak Opioids for Moderate Pain

Drug	Route	Equianalgesic dose (mg)[a]	Peak effect (h)	Duration of effect (h)	Comments
Codeine	PO	200	0.5	3–6	Ceiling for analgesia reached at doses > 240 mg/day orally
	IV/IM	130	0.5	3–6	
Oxycodone	PO	30	0.5	3–6	Parenteral formulation not available
Hydrocodone	PO	NA	0.5	4–6	Available only as fixed combination with acetaminophen or aspirin
Propoxyphene	PO	NA	1.0	4–6	100 mg napsylate = 65 mg hydrochloride salt
Pentazocine	PO	NA	2.0	3	Oral form also available in combination with naloxone; not recommended for treatment of cancer pain
	IV		0.25	1	

[a]Approximate potency relative to 10 mg parenteral morphine. PO, oral; IV, intravenous; IM, intramuscular; NA, not applicable.
Source: Modified from Grossman SA, Gregory E. Management of cancer pain. Cancer Current Therapeutics (Current Medicine) 1994:290–297.

The vast majority of patients can be managed with oral opioids. These are best given "around the clock" to keep pain under control (Table 6). Although tolerance to these agents occurs, tumor progression is the most common reason for increasing opioid requirements. Tolerance can be easily overcome by raising opioid doses. Addiction is extremely rare in cancer patients taking opiates for pain relief. Constipation can be anticipated and should be treated prophylactically. Other opioid side effects can be managed without excessive difficulty.

"Adjuvant" drugs can be beneficial in specific circumstances. Glucocorticoids are effective antiinflammatory agents and reduce the edema associated with brain and epidural metastases. Antidepressants may elevate mood, help with insomnia, and alleviate neuropathic pain. Anxiolytic agents are indicated in selected patients and may potentiate the effect of the opioids. Anticonvulsants, such as carbamazepine and phenytoin, may be effective in neuropathic pain, and amphetamines can decrease opioid-induced sedation. Caution must be exercised in the use of adjuvant drugs with sedative properties: the dose of opioids should not be compromised by the toxicities of these secondary agents.

Patients who present with severe pain should be treated aggressively. Opioids with short half-lives permit rapid oral or intravenous dose escalations. Patient-controlled analgesia is an effective means to titrate opioid doses and toxicities in patients with normal mentation. Once pain is well-controlled, opioid requirements frequently diminish without other intervention. A narcotic equivalency

Table 5 Strong Opiates for Severe Cancer Pain

Drug	Route	Equianalgesic dose (mg)[a]	Peak effect (h)	Duration of effect (h)	Comments
Morphine	PO	30–60	1.5–2.0	4–6	Preferred opiate for management of cancer pain
	PO (SR)	30–60	2.0–3.0	8–12	
	IV/IM	10	0.5–1.0	3–6	
Hydromorphone	PO/PR	7.5	1.0–2.0	3–4	Good choice for SC because of potency
	IV/IM	1.5	0.5–1.0	3–4	
Meperidine	PO	300	1.0–2.0	3–6	Not preferred because of central nervous system toxic metabolite that accumulates in renal failure
	IV/IM	75	0.5–1.0	2–3	
Levorphanol	PO	4.0	1.0–2.0	6–8	Long $T^{1/2}$ (11 h) necessitates slow dose titration; drug accumulation may occur
	IV/IM	2.0	1.0–1.5	6–8	
Fentanyl	TD	0.1(?)	72	≥12	Short $T^{1/2}$ (<1 h); TD dose titration difficult with depot in SC adipose tissue
	IV/IM	0.1	<1.0	0.5–1.0	
Methadone	PO	20	?	4–6	Despite long $T^{1/2}$ (15–150+ h), duration of analgesia is not prolonged; however, drug accumulation can result in toxicities
	IV/IM	10	0.5–1.5	4–6	
Butorphanol	IN	2	1.0	3–4	Mixed agonist-antagonist may precipitate withdrawal in patient previously receiving a pure agonist, thus not generally recommended for cancer pain
	IV/IM	2	0.5–1.0	3–4	

[a]Approximate potency relative to 10 mg parenteral morphine. PO oral; SR, sustained release; IV, intravenous; PO, oral; IV, intravenous; SC subcutaneous; IN, intranasal; TD, transdermal.

Source: Modified from Grossman SA, Gregory E. Management of cancer pain. Cancer Current Therapeutics (Current Medicine) 1994:290–297.

Table 6 Opioid Analgesics: Routes of Administration

Route of administration	Comments	Cost considerations[a]
Oral	Preferred route for cancer pain management	$: D
Buccal/sublingual	Avoids first pass through the liver; otherwise no advantage over oral and unavailable in United States	$: D
Rectal	Available for morphine, oxymorphone, and hydromorphone; dosing considered equivalent to oral, but absorption may be erratic and incomplete	$: D
Transdermal	Available for fentanyl; absorption rates may be affected by subcutaneous fat stores, hypo- or hyperthermia, placement in a radiation port, and ambient temperature; controversial conversion recommendations	$: D
Intranasal	Available for buprenorphine, but not evaluated for management of chronic pain	$: D
Subcutaneous	Bioavailability similar to IV; infection, bleeding, and irritation at injection site may occur	$$$: D, (P), S, Ph, RN, C
Intramuscular	Contraindicated for management of chronic pain	$$: D, S, RN
Intravenous	Indicated only when other routes have failed	$$$: D, P, S, Ph, RN, (SF), C
Epidural/intrathecal	May be useful for avoiding systemic side effects of opiates; usually not effective if systemic treatment has failed	$$$$: D, P, S, Ph, RN, SF, C

[a]Costs: $, overall costs ($, least expensive; $$$$, most expensive). Specific costs for each therapy include D, drug; P, pump rental; S, supplies (tubing, filters, batteries, tape, and heparin); Ph, pharmacy services; RN, nursing services; SF, surgical fee; C, risk of costly complications. Parentheses indicate that the item may or may not be necessary for this route of delivery.

Source: Modified from Grossman SA, Gregory E. Management of cancer pain. Cancer Current Therapeutics (Current Medicine) 1994:290–297.

table should be used to convert patients taking parenteral or short-acting agents to an approximately equianalgesic dose of standard or controlled release oral preparations. Patients with substantial pain who are unable to take oral medications may benefit from parenteral infusions or transdermal opioids. The chronic use of rectal suppositories or injections is usually unnecessary and unacceptable to patients.

Antineoplastic therapy can provide significant analgesia if it reduces the size of lesions invading or compressing normal tissues (15). Radiation therapy is the treatment of choice for most patients with local pain from tumor invasion. It is frequently administered to patients with symptomatic bone, brain, epidural, and plexus metastases. Surgery is effective in relieving pain from intestinal obstruction, pathological fractures, and obstructive hydrocephalus. Chemotherapy can provide substantial pain relief in chemotherapy-sensitive tumors.

Nonpharmacological approaches, such as progressive muscle relaxation, massage, guided imagery, biofeedback, and hypnosis, are useful adjuncts to pain management. Although psychotherapy is indicated for an associated depression, unrelieved pain often results in depression and is best treated with appropriate pain management techniques.

Neurostimulatory techniques, such as transcutaneous electrical nerve stimulation (TENS), peripheral nerve stimulation, dorsal column stimulation, and deep brain stimulation, have been used to treat cancer pain (15). TENS is safe, noninvasive, relatively inexpensive, and easily added to other analgesic approaches. It can provide short-term benefits in cancer patients, and a 2–4 week trial often determines its clinical utility. Peripheral nerve stimulation is invasive, feasible only in the extremities, and of very limited benefit in cancer pain. Dorsal column stimulation is usually performed with an epidural electrode introduced with a Tuohy needle. This may be helpful in mild to moderate neuropathic pain. Deep brain stimulation is rarely used because it requires placement of stimulating electrodes into the internal capsule, thalamus, or hypothalamus. It is ineffective in deafferentation pain.

Regional analgesia can be achieved with long-acting local anesthetics (such as bupivacaine), which provide pain relief for 3–12 h, neurolytic agents (alcohol or phenol), which produce analgesia that can last for weeks to months, or opioids injected into the epidural or subarachnoid space (15). Anesthetic blocks can be used diagnostically or to predict the efficacy and side effects of neurolytic blocks or neurosurgical operations. They can also be useful at "trigger points" in myofascial pain syndromes. Local administration of anesthetic agents is occasionally complicated by hypotension, toxic reactions from accidental intravenous or subarchanoid administration, or pneumothorax following needle placement.

Neurolytic blocks are primarily indicated in patients with localized or regional pain. Subarachnoid and extradural phenol or alcohol destroys nociceptive fibers in the dorsal rootlets, simulating a surgical rhizotomy. This can be useful in thoracic pain in which few motor effects are noted. In cervical and lumbar regions, however, nearly 20% of patients develop motor and/or sphincter dysfunction, which may be permanent. Celiac plexus blocks relieve pain originating in the pancreas, stomach, gallbladder, or other upper abdominal viscera in most patients. Intercostal blocks are helpful in chest or abdominal wall pain. Less commonly used blocks include gasserian ganglion neurolysis (pain in the anterior two-thirds of the head) and brachial plexus blocks (for patients with preexisting limb paralysis). Because neurolytic blocks eventually produce a painful chemical neuropathy, they are limited to patients with advanced disease and a limited life expectancy.

Intraspinal opioids produce analgesia without blocking other sensory, motor, or sympathetic functions. The total daily dose of opioid required with intraspinal administration is 0.1 to 0.01 of an equianalgesic dose of oral or parenteral opioid and is thus associated with fewer systemic toxicities. Chronic epidural or intrathecal opioids are invasive, expensive, and usually ineffective in patients requiring high doses of systemic opioids. Tolerance, pruritus, urinary retention, and nausea and vomiting occur in up to 20% of patients receiving spinal opiates. Respiratory depression is unusual. The addition of low doses of anesthetic agents to intrathecal and epidural opioids may add considerably to pain relief.

Neuroablative procedures are infrequently performed on cancer patients because of the success of more conservative therapies. The open unilateral anterolateral cordotomy, percutaneous cordotomy, and commissural myelotomy are the most commonly performed procedures (15). An open cordotomy is performed through a T2 or T3 laminectomy and produces excellent pain relief in the lower part of the body in 80% of patients. A 5–10% mortality rate and significant morbidity in an additional 15% of patients are reported with this procedure. Hemiparesis, urinary retention, sexual impotence, unmasking pain on the opposite side of the body, and late sensory abnormalities are seen. Bilateral cordotomies are associated with higher complication rates. Percutaneous cordotomy is safer and provides excellent pain relief. However, the pain recurs in about 50% of patients within 3 months. A commissural myelotomy can be considered in selected patients with bilateral pelvic and perineal pain. This involves a laminectomy and surgical division of the crossing fibers of the spinal cord. Although it may result in pain relief with sphincter sparing, there are few neurosurgeons with extensive expertise in this procedure.

V. SUMMARY

Pain occurs in over 70% of patients with cancer and in the vast majority can be well controlled with the currently available treatments. Providing optimal pain relief to cancer patients should be a priority for health care providers, especially in view of mounting data that confirm the undertreatment of cancer pain. A careful and formal pain assessment if required to determine pain intensity, the etiology of the pain, the need for further evaluation, and an appropriate therapeutic plan. Frequent reassessment is required because the underlying malignancy, the antineoplastic therapy, tolerance to opioids, and the patient's psychosocial status change continually during the course of the illness.

SELECTED READINGS

Ad Hoc Committee on Cancer Pain of the American Society of Clinical Oncology. Cancer pain assessment and treatment curriculum guidelines. J Clin Oncol 1992; 10:1976–1982.

Bonica JJ. *The Management of Pain*, 2nd ed. Philadelphia: Lea & Febiger, 1990. This exhaustive reference text contains extensive chapters on cancer pain and the use of anesthetic and neurosurgical procedures that are worth reading.

Foley KM. The treatment of cancer pain. N Engl J Med 1985; 313:84–95. This article offers a complete description of the major issues in cancer pain management.

Foley KM. Controversies in cancer pain: medical perspectives. Cancer 1989; 63:2257–2265. This paper discusses some of the major controversies in the use of drugs, doses, and routes of administration in the treatment of cancer pain.

Grossman, SA. Undertreatment of cancer pain: barriers and remedies. Supportive Care Cancer 1993; 1:74–78. This paper explores the primary reason for the continued undertreatment of cancer pain and suggests practical aproaches to correct these therapeutic inadequacies.

Marks RM, Sachar EJ. Undertreatment of medical inpatients with narcotic analgesics. An Intern Med 1973; 78:173–181. This classic paper is credited with raising the consciousness of clinicians to the undertreatment of pain. It continues to be cited as evidence continues to mount that too little has changed in the treatment of cancer pain in the past two decades.

Portenoy RK. Cancer pain: epidemiology and syndromes. Cancer 1989; 63:2298–2307. This article describes the magnitude of the cancer pain problem and the etiology of common cancer pain syndromes.

REFERENCES

1. Twycross RG. Incidence of pain. Clin Oncol 1984; 3:5–15.
2. Daut RL, Cleeland CS. The prevalence and severity of pain in cancer. Cancer 1982; 50:191–198.
3. Portenoy RK. Cancer pain: epidemiology and syndromes. Cancer 1989; 63:2298–2307.
4. Rodichok LD, Harper GR, Ruckdeschel JC, et al. Early diagnosis of spinal epidural metastases. Am J Med 1981; 70:1187–1188.
5. Grossman SA, Weissman DE, Wang H, et al. Early diagnosis of spinal epidural metastases using out-patient computed tomographic myelography. Eur J Cancer Clin Oncol 1990; 26:495–499.

6. Twycross RG. Relief of pain. In: Sunders CM, ed. The Management of Terminal Disease. Chicago: Yearbook, 1978:65.
7. Foley KM. The treatment of cancer pain. N Engl J Med 1985; 313:84–95.
8. Chapman CR, Casey KL, Dubner R, et al. Pain measurement: an overview. Pain 1985; 22:31.
9. Williams CR. Toward a set of reliable and valid measures for chronic pain assessment and outcome research. Pain 1988; 35:239–251.
10. Cleeland CS. Assessment of pain in cancer. In: Foley KM, Bonica JJ, Ventafridda V, eds. Advances in Pain Research and Therapy, Vol. 6. New York: Raven Press, 1990: 47–55.
11. Fishman B, Pasternak S, Wallenstein S, et al. The Memorial pain assessment card: a valid instrument for the evaluation of cancer pain. Cancer 1987; 60:1151–1158.
12. Grossman SA, Sheidler VR, McGuire DB, et al. A comparison of the Hopkins pain rating instrument with standard visual analogue and verbal descriptor scales in patients with cancer pain. J Pain Symptom Manage 1992; 7:196–203.
13. Bruera E, MacMillan K, Hanson J, et al. The Edmonton staging system for cancer pain: preliminary report. 1989; Pain 37:203–209.
14. Stjernsward J, Teoh N. The scope of the cancer pain problem. Adv Pain Res Ther 1990; 16:7–12.
15. Bonica JJ. The Management of Pain, 2nd ed. Philadelphia: Lea & Febiger, 1990.
16. Grossman SA. Undertreatment of cancer pain: barriers and remedies. Support Care Cancer 1993; 1:74–78.
17. Grossman SA, Sheidler VR. Skills of medical students and house officers in prescribing narcotic medications. J Med Educ 1985; 60:552–557.
18. Grossman SA, Sheidler VR, Swedeen K, et al. Correlations of patient and caregiver ratings of cancer pain. J Pain Symptom Manage 1991; 6:53–57.
19. Angarola RT. National and international regulation of opioid drugs: purpose, structures, benefits and risks. J Pain Symptom Manage 1990; 5:S6–S11.
20. Joranson DE. Federal and state regulation of opioids. J Pain Symptom Manage 1990; 5:S12–S23.
21. Inturrisi CE. Opiate analgesic therapy in cancer pain. Adv Pain Res Ther 1990; 16:133–154.
22. Foley KM. Controversies in cancer pain: medical perspectives. Cancer 1989; 63:2257–2265.

11

Psychiatric and Emotional Problems of Cancer Patients

Darius Razavi
Institut Jules Bordet, Université Libre de Bruxelles, Brussels, Belgium

Friedrich Stiefel
Kantonsspital, St. Gallen, Switzerland

I. INTRODUCTION

An important prevalence of psychiatric disturbances in cancer patients has been reported in many studies. In 1983, the Psychosocial Collaborative Oncology Group observed a prevalence rate of 47% for psychiatric disorders as defined in the Diagnosic and Statistical Manual of Mental Disorders III (DSM-III) in a cohort of cancer patients (inpatient and outpatient populations of three cancer centers). Most importantly, this rate was approximately twice that reported for psychiatric disorders in medical patients and three times the modal estimate appearing in the literature for the general population. As a diagnostic category, adjustment disorders accounted for 68% of all diagnoses. Other diagnoses were major affective disorders (13%), organic mental disorders (8%), personality disorders (7%), and anxiety disorders (4%). In fact, nearly 85% of patients with a positive psychiatric condition presented depression or anxiety as the principal symptom.

Most of these conditions were judged by the authors to be highly treatable disorders (1). In a 1987 study, approximately one in three oncology outpatients assessed with the brief symptom inventory reported moderate to high levels of depression and anxiety (2). A 1989 Swedish study (in Sweden all cases of cancer have been by law notified and recorded since 1958) reported that cancer patients seem to have an increased suicide rate compared with the general population, particularly during the first year after diagnosis, when the rate is multiplied by 15 (3). Last but not least, the high risk of medium- and long-term sequelae of cancer and its treatments has come to light, even if the exact prevalence of these problems remains to be assessed in future prospective research (4). Therefore, the assumption that emotional distress was a foreseeable and ordinary reaction to cancer had to be reviewed, and the need for comprehensive therapeutic models to care for patients who develop psychological disorders was recognized.

Before reviewing recent advances in treating the psychological conditions related to cancer, we must consider three concepts that have a major influence on the current literature: stress, rehabilitation, and quality of life. First, physicians now widely accept the view that cancer and its treatments constitute a stress imposed on a previously healthy individual, involving adjustment efforts (or coping) and possibly adjustment disorders. This stress concept treats psychological disturbances as the consequence of a sustained stressful situation. Several recent articles evaluated the psychosocial disorders associated with cancers in terms of adaptation (5), or adjustment (6).

Second, improvement in cancer treatments and prognosis means that a diagnosis of cancer can no longer be equated with a death sentence. Survivorship, especially in patients with cured hematological malignancies (7), has increased, and with this the need for achieving and maintaining optimal quality of life has become apparent for these patients. Consequently, oncologists are increasingly aware of the patient's needs regarding the return to a normal and useful life, and they therefore are more concerned not only about the short-term psychological effects of their treatments (8) but also about their long-term outcomes in terms of a patient's quality of life (9) and rehabilitation (10). In particular, the psychological distress after surgical treatment of breast cancer is still the center of a controversial debate on partial versus total mastectomy (11, 12). At the same time, surgical and medical treatment decision makers increasingly consider the psychosocial factors predictive of a treatment's success or failure (13).

Rehabilitation of the cancer patient, which seems to be the current leading concept, includes specific support by a multidisciplinary team. From this perspective, psychosocial and psychopharmacological interventions will become a part of large programs oriented toward the rehabilitation and quality of life of cancer patients.

Although most recent articles are related to these promising topics, only a minority investigated ways to make them operational, that is, by the two types of interventions known to be effective for common psychiatric or psychological disorders, which are psychological support and psychotropic medications. The literature of the past years had to be reviewed to provide a valid picture of the current situation in this very new area.

II. ADJUSTMENT DISORDERS

A. Definition and Clinical Presentation

Cancer and its treatments are stressful life events producing an acute stress reaction or a significant life change leading to continued unpleasant circumstances, which may result in an adjustment disorder (AD). AD are thought to arise as a direct consequence of stress or trauma. It is assumed that AD would not have occurred without the impact of cancer stress or trauma.

As discussed in the World Health Organization International Classification of Diseases, AD should be differentiated from acute stress reactions, which are transient disorders of significant severity. This disorder usually subsides within hours or days. Symptoms of acute stress reactions usually appear within minutes of the impact of the stressful event (cancer diagnosis, for example) and disappear within 2 or 3 days: inattention, daze, numbness, inability to comprehend stimuli is the first phase, followed by withdrawal, agitation, or anxiety.

AD are states of subjective distress and emotional disturbance interfering with social functioning and performance. The onset of AD is usually within 1 month of the occurrence of a stressful event, and the duration does not usually exceed 6 months. The manifestations are depressed mood, anxiety, feeling of inability to cope, loss of control, and low self-esteem.

AD should also be differentiated from posttraumatic stress disorder, which occurs as a delayed or protracted response to a stressful event or situation. Typical symptoms include episodes of repeated reliving of the trauma in intrusive memories, dreams, and nightmares and avoidance of activities and situations reminiscent of the trauma or its causes. Commonly there is thus fear and avoidance of reminders of the original trauma. Moreover, patients may also avoid situations to which they attribute the stressful event. There may be also acute outbursts of fear, panic, or aggression. Anxiety and depression are also common. There is support for conceptualizing events in the life of the cancer patients as analogous to physical traumas, such as natural disaster or victimization. Cancer-related events are often of sudden onset and frequently unexpected. They are also associated with physical discomfort and experience of helplessness (14).

It might be useful to recall that postchemotherapy nausea and vomiting often associated with helplessness may led to the development of anticipatory nausea and vomiting. During the course of chemotherapy, an important percentage of patients become sensitized to treatment, reporting anxiety, depression, and nausea in anticipation of chemotherapy (conditioned symptoms). For these reasons chemotherapy may be considered a severe stressor, and it can be useful to assess psychological and pharmacological interventions designed to reduce, retard, or prevent these consequences.

B. Etiology

Patients experience periods of extreme stress. Hospitalization, illness, surgery, and nonoperative procedures are stressful to all patients and may produce AD, because coping with pain, disability, or death challenges human adaptation.

Stressors not related to medical problems, such as marital or job difficulties and financial problems, can also contribute to the development of AD.

The number and significance of psychosocial stressors related or not to cancer in a patient's life are important factors in determining the degree of disability. The more stressors the patients experiences at one time and the more disturbing the stressors are to the patient, the greater the effect on the patient's ability to adjust.

Vulnerability factors are unfortunately not available to help predict which patients will develop AD. Even if it has not been clearly demonstrated, patients with a previous history of AD or complicated prolonged psychological reaction to stressors may be at increased risk for developing these disorders.

C. Major Diagnostic Procedures

The medical interview is the major means of establishing a diagnosis of AD and a therapeutic relationship with the patient. The interview allows definition of past and present problems.

A diagnosis of AD should be considered in patients who have symptoms of anxiety or depression who are experiencing a major psychosocial stressor and who do not meet the criteria for an anxiety disorder, a depressive disorder, or a posttraumatic stress disorder.

It can be argued that the training of health care professionals may be a way to improve the early detection and recognition of psychological problems or psychiatric disorders. This is probably true, but considering that traditional standardized interviews leading to early detection are time consuming (15,16), it is not reasonable to assign all specialized staff to this procedure. A balance should be found between time allocated to interviews, on the one hand, and to treatment or support on the other. The type of health care available and the skills of the health care provider are important factors affecting health policy in this area.

That effective methods of treatment are available for several psychological problems and psychiatric disorders associated with cancer is another argument that justifies the cost of the development and implementation of a screening procedure.

The question of whether screening for the need of psychosocial interventions may be harmful to an individual should also be considered (17). Screening for the need for psychosocial interventions in a cancer population is certainly quite difficult compared with other psychiatric screening. In traditional psychiatric screening, it has been argued that the stigma of a psychiatric label may have negative consequences for the patient in terms of income (18), friendships, and social interaction (19). Moreover, referral to mental health specialists is poorly accepted by some patients (20). For cancer patients, the same arguments fall short. First, one study showed that 85% of cancer patients who reported significant emotional problems said they definitely or probably would go to a mental health professional if they were referred by a medical staff member, and 72% responded positively to meeting a mental health professional together with their families (21). These results confirm previous studies (22).

Moreover, for cancer patients it could not be argued that the stigma of a psychiatric label might have a harmful effect on a condition in which the stigma of being a cancer patient is already quite distressing and full of psychosocial consequences. It also seems that psychosocial studies are viewed by most patients as a helpful extension to treatment (23).

Are specific and sensitive screening methods available at a reasonable cost? The performance of screening methods is beginning to be studied in psychosocial oncology. Most of the methods tested have been self-administered questionnaires because standardized research interviews require time and training. Beck's depression inventory (24), Zung's self-rating depression scale (25), the general health questionnaire (26), Hopkins symptom checklist (27), the Rotterdam symptom checklist (28), and the hospital anxiety and depression scale (29) are the most frequently used screening methods in psychiatry for depression or for general psychopathology. These screening instruments generally take less than 15 minutes to complete and have proven to be quite acceptable to most patients. Most of these questionnaires have been tested in oncology and in primary care settings. The validity of the oral administration of some of these scales for inpatients has also been studied (30).

The orally administered questionnaire allows patients who have difficulty in writing or who have organic mental disorders to participate. The determination of optimal cutoff points is a major issue for screening instruments. The optimal cutoff point curve is generally determined by a cost-benefit analysis.

Cost and benefit should be objective. One must take into account the medical costs implicated in the decision to screen for a given condition and the benefits in terms of quality of life. The medical costs include the expenses related to the screening method and the optimal treatment of the disorders screened. The benefits derive from the improvement of quality of life for patients and their families. This issue is closely related to the effectiveness of the interventions designed for the treatment of the disorders.

At this point, most research efforts have focused on the screening of anxiety and depression, which are the most frequent symptoms of adjustment disorders and anxiety and affective disorders associated with the diagnosis of cancer and its treatment and evolution. For these conditions, self-administered anxiety and depression questionnaires are methods with sufficient sensitivity and specificity to be used for screening. The few studies that assess the performance of the screening methods report a sensitivity and specificity of around 75% (31, 32).

D. Therapy

In this chapter, the term "psychological support" includes all the psychosocial interventions relevant to oncology. Psychological support may thus range from the information provided by the general practitioner who suspects a diagnosis of cancer to the use of sophisticated techniques performed by well-trained oncologists and psychiatrists. Evidence has been found that cancer psychologically affects not only the patients, but also their relatives and the health professionals dealing with them (33). Family interventions and psychological training or support for health professionals should thus also be included in psychological support programs (34).

Not surprisingly, therefore, the literature includes various techniques, more or less explicitly described, dealing with this question: What can we do, without medications, to help the cancer patient cope? Despite the multiplicity of approaches and the objectives they openly declare (to reduce psychological morbidity, enhance quality of life, improve communication, provide information, and teach skills), their purpose can be summarized as optimization of the patient's adaptation to the consequences of the disease. Although techniques constantly overlap in clinical practice, they can be divided schematically according to (1) their degree of directivity, such as nondirective versus directive and (2) their form, including individual, family, or group (Table 1).

Table 1 Common Psychological Support Techniques in Oncology

Nondirective techniques	Directive techniques
Individual	Individual
Information	Behavior therapy
Counseling	Hypnosis
Psychotherapy (supportive or psychodynamic)	Relaxation
Group	Progressive muscle relaxation training
Self-help	Electromyographic biofeedback
Supportive psychotherapy	Guide imagery
Family: supportive psychotherapy	Systematic desensitization
	Distraction
	Cognitive therapy
	Group
	Behavior therapy
	Hypnosis
	Relaxation
	Cognitive therapy

1. Directive Psychological Support Techniques

Behavioral therapies are based on conditioning theories. They involve precise observation of behavior and use directive methods to achieve determined goals. Their results can be directly observed by the disappearance or persistence of the symptom. The positive effects of the behavioral techniques in treating adverse reactions are rather well documented by controlled studies. These techniques are especially effective for anticipatory nausea and vomiting related to cancer chemotherapy (35). They are also proposed for controlling and treating psychological reactions secondary to painful procedures and acute pain and adverse reactions to surgery, radiotherapy, and hyperthermia treatment. Recently they have been proposed for treating postprostatectomy urinary incontinence (36) and also for anxiety and depression in patients with early breast cancer (37). These uses represent a considerable and promising increase in indications for the use of behavioral techniques.

Cognitive therapy deals with present problems and tries to identify maladaptive thoughts, irrational beliefs, and inner factors that are responsible for psychological or somatic symptoms. Once identified, these thoughts are confronted with reason and reality. Self-monitoring automatic thoughts, restructuring, and learning coping strategies are commonly used with cancer patients. No recent article related to this topic was found.

2. Nondirective Psychological Support Techniques

Providing information is the first step in helping patients cope with cancer. Information on diagnosis, prognosis, treatment, and long-term sequelae is given by oncologists and general practitioners in the first line but can be further delivered by other medical staff members and completed by members of self-help groups, either alone or in groups. Information can be provided to the patient alone, to the patient in the presence of family members, or even to family members apart from the patient. As reported recently, perception of information by the patient or family may be distorted by intellectual and psychological factors, especially in the case of negative information (38). Another bias may be the patient's inability or unwillingness to attend to all presented information.

Counseling is a special form of help performed by more or less trained persons whose purpose is to listen to the patients, help them express and understand their feelings about cancer, and encourage them to cope with their current situation. Counselors can be specialized nurses, veteran patients, or even volunteers (39). Counseling is a rather ubiquitous term, but this technique is an attempt to provide cancer patients with first-line support and continuity when no other more specialized help is available.

Psychotherapy is the development of a trusting relationship that allows free communication between patient and specialized therapist. Two models of psychotherapy are used with the cancer patient: supportive and dynamic.

Supportive psychotherapy is based on a short-term, crisis intervention model. This technique is useful in restoring or maintaining the status quo in crisis situations. Individuals, families, or groups can be treated. However, a recent article concluded that although group support was effective in providing information and new friends, it did not help patients cope better with cancer (40). Dynamic psychotherapy, based on the psychoanalytical model, is useful when patients desire to explore further their reactions and feelings to promote personality changes and when un- or preconscious conflicts are responsible for a large part of the psychic symptoms presented. Because its duration can be long, it is indicated for cancer patients with good prognoses.

Recent literature indicates that nondirective therapies achieve their supposed wide field of action at great cost: no definite conclusion can be drawn on their efficiency because of methodological deficiences, such as terms that are too broad and include different techniques, lack of fully completed interventional descriptions, the vague determination of which patients could benefit from these interventions, the nonhomogeneous constitution of the patient groups studied, and the absence of control groups or randomization in most studies. One author counted only seven randomized controlled trials in the field of psychotherapy (41). Another author, considering the benefits of counseling, noted that such interventions have failed to provide unequivocally positive results in oncology (39). Not so surprisingly, despite the unanimous regrets of these authors regarding methodology, general agreement still exists, supported by clinical experience, on the effectiveness of nondirective therapies and their feasibility in a cancer setting.

3. Psychotropic Medications

Clinical experience supports the need and usefulness of psychotropic medications in oncological settings. However, because psychotropic medications have been too rarely tested rigorously in oncology, any advances in the treatment of psychological disturbances remains dependent on progress in the clinical psychiatric research. With the exception of treatment for pain, which is discussed elsewhere, very few psychotropic medications have been tested in oncology: mianserin (42) and methylphenidate (43) have been tested for treating depression, and alprazolam (44,45) and lorazepam (46) have been tested for treating phobic nausea and vomiting related to chemotherapy.

The effectiveness of mianserin versus placebo has been tested in a double-blind design. The doses used were 10 mg/day, three times in the first week, and 20 mg/day, three times in the following weeks; 28 patients in the mianserine groups and 18 in the placebo groups benefited from the treatment.

It may be useful to recall that alprazolam has been already tested to treat aversion to CT and adjustment disorders. Greenberg et al. demonstrated in a double-blind crossover design study that alprazolam significantly reduced nausea before and vomiting during and after CT in patients who had developed an aversive syndrome (44). Patients receiving the active agent typically took 0.25 mg at dinner, 0.5 mg at bedtime, 0.5 mg on morning awakening, and 1.0 mg at noon before chemotherapy. Following chemotherapy they continued 0.5 mg four times daily as tolerated for an additional 2 days.

Both alprazolam and relaxation reduce cancer-related anxiety and depression (mostly adjustment disorders) (45). Although both treatment arms were effective, patients receiving alprazolam (0.5 mg three times a day) showed a slightly more rapid decrease in anxiety and greater reduction in depressive symptoms.

In 1988, an uncontrolled pilot study in which imipramine "or its equivalent" was used suggested the efficacy of antidepressants in treating major depression in cancer patients (47). Regretfully, for our review we found no recent, controlled double-blind study related to this subject. The lack of controlled studies on psychotropic compounds in oncology is explained in part by the lack of recognition of psychiatric disturbances in oncology. Another factor is the relatively small number of psychiatrists specializing in this field. Moreover, the assumption that trials are difficult to conduct because of possible drug interactions and altered pharmacokinetics as a result of medications prescribed for the malignancy is irrelevant, especially for the psychotropic drugs, which are generally well tolerated. Table 2 reviews the principal psychotropic drugs currently admitted to be effective in oncology.

III. ANXIETY DISORDERS

A. Definition and Magnitude of the Problem

Anxiety can be classified following the Diagnostic and Statistical Manual of Mental Disorders (48). These definitions are of help for research purposes but not for daily clinical work, because anxiety may be caused by different events in cancer patients than in the psychiatric setting (49). Using DSM-III criteria, anxiety appears most frequently as a symptom of adjustment disorders (see Sec. II) but could be related in some cases to an anxiety disorder.

However, anxiety is a very prominent symptom of cancer patients: it serves as a physiological reaction to signalize danger to human beings and is therefore in a way part of the somatic disease. In this section, anxiety is reviewed with special emphasis on the different causes that may produce anxiety in cancer patients.

As already mentioned, anxiety disorders, such as generalized anxiety, phobias, or panic disorders, are rare and often predate cancer diagnosis. Anxiety is known by every human being, and the clinical presentation, with anxious mood, increased attention, fearfulness, inability to concentrate, and restlessness, is easy to diagnose. However, the associated somatic symptoms, including

Table 2 Commonly Prescribed Psychotropic Medications in Oncology

Psychotropic agent	Dosage: Initial[a] (mg/day)	Dosage: Range[b] (mg/day)
Antidepressants		
Tricyclics		
Amitryptiline[c]	25	50 – 150
Imipramine	25	50 – 150
Nortryptiline	10	25 – 75
Desipramine	25	50 – 150
Doxepin[c]	25	50 – 150
Second-generation antidepressants		
Maprotiline	25	50 – 150
Mianserin	10	10 – 30
Trazodone	50 mg 3 × daily	150 – 300
Fluoxetine	20	20 – 60
Monoamine oxidase inhibitors		
Isocarboxazid	10 mg 2 × daily	20 – 40
Phenelzine	15 mg 2 × daily	30 – 60
Tranylcypromine	10 mg 2 × daily	20 – 40
Moclobemide	150 mg 2 × daily	300 – 450
Triazolobenzodiazepine		
Alprazolam	0.25 mg 3 × daily	0.75– 6
Stimulants		
Dextroamphetamine	2.5 in the a.m.	5 – 10
Methylphenidate	5 in the a.m.	10 – 20
Lithium		
Lithium carbonate	250 mg 3 × daily	750 –1250
Anxiolytics		
Long half-life benzodiazepines		
Diazepam[c]	5 mg 3 × daily	15 – 30
Clorazepate[c]	5 mg 3 × daily	15 – 30
Short half-life benzodiazepines		
Lorazepam[c]	1 mg 3 × daily	3 – 7.5
Oxazepam	15 mg 3 × daily	45 – 90
Alprazolam	0.25 mg 3 × daily	0.75– 6
Antipsychotics		
Phenothiazine		
Thioridazine	25 mg 3 × daily	75 – 300
Butyrophenone		
Haloperidol[c]	1 mg 3 × daily	3 – 30

[a]Suggested oral dosage, administered once daily at bedtime unless otherwise noted.
[b]Suggested oral dosage.
[c]Available for parenteral use.

dyspnea, tremor, palpitations or sweat, can also be caused by the cancer or its treatment and are therefore less reliable for the diagnosis of anxiety.

B. Etiology

Anxiety can be reactive to a stressor and may also be a consequence of an underlying somatic process or a symptom of a psychiatric disturbance. The following classification is arbitrary and incomplete, but it may help to conceptualize states of anxiety in cancer patients and may serve as a beginning for differential diagnostic considerations.

Anxiety as a reaction to a cancer-related stress is the most common form in oncology. In the DSM-IIIR (revised) classification, this is called an adjustment disorder with anxious mood, alone or in combination with depressed mood. Anxiety as a reaction to cancer is covered in elsewhere (see Sec. II).

Less often, anxiety may arise as phobias activated by aspects of medical care, panic, and generalized anxiety disorders. Phobias, like claustrophobias, may complicate medical procedures and even result in the refusal of a necessary medical intervention. These patients have insight that their fears are unrealistic and are compliant with psychopharmacological or behavioral interventions to help them to overcome their difficulties. Panic disorders, sudden attacks of intense discomfort and fear with such physical symptoms as shortness of breath and palpitations, may be difficult to differentiate from somatic disorders; a history of panic disorders is usually recognized by the family or the patient. Generalized anxiety disorders can arise in patients who have had this problem before or can be a consequence of repressed fears surrounding the diagnosis of cancer.

Anxiety is also a prominent symptom of delirium (acute confusional states): up to 50% of delirious patients express anxiety as one of the main symptoms (50). Withdrawal from alcohol and benzodiazepines is also very often associated with anxiety. Other psychiatric disorders, such as depressive disorders, may include in their clinical presentation mild to severe anxiety.

Different somatic processes can cause anxiety in cancer patients. Acute pain is one of the most common causes of anxiety, but hypoxia or metabolic disorders like hypercalcemia can also be associated with anxiety. A variety of drugs provoke anxiety as known side effects: corticosteroids (and corticosteroid withdrawal), morphine by inducing hallucinatory states, and others (51). Akathisia, a side effect of neuroleptics often used as antiemetics, is commonly misdiagnosed as anxiety and can be very discomforting to the patient.

There are many other forms of anxiety in cancer patients, and some of them have a spiritual and existential dimension. It is beyond the scope of this chapter to include these dimensions, but their mention illustrates that not all anxious states are the domain of the medical doctor or the psychiatrist, and practitioners should be aware of their own possibilities and limitations.

C. Major Diagnostic Procedures

To assess anxiety, the main diagnostic tool remains the dialogue with the cancer patient and significant others. Possible misconceptions, unrealistic fears, psychiatric disorders, and somatic complaints can be questioned, and if an organic cause is suspected to provoke anxiety, additional medical examinations and laboratory work-up, as well as a chart review for side effects of administered drugs, are required. Repeated examinations of cognitive functions is often neglected, and delirium in cancer patients is often not diagnosed. To assume that an anxious patient has "the right to be anxious, since he has cancer" is probably the most common obstacle to diagnosis and appropriate treatment.

D. Therapy

Any therapeutic approach requires a discussion with the patient to understand possible reasons for anxiety. A discussion on how the patient thinks about the illness and the future, how he or she copes with the situation, and what physical symptoms he or she suffers is necessary for proper treatment and in itself therapeutic. Often the dialogue with the treating physician, in which a patient is allowed to express feelings and possible misconceptions and unrealistic fears can be clarified, is the best therapeutic procedure. If organic causes or psychiatric disturbances as source of anxiety are ruled out and psychotherapeutic interventions and spiritual support are not successful, symptomatic treatment with psychotropic medication is indicated.

Benzodiazepines and sometimes low doses of neuroleptics are frequently and successfully utilized for symptomatic treatment of anxious states in cancer patients. Benzodiazepines (such as diazepam) with long half-lives and active metabolites can cause profound and prolonged sedation and should therefore be used with caution (52); newer benzodiazepines with short half-lives, such as lorazepam, are therefore more suited to treat anxiety in cancer patients. In the elderly patient, benzodiazepines can sometimes induce paradoxical excitement, and low-dose neuroleptics may be the better choice (53).

IV. DEPRESSIVE DISORDERS

A. Definition and Clinical Presentation

The frequency of depression in cancer patients ranges from 4.5 to 58% in different studies (53). A study (1) using DSM-III criteria reported a rate of 13% of cancer patients with a major affective disorder (unipolar and bipolar depression, atypical depression, and dysthymic depression) among patients who met the criteria for psychiatric disorder.

The clinical presentation includes psychological and somatic symptoms:

dysphoric and diurnal mood changes, feelings of hopelessness and helplessness, suicidal ideation, guilt, poor concentration and, rarely, delusional thoughts; somatic symptoms, such as constipation, insomnia, pain, fatigue, anorexia, and psychomotor retardation or agitation, are not reliable signs in cancer patients, because they can be caused by the tumor or its treatment (51).

B. Etiology

Patients with a family or a personal history of depression are certainly at greater risk to develop a depression during the course of cancer. As in the general population, alcohol abuse is also a risk factor for depression, which is also illustrated by the higher incidence of depression in patients with head and neck cancer (54). Patients with pancreatic cancer also have a higher risk for depression (55); the causes for this phenomenon is unknown, but a paraneoplastic syndrome is suspected (56). Other common causes for depression in cancer patients include chronic unreliefed pain, medications (corticosteroids, vincristine, interferon, cimetidine, and others), metabolic alterations (like hypercalcemia), or damage to the central nervous system by the tumor or its treatment (52,57).

C. Major Diagnostic Procedures

Clinical evaluation includes a careful assessment of the symptoms just described; that depression in cancer patients remains undiagnosed is often related to the fear of treating physicians to ask direct questions about the feelings of their patients. However, daily clinical experience with cancer patients demonstrates that patients do not believe such questions to be stressful as long as they are posed in an emphathetic way. On the contrary, most cancer patients are relieved to talk about their feelings.

The differential diagnosis of depression includes sadness, adjustment disorders with depressed mood, grief, and delirious states with depressed affect. If the psychological symptoms described earlier are present and the cognitive state of the patient is not altered, then the diagnosis of depression is likely and a treatment should be considered. It may sometimes be very difficult to diagnose depression in cachectic cancer patients with advanced disease, and confirmation of the diagnosis by a consultation-liaison psychiatrist may become necessary.

Criteria have been suggested for diagnosing major depressive syndromes in medical patients (58). Somatic items of DSM-III criteria, such as problems with appetite, with sleep, fatigue, and complaints about lessened concentration, could be replaced by psychological items, such as fearfulness or depressed appearance, social withdrawal or decreased talkativeness, brooding self-pity, and pessimism.

D. Therapy

Once the cause of depression has been established and a causal therapeutic approach (treatment of hypercalcemia, for example) is not possible, short-term psychotherapy supporting past strengths and successful coping strategies becomes necessary. If possible and helpful, the inclusion of family members in the therapy may be beneficial. Severe depressive states usually also requires treatment with psychotropic drugs. Antidepressants utilized in cancer patients include the tricyclic and second-generation antidepressants started in low doses, monoamine oxidase inhibitors, benzodiazepines, and stimulants (e.g., dextroamphetamine). Cancer patients respond to lower doses of psychotropic medications because of an altered metabolism and may be more sensitive to side effects (52). Second-generation antidepressants may therefore be more appropriate for cancer patients because they have fewer anticholinergic side effects than tricyclic antidepressants.

One of the reasons for underutilizing antidepressants is the importance given to interference with cytotoxic drugs, morphinics, sterroids, and anticoagulants. The limited use of antidepressants is also a result of some badly tolerated side effects, particularly in elderly patients. There are some cardiovascular risks (conduction disorders and low blood pressure), neurological risks (sedation, confusion, and seizure), and risks of the development of visual disorders, constipation, and urinary retention. In elderly patients with cardiac disorders, electrocardiograph, monitoring of arterial pressure, and plasmatic dosage of antidepressants are usually required (59).

As with the anxiety disorders, a major setback to effective treatment is that depression often remains unrecognized and, if recognized, remains untreated (52). Knowledge of psychiatric complications in medically ill patients is unfortunately not extensive among nonpsychiatrists, and future medical education should include these subjects during training.

V. DELIRIUM IN CANCER PATIENTS

A. Definition and Clinical Presentation

Delirium (acute confusional states) is a common psychiatric complication of patients with cancer (60). It is the most common neglected psychiatric syndrome, partly because it is a psychiatric syndrome mainly seen by nonpsychiatric physicians (61). Since Engel and Romano's classic studies investigating delirium (62), there has been a lack of research into classification, epidemiology, pathophysiology, etiology, clinical presentation, diagnostic procedure, treatment, and prevention of delirium (50). With this in mind, this section is devoted to a brief overview of the current literature of delirium in cancer patients.

Early symptoms of delirium are often unrecognized or misdiagnosed as depression or dementia (63). Delirium usually has an acute onset and is of brief duration; three clinically distinctive types can be distinguished: the hyperactive-hyperalert, mixed, and hypoactive-hypoalert (64). It is unfortunate that most of the published literature consists of reviews of the clinical syndrome, but none of the papers address the issue of to what extent the clinical criteria are valid and reliable in the diagnosis of delirium (65).

Delirium is by definition a reversible syndrome, but the clinical course and consequences of delirium (mortality and length of hospitalization) are not well elucidated. However, the onset of delirium is always a serious sign of a dangerous underlying somatic process and can serve as a predictor of shortened survival (66).

Lipowski, who is devoted to the elucidation of this syndrome and edited the most comprehensive book on this subject (67), described the core features as "disorders of cognition, attention, sleep-wake cycle, and psychomotor behavior" (68). However, the criteria for delirium according DSM-IIIR were all based on extensive clinical experience, particularly that of the general hospital psychiatrist, but without data from field testing or clinical research, which only recently were undertaken and will be of interest for future diagnostic criteria in DSM-IV (50,65).

The magnitude of the problem can be concluded from different studies on the prevalence of delirium in cancer patients, which has ranged from 5 to 25% (63). In one study, 85% of terminally ill cancer patients suffered from delirium (69). These differences are based on variations in the population sampled and are largely dependent on age, level of physical disability, and stage of disease, which are all risk factors of delirium in cancer patients (70).

B. Etiology

Different hypotheses for the etiology of delirium exist in the literature, and it may be that different mechanisms contribute simultaneously to a delirious state in a cancer patient or that the pathophysiology may differ according to the underlying etiology.

The following and other hypotheses have been posited to explain the onset of delirium (50,60):(1) any factor that reduces cerebral oxidative metabolism can lead to changes in the functional metabolism of cerebral neurons; (2) imbalance of neurotransmitter (imbalance between acetylcholine and dopamine caused by anticholinergic drugs or other reasons); (3) hypercortisolism caused by stress or external agents; (4) neuroanatomical models (brain metastases); and (5) changes in endorphine levels.

A range of factors cause delirium in cancer patients. They can be classified as direct and indirect effects on the central nervous system (see Table 3) (71). Direct effects are those related to primary brain tumor or metastatic spread;

Table 3 Causes of Delirium in Cancer Patients

Direct effects
Primary tumor
Metastatic lesions by local extension, hematogenous, or lymphatic routes
Indirect effects
Metabolic problems (organ failure and electrolyte imbalance)
Treatment effects (chemotherapeutic agents, radiation, medications)
Infections (pneumonia) and systemic infections
Vascular complications (thromboembolic cerebral infarction, intracranial hemorrhage)
Hematological abnormalities (anemias, coagulopathies)
Nutritional deficits (general malnutrition and vitamin deficits)
Paraneoplastic syndromes

Source: Modified from Posner, 1978.

indirect effects are far more frequent and are caused by infections, vascular complications, metabolic abnormalities, hematological complications, nutritional deficiencies, treatment side effects, and paraneoplastic syndromes.

The following causes of delirium in cancer patients are most important (70): metabolic abnormalities (organ failure and electrolyte imbalance), infections (pneumonia and sepsis), vascular complications (thromboembolic cerebral infarction), metastatic brain disease, and treatment effects. Among treatment side effects, corticosteroids, narcotic analgesics, psychotropics and other drugs with anticholinergic properties, and chemotherapeutic agents are the most common causes of delirium in cancer patients (63,70,72).

Patients with cancer who are seriously ill often have multiple causes for delirium. In a study of patients with advanced and terminal disease (69), in only 1 of 11 patients with delirium was a single cause established. The remaining patients' delirium was attributed to multiple factors. In a retrospective study on cognitive failure in cancer patients with advanced disease (60), the causal agent remained unknown in 75%. This may be because an extensive work-up in terminally ill patients is rarely appropriate.

C. Major Diagnostic Procedures

The diagnosis of delirium relies heavily upon the history and presence of an altered mental state, with identification of the cognitive impairment; clinical examination, laboratory data, and other investigations assist in establishing etiology and diagnosis (70). Unlike other medical patients, many cancer patients are faced with dealing with a fatal disease, and normal stress reactions, depression, and other psychiatric disturbances may be difficult to differentiate. Subtle changes in mental status and behavior are therefore apt to go unnoticed or to be attributed to the stress of cancer diagnosis. A close watch of mental functions and comparison with its prior level (history by family members and chart review) help to differentiate delirium from a normal stress reaction, an adjustment disorder, or an early dementia.

D. Therapy

Management of delirium is first directed toward determining the underlying cause and toward treatment, when possible, of the etiology agent to reverse the condition. However, because this is rarely possible, symptomatic treatment becomes necessary. General supportive and nonspecific treatments may help in milder forms of delirium: environmental manipulation with a clock at bedside to help the patient's orientation are staff instructions to minimize the number of different members involved in the care of the patient are examples (70).

More often, acute confusion with hallucinations, delusions, anxiety, agitation, and disruptive behavior requires symptomatic treatment with psychotropic drugs. The cornerstones of symptomatic psychotropic therapy are the neuroleptic and benzodiazepine drugs.

Haloperidol is a commonly prescribed antipsychotic drug in the cancer setting because of its low incidence of cardiovascular and anticholinergic effects (52). Hospitalized cancer patients usually respond to low doses of psychotropic medication, such as 0.5 mg haloperidol given two or three times daily; acute extrapyramidal side effects, although not common at these dose levels, are usually controlled by diphenhydramine or benztropine twice a day (70). The addition of lorazepam for sedation or a continuous subcutaneous infusion of midazolam in severe cases is being increasingly used (57,67).

It is very unfortunate that there are virtually no studies comparing benzodiazepines with neuroleptics in the treatment of delirium, and any suggestions from the literature remain on empirical grounds.

VI. CONCLUSIONS

First, it is important to recall that a precise and comprehensive assessment of the psychological and psychiatric problems and a good understanding of the social situation are of the utmost importance for any reasonable therapeutic intervention. Developing specific assessment methods is still necessary, as are simple, reliable, and valid tools for the early screening of psychological disturbances in an oncology population. Early detection of mild psychological distress may identify patients who could be helped with psychosocial interventions. Moreover, even if no data are available stating that early treatment could have therapeutic results superior to those of delayed treatment, early treatment obviously has a positive effect on quality of life. Along the same lines, early recognition of distress among family members and caretakers is another promising subject of research to improve the quality of support.

Second, lack of precise, uniform description for most psychological interventions remains an obstacle to any progress in this field. Especially for nondirective techniques, the indications for and purposes of psychological support remain unclear. The type of cancer and treatment, the time in the illness course, the patient's personality, gender, and age, and the quality of social support are all factors that should be taken into account to increase the relevance and validity of research in this area. Most interestingly, the question of whether appropriate psychological support has a positive influence on cancer patient survival has recently come to the fore. This topic requires careful examination and further controlled studies (73).

Third, it is unfortunate that the qualifications of the person performing the therapy are hardly defined. Should a general practitioner, an oncologist, a nursing staff member, a mental health professional (e.g., psychiatrist, psychologist, or trained therapist), or a nonprofessional (e.g., veteran patient or voluntary organization member) intervene? Specific training should be designed and organized for each of these categories (34,74). More research comparing the efficacy of same treatments performed by differently trained persons must be done, not only to provide patients with the most effective therapy but also to take into account its cost and feasibility in a cancer setting. In conclusion, without rigorous research and controlled studies, psychological support will continue to be suspected of empiricism, although its efficacy as adjuvant therapy in oncology can no longer be questioned (75).

Despite recognition of the high prevalence of psychiatric and psychosocial disturbances associated with cancer and its treatment and inclusion of the psychosocial factors in quality of life assessments and rehabilitation programs, very few articles rigorously investigate what can actually be done to prevent and alleviate these disturbances. In particular, research should be encouraged in the newly identified class of adjustment disorders that occur so frequently in oncology; new concepts to understand and treat them are dramatically needed. The respective indications of psychological support, psychotropic medications, or both are based on clinical experience and rarely controlled in large prospective studies. A first step should be to recognize the respective usefulness of single psychological interventions and single medical agents in specific situations. A second step should be to compare different techniques for their efficacy, cost, and feasibility in a cancer setting. A third step should be to test for the possible superior effectiveness of combinations, such as nondirective technique with directive technique, individual psychological support with family support, psychological support with psychotropic medication, and antidepressant with benzodiazepine.

Because the psychiatric conditions found in cancer patients are reported to be quite different from those encountered in the general population and in other medically ill patients, further development of specific tools is needed to assess psychiatric morbidity in oncology. Controlled studies must test the usefulness of psychotropic agents for major depressive disorders, delirium, and insomnia. The complete lack of controlled studies in the field of adjustment disorders must be addressed without delay. The feasibility and effectiveness of using specific classes of psychotropic medications for preventing psychological and psychiatric disorders in cancer patients should be evaluated in prospective studies at each phase of the illness course. For example, concepts and research about the preventive use of psychopharmacotherapy for patients undergoing stressful medical procedures or treatment (chemotherapy, for example) is in its infancy, so that at present only tentative guidelines can be offered to oncologists (76). The goals of a preventive treatment should be the reduction of psychological and psychiatric morbidy and reduction in the delay of symptom control when some symptoms may be frequent and expectable (such as sleeping problems, conditioned symptoms, and adjustment disorders). More studies are needed to find the most effective drug combinations, optimal drug dosage, and treatment duration. The ideal evaluation of the efficacy of prevention programs requires randomized controlled trials that compare not only prevention in normal clinical follow-up but also in early detection and early treatment. Finally, more research on the development of the most frequent psychological or psychiatric conditions encountered in oncology will allow to select on a less empirical basis which drugs should be combined for preventive use.

The important prevalence of psychosocial problems and psychiatric disturbances that have been reported in oncology emphasizes the need for a comprehensive psychosocial support of cancer patients and their families. Psychosocial support is designed to preserve, restore, or enhance quality of life. Quality of life refers not only to psychosocial distress and adjustment-related problems but also to the management of cancer symptoms and treatment side effects. Psychosocial interventions designed for this purpose should be divided in five categories: prevention, early detection, restoration, support, and palliation. Preventive interventions are designed to avoid the development of predictable morbidity secondary to treatment and/or disease. Early detection of a patient's needs or problems anticipates that early interventions could have therapeutic results superior to those of delayed support, for both quality of life and survival. Restorative interventions are used when a cure is likely, the aim being the control or elimination of residual cancer disability. Supportive rehabilitation is planned to lessen disability related to chronic disease characterized by numerous cancer illness remission, progression, and active treatment. Palliation is required when curative treatment is likely to be no longer effective and when maintaining or improving comfort becomes the main goal.

Psychosocial interventions are often multidisciplinary, with a variety of content. The content of psychological interventions range from information and education to more sophisticated support program, including directive (behavioral or cognitive) therapies and nondirective (dynamic or supportive) therapies. Social interventions usually include financial, household, equipment, and transport assistance, depending on individual and family needs and resources. These interventions may be combined with the prescription of pharmacological (e.g., psychotropic or analgesic), physical, speech, or occupational therapies, especially in rehabilitation programs. Health care services devoted to deliver these interventions are hospital, hospice, or home based and organized very differently depending on already available community resources and needs.

REFERENCES

1. Derogatis LR, Morrow G, Fetting J, et al. The prevalence and severity of psychiatric disorders among cancer patients. JAMA 1983; 249(6):751–757.
2. Stephanek ME, Derogatis LP, Shaw A. Psychological distress among oncology outpatients. Psychosomatics 1987; 28:530–539.
3. Allebeck P, Bolund C, Ringbäck G. Increased suicide rate in cancer patients: a cohort study based on the Swedish Cancer-Environment Register. J Clin Epidemiol 1989; 42:611–616.
4. Loescher L, Welch-McCaffrey D, Leigh S, Hoffman B, Meyskens F. Surviving adult cancers. Part 2. Psychosocial implications. Ann Intern Med 1989; 111:517–524.
5. Eil K, Nishimoto R, Morvay T, Mantell J, Hamovitch M. A longitudinal analysis of psychological adaptation among survivors of cancer. Cancer 1989; 63:406–413.
6. Vinokur A, Threatt B, Caplan R, Zimmerman B. Physical and psychosocial functioning and adjustment to breast cancer: long-term follow-up of a screening population. Cancer 1989; 66:394–405.
7. Lesko L, Holland J. Psychological issues in patients with hematological malignancies. Recent Results Cancer Res 1988; 108:243–270.
8. Love R, Leventhal H, Easterling D, Nerenz D. Side effects and emotional distress during cancer chemotherapy. Cancer 1989; 66:604–612.
9. Ochs J, Mulheim R, Kun L. Quality-of-life assessment in cancer patients. Am J Clin Oncol 1988; 11:415–421.
10. Kurtzman S, Gardner B, Kellner W. Rehabilitation of the cancer patient. Am J Surg 1988; 155:791–801.
11. Kemeny M, Wellisch D, Schain W. Psychosocial outcome in a randomized surgical trial for treatment of primary breast cancer. Cancer 1988; 62:1231–1237.
12. Wolberg W, Romsaas E, Tanner M, Malec J. Psychosexual adaptation to breast cancer surgery. Cancer 1989; 66:1645–1655.
13. Salmon S. Factors predictive of success or failure in acquisition of esophageal speech. Head Neck Surg 1988; 10:5105–5109.
14. Cella D, Mahon S, Donovan M. Cancer recurrence as a traumatic event. Behav Med 1990; 15–21.

15. Hamilton M. The assessment of anxiety states by rating. Br J Med Psychol 1959; 32:50–58.
16. Wing JK, Cooper JE, Sartorius N. The Measurement and Classification of Psychiatric Symptoms. London: Cambridge University Press, 1974.
17. Ford DE. Principles of screening applied to psychiatric disorders. Gen Hosp Psychiatry 1988; 10:177–188.
18. Link B. Mental patient status, work and income: an examination of the effects of a psychiatric label. Am Sociol Rev 1982; 47:202–215.
19. Phillips D. Public identification and acceptance of the mentally ill. Am J Public Health 1966; 56:755–763.
20. Bursztajn H, Barsky AJ. Facilitating patient acceptance of a psychiatric referral. Arch Intern Med 1985; 145:73–75.
21. Houts P, Lipton A, Harvey H, Simmonds M, Cadieux R, Bartholomew M. Willingness to use mental health services by cancer patients with emotional problems. International Conference on Supportive Care in Oncology. Abstracts. Princeton: Symedco, 1988:182.
22. Worden JW, Weisman AD. Do cancer patients really want counseling? Gen Hosp Psychiatry 1980; 2:100–103.
23. Fallowfield L. Do psychological studies upset patients? In: Holland JC, Massie MJ, Lesko LM, eds. Current Concepts in Psycho-Oncology and AIDS. Syllabus of the Postgraduate Course/Memorial Sloan-Kettering Cancer Center, New York, 1987:335.
24. Beck AT, Beck RW. Screening depressed patients in family practice. Postgrad Med J 1972; 52:81–85.
25. Zung WWK. A self-rating depression scale. Arch Gen Psychiatry 1965; 12:63–70.
26. Goldberg DP. A Technique for the Identification and Assessment of Nonpsychotic Psychiatric Illness. London: Oxford University Press, 1972.
27. Derogatis DL. The SCL-90 Administration, Scoring and Procedures Manual I. Baltimore: Clinical Psychometric Research, 1977.
28. Haes De JCJM, Pruyn JFA, Knippenberg FCE. Klachtenlijst voor kankerpatienten, eerste ervaringen. Ned Tijdschr Psych 1983; 38:403–422.
29. Zigmond AS, Snaith RP. The hospital anxiety and depression scale. Acta Psychiatr Scand 1983; 67:361–370.
30. Griffin P, Kogut D. Validity of orally administered Beck and Zung depression scales in a state hospital setting. J Clin Psychol 1988; 44:756–759.
31. Razavi D, Delvaux N, Farvacques C, Robaye E. Screening for adjustment disorders and major depressive disorders in cancer in-patients. Br J Psychiatry 1990; 156:79–83.
32. Razavi D, Delvaux N, Brédart A, et al. Screening for psychiatric disorders in a lymphoma out-patient population. Eur J Cancer 1992; 28A(11):1869–1872.
33. Delvaux N, Razavi D, Farvacques C. Cancer care—a stress for health professionals. Soc Sci Med 1988; 27:159–166.
34. Razavi D, Delvaux N, Farvacques C, Robaye E. Immediate effectiveness of brief psychological training for health professionals dealing with terminally ill cancer patients: a controlled study. Soc Sci Med 1988; 27:369–375.

35. Morrow GR, Morrel C. Behavioral treatment for the anticipatory nausea and vomiting induced by cancer chemotherapy. N Engl J Med 1982; 307:1476–1480.
36. Burgio K, Stutzman R, Engel B. Behavioral training for post-prostatectomy urinary incontinence. J Urol 1989; 141:303–306.
37. Bridge L, Benson P, Pietroni P, Prest R. Relaxation and imagery in the treatment of breast cancer. BMJ 1988; 297:1169–1172.
38. Mackillop W, Stewart W, Ginsburg A, Stewart S. Cancer patient's perceptions of their disease and its treatment. Br J Cancer 1988; 58:355–358.
39. Fallowfield L. Counseling for patients with cancer. BMJ 1988; 297:727–728.
40. Deans G, Bennett-Emslie J, Weir J, Smith D, Kaye S. Cancer support groups—who joins and why? Br J Cancer 1988; 58:670–674.
41. Greer S. Can psychological therapy improve the quality of life of patients with cancer? Br J Cancer 1989; 59:149–151.
42. Costa D, Mogos I, Toma T. Efficacy and safety of mianserin in the treatment of depression of women with cancer. Acta Psychiatr Scand 1985; 72:85–92.
43. Fernandez F, Adams F, Holmes VF. Methylphenidate for depressive disorders in cancer patients. Psychosomatics 1987; 28:455–461.
44. Greenberg DB, Surman OS, Clarke J, Baer L. Alprazolam for phobic nausea and vomiting related to cancer chemotherapy. Cancer Treat Rep 1987; 71(5):549–550.
45. Holland JC, Morrow GR, Schmale A, et al. A randomized clinical trial of alprazolam versus progressive muscle relaxation in cancer patients with anxiety and depressive symptoms. J Clin Oncol 1991; 9(6):1004–1011.
46. Greenspoon J, Leuchter RS, Semrad N. Lorazepam for chemotherapy-induced emesis. Arch Intern Med 1984; 144:2432–2433.
47. Evans DL, McCartney CF, Haggerty JJ, et al. Treatment of depression in cancer patients is associated with better life adaptation: a pilot study. Psychosom Med 1988; 50:72–76.
48. Othmer E, Othmer SC. The Clinical Interview using DSM-III-R. Washington, DC: American Psychiatric Press, 1989.
49. Stiefel F. Angst und terminale Tumorerkrankung. Schweiz Rundschau Med (Praxis) 1993; 82(2):41–44.
50. Stiefel F. Age and the Syndrome of Delirium—Ein Workshop des National Institut of Mental Health, Washington, DC, June 1989. Schweiz Rundschau Med (Praxis); 78:1329.
51. Massie MJ. Depression. In: Holland JC, Rowland JH, eds. Handbook of Psychooncology. New York: Oxford University Press, 1989:300–309.
52. Stiefel F, Kornblith A, Holland J. Changes in the prescription patterns of psychotropic drugs for cancer patients during a 10-year period. Cancer 1990; 65:1048–1053.
53. Massie MJ. Anxiety, panic and phobias. In: Holland JC, Rowland JH, eds. Handbook of Psychooncology. New York: Oxford University Press, 1989:300–309.
54. Baile WF, Gibertini M, Scott L, Endicott J. Depression and tumor stage in cancer of the head and neck. Psycho-Oncology 1992; 1:15–24.
55. Holland JC, Hughes AH, Tross S, Silberfarb P, Perry M, Comis R. Oster M. Comparative disturbance in patients with pancreatic and gastric cancer. Am J Psychiatry 1986; 143:982–986.

56. Pomara NP, Gershon S. Treatment-resitant depression in an elderly patient with pancreatic carcinoma. J Clin Psychiatry 1984; 45:439–440.
57. Stiefel F, Volkenandt M, Breitbart W. Suizid und Krebserkrankung. Schweiz Med Wocherschr 1989; 119:891–895.
58. Endicott J. Measurement of depression in patients with cancer. Cancer 1984; 53(10):2243–2248.
59. Razavi D, Mendlewicz J. Tricyclics antidepressant plasma levels: the state of the art and clinical prospect. Neuropsychobiology 1982; 8:73–95.
60. Stiefel F, Fainsinger R, Bruera E. Acute confusional states in patients with advanced cancer. J Pain Symptom Manage 1992; 7:25–29.
61. Levine PM, Silberfarb PM, Lipowski ZJ. Mental disorders in cancer patients. A study of 100 psychiatric referrals. Cancer 1978; 42:1385–1391.
62. Engel GL, Romano G. Delirium, a syndrome of cerebral insufficiency. J Chron Dis 1959; 9:260–277.
63. Lesko LM, Massie MJ, Holland JC. Oncology. In: Principles of Medical Psychiatry, New York: Grune and Stratton, 1987:501–503.
64. Stiefel F, Bruera E. Psychostimulants for hypoactive-hypoalert delirium? J Palliat Care 1991; 7(3):25–26.
65. Liptzin B, Levkoff SE, Clearly PD, et al. An empirical study of diagnostic criteria for delirium. Am J Psychiatry 1991; 148:454–457.
66. Bruera E, Miller MJ, Kuehn N, MacEachern T, Hanson J. Estimate of survival of patients admitted to a palliative care unit: a prospective study. J Pain Symptom Manage 1992; 7:82–86.
67. Lipowski ZJ. Delirium: Acute Confusional States. New York: Oxford University Press, 1990.
68. Lipowski ZJ. Transient cognitive disorders (delirium, acute confusional states) in the elderly. Am J Psychiatry 1983; 140:1426–1436.
69. Massie MJ, Holland J, Glass E. Delirium in terminally ill cancer patients. Am J Psychiatry 1983; 140:1048–1050.
70. Stiefel F, Holland J. Delirium in cancer patients. Int Psychogeriatrics 1991; 3(2):333–336.
71. Posner JB. Neurologic complications of systemic cancer. Dis Mon 1978; 25:1–60.
72. Stiefel F, Breitbart W, Holland J. Corticosteroids in cancer: neuropsychiatric complications. Cancer Invest 1989; 7:479–491.
73. Spiegel D, Kraemer H, Bloom J, Gottheil E. Effects of psychosocial treatment on survival of patients with metastatic breast cancer. Lancet 1989; 2:888–891.
74. Razavi D, Delvaux N, Farvacques C, Robaye E. Brief psychological training for health care professionals dealing with cancer patients: a one-year assessment. Gen Hosp Psychiatry 1991; 13:253–260.
75. Moorey S, Greer S. Psychological Therapy for Patients with Cancer: A New Approach. Oxford: Heinemann Medical Books, 1989.
76. Razavi D, Delvaux N, Farvacques C, et al. Prevention of adjustment disorders and anticipatory nausea secondary to adjuvant chemotherapy: a double-blind placebo controlled study assessing the usefulness of alprazolam. J Clin Oncol 1993; 11:1384–1390.

12

Obstructive Syndromes

Martin H. N. Tattersall
University of Sydney, Sydney, New South Wales, Australia

J. Norelle Lickiss
Royal Prince Alfred Hospital, Sydney, New South Wales, Australia

I. INTRODUCTION

Symptoms and signs caused by organ obstruction are relatively common in cancer patients, and their early identification and appropriate management play a significant part in total patient care. Some obstructive syndromes in cancer patients may be regarded as medical emergencies because early treatment may avert major morbidity (e.g., cord compression leading to paraplegia or mediastinal obstruction leading to respiratory failure). In other contexts, early identification of an obstructive syndrome (symptom complex) may lead to improved patient welfare even if the obstructive syndrome is not completely reversible.

Obstructive symptoms may be the presenting feature of patients with cancers of several sites, but more commonly these symptoms develop in patients with previously diagnosed cancer. Whatever the context of the patient's symptoms, it is crucial to establish exactly the major symptoms and to determine whether an obstruction is responsible for the symptoms. The pattern of evolution of the symptoms and the rate of change are important determinants of the biology of the obstruction. The background against which these symptoms have appeared is also a crucial element in decision making about interventions. For example, are the symptom complexes an isolated problem or the last straw in a patient with far advanced malignant disease? In assessing the patient with obstructive symptoms, it is important to clarify on clinical grounds the most likely site of the obstruction and the most likely cause of the obstruction.

Before undertaking investigations to clarify the site and cause of the obstruction, it is important to determine the options that are realistically available to reverse any obstruction that may be detected. What are the particular pros and cons of each option for the particular patient at the time? For example, in a patient with pelvic malignancy who is found to have become uremic, it is important to decide whether investigations to establish the cause of the uremia are merited, particularly if the patient is asymptomatic, because these investigations may inconvenience the patient and/or have morbidity of their own. In a symptomatic patient there still may be a case to relieve the symptoms, care for the patient, and "let the obstruction be." Although all efforts must focus on symptom control in patients presenting with obstructive syndromes, it may not always be appropriate to identify precisely the site or cause of the obstruction, particularly if efforts will not be directed at alleviating the obstruction but rather at treating symptoms.

Good communication between patient and doctor and understanding of the patient's overall situation are important components of decision making as soon as a patient presents with obstructive symptoms and/or is found to have organ dysfunction likely caused by obstruction. Table 1 outlines the decision making

Table 1 Decision Points in the Approach to Management of Patients Presenting with Obstructive Syndromes

What are the presenting symptoms and signs, and what is the length of history or rate of change?

↓

Is the syndrome an isolated problem or the last straw?

↓

What is the likely cause and site of the syndrome
- Cancer
- Treatment
- Other

↓

What options are available to reverse or bypass the obstruction? What are the *pros* and *cons* of each option for this patient, and which is recommended and in accord with the patient's preferences and welfare?

↓

What further investigations are justified to clarify the details of treatment?

↓

Confirm the preferred management option in light of the preceding.

↓

Institute treatment with clear objectives.

↓

Evaluate effectiveness as planned or promised, and be prepared to cease treatment.

↓

Continue all symptomatic measures in a context of comprehensive care.

required before embarking on any invasive investigations and/or attempts to bypass obstruction in cancer patients who present with obstructive syndromes.

After determining that further investigations are indicated, it is necessary to consider which investigations are most appropriate to define the cause and site of obstruction. A variety of technologies are available to examine organ function and disordered anatomy, but it is rarely necessary to undertake the full gamut of investigations but rather to select from the range of possibilities the investigation that will provide the necessary information for appropriate patient management. While these investigations are in progress, attention to controlling the patient's symptoms is important, as is emergency care if required to maintain physiological function as much as possible.

Having clarified the site and cause of an obstruction in a cancer patient, decisions must be made about the goals of any treatment to be recommended. The objectives of this treatment must be set in consultation with the patient in the light of what is reasonably possible. It is important that clinicians recommending treatment or interventions be aware of the morbidities of these interventions because, not uncommonly, the person undertaking the actual procedure is not known to the patient and is not necessarily familiar with all aspects of the case history, for example.

After treatment has been embarked upon, it is appropriate to evaluate its effectiveness. If treatment is not initially effective and additional interventions are required, again it is important to clarify their objectives and determine whether these additional investigations and/or interventions are justified.

If a patient with an obstructive syndrome does not improve in a life-threatening situation, it is appropriate to ensure that the patient has access to as competent and specialized terminal care as was the access to treatment directed at relieving obstruction. The clinical expertise required for palliation of symptoms must be at least equal that required to offer sound and appropriate chemotherapy or radiotherapy advice to patients with advanced cancer. There is no place for the patient ever to consider the treatment has failed; rather there are situations in which treatment must be changed to achieve new goals agreed on with the patient.

II. TREATMENT APPROACHES DIRECTED TOWARD RELIEF OF SYMPTOMS AT ANY SITE

When obstruction is caused directly by tumor infiltration, the choice is between direct antitumor measures (radiotherapy and chemotherapy) and, less commonly, surgical excision, mechanical devices designed to reconstitute the passage, or surgical or other techniques to bypass the obstruction. The choice is influenced by such factors as demonstrated known or probable chemosensitivity or resistance of the tumor to available treatment; the fitness of the patient for surgical procedures and the availability of the necessary surgical expertise; the availability of radiotherapy and the likely effectiveness of that treatment; and the overall condition of the patient (obstruction as an isolated problem or the last straw), as discussed.

In the nonsurgical approaches, there is a place for concurrent or prescriptive treatment with corticosteroids to induce rapid functional improvement and symptom relief by edema reduction while awaiting the effects of any antitumor treatment that is instituted (1). Care must be taken to avoid drugs that may aggravate the obstruction or symptoms arising from it. For example, gastrokinetic antinauseants may worsen nausea, vomiting, and colic (if present).

III. ALIMENTARY TRACT OBSTRUCTION

The incidence of alimentary tract obstruction in cancer patients varies greatly depending upon the site of the primary tumor, which in turn is influenced by the patient's race and environment. Large bowel obstruction is a relatively common presenting symptom in patients with large bowel cancer, the most common tumor in the developed world. On the other hand, in Asia, esophageal cancer and gastric cancer are much more frequent than large bowel cancer, and upper alimentary tract obstruction is more common. The symptoms associated with the alimentary tract obstruction vary with the site of the obstruction (Table 2).

The cause of the obstruction is commonly directly related to cancer, but in some circumstances, prior surgery leading to adhesions or widespread intraabdominal spread may cause a multisite obstructed bowel. It is particularly important when opiate analgesics are being utilized to recognize the high prevalence of constipation related to these treatments, and patients must not be

Table 2 Alimentary Tract Obstruction

Site	Symptoms	Investigation
Pharyngeal	Choking, pain dysphagia	Direct vision
Oesophageal	Dysphagia, weight loss, cough, regurgitation	Oesophagoscopy, Barium swallow
Gastroduodenal	Fullness, vomiting, nausea, dehydration	Gastroscopy, Barium studies
Biliary	Jaundice, pain, diarrhoea	ERCP, PTHC, CT scan
Small Bowel	Colicky pain, vomiting	Barium swallow
Large Bowel	Constipation, thin feces, colic	Barium enema, colonoscopy, CT scan
Anorectal	Tenesmus, constipation, pain	Sigmoidoscopy

assumed to have obstructive symptoms caused by cancer without major efforts being made to clear the intestinal tract of constipated feces (2).

A variety of investigations are available to identify the site of alimentary tract obstruction, and these vary greatly in their morbidity, cost, and specificity. In the upper alimentary tract, endoscopy sometimes coupled with barium studies often clarifies the site of an obstruction, and biopsy via the endoscope may establish the cause. Within the small and upper large bowel direct examination by the endoscope is difficult, and barium studies, although widely used, are not easily or necessarily correctly interpreted. Laparotomy may not only be diagnostic, but also the means by which bypass of the obstruction is achieved.

In the biliary tract, percutaneous transhepatic cholangiography, computed tomography (CT) scanning, or ERCP may identify the site of the obstruction and/or provide a means to relieve the obstruction by the passage of a stent draining internally or externally.

When the alimentary tract obstruction is caused by tumor, the treatment choice is between direct antitumor treatment (radiotherapy, chemotherapy, and less commonly surgical excision), and mechanical devices designed to reconstitute the passage, by either surgical bypass procedures or stents. The choice of management is influenced by such factors as the demonstrated known or probable chemosensitivity to available cytotoxics; the fitness for surgical procedures and the availability of necessary expertise; the availability of radiotherapy and the probable sensitivity to ionizing radiation; and the overall condition of the patient (obstruction an isolated problem or the last straw).

In the nonsurgical approaches, corticosteroids may induce rapid functional improvement (and symptom relief) in edema reduction while awaiting antitumor effects of chemotherapy and/or radiotherapy.

Drugs that may aggravate the obstruction or symptoms arising from it should be avoided. There may be a place for a trial of corticosteroids for a few days in pharyngeal, esophageal, or intestinal obstruction to assess how much benefit may be obtained by this approach alone (repeated every few weeks in a very compromised patient), but normally, especially in pharyngeal obstruction, radiotherapy if available should be instituted if any antiobstruction treatment is justified.

If swallowing is impossible or vomiting is still problematical despite the institution of appropriate symptomatic measures with specialist assistance as necessary, and in a context of optimism concerning the outcome of measures to relieve the obstruction, there is a place for the temporary use of parenteral fluid. Rather than resort to intravenous measures, subcutaneous infusion is convenient and effective. It is to be stressed that in irreversible end-stage alimentary tract obstructions, infusions are not necessary. Advances in therapeutics have led to the feasibility of obtaining comfort and dignity without such measures (3). Relative dehydration has in fact much advantaged patients with end-stage intestinal obstruction, and attempts to maintain such patients in fluid balance are a potent cause of difficulty in controlling vomiting. Mouth care is crucial.

The care of patients whose intestinal obstruction is unrelieved or best left alone involves due consideration of the available options, which include the following measures:

1. *Management of colic*. Stopping of gastrokinetic or stimulative laxative drugs or instituting regular subcutaneous morphine in small doses (10–20 mg/day) may be sufficient (in four hourly doses or by infusion). The use of antispasmodics (hyoscine butylbromide, 30–60 mg/day) by subcutaneous injection of four hourly doses or by infusion may also be helpful.
2. *Control of nausea*. Centrally acting antinauseants, such as haloperidol (3–5 mg once or twice daily) subcutaneously or by infusion or cyclizine (50–100 mg) by subcutaneous injection, are often effective. Rectal prochlorperazine (25–75 mg/day) may be of assistance if other measures are inconvenient. Metoclopramide may make vomiting (and colic) worse in patients with high obstruction and is probably best avoided except in specialist units. Hyoscine hydrobromide and, in some patients, also octreotide are of value in reducing gastric secretions and thereby alleviating vomiting. Patients are welcome to drink (and eat a little if they wish), but parenteral fluids are not used, and some degree of dehydration is beneficial, as previously mentioned, provided mouth care is of high quality (with care concerning cleanliness and candidiasis) and ice occasionally offered to suck (3).

In most cases these measures are highly successful but require care and experience. In a small minority of patients with gastroduodenal obstruction, a nasogastric tube is necessary (and in very occasional patients stenting gastroscopy may be of benefit), but neither of these measures should be considered before an adequate trial of competent conservative management has been undertaken.

Biliary tract obstruction may be bypassed endoscopically or by percutaneous passage of a stent. The case for surgical bypass in malignant obstructive jaundice has been called into question by the results of recent randomized trials that revealed that endoscopically introduced endoprotheses were as effective as operative bypass (4). The selection of stent may be influenced by the patient's life expectancy, but recent studies indicate a prolonged patency of metal stents compared with polyethylene stents (273 versus 176 days) (5). The major causes of stent dysfunction were tumor ingrowth of the metal stent group and sludge deposition in the polyethylene stent group. Symptomatic measures that may be helpful in patients with biliary obstruction include cholestyramine sachets to minimize itch, although sometimes they cause significant diarrhea, pancreatic enzyme replacements in patients with uncontrolled diarrhea, and continuous antibiotics in those with biliary stents.

IV. RESPIRATORY OBSTRUCTION

Respiratory obstruction is a much feared development in relevant patients. Obstruction may be in the larynx, trachea, or bronchi, and the etiology may be directly related to tumor with or without difficulty in clearing secretions and/or the presence of a foreign body. Relief of the obstruction may be achievable in many instances by radiotherapy (6), but there has been much recent attention devoted to the use of endoscopically placed bronchial stents, laser therapy, and even brachytherapy (6–8).

Laryngeal obstruction is seen most commonly in patients with primary tumors in the larynx and occasionally in patients who develop bilateral recurrent laryngeal palsies. Emergency tracheostomy may sometimes be necessary, although in patients with laryngeal tumors this is frequently performed as an elective procedure before local treatment. In those patients in whom clearance of secretions is the major cause of acute respiratory obstruction, mucolytics, moisturizers of inhaled air, and active physiotherapy may minimize distress and alleviate recurrent symptoms. In those cases in whom no major intervention to overcome the obstruction is considered justifiable, a careful and compassionate sedation to render the patient asleep until they die may be correct in some circumstances, normally within a patient-doctor relationship characterized by respect, competence, and trust. Midazolam (5–10 mg subcutaneously) followed by infusion (20–50 mg/day) or intravenous or rectal diazepam (10–20 mg) or clonazepam (1 mg SCI bd) is usually effective. Clearly, the context must be that of quiet competent support for patient and family and for professional staff.

It is important to consider the possibility of an endobronchial obstruction in patients with dyspnea but no apparent radiographic cause. In one series no radiographic signs of obstruction were found in 44% of patients having bronchoscopy who had complete endobronchial obstruction with normal chest x-rays (9). Segmental bronchial obstruction was more likely to be undetectable than obstruction of the more proximal airways, and chest radiographs were judged completely normal in 16% of patients. Silicon and expandable metallic stents are now available for palliation of patients with obstructing lesions of the central bronchial tree. Both sorts of stents appeared to be effective in achieving immediate relief of dyspnoea, but the expandable stents woven of metallic wire seemed to be preferred (10). Endoscopic relief of malignant airway obstruction may be achieved simply by coring out the obstructing neoplasm, but laser bronchoscopy has also been found to be affective (7,11).

In centers where these techniques are not available, radiotherapy with steroid and vigorous physiotherapy is often effective in relieving acute tracheal or bronchial obstruction, and recent randomized trials indicate that high-dose single-fraction treatment may have similar effects and reduced cost and morbidity than more protracted courses of radiotherapy (12).

When tracheo-bronchial obstruction is a component of mediastinal obstruction, treatment approaches should be similar. In the absence of major airway obstruction, mediastinal compression (superior vena caval syndrome) is not a medical emergency even though the patient's appearance may be distressing.

V. OBSTRUCTION OF THE URINARY TRACT

Obstruction may occur in several locations from renal pelvis to urethra, with varying clinical manifestations, usually permitting a confident clinical diagnosis that is easily verifiable.

Obstruction of both ureters may present a complex clinical problem with a variety of presenting features. Considerable information and reflection is necessary to reach a wise management approach, particularly in patients with locally recurrent rectal, bladder, or cervical cancers. The presenting symptoms may vary, and an ambulant patient with anorexia and some nausea may prove to have grossly raised serum creatinine and potassium. Minor discomfort may be felt in the back, and mental changes may be absent or subtle, but oliguria or anuria may have been noted but not mentioned. In other patients, especially if infection is also present, the patient may be gravely ill, even in extremis.

The diagnosis of uremia is readily established by simple investigation. Abdominal ultrasound may demonstrate bilateral hydronephrosis, and sometimes the site of obstruction is apparent without resorting to retrograde pyelography or CT scan. It is important to establish whether the patient has recurrent cancer as a cause of the ureteric obstruction, and screening for other sites of metastasis is an important component of this evaluation. The frequency of ureteric obstruction caused by radiotherapy after complex surgery varies in different reports, but certainly ureteric obstruction on the basis of a benign cause is reported in a significant proportion of patients with pelvic malignancy treated surgically and/or by radiotherapy (13).

The management approach for bilateral ureteric obstruction depends upon the goals of therapy. The management approach may be to refrain from any attempt to correct the obstruction and allow the patient to die from the biochemical derangement. This may be appropriate when the patient is irreversibly ill and clearly is dying. This may also be also the correct course of action in a patient in whom a crisis was anticipated and who, when the approach to be taken was discussed, preferred the conservative management.

When such discussions have not occurred—when the complication had developed suddenly or at least unexpectedly and the patient's condition on other grounds is reasonable—then there is a case for urgent action to try to reverse the biochemical lesions (especially the raised serum potassium) and bypass or reverse the obstruction. Dialysis may be essential in the first instance, but other measures may be used, including insulin and glucose or Resonium A (sodium polystyrene sulfonate). In some patients, the ureteric obstruction can be overcome at least temporarily by moderate doses of corticosteroids given for a few days (e.g., dexamethasone at 8 mg/daily, intravenously, subcutaneously, or orally). In most patients a stenting procedure is appropriate (ureteric stenting if successful is more acceptable) but percutaneous nephrostomy is more appropriate at least as a first measure in some patients. The use of self-expanding metal stents for the palliative treatment of malignant ureteral obstruction was recently advocated as providing a higher rate of patency over time (14). However, the cost of these stents is considerable.

These stenting procedures are not without emotional and medical cost. Complications associated with mechanical failures, leaking, infection, and local discomfort in a nephrostomy site can significantly reduce the quality of life and increase the complexity of care. Also, the local tumor may advance to produce new symptoms. Should the obstruction be likely to recur and certainly when urgent measures have been taken to relieve obstruction in an unexpected situation, the opportunity must be found for a careful discussion with the patient, preferably in the presence of a family member or advocate. The management plan must be constantly reviewed in this way in the light of changing circumstances, in such a manner that the patient knows that he or she is listened to and understood. The doctor must make the final decision and take responsibility for it after the consultation, but the patient's wishes should normally prevail. As in other situations in which the patient is not in a position to give consent to instrumental treatment, the doctor is bound to act in the best interests of the patient.

Irrespective of decisions concerning attempts to reverse obstruction by instrumentation or by any other measures, the patient should receive support, good quality symptom management, and comprehensive palliative care.

When ureteric obstruction is unilateral and the patient has no symptoms and a normal creatinine, a case for ureteric stenting can sometimes be made, although in many cases the morbidity of the procedure does not justify the intervention.

In patients with urethral obstruction (prostatic obstruction), whose prognosis is otherwise reasonable, permanent catheterization or suprapubic cystostomy may be appropriate.

VI. VASCULAR OBSTRUCTION

Obstruction of the vena cava associated with mediastinal tumor contributes to a variety of symptoms, depending upon the precise site of obstruction. Venous obstruction in the pelvis may cause chronic leg edema and/or be complicated by recurrent pulmonary embolism. Venous obstruction commonly coupled with lymphatic obstruction may complicate axillary surgery and/or radiotherapy, and massive arm edema may be a major cause of patient inconvenience and distress. Renal vein thrombosis may complicate retroperitoneal tumor and give rise to renal failure and/or hypoproteinemia.

The appropriate intervention in patients with venous obstruction (thrombosis) caused by malignant disease depends on the site of the obstruction and the patient's context. Superior vena caval obstruction may be a presenting sign in patients who subsequently prove to have lung cancer, lymphoma, or germ cell tumors of the mediastinum. Under these circumstances, a tissue diagnosis is sometimes not achievable without major risk to the patient because of airway compression. When no tissue diagnosis has been made and if time allows, it may be appropriate to organize a bone marrow aspiration while commencing high-dose steroid and making arrangements for local radiotherapy.

Clearly, in patients in whom a diagnosis of cancer has already been made, the treatment approach depends upon the likely responsiveness of the tumor to treatment, and in some cases primary chemotherapy may be preferred. In any event, the use of anticoagulation and high-dose steroid is commonly advocated. Several recent papers have described the use of superior vena caval self-expanding stents, but no randomized trial has yet demonstrated whether these high-technology procedures have advantages compared to treating the cause of the obstruction and anticoagulation, for example (15).

In patients with venous obstruction in the pelvis or axilla associated with recurrent tumor or postsurgery and radiotherapy fibrosis, anticoagulation, often with massage to enhance lymphatic drainage, can assist in palliating symptoms. Compression bandages and/or stockings to minimize the reaccumulation of fluid after effective massage have substantially improved the symptomatic management of patients with these complications.

Venous obstruction complicating the use of venous access devices is increasingly reported in patients in whom these devices have been implanted to assist in the delivery of chemotherapy. Expertise in the management of these devices minimizes this risk. However, in patients who develop venous access complications associated commonly with recurrent infection, removal of the device with anticoagulation and systemic antibiotic treatment is usually effective.

Arterial obstruction complicating cancer is an unusual development in clinical practice. Most reports are in patients with promyelocytic leukemia who develop peripheral arterial occlusion associated with high peripheral white cell counts (16). Embolic obstruction of arteries may also occur associated with radiation damage or tumor infiltration to blood vessels in the neck (17). Anticoagulation is the only treatment known to be effective in the latter setting, and treatment of leukemia combined with allopurinol and high fluid volumes to minimize the tumor necrosis syndrome may be effective in the leukemic setting.

VII. NEUROLOGICAL OBSTRUCTION

Obstructive hydrocephalus, spinal cord compression, compression of the cauda equina, and nerve route compression frequently complicate the course of cancer patients. The management of obstructive hydrocephalus may require immediate treatment by steroid or osmotic approaches if subsequent surgical or radiotherapeutic interventions are possible. The case for shunting depends very much on the patient's status and whether antitumor treatment has already been given. In many cases in whom obstructive hydrocephalus develops late in the course of disease, symptomatic measures only may be preferred. However, in patients with posterior fossa tumors diagnosed at the time of presentation with obstructive hydrocephalus, emergency measures to minimize edema and shunting are appropriate.

Spinal cord compression (obstruction) is a common complication of malignant disease and a source of much distress not only to patients but also to staff because of the severity of the impact of this complication on the quality of life of patients and their carers and the poor outcome of treatment in most cases (18).

Epidural spinal cord compression occurs in many patients who die of cancer, and if untreated it inexorably progresses, leading to paralysis, sensory loss, and sphincter incontinence. Because the most important factor determining outcome is the level of neurological function at the beginning of therapy, the clinical challenge is to diagnose the condition and begin treatment before major neurological injury occurs (19).

Metastases to the spine are far more common than primary spinal neoplasms. Epidural metastases are also much more common than leptomeningeal or intramedullary spread. Approximately 50% of the cases of metastatic epidural compression in adults arise from breast, lung, or prostate cancer, but other frequent primary tumors include lymphoma, melanoma, renal cancer, sarcoma, and multiple myeloma. In children, the most common tumors are sarcoma, neuroblastoma, and lymphoma. The development of spinal cord compression occurs most commonly in the setting of disseminated cancer, and the compression is at the thoracic level in approximately 70% of cases, lumbar in 20%, and cervical in 10% (20%).

Several studies have shown that metastatic epidural compression occurs at multiple noncontiguous levels in up to a third of cases. The tumor usually occupies the anterior or anterolateral spinal canal.

The initial symptom of metastatic epidural compression is often pain, usually in the back but occasionally referred or radicular in distribution (18). The pain is usually aggravated by movement, straight leg raising, and neck flexion. Sensory loss and incontinence develop after the first appearance of pain but may precede it. Once a neurological deficit appears, it can evolve rapidly to paraplegia over a few hours to days. Trivial neurological signs, such as a hesitant or equivocal plantar response, may be present in a patient with significant spinal cord compression: to wait for "hard" neurological signs in a patient with backache (especially thoracic), even if the pain is controllable by analgesics, may be to wait too long.

The diagnostic steps to clarify the cause of backache in a patient with cancer, whether or not they have neurological signs, is the subject of some controversy. Radiographs reveal vertebral metastasis in approximately 85% of adults with metastatic epidural compression (20). The frequency of bony abnormality is influenced by the primary tumor, only one-third of patients with lymphoma or children with cancer having abnormal radiographs. Until recently, myelography was the procedure recommended for the spinal canal to diagnose metastatic epidural compression (21). However, magnetic resonance imaging (MRI) is reported to be equally sensitive in most cases and to be preferred in centers where MRI readily available. Myelography should be performed, however, when MRI is not available or the quality of the pictures is poor. The decision to proceed to MRI or CT myelogram is exceedingly difficult.

The care of patients with backache, normal neurological examination, and evidence of metastatic disease on conventional radiographs is controversial: if the backache has been very severe (even if relieved) and the patient expresses a sense of a progressing scenario, with even trivial neurological signs and subjective sense of "change in legs," the case is far stronger to investigate quickly. The advantage of definitive imaging is that unexpected epidural disease may be identified outside what otherwise might be the planned radiotherapy ports. The disadvantages are the expense of the imaging and the possible delay in commencing treatment. In patients undergoing lumbar puncture and myelography, it is important to monitor neurological signs after the procedure because not uncommonly there may be a rapid deterioration possibly related to changing fluid dynamics.

The management of spinal cord compression involves corticosteroids and radiation therapy, but excellent results may also be achieved with anterior decompression in selected patients. Chemotherapy may also be effective in tumors that are exceedingly chemosensitive. Clinical and laboratory studies demonstrate that corticosteroids improve neurological function and alleviate pain in the short term, but their contribution to ultimate neurological recovery is not clear. Corticosteroids should be administered immediately to patients in whom the clinical manifestations of cord compression have been confirmed by diagnostic imaging or in whom compression is strongly suspected on clinical grounds.

The dosage of dexamethasone most commonly recommended is 4 mg four times per day, but some studies have shown a dose-related benefit with dexamethasone leading to clinical use of loading doses of 100 mg, followed by 24 mg four times per day in some settings (18,22).

Several retrospective studies and one small prospective study have demonstrated no difference in neurological outcome between radiotherapy alone and laminectomy followed by radiotherapy (23). Radiotherapy initiated promptly after diagnosis has therefore become the primary definitive treatment for most patients, and radiation ports are best defined by MRI.

Although surgical indications need to be defined, it has been suggested that surgical decompression should be considered in patients in whom the diagnosis of the spinal lesion is in doubt, those with a neurological deterioration caused by metastatic compression at a previously irradiated level, and in those who have progressive neurological deterioration during radiotherapy despite large doses of steroids. Surgery may also be considered in patients with radioresistant tumors and intractable pain.

Pain management in patients with spinal cord compression should include nonsteroidal antiinflammatory drugs (NSAID; if not contraindicated) and opioids if necessary. Paracetamol is helpful as an alternative to NSAID, although possibly less effective. Although experimental studies have indicated that opiates may have deleterious effects on neurological recovery, symptomatic control is clearly an essential component of the management of spinal cord compression.

Nerve root compression and nerve compression may cause significant symptoms in patients with cancer. Local decompression or radiotherapy in sensitive tumors may relieve symptoms and achieve return of function. In many settings, however, particularly in patients with Pancoast's syndrome or pelvic plexopathy caused by cancer, local treatments are not able to control the tumor and/or relieve the symptoms. Even while radiotherapy is proceeding, drugs relevant to neuropathic pain, according to type, should be used. If the pain is lancinating, corticosteroids with or without anticonvulsants, such as valproate, carbamezepine, or clonazepan, or oral local anesthetics, such as Mexiletine, may be useful, but all are potentially toxic and caution is necessary with due regard to contraindications. Tricyclic antidepressants should be introduced if pain is dysesthetic or burning in quality, again with due regard to hazards. Nonsteroidal antiinflammatory drugs may also achieve some palliation, especially if bone involvement is associated with the plexopathy.

REFERENCES

1. Twycross RG. Corticosteroids in advanced cancer. If they are not working stop them. BMJ 1992; 305:969–979.
2. Twycross RG, Lack SA. Control of alimentary symptoms in far advanced cancer. Edinburgh: Churchill Livingstone, 1986.
3. Baines M, Oliver DJ, Carter RC. Medical management of intestinal obstruction in patients with advanced malignant disease: a clinical and pathological study. Lancet 1985; 2:990–993.
4. Andersen JR, Srensen SM, Kruse A, et al. Randomised trial of endoscopic

endoprosthesis versus operative bypass in malignant obstructive jaundice. Gut 1989; 30:1132–1135.

5. Davids PH, Groen AK, Rauws EA, et al. Randomised trial of self-expanding metal stents versus polyethylene stents for distal malignant biliary obstruction. Lancet 1992; 340:1488–1492.
6. Chetty KG, Moral EM, Sassoon CE, et al. Effect of radiation therapy on bronchial obstruction due to bronchogenic carcinoma. Chest 1989; 95:582–584.
7. Beamis JF, Vergos K, Rebeiz EE, Shapshay SM. Endoscopic laser therapy for obstructing tracheobronchial lesions. Ann Otol Rhinol Laryngol 1991; 100:413–419.
8. Mehta M, Shahabi S, Jarjour N, et al. Effect of endobronical radiation therapy on malignant bronchial obstruction. Chest 1990; 97:662–665.
9. Shure D. Radiographically occult endobronchial obstruction in bronchogenic carcinoma. Am J Med 1991; 91:19–22.
10. Breyer G, Haussinger K. Tracheobronchial stents indications and possibilities. Pneumonologie 1991; 45:997–1003.
11. Mathisen DT, Gritto HC. Endoscopic relief of malignant airway obstruction. Ann Thorac Surg 1989; 48:469–475.
12. Bleehen NM, Girling DJ, Machin D, et al. A. Medical Research Council randomised trial of palliative radiotherapy with two fraction or a single fraction in patients with inoperable non small cell lung cancer and poor performance status. Br J Cancer 1992; 65:934–941.
13. Parliament M, Genest P, Girand A, et al. Obstructive ureteropathy following radiation therapy for carcinoma of the cervix. Gynecol Oncol 1989; 33:237–240.
14. Lugmayr H, Pauer W. Self expanding metal stents for palliative treatment of malignant ureteral obstruction. Am J Roentgenol 1992; 159:109–114.
15. Oudkerk M, Heysttraten FM, Stoter G. Stenting in malignant vena canal obstruction. Cancer 1993; 71:142–146.
16. Fass R, Haddod M, Zaizov R, et al. Recurrent peripheral arterial occlusion by leukaemic cells sedimentation in acute promyelocytic leukaemia. J Paediatr Surg 1992; 27:665–667.
17. Kearsley JH, Tattersall MHN. Cerebral embolism in cancer patients. Q J Med 1982; 203:1–13.
18. Byrne TN. Spinal cord compression from epidural metastases. N Engl J Med 1992; 327:614–619.
19. Kim RY, Spencer SA, Meredith RF, et al. Extradural spinal cord compression: analysis of factors determining functional prognosis—prospective study. Radiology 1990; 176:279–282.
20. Stark RJ, Henson RA, Evans SJW. Spinal metastases: a retrospective survey from a general hospital. Brain 1992; 105:189–213.
21. Zimmerman RA, Bilaniuk LT. Imaging of tumors of the spinal canal and cord. Radiol Clin North Am 1988; 26:965–1007.
22. Posner TB. Backpain and epidural spinal cord compression. Med Clin North Am 1987; 71:185–205.
23. Young RF, Post EM, King GA. Treatment of spinal epidural metastases: randomised prospective comparison of laminectomy and radiotherapy. J Neurosurg 1980; 53:741–748.

13

Management of Malignant Effusion

Kenji Eguchi
National Cancer Center Central Hospital, Tokyo, Japan

I. MALIGNANT PLEURAL EFFUSION

A. Etiology

The pleural space consists of a continuous serosal lining. The side of the surface toward the lung is the visceral pleura and the other side, which covers the chest wall, is the parietal pleura. In the parietal pleura, a single sheet of the mesothelial cells lies on a connective tissue layer. The endothoracic fascia consists of the outer part of the parietal pleura adjacent to the muscle layer of the chest wall. The single layer of mesothelial cells, the thin layer of connective tissue, the chief layer of connective tissue rich in collagen and elastic fibers, and the vascular layer adjacent to the limiting membrane of the lung parenchyma constitute the structure of the visceral pleura.

Normally the pleural space contains approximately 5–20 ml fluid with a protein content of less than 2 g/dl. The physiological mechanism of the formation and clearance of pleural fluid can be described by the Starling equation. The equation factors consist of the capillary hydrostatic pressure, the interstitial hydrostatic pressure, the plasma protein osmotic pressure, and the interstitial protein osmotic pressure. The hydrostatic-oncotic pressures of the capillaries of the parietal pleura make fluid move into the pleural space, and 80–90% is reabsorbed by the pulmonary venous capillaries of the visceral pleural. About 10–20% of the fluid is reabsorbed by the pleural lymphatic. About 5–10 liters fluid is said to move through the pleural space per day.

The mechanisms of malignant pleural effusion are thought to be as follows:

(1) increased capillary permeability as a result of inflammation and/or disruption of the capillary endothelium, (2) impaired lymphatic drainage and/or decreased drainage in pulmonary vein secondary to obstruction by tumor, (3) direct invasion of the pleural space by tumor, (4) hypoalbuminemia caused by the malnourished state of cancer patients, and (5) chylous pleural effusion arises from obstruction of thoracic duct.

The types of cancer causing malignant pleural effusions are lung, breast, lymphoma, and gastrointestinal and genitourinary malignancies. The prognosis of malignant pleural effusions depends on the type of the tumor; gastric cancer has one of the worst prognoses and breast cancer the best. In patients with primary lung cancer, pleural effusion is sometimes revealed to be benign, especially in epidermoid histology. According to a large-scale study of prognostic factors in patients with small cell and non–small cell lung cancer by the Veterans Administration Lung Group and the Eastern Cooperative Oncology Group, pleural effusions were not the independent prognostic factors for survival.

B. Clinical Manifestation and Examination

Dyspnea, cough, and chest pain are three common symptoms in patients with pleural effusion. Dry cough when the patient changes the position or progressive shortness of breath on exertion are the symptoms suggestive of pleural effusion. Patients with pleural effusion sometimes complain of chest oppression or dull back pain. Mechanical disturbance of lung expansion and compression atelectasis by the massive pleural effusion cause respiratory symptoms. Some patients present with severe progressive dyspnea because of malignant pleural effusion accompanied by disseminated carcinomatous lymphangitis of the lung.

The symptoms caused by the pleural effusion may sometimes be the initial manifestation of malignancy. Only one-fourth of patients with pleural effusion are asymptomatic at presentation. Decrease in breath sounds, increased dullness in percussion, and undetectable diaphragmatic excursion are the common physical findings.

The chest x-ray is the most practical method for assessment of the presence of pleural effusion. The ground-glass appearance of a fluid collection blurring the costophrenic angle and the diaphragm is the typical x-ray finding of pleural effusion. In massive effusion one side of the lung shows complete opacity on a chest x-ray film. X-ray can differentiate massive pleural effusion from complete atelectasis of the one-sided lung with the findings of reduction in the volume of the hemithorax. The shift of the mediastinal structure to the opposite side, expansion of the intercostal space, and downward shift of an intestinal or stomach air bubble are the x-ray findings for increased volume of the hemithorax with massive pleural effusion. The lateral decubitus view is useful to find small amounts of free pleural fluid. These x-ray findings are easily observed using computed tomography (CT) of the thorax. Compared with conventional x-ray film, CT scan is a powerful tool to identify the solid mass or collapsed lung in massive pleural effusion. Ultrasonography is also very useful to differentiate free pleural effusion from organized thickening of the pleura and to detect minimal free effusion. One can see the movement of reactive fibrous strings floating in the pleural effusion and surmise the contents of the effusion.

C. Diagnosis

If pleural effusion arises in a cancer patient, it is important to find the definitive cause. There are many causes of nonmalignant pleural effusion in patients who also have malignancies, such as cardiogenic, infection related, from pulmonary infarction, or as a result of cirrhosis of the liver.

Thoracentesis is the first and most productive diagnostic procedure (Fig. 1). Chest x-ray films or ultrasonography is useful to determine the puncture site. The procedure should be performed with the patient sitting erect or lying on the bed. One should be careful to observe even minimal changes in the physical findings of the patient during the procedure, and the vital signs should be monitored by nursing staff. All procedures should be done using sterilized

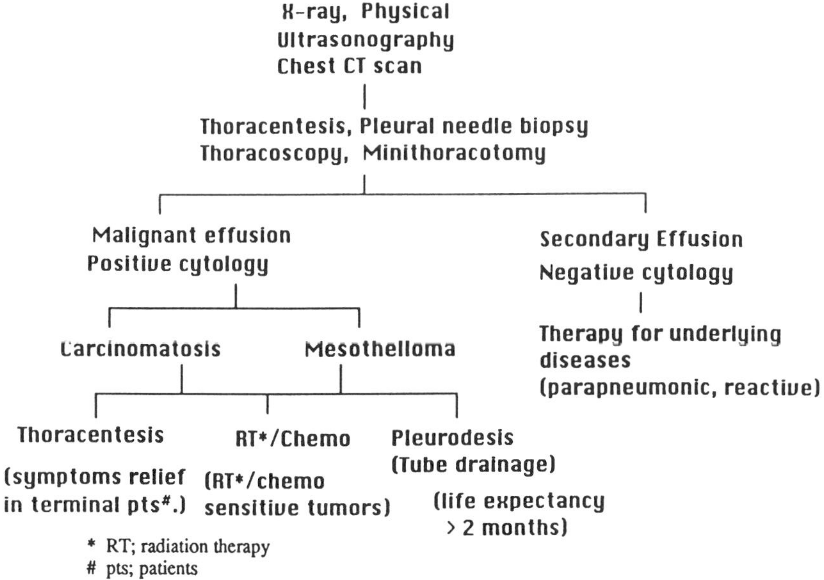

Figure 1 Management of pleural effusion in patients with malignancy. (Modified from Rusch VW, Harper GR.)

techniques. Following local anesthesia, a 14–18 gauge elastic needle attached to a syringe through a three-way stopcock is inserted into the desired puncture site. To avoid injury of the intercostal artery or nerve, one should choose the puncture site over the lower rib. When the tip of the needle reaches the parietal pleura and the pleural cavity, one can feel the subtle sense of resistance of the tissue through the needle. To avoid excessive pain, it is wise to give sufficient local anesthesia, especially in the area of the parietal pleura. "Pleural shock," severe bradycardia, and hypotension may occur as irritable reactions of the vagal nerve in the parietal pleura. A thoracentesis is contraindicated in a patient who has a hemorrhagic diathesis. The complications of the thoracentesis are very rare if the procedure is done carefully. In minimal effusion or compartmentalized effusion, ultrasonography is very helpful to determine the puncture site.

Bloody effusion dose not always mean malignancy, and vice versa. It is helpful to determine whether the pleural fluid is a transudate or an exudate. Transudative effusion is caused primarily by an increased leakage of water. The abnormal accumulation of protein in the pleural space results in exudative effusion. Malignancy is the most frequent cause of exudative effusions. A pleural fluid protein level of 3.0 g/dl was used to separate transudates from exudates. Useful criteria for exudative effusion are (1) a ratio of pleural fluid protein to serum protein greater than 0.5, (2) a ratio of pleural fluid lactic acid dehydrogenase (LDH) to serum LDH greater than 0.6, and (3) an LDH value greater than 200 mg/dl.

There are many laboratory examinations for specimens of effusion to differentiate malignant effusion from others, such as LDH, adenosine deaminase, and glucose; however, none of them are definitive. Among the tumor markers, elevation in carcinoembryonic antigen (CEA) is indicative of malignant effusion. Values from 2.5 to 12.5 ng/ml have been used to separate benign from malignant, and the reported sensitivities in malignant pleural effusion range from 25 to 57% using these values as a cutoff level. The pleural fluid of chylothorax can be diagnosed by its milky appearance, positive fat staining, and elevated triglyceride level (>110 mg/dl).

Cytology is the best means for diagnosis of malignant effusion. Using thoracentesis, a cytological diagnosis of malignancy can be made and more than 60% of patients are found to have malignant pleural effusion. Chromosomal analysis of cells found in the pleural space is reported to be useful in patients with lymphoma and leukemia. A chromosomal abnormality indicates a high probability that the effusion is malignant.

Pleural biopsy with Cope's or Abram's needle sometimes gives more information than the results of thoracentesis (Fig. 2). The combination of percutaneous pleural biopsy with cytological examinations correctly diagnoses about 80% of malignant pleural effusions.

The diagnostic role of thoracoscopy was recently reevaluated. Television-

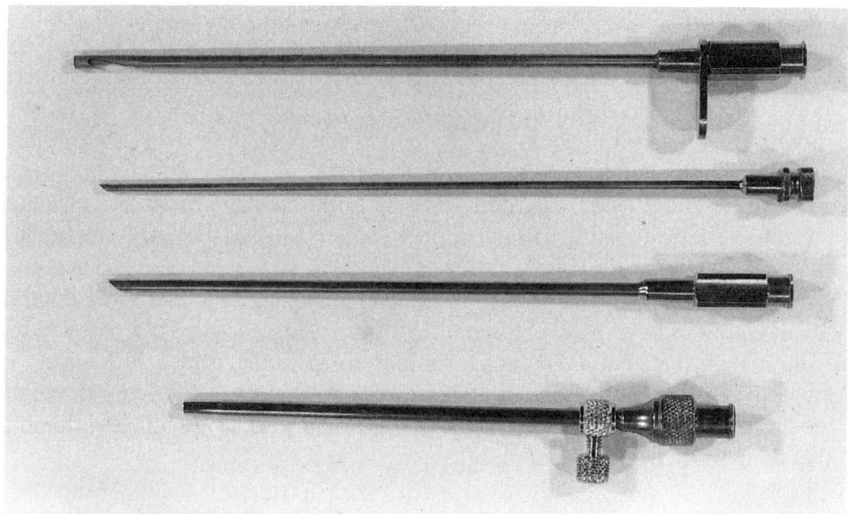

(A)

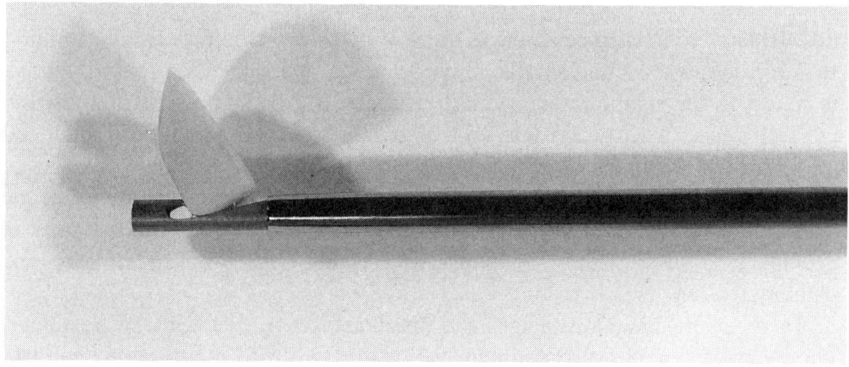

(B)

Figure 2 Needle biopsy of the pleura. (A) Cope pleural needle: hollow, blunt-tipped, hooked biopsy trocar, obturator or stylet, hollow-beveled trocar, and outer cannula. (B) The parietal pleura is hooked with the hollow, blunt-tipped biopsy trocar. The biopsy specimen is obtained by advancing the outer cannula with a rotary motion to sever the engaged piece of pleura.

guided thoracoscopic surgery is applied for this purpose. Thoracoscopy is a high-yield procedure compared with thoracentesis or pleural needle biopsy, but the need for general anesthesia makes this procedure less indicative. Thoracoscopy is contraindicated for obliteration of the pleural space by adhesions. Thoracotomy is generally considered the final approach in those patients whose diagnosis cannot be made with other methods.

There is no definitive diagnostic method to differentiate malignant effusion accompanied by primary malignant mesothelioma from that with metastatic tumors. Elevation in the concentration of hyaluronic acid in effusion and negative values of CEA tend to be higher in primary malignant mesothelioma than in other conditions. Using the immunohistochemistry, a negative stain reaction for epithelial mucin, that is, a negative diastase–periodic acid-Schiff stain, is suggestive of mesothelioma. In patients with both metastatic adenocarcinoma and mesothelioma, cytokeratin may be positive, and weak or absent CEA staining may be indicative of mesothelioma.

D. Treatment

1. Consideration of the Indications for Treatment Methods

For patients with chemoendocrine therapy or chemotherapy-sensitive tumors, such as breast cancer and small cell lung cancer, systemic treatment is effective in relieving the symptoms of pleural effusion. If a patient who suffered from refractory pleural dissemination, such as postoperative relapse of non–small cell lung cancer, complains of severe chest wall pain caused by direct invasion of tumor to the chest wall, external irradiation may be a choice as palliative therapy to lessen severe pain. Another possible indication for external irradiation is in patients who suffer from lymphoma with mediastinal lymphadenopathy and pleural effusion.

There are potential advantages and disadvantages to each form of treatment. The relief of symptoms to maintain the quality of life is the goal of treatment for malignant pleural effusion. Median survival after treatment for malignant pleural effusion has varied from 3 to more than 12 months. Some patients with breast cancer and well-differentiated adenocarcinoma of the lung survive more than 1 year after treatment for malignant pleural effusion.

2. Thoracentesis

Thoracentesis is a tentative treatment to reduce malignant pleural effusion. In patients of poor performance status with refractory tumors or with bilateral malignant effusion, tube drainage is often difficult to manage and excessively burdens the patient. In this case thoracentesis is a good alternative. However, the effect of thoracentesis is temporary and it is often necessary to repeat it. The efficiency in removing effusion is diminished after repeated thoracentesis.

Pneumothorax, bleeding, and "pleural shock" are possible complications of thoracentesis.

3. Tube Drainage

Tube drainage is a popular maneuver to relieve respiratory symptoms. The disadvantages of the procedure are similar to those of thoracentesis. Local anesthesia and disclosure of the insertion route using a hemostat through the chest wall before insertion of the tube make the procedure safe and easy without excessive patient trauma. Because significant force is required to insert the trocar, operative tube thoracostomy is probably safer than trocar tube thoracostomy. A 16–20F double-lumen catheter is used to remove effusion to avoid obstruction and to instill sclerosing agents (Fig. 3). Recently, a small-bore silastic catheter has been used as the substitution for larger catheters. Safer insertion of the drainage tube can be done using ultrasonography or x-ray fluoroscopy.

The care of a chest tube to maintain efficient drainage is as follows: (1) Is there bubbling through the water-seal bottle or the water-seal chamber on the disporsable unit? (2) Is the tube functioning? (3) What are the amount and type of drainage from the tube? These are important check points to find air leakage from the lung, disconnection of the tube, or decreased patency of the tube. The amount and character of the drainage fluid should be recorded for each 24 h period. The tube can be removed when the drainage volume of effusion is reduced below 100 ml per day. Tube drainage alone is effective in reducing pleural effusion in few cases.

The adverse complications of tube drainage are similar to those of thoracentesis. Circulatory disturbances, such as hypotension, after rapid reduction of massive pleural effusion and reexpansion pulmonary edema are rare complications of tube drainage. During prolonged tube drainage and repeated instillation of drugs, the chance of infection increases. The local implantation of tumor in the chest wall may occur along the tube, probably because of leakage of effusion.

4. Thoracoscopy

Video-assisted thoracoscopy has become popular in thoracic surgical oncology (Fig. 4). There have been some studies on the application of the thoracoscope as a useful tool for the instillation of a sclerosing agent, such as talc. Direct observation of the thoracic cavity and many techniques to obtain biopsy specimens and to instill agents are the advantages of thoracoscopy. However, general anesthesia and the cost of the maneuver are disadvantages compared with tube drainage.

5. Instillation Therapy

There have been many studies on the efficacy of sclerosing and nonsclerosing agents for controlling malignant effusion. The most common agents are tetracycline, bleomycin, and talc (Table 1). The dosages for instillation therapy are 500 mg for tetracycline and 15–240 mg for bleomycin. These agents are administered

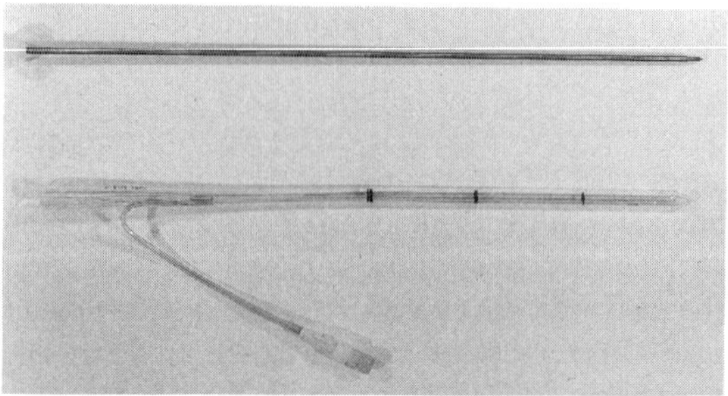

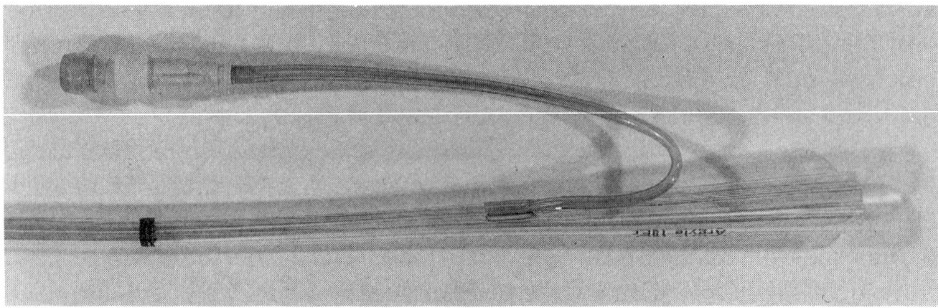

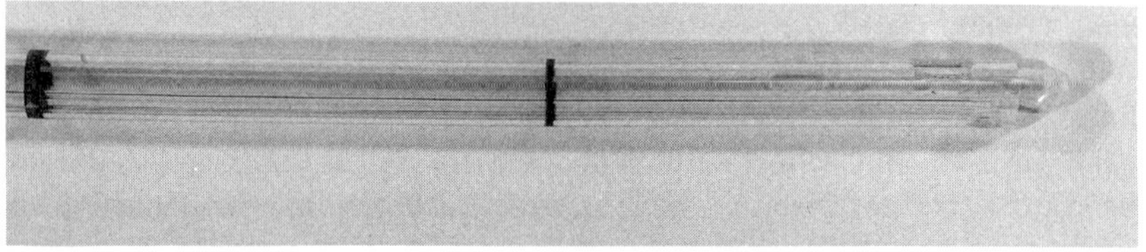

(A)

Figure 3 Pleural drainage systems: (A) double-lumen catheter; (B) suction and three-bottle collection system (Pleur-evac). There are four kinds of available drainage systems, such as one-way valve (Heimlich valve, a one-way flutter valve assembly), one-bottle collection system, two-bottle collection system, and suction control, water-seal, collection system.

with 40–100 ml normal saline and sometimes are mixed with local anesthetics, such as procaine hydrochloride. Following administration of the agent, a drainage tube is usually clamped for a few hours and then suction is restarted. Pain and fever are common side effects of instillation therapy that can be prevented with nonnarcotic analgesics, such as indomethacin, or more potent analgesics, such as pentazocine and morphine sulfate. Careful explanation of the pain associated with instillation therapy to the patient before administration of the agent and full premedication against pain may very effectively relieve the patient's fear of severe pain. Like the systemic administration of antineoplastic agents, mild to

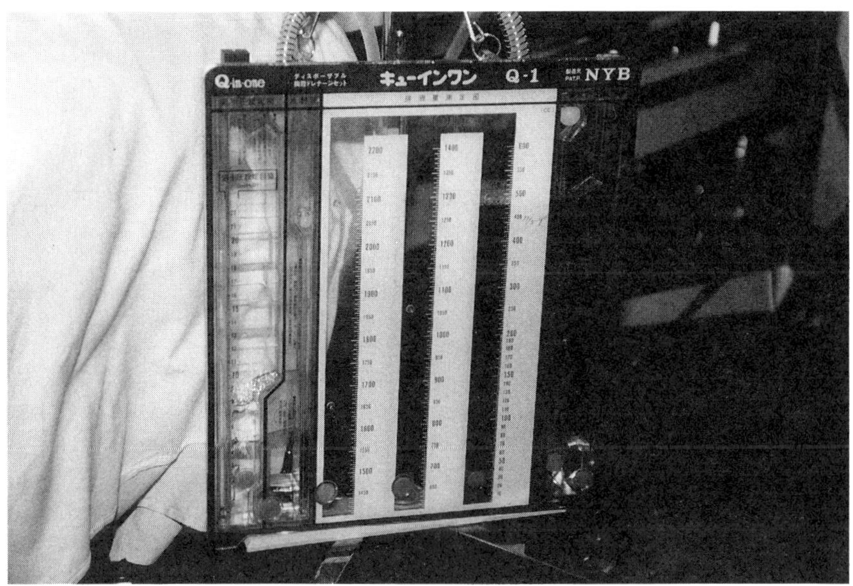

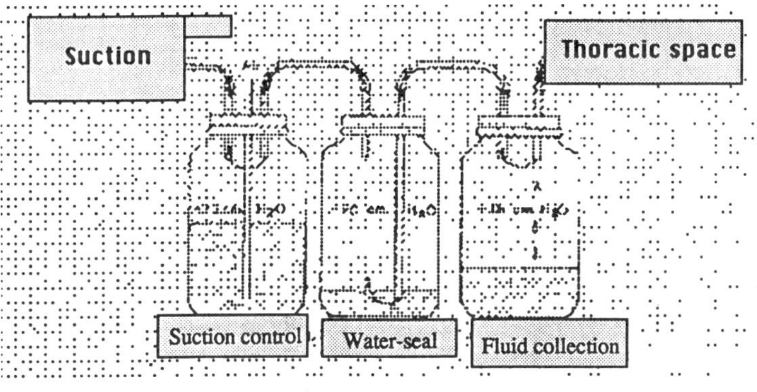

(B)

moderate myelosuppression, nausea, vomiting, and hair loss may occur after the instillation of anticancer agents.

The results of randomized control trials of sclerosing therapy are shown in Tables 2 and 3. Although the criteria for response were different, most results showed a high response rate. However, there was no evidence of a survival advantage in choosing any of these agents. The superiority of anticancer agents, such as Adriamycin, mitomycin, and cisplatin, to control malignant effusion, comparing with other sclerosing agents has not yet been confirmed. There have

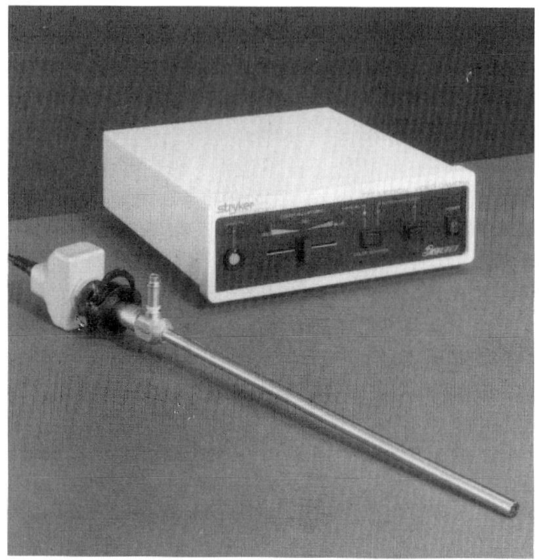

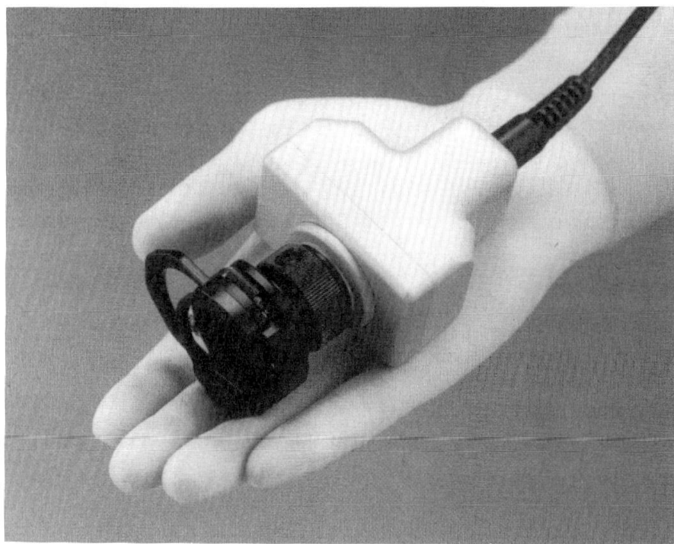

(A)

Figure 4 Video-assisted thoracoscopy (A) thoracoscopic and surgery (B) under general anesthesia. (Courtesy of Dr. Tsuguo Naruke.)

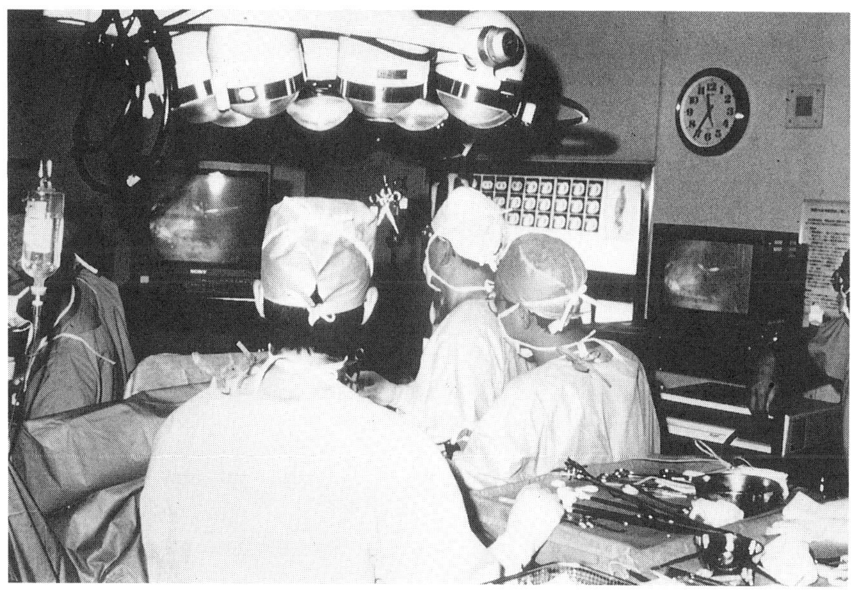

(B)

been several clinical trials on the efficacy of biological response modifiers, including recombinant cytokines (Table 4). According to the results of trials with recombinant human interleukin-2 (rh IL-2) and interferon (IFN), fever and flu-like syndrome were observed as adverse effects but were mild and tolerable. To date, no superiority in antitumor or sclerosing effect of these recombinant products has been clearly demonstrated compared with conventional treatment.

II. MALIGNANT PERICARDIAL EFFUSION

A. Etiology

The pericardial sac normally contains a small amount of fluid. The fluid is produced in the myocardium and diffuses through the mesothelial tissue of the visceral pericardium into the sac. Most of the fluid is reabsorbed by the parietal lymphatics at the base of the heart and drains into the thoracic duct. Some of the fluid may be reabsorbed by the visceral pericardial lymphatics and capillaries connected to the coronary sinus. Because of its anatomical characteristics, the lymphatic drainage of the heart and pericardium has a narrow zone. Metastatic tumors may block lymphatic drainage progressively without the development of collateral flow. Malignant pericardial effusion occurs by direct infiltration and hematogenous and lymphatic spread of tumors. Bulky involvement of mediastinal

Table 1 Overall Results of Controlled Trials of Intracavitary Therapy for Malignant Pleural Effusions

Number of Patients	Treatment[a]	Response (%)	Research group
67	Drainage	44	Izbicki et al. 1975 (Ref. 1)
	Drainage + ^{32}P	61	
38	Drainage	11	Mejer et al. 1977 (Ref. 2)
	Quinacrine	64	
	Thio-TEPA	27	
20	Tetracycline	80	Bayly et al. 1978 (Ref. 3)
	Quinacrine	60	
18	Mustine hydrochloride	45	Millar et al. 1979 (Ref. 4)
	Corynebacterium parvum	100	
29	Drainage	36	O'Neil et al. 1980 (Ref. 5)
	Tetracycline	72	
25	Bleomycin	54	Gupta et al. 1980 (Ref. 6)
	Tetracycline	58	
22	pH 2.8	11	Zaloznik et al. 1983 (Ref. 7)
	Tetracycline	69	
37	Mustine hydrochloride	53	Fentiman et al. 1983 (Ref. 8)
	Talc	90	
53	ADM	48	Urata et al. 1983 (Ref. 9)
	ADM + OK432	72	
62	Bleomycin	87	Johnson et al. 1984 (Ref. 10)
	Tetracycline	56	
21	Drainage	58	Sorenson et al. 1984 (Ref. 11)
	Talc	100	
32	Tetracycline[b]	56	Leahy et al. 1985 (Ref. 12)
	Tetracycline[c]	86	
	C. parvum	88	
30	Mustine hydrochloride	44	Kefford et al. 1986 (Ref. 13)
	Adriamycin	73	
	Tetracycline	70	
33	Tetracycline	48	Fentiman et al. 1986 (Ref. 14)
	Talc	92	
31	Tetracycline	65	Kessinger et al. 1987 (Ref. 15)
	Bleomycin	62	
50	Tetracycline, Single	84[d]	Landvater et al. 1988 (Ref. 16)
	Repeated	84[d]	
44	Bleomycin	72	Ostrowski et al. 1989 (Ref. 17)
	C. parvum	47	
85	Bleomycin	70[d]	Ruckdeshel et al. 1991 (Ref. 18)
	Tetracycline	47[d]	

[a]ADM, Adriamycin (doxorubicin HCl); OK432 is a streptococcal preparation.
[b]Through needle.
[c]Using tube drainage.
[d]Rate of no relapse (within 90 days).

Table 2 Results of Trials of Intracavitary Therapy for Pleural Effusions Secondary to Breast Cancer

Number of Patients	Treatment	Response (%)	Research group
52	Drainage	50	Izbicki et al. 1975 (Ref. 1)
	Drainage + ^{32}p	54	
10	Drainage	33	Mejer et al. 1977 (Ref. 2)
	Quinacrine	75	
	Thio-TEPA	67	
10	Tetracycline	71	Bayly et al. 1978 (Ref. 3)
	Quinacrine	67	
37	Mustine hydrochloride	53	Fentiman et al. 1983 (Ref. 7)
	Talc	90	
12	Tetracycline	40	Zaloznik et al. 1983 (Ref. 8)
	pH 2.8	43	
33	Tetracycline	48	Fentiman et al. 1986 (Ref. 14)
	Talc	92	
22	Bleomycin	67[a]	Hamed et al. 1989 (Ref. 19)
	Talc	100[a]	

[a]Rate of no reccurence.

lymph nodes may be a cause of retrograde lymphatic spread. Obstruction of lymphatic drainage and blood vessels of the heart disrupts the equilibrium between capillary filtration and osmotic pressure. As a result the pericardial effusion appears in the pericardial sac. Disseminated tumors on the pericardial surface cause exudation. The consequences of the accumulation of pericardial effusion partly depend on the rate of exudation and the compliance of the pericardial cavity. A rapid accumulation of fluid and a thickened pericardium with tumor infiltration or fibrosis cause cardiac tamponade. The elevation of intrapericardial pressure interferes with ventricular movement, and the cardiac output decreases. The increased ventricular diastolic pressure results in right-sided cardiac failure. Tachycardia and increased peripheral vascular tone are signs of hemodynamic crisis caused by cardiac tamponade. Shock and cardiac arrest occur if these compensatory responses fail. A thickened pericardium with tumor infiltration causes constrictive pericarditis, and cardiac tamponade may occur without fluid accumulation.

Pericardial involvement is not rare in patients with lung cancer, breast cancer, melanoma, lymphoma, and leukemia. Occasionally, cardiac tamponade may be the first manifestation of leukemia or metastatic cancer, such as primary adenocarcinoma of the lung.

Table 3 Results of Controlled Trials of Intracaviatry Therapy for Pleural Effusions Secondary to Lung Cancer

Number of Patients	Treatment	Response (%)	Research group
16	Drainage	0	Mejer et al. 1977 (Ref. 2)
	Quinacrine	40	
	Thio-TEPA	29	
5	Tetracycline	75	Bayly et al. 1978 (Ref. 3)
	Quinacrine	0	
16	Mustine hydrochloride	44	Millar et al. 1979 (Ref. 4)
	C. parvum	100	
11	pH 2.8	20	Zaloznik et al. 1983 (Ref. 7)
	Tetracycline	67	
34	ADM or MMC[a]	62	Sajio et al. 1983 (Ref. 20)
	ADM or MMC + *N*-CWS[b]	83	
68	ADM or MMC[a]	60	Yamamura et al. 1983 (Ref. 21)
	ADM or MMC + *N*-CWS[b]	86	
53	OK432[c]	88	Luh et al. 1992 (Ref. 22)
	MMC	67	

[a]ADM, Adriamycin (doxorubicin HCl); MMC, mitomycin.
[b]N-CWS, *Nocardia rubra* cell wall skeleton.
[c]OK432, streptococcal preparation.

B. Clinical Manifestation

Patients with cardiac and pericardial invasion of tumor may be asymptomatic unless the pericardial effusion accumulates more than 200–300 ml. Cardiac enlargement on percussion, engorgement of the cervical veins, enlargement of the liver, and increased venous pressure are common findings of pericardial effusion. Such symptoms as a precordial oppressive feeling, appetite loss, chest pain, dyspnea, nausca, casy fatigability, and epigastralgia are frequently observed in patients with pericardial effusion. The symptoms of pericardial effusion and cardiac tamponade may be similar to those of generalized carcinomatosis, and one should be cautious not to overlook them in routine follow-up after the initial treatment of malignancy. Dyspnea on exertion, edema of the lower extremities, dilatation of jugular vein, oliguria, arrhythmias, and hepatomegaly are the symptoms and signs of right-sided heart failure caused by pericardial effusion. Bilateral pleural effusion is sometimes associated with pericardial effusion as a consequence of cardiac dysfunction. Pericardial friction rub may be audible. The rapid development of a pericardial effusion can lead to cardiac tamponade. Orthopnea is frequently seen in patients with cardiac tamponade. Without

Table 4 Recent Results of Nonrandomized Trials of Intracavitary Therapy for Malignant Pleural Effusions

Number of Patients	Treatment	Response (%)	Research group
50	*C. parvum*	100[a]	Casali et al. 1988 (Ref. 25)
50 Breast	*C. parvum*	100[a]	Contegiacomo et al. 1987 (Ref. 23)
25	Tetracycline	15[a]	Gravelyn et al. 1987 (Ref. 24)
37	Cisplatin + cytarabine	49	Rusch et al. 1991 (Ref. 26)
34	Iodized talc	100[a]	Webb et al. 1992 (Ref. 27)
29	Natural IFN-β ($5-20 \times 10^6$ U)	27[a]	Rosso et al. 1988 (Ref. 28)
10	rhIL-2 (1×10^3 U/day)	30[a]	Suzuki et al. 1989 (Ref. 30)
4	rhIFN-β ($3 \times 10^6-1.8 \times 10^9$ U)	75	Tanaka 1988 (Ref. 29)
35 Lung	rhIL-2 (1×10^3 U/day)	37[a]	Yasumoto et al. 1991 (Ref. 31)
14 Lung	IFN-α (2×10^6 U)	79	Tercelj-Zorman et al. 1991 (Ref. 32)
22	rhIL-2 ($3-24 \times 10^6$ U)	45	Astoul et al. 1993 (Ref. 33)

[a]Complete response.

emergency treatment cardiac tamponade causes sudden death. Venous distension, distant heart sounds, paradoxical pulse, and oliguria are common findings in rapidly progressing cardiac tamponade. A paradoxical pulse is one that diminishes in amplitude during inspiration, and the width of the pulse pressure is narrowed.

C. Diagnosis

1. *Electrocardiography*

Nonspecific electrocardiographic changes, such as low voltage, sinus tachycardia, elevation of the ST segment, and T wave changes, are common findings in patients with pericardial effusion. Electrical alternans with alterations in the P wave as well as the QRS-T complex is seen in pericardial effusion with a stiff pericardium.

2. *Radiography*

An enlarged cardiac silhouette (a globular or ice bag appearance) is common finding in pericardial effusion on plain x-ray film. Serial comparison of the x-ray film with the previous film makes the diagnosis easier. In some patients

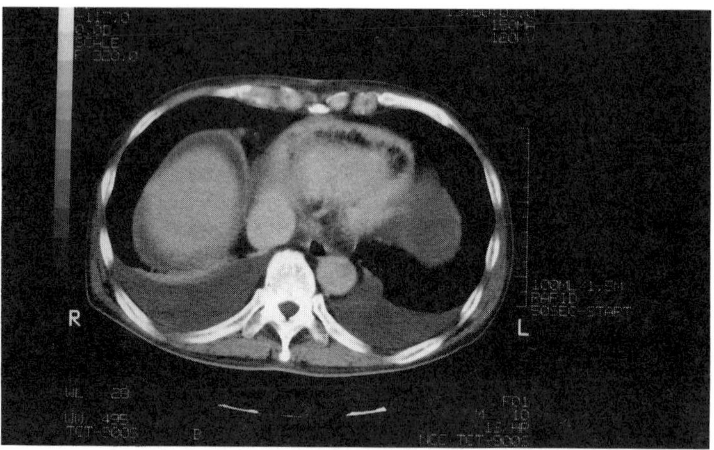

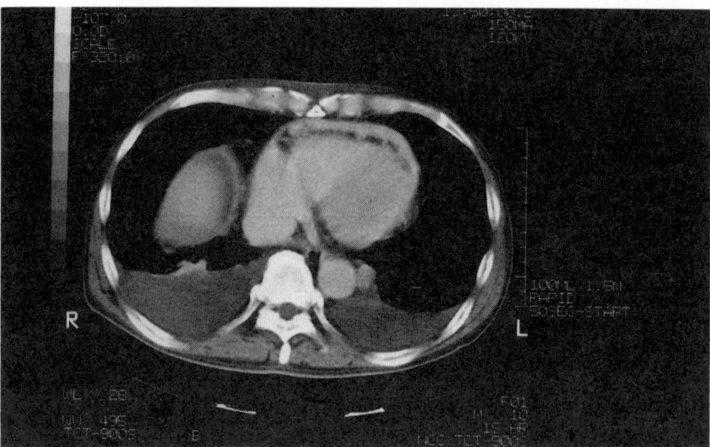

(A)

Figure 5 Diagnosis of pericardial effusion and cardiac tamponade. (A) CT findings of pericardial invasion of tumor. This patient received tube drainage through subxyphoid pericardiectomy for malignant pericardial effusion caused by advanced renal cancer. Chest CT scan reveals irregularly thickened pericardium, bilateral pleural effusion, and ascites. (B) Ultrasonographic findings of pericardial effusion: PE, pericardial effusion; LA, left atrium; LV, left ventricle; RV, right ventricle; AO, aorta.

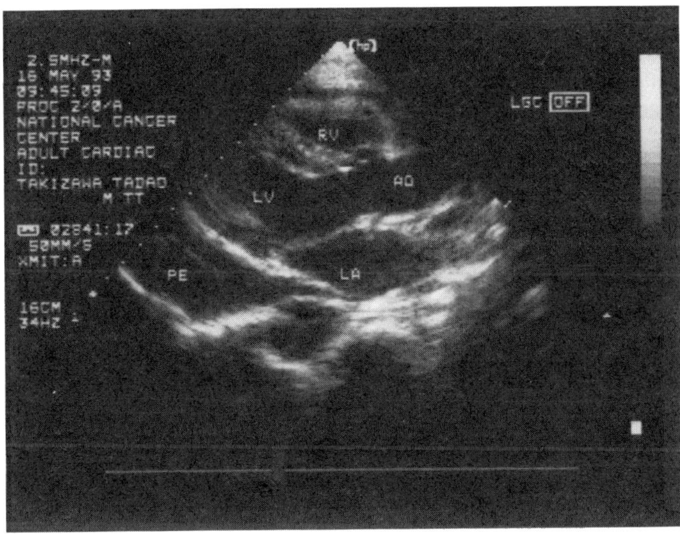

(B)

pericardial effusion may be accompanied by pleural effusion. In cardiac failure the vascular markings of both lung fields are blurred. Using CT scan of the chest, a double contour with low attenuation around the heart is the typical finding in pericardial effusion (Fig. 5A). Asymptomatic pericardial effusion can be identified by thoracic CT scan.

3. *Echocardiography*

Echocardiography is a simple and sensitive method for the diagnosis of pericardial effusion with safe and noninvasive features (Fig. 5B). If two distinct echoes, one from the pericardium and another from the posterior heart border, are observed, the space between these echoes indicates the presence of pericardial effusion or the pericardial thickness. Abnormal motion of the mitral leaflet may suggest the presence of cardiac tamponade. Two-dimensional echocardiography may differentiate a solid mass from pericardial effusion.

4. *Pericardiocenthesis*

To clarify the cause of pericardial effusion or pericarditis in cancer patients is important because these patients may have nonmalignant effusion of various etiologies. The differential diagnosis between chronic radiation-induced pericarditis and progressive malignant involvement of the pericardium is difficult, especially in a patient with prior radiation therapy. Pericardiocentesis is useful for the diagnosis of malignancy. The common puncture site is the joint portion of the lowest costal cartilage and the sternum just to the left of the xyphoid process. Ultrasonography is used to find the appropriate site of puncture. All procedures should be performed under sterilized conditions. Following the insertion of the needle at the site of local anesthesia and proceeding underneath the xyphoid process, the needle should be directed toward the apex of the left shoulder. Electocardiographic and blood pressure monitoring should be done during the pericardiocentesis. The complications of pericardiocentesis include cardiac arrythmias caused by trauma to the myocardium; hemorrhage, pneumothorax, and sudden death may occur. Because the presence of pericardial effusion does not necessarily mean it is malignant, even in patients with malignancy, most important is the confirmation of the malignant origin of the pericardial effusion.

D. Treatment

Indications for initial systemic chemotherapy and radiotherapy are limited in patients with malignant pericardial effusion (Fig. 6). For chemosensitive, previously untreated tumors, such as lymphoma and breast cancer, induction chemotherapy may be effective for pericardial effusion. Radiotherapy is the only treatment choice in patients with chemorefractory and radiosensitive tumors, such as lymphoma, leukemia, testicular cancer, and small cell lung cancer. Patients at poor risk for surgery may also be candidates for radiotherapy. Such surgical approaches as the formation of a pericardial pleural window are well-tolerated; however, they sometimes fail to obtain prolonged palliation. The overall survival of patients after treatment for malignant pericardial effusion is 2–6 months, and very limited numbers of patients have a longer life expectancy, beyond 1 year.

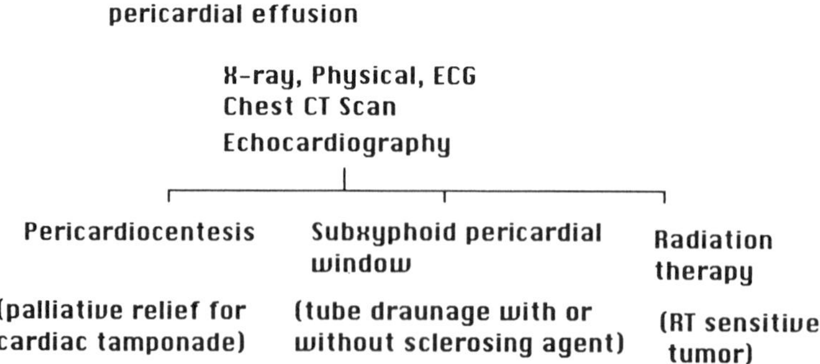

Figure 6 Management of malignant pericardial effusion. (Modified from Graeber GM.)

The prognosis of patients who have malignant pericardial effusion is poor even after the control of effusion because of decreased cardiac function with local and systemic dissemination of tumor. It is not rare to find diffuse sclerosis of the pericardium with tumor infiltration and constrictive pericarditis in autopsy of patients who received treatment for malignant pericardial effusion.

1. Pericardiocentesis

Pericardiocentesis is performed as an emergency treatment for the palliative relief of symptoms of cardiac tamponade. The initial removal of the effusion frequently obtains dramatic relief of circulatory symptoms, but recurrent pericardial effusion is common without additional treatment. Electrocardiographic and blood pressure monitoring are necessary during the procedure. The procedure should be performed with careful supportive treatment, such as intravenous fluid supplements and nasal oxygen, and pericardiocentesis has the risk of complications. These include cardiac arrythmias caused by trauma to the myocardium, hemorrhage, and sudden death.

2. Tube Drainage

Tube drainage is the standard procedure for symptomatic pericardial effusion, including cardiac tamponade. Subxyphoid pericardiectomy is a common procedure for tube drainage. The operation can be performed in 30–60 minutes under local anesthesia. There have been many reports of intrapericardial instillation therapy, such as tetracycline, talc, bleomycin, and radioactive isotopes. The dosage of tetracycline hydrochloride is 500–1000 mg in 20 ml sterile saline. Tetracycline is readministered daily until pericardial sclerosis occurs. The disadvantages of these sclerosing and antineoplastic agents include limited efficacy despite severe local pain or myelosuppression. No controlled trials have been performed for the treatment of malignant pericardial effusion. During the drainage period the cardiac silhouette on the chest x-ray may not show much improvement in size. The tube can be removed if the volume of drainage fluid decreases to less than 10 ml/day. Empirically, many of pericardial effusions can be controlled within 1–2 weeks using tube drainage without sclerosing agents.

III. MALIGNANT ASCITES

A. Etiology

Malignant ascites occurs as a result of subdiaphragmatic lymphatic obstruction and increased production of intraperitoneal fluid. In patients with gastric, large bowel, and pancreatic cancer, a direct extension through the visceral layer of the peritoneum may occur. The affected parts of the intestine become adherent to adjacent organs. Sometimes the affected lesion may lead to intraabdominal fistulas, volvulus formation, and complete obstruction. In patients with rapid growing tumors, such as ovarian and gastric cancer, invasion of tumor cells tends to be transcoelomic dissemination. Small lumps of tumor cells become suspended in the ascites fluid. Increased capillary permeability caused by damaged capillary vessels, with generalized carcinomatosis and increased venous pressure from local obstruction, results in changes in the clearance of peritoneal fluid. Hypoalbuminemia associated with malignancy may also exacerbate ascites. Chylous ascites may arise as a result of disturbance of a major lymphatic drainage, such as obstruction of the thoracic duct in patients with lymphoma.

Ovarian, endometrial, breast, colonic, gastric, and pancreatic cancer are common tumors that may be associated with malignant ascites.

B. Clinical Manifestation

Ascites may result in anorexia, indigestion, heartburn, or respiratory disturbance, such as tachypnea and orthopnea, caused by the increase in intraperitoneal pressure and restriction of the movement of the diaphragm. The most common signs are abdominal distension, weight gain, and general discomfort. A functional or organic decrease in bowel movement may occur because of carcinomatous peritonitis, metastasis to the bowel wall, and ascites. On physical examination, a fully distended abdomen with stretched skin is common, and the shifting of fluid waves and flank dullness, depending on the position of the patient, are notable.

C. Diagnosis

Abdominal plain x-ray film reveals opacity on the outer side of the abdomen along the flank stripe and blurring of the contour of the psoas muscles and the kidneys. The gas bubbles in the bowel gather in the central portion of abdomen on the film in a supine position. Ultrasonography and abdominal CT scan are useful to find not only ascites but also intraabdominal and retroperitoneal tumor spread. Because the details of the ultrasonographic findings may occasionally be obscured by the gas in the intestines, an abdominal CT scan is more helpful in evaluating the extent of the disease.

Because there may be a possibility of nonmalignant ascites in cancer patients, paracentesis is a very important procedure to identify the etiology of ascites. In malignant effusion three-fourths of patients have ascites protein values greater than 2.5 g/ml. Tumor markers, such as CEA, are helpful in disclosing malignancy. CEA levels greater than 12 ng/ml are suggestive of malignant ascites. Cytological examination is necessary for the definitive diagnosis of malignant effusion.

D. Treatment

Diuretics are ineffective for most patients with massive malignant ascites, and their use without precautions may induce water imbalance (Fig. 7). Paracentesis

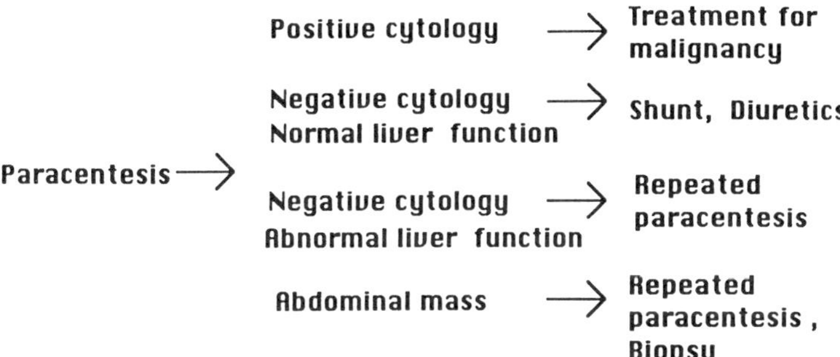

Figure 7 Management of ascites. (Modified from Lacy JH, Shively EH.)

is also not effective in controlling ascites, and the repeated procedure causes a rapid loss of protein and progressive dehydration.

Intraperitoneal administration of radioactive isotopes, such as ^{198}Au, has been shown to be effective in controlling malignant ascites. However, these agents can be troublesome if leakage or spillage occurs. Intracavitary treatment with chemotherapeutic agents may be effective if the tumor is sensitive to chemotherapy as in patients with ovarian or breast cancer. There have been trials of the intracavitary instillation of platinum-based agents. Reviewing the pathological complete response (CR) reported in ovarian cancer patients undergoing second-line intraperitoneal therapy using various chemotherapeutic agents, about 10% of patients achieved pathological CR. The intracavitary instillation of anticancer agents, such as 5-fluorouracil, bleomycin, and thio-TEPA, resulted in about a 30–35% response. Mild to moderate myelosuppression may occur after intracavitary treatment with anticancer agents. Devices for delivering chemotherapeutic agents have been developed, such as the Tenckhoff catheter and the Port-A-Cath (Fig. 8). The complications from implanting these devices were bowel perforation, bleeding, ileus, and leakage of fluid. The incidence was less than 10%, and even less with the Port-A-Cath. Problems with the functioning of these devices included outflow obstruction, inability to drain, and inflow obstruction; the rate of complication was less than 30%. Intraabdominal infection was reported in 5–8% of the patients.

Recently the intracavitary instillation of various immunopotentiators, including recombinant cytokines, has been reported, as shown in Table 5. Some were expected to have both a sclerosing effect for the pleura and an antitumor effect against cancer cells in the ascites through immunological reaction. However, the efficacy of these agents in achieving long-term palliation have not yet been confirmed.

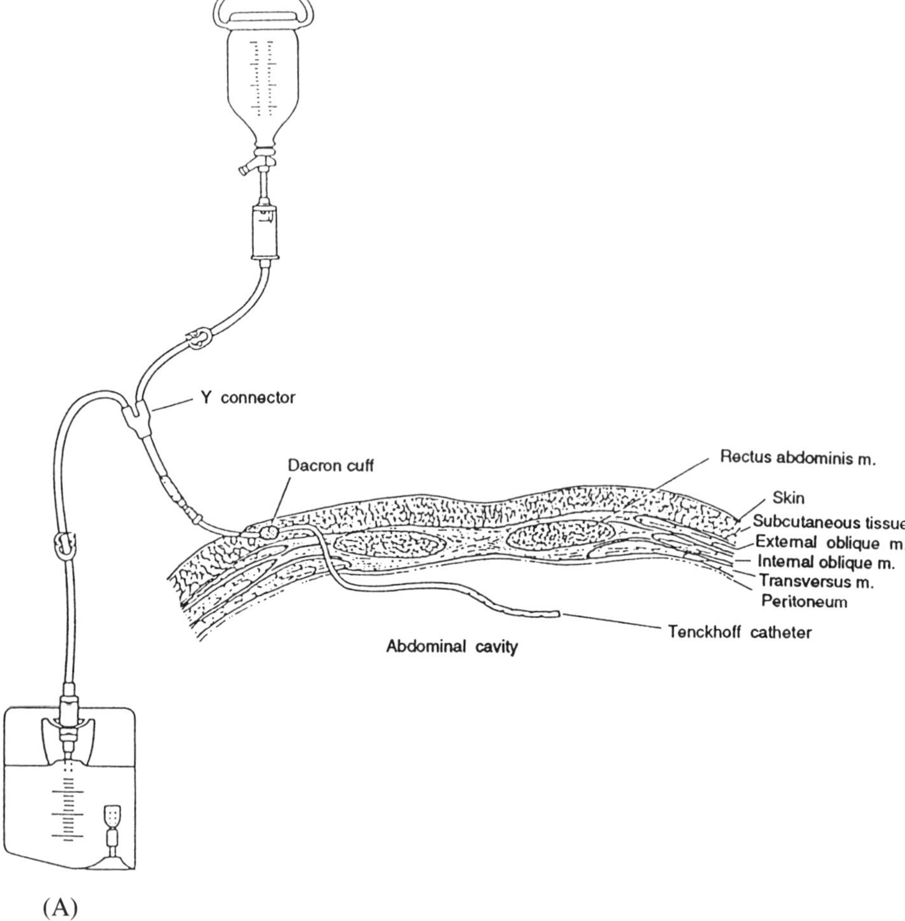

(A)

Figure 8 (A) Tenckhoff catheter and (B) Port-A-Cath. (Modified from Piccart MJ, Muggia F, et al.)

Portovenous shunting is a common procedure for surgical relief of malignant ascites. The LeVeen shunt drains fluid from abdominal cavity into the superior vena cava. This kind of treatment has shown long-term palliation, longer than 3 months, with minimal operative risk. The complications of the shunt revealed obstruction with clotting in bloody ascites and the increased risk of disseminated intravascular coagulation. The Denver shunt has a valve mechanism, and the system can be flushed and controlled by manipulation. The Denver shunt showed a lower failure rate than the LeVeen shunt; however, both were palliative treatments with the risk of fatal coagulopathy.

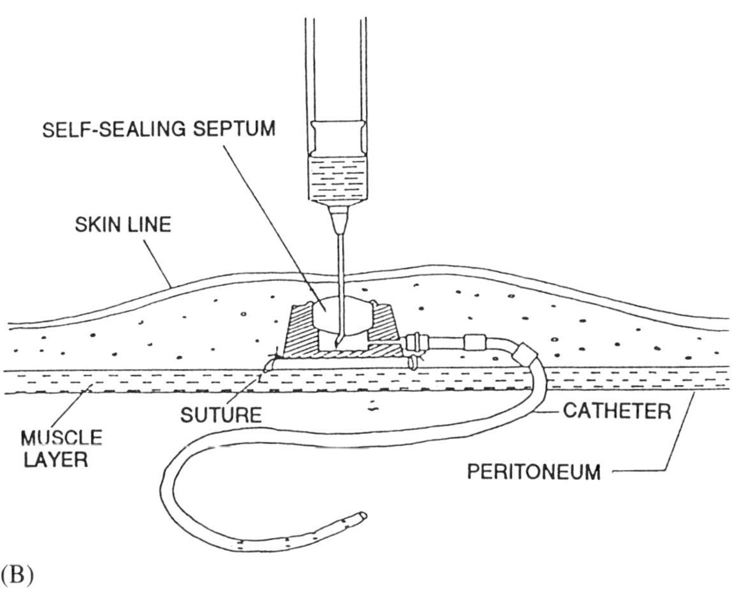

(B)

Table 5 New Agents for Intraperitoneal Instillation in Patients with Malignant Ascites

Number of Patients	Treatment	Response (%)	Research group
14 Ovarian	rhIFN-α (5–50 × 10^6 U)	36[a]	Berek et al. 1985 (Ref. 34)
7 Ovarian	rhIL-2 (1 × 10^5–5 × 10^7 U)	None (1 × 10^6 U twice per week)	Champman et al. 1988 (Ref. 35)
8 Gastric, uterine	OK-432	25	Kato et al. 1989 (Ref. 36)
19 Ovarian	rIFN-α (5–15 U/m^2 twice per week)	36	Bezwoda et al. 1991 (Ref. 37)
29	rTNF-α (40–350 Âg/m^2/week)	76	Räth et al. 1991 (Ref. 38)

[a]Complete response.

SELECTED READING

Muach P, Ultmann JE. Treatment of malignant pericardial effusion, treatment of malignant pleural effusion, treatment of malignant ascites. In: Devita VT, Hellman S, Rosenberg SA, eds. Cancer Principles and Practice of Oncology. Philadelphia: J. B. Lippincott, 1985:2141–2153.

Light RW. Pleural Diseases. Philadelphia: Lea & Febiger, 1983.

Vladutu AO. Pleural Effusion. New York: Futura, 1986.

Jones JSP. Pathology of the Mesothelium. London: Springer-Verlag, 1987.

Rusch VW, Harper GR. Pleural effusions in patients with malignancy. In: Roth JA, Ruckdeschel JC, Weisenburger TH, eds. Thoracic Oncology. Philadelphia: W. B. Saunders, 1989:594–605.

Graeber GM. Complications of therapy of malignant tumors involving the pericardium. In: Roth JA, Ruckdeschel JC, Weisenburger TH, eds. Thoracic Oncology. Philadelphia: W. B. Saunders, 1989:504–512.

Fentiman IS. Diagnosis and treatment of malignant pleural effusion. Cancer Treat Rev 1987; 14:107–118.

Ruckdeschel JC. Management of malignant pleural effusion; an overview. Semin Oncol 1988; 15:24–28.

Press OW. Management of malignant pericardial effusion and tamponade. JAMA 1987; 257(8):1088–1092.

Theologides A. Neoplastic cardiac tamponade. Semin Oncol 1987; 5:181–192.

Lacy JH, Shively EH. Management of malignant ascites. Surg Gynecol Obstet 1984; 159:397–412.

Piccart MJ, Muggia F, et al. Intraperitoneal chemotherapy; technical experience at five institutions. Semin Oncol 1985; 12(3):58–62.

REFERENCES

1. Izbicki R, Weyhing BT, Baker L, et al. Pleural effusion in cancer patients. A prospective randomized study of pleural drainage with the addition of radioactive phosphorus to the pleural space vs. pleural drainage alone. Cancer 1975; 36:1151–1518.
2. Mejer J, Mortensen KM, Hausen HH. Mepacrine hydrocloride in the treatment of malignant pleural effusions. Scand J Resp Dis 1977; 58:319–329.
3. Bayly TC, Kisner DL, Sybert A, et al. Tetracycline and quinacrine in the control of malignant pleural effusions: a randomized trial. Cancer 1978; 41:1188–1192.
4. Millar JW, Hunter AM, Horne NW. Intrapleural immunotherapy with *Corynebacterium purvum* in recurrent malignant pleural effusions. Thorax 1979; 35:856–858.
5. O'Neil W, Spurr C, Moss H, et al. A prospective study of chest tube drainage and tetracycline sclerosis versus chest tube drainage in the treatment of malignant pleural effusions. Proc Am Soc Clin Oncol 1980; 21:349.
6. Gupta N, Opfell RW, Padova J, et al. Intrapleural bleomycin versus tetracycline for control of malignant pleural effusion: a randomized study. Proc Am Assoc Cancer Res 1980; 21:366.

7. Zaloznik AJ, Oswald SG, Langin M. Intrapleural tetracycline in malignant pleural effusions: a randomized study. Cancer 1983; 51:752–755.
8. Fentiman IS, Rubens RD, Hayward JL. Control of pleural effusions in patients with breast cancer: a randomized trial. Cancer 1983; 52:737–739.
9. Urata A, Nishimura Y, Ohta K, et al. Randomized controlled study of OK-432 in the treatment of cancerous pleurisy. Gan to Kagaku Ryohou 1983; 10:1497–1503 (Abstract in English).
10. Johnson CE, Curzon PG. Comparison of intrapleural bleomycin and tetracycline in the treatment of malignant pleural effusions. Proc Brit Thor Soc 1984; S:6.
11. Sorenson PG, Svendsen TC, Enk B. Treatment of malignant pleural effusion with drainage with or without installation of talc. Eur J Respir Dis 1984; 65:131–135.
12. Leahy BC, Honeybourne D, Brear SG, et al. Treatment of malignant effusions with intrapleural *Corynebacterium parvum* or tetracycline. Eur J Respir Dis 1985; 66:50–54.
13. Kefford RF, Woods RL, Fox RM, et al. Intracavitary adriamycin nitrogen mustard and tetracycline in the control of malignant effusions, a randomized study Med J Aust 1986; 2:447–448.
14. Fentiman IS, Rubens RD, Hayward JL. A comparison of intracavitary talc and tetracycline for the control of pleural effusions secondary to breast cancer. Eur J Clin Oncol 1986; 22:1079–1081.
15. Kessinger A, Wigton RS. Intracavitary bleomycin and tetracycline in the management of malignant pleural effusions: a randomized study. J Surg Oncol 1987; 36:81–83.
16. Landvater L, Hix WR, Mills M, et al. Malignant pleural effusion treated by tetracyline sclerotherapy: a comparison of single vs. repeated instillation. Chest 1988; 90:1196–1198.
17. Ostrowski MJ, Houston PT, Martin WNC. A randomized trial of intracavitary bleomycin and *Corynebacterium parvum* in the control of malignant pleural effusions. Radiotherapy and Oncology 1989; 14:19–26.
18. Ruckdeshel JC, Moores D, Lee JY, et al. Intrapleural therapy for malignant pleural effusions, a randomized comparison of bleomycin and tetracycline. Chest 1991; 100:1528–1535.
19. Hamed H, Fentiman IS, Chaudary MA, et al. Comparison of intracavitary bleomycin and talc for control of pleural effusions secondary to carcinoma of the breast. Br J Surg 1989; 76:1266–1267.
20. Saijo N, Eguchi K, Tominaga K, et al. Effect of *Nocardia Rubra* cell wall skeleton against pleuritis carcinomatosa in adenocarcinoma of the lung. Gan to Kagaku Ryohou 1983; 10(2):290–295 (Abstract in English).
21. Yamamura Y, Sakatani M, Ogura T, et al. Clinical effect of *Nocardia Rubra* cell wall skeleton (N-CWS) on lung cancer with malignant pleural effusion. Gan to Kagaku Ryohou 1983; 10:63–70 (Abstract in English).
22. Luh K-T, Yang P-C, Kuo S-H, et al. Comparison of OK-432 and mitomycin C pleurodesis for malignant pleural effusion caused by lung cancer: a randomized trial. Cancer 1992; 69:674–679.
23. Contegiacomo A, Fiorillo L, De Placido S, et al. The treatment of metastatic pleural effusion in breast cancer: report of 25 cases. Tumori 1987; 73:611–616.

24. Gravelyn TR, Michelson MK, Gross BH et al. Tetracycline pleurodesis for malignant pleural effusions, a 10-year retrospective study. Cancer 1987; 59:1973–1977.
25. Casali A, Gionfra T, Rinaldi M, et al. Treatment of malignant pleural effusions with intracavitary *Corynebacterium parvum*. Cancer 1988; 62:806–811.
26. Rusch VW, Figlin R, Godwin D, et al. Intrapleural cisplatin and cytarabine in the management of malignant pleural effusions: a Lung Cancer Study Group Trial. J Clin Oncol 1991; 9:313–319.
27. Webb WR, Ozmen V, Moulder PV, et al. Iodized talc pleurodesis for the treatment of pleural effusions. J Thorac Cardiovasc Surg 1992; 103:881–886.
28. Rosso R, Rimoldi R, Salvati F, et al. Intrapleural natural beta interferon in the treatment of malignant pleural effusions. Oncology 1988; 45:253–256.
29. Tanaka N, Matsui T, Yamada J, et al. Local administration of recombinant interferon-beta to patients with cancer-associated body cavity fluids. Gan to Kagaku Ryohou 1988; 15(2):237–241. (Abstract in English).
30. Suzuki H. Experimental and clinical studies on intrapleural instillations of interleukin-2(IL-2) in patients with malignant pleural effusion. Nippon Geka Gakkaishi 1989; 90(11):1922–1931. (Abstract in English).
31. Yasumoto K, Ogura T. Intrapleural application of recombinant interleukin-2 in patients with malignant pleurisy due to lung cancer: a multi-institutional cooperative study. Biotherapy 1991; 3:345–349.
32. Tercelj-Zorman M, Mermolja M, Jereb M, et al. Human leukocyte interferon alpha (HLI-a) for treatment of pleural effusion caused by non-small cell lung cancer. Acta Oncologica 1991; 30(8):963–965.
33. Astoul P, Viallat J-R, Laurent JC, et al. Intrapleural recombinant IL-2 in passive immunotherapy for malignant pleural effusion. Chest 1993; 103:209–213.
34. Berek JS, Hacker NF, Lichtenstein A, et al. Intraperitoneal recombinant alpha-interferon for "salvage" immunotherapy in stage III epithelial ovarian cancer: a Gynecologic Oncology Group Study. Cancer Res 1985; 45:4447–4453.
35. Chapman PB, Kolitz JE, Hakes TB, et al. A phase I trial of intraperitoneal recombinant interleukin 2 in patients with ovarian carcinoma. Invest New Drugs 1988; 6:179–188.
36. Kato H, Yamamura Y, Kin R, et al. Treatment of malignant ascites and pleurisy by a *Streptcoccal* preparation OK-432 with fresh frozen plasma: a mechanism of polymorphonuclear leukocyte(PMN) accumulation. Int J Immunopharmacol 1989; 11(2):117–128.
37. Bezwoda WR, Golombick T, Dansey R, et al. Treatment of malignant ascites due to recurrent/refractory ovarian cancer: the use of interferon-alpha or interferon-alpha plus chemotherapy in vivo and in vitro. Eur J Cancer 1991; 27(11):1423–1429.
38. Räth U, Kaufmann M, Schmid M, et al. Effects of intraperitoneal recombinant human tumor necrosis factor alpha on malignant ascites. Eur J Cancer 1991; 27(2):121–125.

14

Organ Failure from Cancer or Its Therapy

Louis E. Schroder
University of Cincinnati Medical Center, Cincinnati, Ohio

Nicholas J. Vogelzang
University of Chicago, Chicago, Illinois

I. INTRODUCTION

Individuals who die from progressive cancer often experience organ failure as a terminal event. This chapter addresses those circumstances in which organ failure occurs earlier in the course of cancer, either at diagnosis or during active therapy or follow-up. It focuses on the kidney, heart, lung, liver, and adrenal gland. Discussion includes organ failure caused by (1) direct cancer invasion, (2) paraneoplastic effects (when applicable), and (3) drug therapy.

Causes of organ failure that are not discussed here include radiation therapy, surgery, high-dose chemotherapy and bone marrow transplant, and infections. Radiation therapy as delivered at the present time is an uncommon cause of organ failure except in endocrine failure of the thyroid following neck irradiation. Radiation may be a contributing factor, however, in certain situations of organ compromise, such as anthracycline-induced cardiac damage. Organ failure following high-dose chemotherapy and bone marrow transplantation is a major topic itself and is not considered here. Various infections in the cancer patient may result in organ failure caused by the infection itself or by the drugs used in treating the infection. Specific infections are not addressed here, but antibiotics used frequently in cancer patients are covered in the discussion of renal toxicity caused by drugs.

II. RENAL FAILURE

A. Direct Cancer Invasion

Renal failure in patients with cancer may occur as a result of a wide variety of cancer-related etiologies (1,2). These include *prerenal* causes, such as volume depletion (caused by poor intake, vomiting, diarrhea, bleeding, excessive diuresis as a result of diuretics or hypercalcemia, or frequent large-volume paracenteses), functional volume depletion (caused by sepsis), myocardial dysfunction (from an anthracycline, such as doxorubicin), or pericardial tamponade (as a result of malignant pericardial effusion). Prerenal failure is generally mild, but it may predispose to more severe forms of renal failure, such as contrast-induced acute renal failure. *Postrenal* (obstructive) causes of renal failure include bladder outlet or bilateral ureteral and pelvic obstruction. (See Chap. 12.)

One of the more common *renal* causes of renal failure is acute tubular necrosis (vasomotor nephropathy) caused by sepsis in the neutropenic patient. Table 1 lists the renal causes of renal failure, excluding sepsis and acute tubular necrosis and excluding drugs.

Neoplastic infiltration of the kidney is relatively common, but renal failure as a result of infiltration is rare. In Richmond et al.'s large series (3), 33.5% of

Table 1 Causes of Renal Failure in Cancer Patients[a]

I. Cancer infiltration
   A. Leukemias
   B. Lymphomas
   C. Solid tumors
II. Tumor by-products, deposition diseases
   A. Hypercalcemia
   B. Hyperuricemia
   C. Hyperphosphatemia, tumor lysis syndrome
   D. Multiple myeloma, paraproteinemias
   E. Amyloidosis
   F. Mucoprotein deposition
III. Paraneoplastic
   A. Glomerulopathies
   B. Hemolytic uremic syndrome (HUS), thrombocytopenic purpura (TTP)
   C. Hepatorenal syndrome

[a](Excluding prerenal and postrenal causes and excluding acute renal failure from sepsis or acute tubular necrosis or drugs).

autopsied lymphoma patients had renal involvement but only 13% of those with renal involvement had blood urea nitrogen > 25 mg% attributable primarily to the renal infiltration. Only 5 of 696 patients in Richmond's series had renal failure from parenchymal infiltration implicated as the main cause of death. In other series, 6–60% of autopsied patients had renal involvement. Lymphoma in the kidneys is more often nodular (Fig. 1) than diffuse (3). In patients developing renal failure, diffuse infiltration and enlargement of the kidneys appear to be more common. When renal failure is caused by lymphomatous infiltration, the histology is usually a non-Hodgkin's lymphoma, most commonly diffuse histiocytic (large cell) lymphoma (4). Note that massively enlarged kidneys from lymphoma have occurred without significant renal functional impairment and that renal failure as a result of lymphomatous infiltration has occurred in kidneys of normal size. Lymphoma *presenting* as renal failure has occasionally been reported (5,6), and in at least two cases the kidney appeared to be the sole site of lymphoma (5). In series of acute and chronic leukemia patients, 30–50% have evidence of renal involvement (7). As with lymphoma patients, renal failure as a result of infiltration is rare (8).

The kidney is frequently a metastatic site for cancers originating elsewhere. Bronchogenic carcinoma metastatic to the kidney is approximately twice as common as primary renal carcinoma. Five patients have been reported (9–13) who had renal failure caused by solid tumor infiltration of the kidney (two non-small cell lung, one head and neck, one gastric, and one seminoma), and only in the seminoma patient (13) was renal failure present at the time of initial cancer diagnosis.

In patients with responsive tumors (e.g., lymphoma or seminoma), treatment of the cancer with chemotherapy or local radiation to the kidneys has resulted in improvement or normalization of renal function.

B. Tumor By-products and Deposition Diseases

Renal failure caused by hyperuricemia or tumor lysis syndrome can generally be prevented by prophylactic treatment with allopurinol, hydration, and other

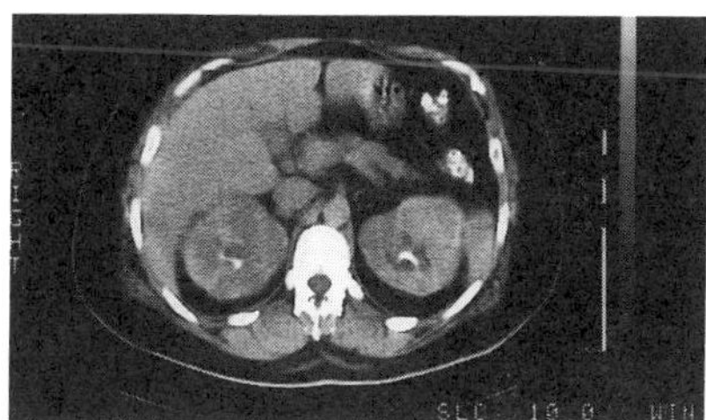

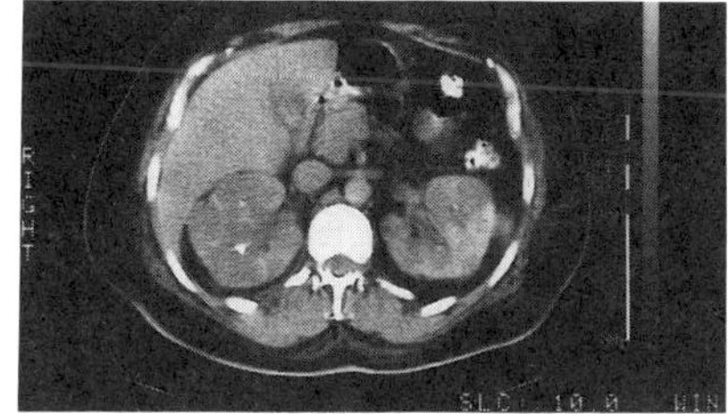

Figure 1 Nodular irregularities are present in both kidneys of this 43-year-old man with large cell lymphoma. The abnormalities completely resolved with chemotherapy. Renal function was normal throughout.

supportive measures, as discussed in Chapter 16. Hypercalcemia can usually be effectively managed, at least in the short term. (See Chaps. 16 and 17.)

Multiple myeloma and other paraproteinemias may cause renal failure by a variety of mechanisms (14). These include hypercalcemia, cast nephropathy (myeloma kidney), light-chain deposition disease, and amyloidosis. A major cause of renal insufficiency in myeloma patients is cast nephropathy, with hypercalcemia as a contributing cause. A critical time for cast nephropathy in myeloma patients is at diagnosis or soon thereafter, before the urinary excretion of protein has decreased in response to treatment. When patients present with renal insufficiency, correction of hypercalcemia, vigorous hydration, and initiation of chemotherapy are the most important management strategies (15). Plasmapheresis may be beneficial, especially in patients without severe cast nephropathy (15,16). Renal function will return to normal in about 50% of patients, most frequently in those with initially mild renal impairment (17). The stress of dehydration or radiographic contrast administration may precipitate renal failure in a previously stable patient. Note, however, that in well-hydrated myeloma patients the absolute risk of acute renal failure following radiographic contrast procedures is probably no greater than 1% (18). Light-chain deposition disease (14) occurs in 5–10% of patients with myeloma and renal insufficiency. Light-chain deposition in the kidney was first described in 1973 (19). It is characterized pathologically by ribbonlike thickening of the tubular basement membrane (as a result of light-chain deposition) and mesangial expansion with formation of intercapillary nodules (also caused by light chains). Patients may have nephrotic syndrome; the renal failure is usually rapidly progressive and severe. If treatment for the myeloma is instituted early, however, renal function may stabilize or improve. Light-chain deposition may occur systemically and has many clinical similarities to light-chain amyloidosis (20).

Amyloidosis is a more chronic cause for renal failure that may occur in the setting of myeloma or secondary to other malignancies. Amyloidosis occurs in approximately 10% of multiple myeloma patients, 4% of Hodgkin's disease patients, 1% of other lymphomas, and occasionally in carcinoma (21). Renal, renal pelvis, bladder, cervical, biliary tract, and bronchogenic cancers have been associated with amyloidosis, renal carcinoma being the most frequent (21, 22). Light-chain amyloidosis as seen in myeloma and amyloid A protein (an apolipoprotein) amyloidosis as seen in Hodgkin's disease and some solid tumors may have renal involvement (21–23). There is no satisfactory treatment to reverse amyloidosis-induced renal failure.

There is a report in the literature documenting a cast nephropathy secondary to mucoproteins (24). The patient, who had a mucin-secreting pancreatic carcinoma and ascites, presented with oliguric renal failure. A renal biopsy and subsequent autopsy confirmed a cast nephropathy caused by a mucoprotein identical to that in tumor extract. Maintaining good hydration presumably would minimize this problem.

C. Glomerulonephropathies

The glomerulonephropathies in cancer patients are usually either minimal change disease, as seen in Hodgkin's disease, or membranous glomerulopathy, as seen in solid tumor patients (25). The glomerulopathies are usually recognized clinically as nephrotic syndrome and may precede, coincide with, or follow a diagnosis of cancer. Minimal change disease and membranous glomerulopathy are usually associated with normal renal function. Most patients with renal failure have crescentic glomerulonephritis (26) or another less common histology. Approximately 60% of patients with nephrotic syndrome and Hodgkin's disease have minimal change disease on renal biopsy. The renal lesion is believed secondary to disordered T cell function. Approximately 70% of patients with nephrotic syndrome and carcinoma have membranous glomerulopathy related to immune complex deposition. Non-Hodgkin's lymphoma patients with nephrotic syndrome do not have one dominant histological pattern on renal biopsy. Treatment of the malignancy by resection or chemotherapy can reverse the nephrotic process and is the treatment of choice. Patients with frank renal failure are less likely to improve despite treatment of their cancer.

D. HUS or Hepatorenal Syndrome

Hemolytic uremic syndrome (HUS)/thrombotic thrombocytopenic purpura (TTP) is a rare cause of renal failure in cancer patients. It occurs most commonly as a complication of mitomycin C chemotherapy (see later). A few reports, however, have documented that HUS may occur as a direct complication of cancer (27, 28).

Hepatorenal syndrome may occur as a result of primary or secondary tumor in the liver if the liver is extensively replaced by tumor (29). As in other settings, it is usually fatal.

E. Drugs

Drugs are a frequent cause of renal failure in cancer patients (30,31). Table 2 lists the drugs responsible for most nephrotoxicity in cancer patients. Early in its development as an antineoplastic agent, platinum was noted to cause renal failure. Adequate hydration with or without mannitol diuresis was found largely to prevent this complication (32). Patients at greatest risk at present are those in whom hydration and diuresis are not maintained, those who receive several simultaneous nephrotoxins (e.g., aminoglycoside plus platinum), or those with prior renal disease. Various renal "protectors" have been studied (31,33), but none have a proven role. Circadian dosing appears to reduce nephrotoxicity, but it has not found widespread acceptance clinically (31).

Hydration and alkalinization usually prevent high-dose (i.e., g/m^2) methotrex-

Table 2 Drug-Related Causes of Renal Failure in Cancer Patients

I. Chemotherapy
   A. Platinum
   B. High-dose methotrexate
   C. Mitomycin C
   D. Nitrosoureas, including streptozocin
   E. Ifosfamide
   F. Gallium
II. Antibiotics
   A. Aminoglycosides
   B. Amphotericin B
   C. Acyclovir
   D. Foscarnet sodium
III. Biologic response modifiers
   A. Interferon
   B. Interleukin-2
IV. Immunosuppressives: cyclosporine
V. Analgesics: nonsteroidal antiinflammatory agents
VI. Contrast agents

ate from causing renal failure. Mitomycin C, and occasionally other drugs, may cause renal failure, with microangiopathic hemolytic anemia and thrombocytopenia (HUS), or it may cause a more complete TTP syndrome with neurological changes (34). Plasma perfusion over a protein A column may induce remissions (34). Durable remissions are most likely to occur if the patient is in complete remission at the time the syndrome develops. Streptozocin, a nonmyelosuppressive nitrosourea, is frequently nephrotoxic. Other nitrosoureas and ifosfamide are occasionally nephrotoxic. Gallium nitrate, a heavy metal, is a relatively new agent being used for cancer patients. Although it has clinical activity against lymphoma and bladder cancer, it has been approved in the United States for treatment of hypercalcemia. Its dose-limiting toxicity is proteinuria, but nephrotoxicity may occur at recommended doses. As with platinum, adequate hydration and avoidance of other nephrotoxins largely eliminate significant nephrotoxicity.

Aminoglycosides are frequently used in patients with malignancy during periods of neutropenic fever. Careful attention to drug levels reduces the incidence of renal toxicity. Avoiding aminoglycosides in patients receiving other renal toxins (such as amphotericin or platinum) is desirable if the clinical situation allows.

Biological agents may cause renal failure, most notably interferon (35) and interleukin-2 (36–38).

Other agents, as noted in Table 2, may also cause renal failure in cancer patients. The list is not exhaustive but includes the agents most commonly associated with renal toxicity. These include amphotericin, acyclovir, foscarnet, cyclosporine, nonsteroidal antiinflammatory agents, and radiographic contrast agents. In regard to the last, adequate hydration usually prevents renal problems.

In summary, acute renal failure may occur from a variety of cancers or cancer-related etiologies. An understanding of these entities and appropriate preventive or management strategies can minimize the renal problems experienced by cancer patients.

III. LUNG FAILURE

A. Cancer

Individuals who are known to have cancer and present with dyspnea are evaluated carefully for the possibility that metastatic disease is causing the symptoms. When cancer is present but undiagnosed, patients with dyspnea and non-diagnostic x-rays may experience a significant delay in diagnosis. Occasionally, diagnosis is not made until autopsy. Physicians should be aware of the less common pulmonary manifestations of cancer that may be presenting findings or develop during the course of illness in a patient with known cancer.

Several patients with prostate cancer (39) have been described who presented with progressive shortness of breath and bilateral reticular infiltrates on chest x-ray that proved to be lymphangitic metastases from prostate cancer. Although the presentation is unusual, patients may respond dramatically to hormonal therapy. Other cancers may occasionally present in a similar fashion, and some, such as breast cancer, may also be responsive to therapy. Although some form of lung involvement is present in 12% of Hodgkin's disease patients and 4% of non-Hodgkin's lymphoma patients at presentation (40), respiratory insufficiency is very uncommon. There is one report of a patient developing rapidly progressive respiratory failure caused by diffuse alveolar infiltrates, which were shown on open-lung biopsy to be a high-grade T cell lymphoma (41).

In patients with underlying chronic obstructive pulmonary disease (COPD), lymphangitic metastases (or other forms of pulmonary metastases) may be the cause of COPD exacerbation.

A less obvious cause of dyspnea (usually in patients with known cancer) is *tumor* emboli. These can be large and involve pulmonary arteries or large segmental branches (perhaps most often in renal carcinoma) but more commonly are microscopic, involving the small arteries or arterioles (42). Patients may complain of dyspnea in the face of a normal physical examination and chest x-ray. The primary site of cancer varies, and patients with solid tumors and lymphomas have been reported to experience this complication. Patients with tumor emboli are to be distinguished from patients with pulmonary *thromboemboli* secondary to venous thrombosis associated with malignancy.

One of the most dramatic examples of cancer presenting as respiratory failure is the "choriocarcinoma syndrome" in men with testis cancer (43,44). The patient with pure or predominant choriocarcinoma is uncommon. Fewer than 1% of men with testis cancer present with this syndrome. Patients present with shortness of breath and hemoptysis. The chest x-ray generally shows bilateral diffuse infiltrates and sometimes a near "whiteout" (Fig. 2). Choriocarcinoma in women can have a similar presentation (45). Chemotherapy should be instituted promptly at diagnosis in an effort to minimize the need for mechanical ventilation. Mechanical ventilation and its attendant complications (Fig. 3) may exacerbate

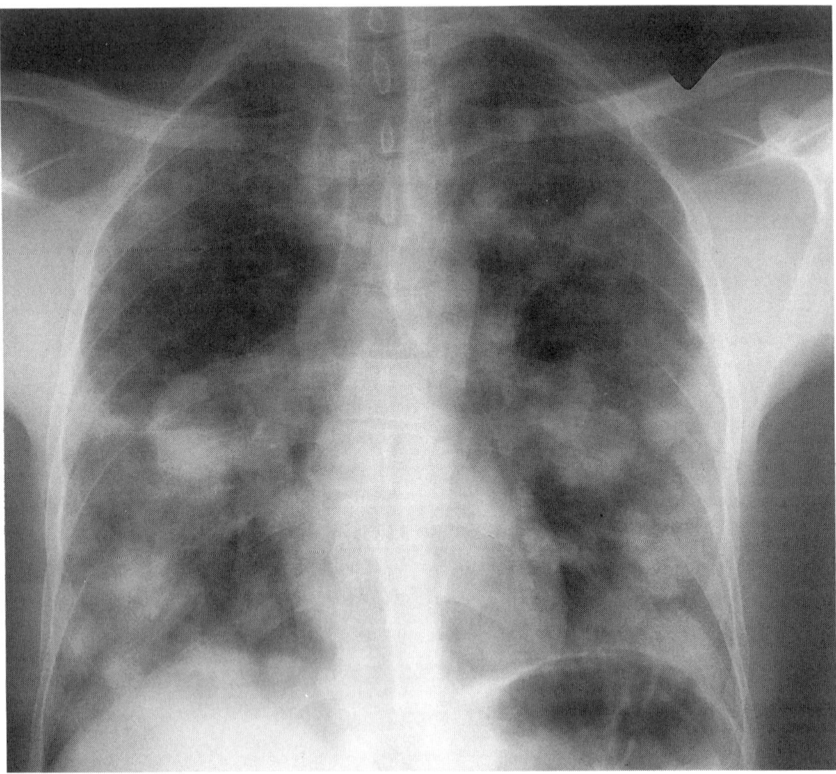

Figure 2 This 31-year-old man with mixed germ cell tumor presented with a "choriocarcinoma syndrome": dyspnea, hemoptysis, and β-hCG of 5660 milli International Units (MIU)/ml.

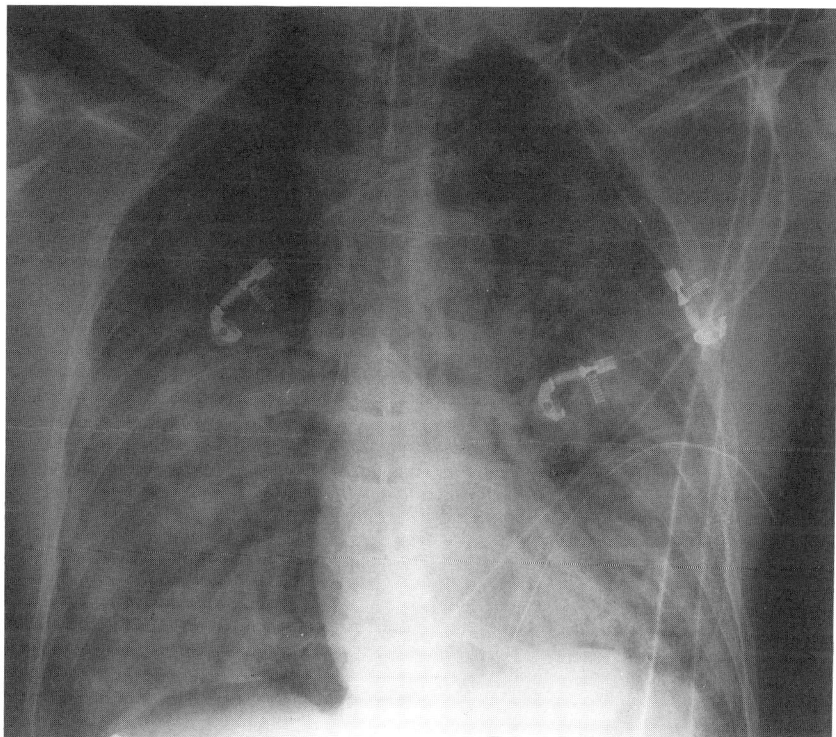

Figure 3 Same patient as Figure 2, 2 weeks later. He became increasing dyspneic after initiation of chemotherapy. Respiratory deterioration necessitated intubation and mechanical ventilation. This x-ray, taken 2 days before the patient's death, shows worsening infiltrate and a small right apical pneumothorax.

pulmonary dysfunction and lead to progressive respiratory failure and death (46). Despite the far advanced cancer in these patients, some are cured, as illustrated in Figures 4 and 5.

An unusual cause of cancer-related respiratory failure is bilateral vocal cord paralysis caused by bilateral involvement of the laryngeal nerves (47). Such patients present with upper airway obstruction, necessitating intubation and laryngeal surgical procedures. More obvious causes of respiratory failure include extensive parenchymal lung metastases or large pleural effusions. For extensive lung metastases, chemotherapy is generally the only treatment option. For effusions, thoracentesis, with or without pleurodesis, usually provides symptomatic relief. (See Chap. 13.)

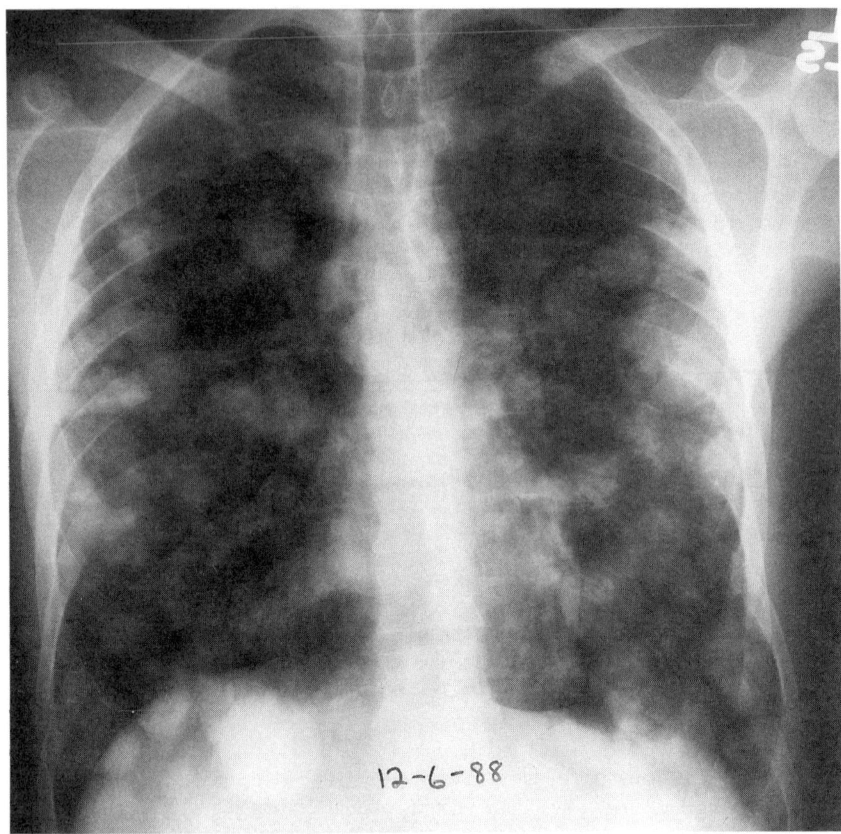

Figure 4 This 28-year-old man had a mixed germ cell tumor with a β-hCG of 660,000 MIU/ml, signifying a major choriocarcinoma component. He had dyspnea but no hemoptysis.

B. Drugs

Pulmonary toxicity secondary to drugs used in the cancer patient is predominantly pulmonary toxicity secondary to chemotherapy. Several recent reviews of this topic have been published (48–50). Table 3 lists the drugs most commonly implicated in pulmonary toxicity.

The chemotherapeutic agent most frequently causing pulmonary toxicity is bleomycin. This drug is believed, by some, to be an essential ingredient in curative chemotherapy regimens for men with testis cancer and is frequently used in combination regimens for lymphoma patients. Symptomatic pulmonary toxicity at doses < 400 units occurs in 3–5% of patients, and 1% of patients

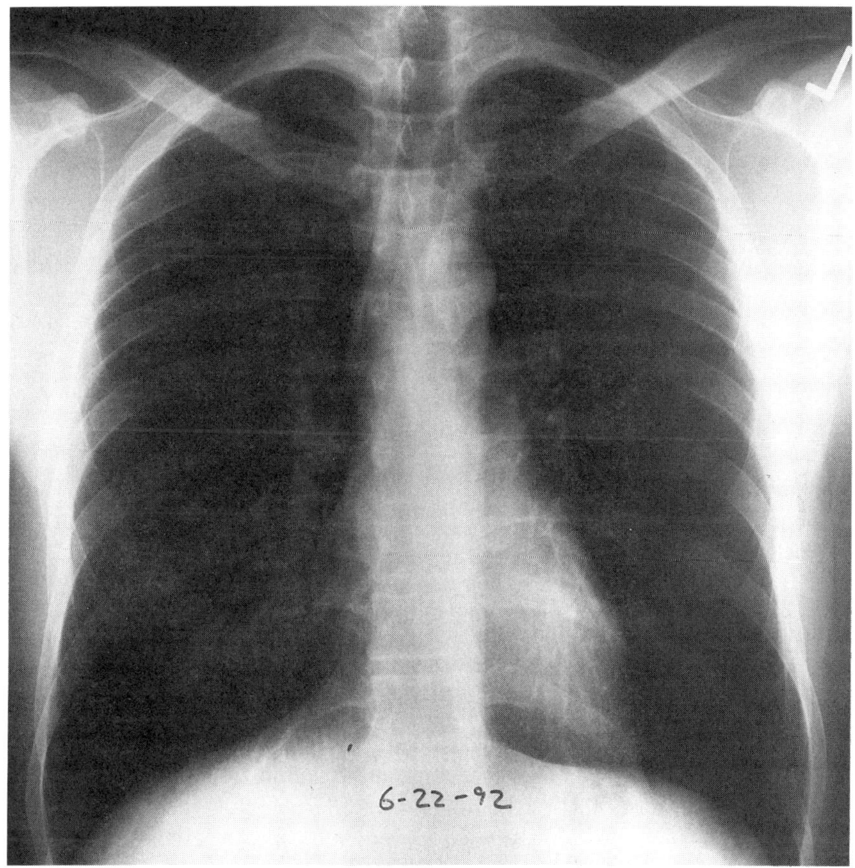

Figure 5 Follow-up chest x-ray on the same patient as in Figure 4. He remains in complete remission $3^1/2$ years later after four cycles of chemotherapy with platinum, VP-16-213 (etoposide), and bleomycin.

Table 3 Chemotherapy Agents Commonly Associated with Pulmonary Toxicity

Bleomycin
Nitrosourea (especially carmustine, BCNU)
Mitomycin C
Methotrexate
Busulfan
β-cytosine arabinoside (cytarabine)

receiving these doses may die from pulmonary toxicity. Patients who appear to be at high risk for pulmonary toxicity include those who have received a total dose > 400 units, concomitant chest irradiation, age great than 70, and renal dysfunction. There is no test that will always predict an impending pulmonary toxic event. Nonetheless, a carbon monoxide oxygen diffusing capacity (DLCO) fall to ≤0.4 of a baseline level signals a high-risk patient, and bleomycin should be stopped (51). The onset of toxicity often occurs 1–3 months after completion of therapy, but it may occur during treatment or shortly thereafter. Once pulmonary toxicity is manifest, it either responds to steroids and the patient improves or it does not respond and the patient dies of pulmonary failure.

Occasionally following bleomycin therapy, vague nodular densities may be apparent on chest x-ray (52). Although recurrent tumor must be considered in the differential diagnosis, these findings are frequently only a manifestation of the prior bleomycin exposure. The abnormalities may regress over time.

Patients with current or recent bleomycin therapy are considered in a high-risk category for a postoperative adult respiratory distress syndrome (ARDS). The 5 patients who developed ARDS in Goldiner et al.'s original report (53) had received a fraction of inspired oxygen (FI_{O2}) of 35–42%, whereas none of a prospective group of 12 patients who received FI_{O2} of 22–26% developed the syndrome. Fluid management also differed between the groups, and some have questioned whether FI_{O2} is a critical factor. Nevertheless, current practice is to use the lowest FI_{O2} (<30% if possible) that provides adequate O_2 saturation. Risks appear to be greatest during prolonged, complicated surgical procedures. A review of perioperative considerations for bleomycin-treated patients was recently published (54).

Details of toxicity from the other drugs are found in the referenced reviews, but it should be noted that of the drugs listed in Table 3 as relatively frequent causes of pulmonary toxicity, steroids are not uniformly beneficial in reversing toxic effects. The pulmonary toxicity from bleomycin, mitomycin C, methotrexate, and Ara-C (cytarabine) are frequently steroid responsive. Steroids are of less certain benefit for busulfan pulmonary toxicity, and they rarely seem to influence nitrosourea-induced pulmonary complications.

IV. HEART FAILURE

A. Cancer

Metastatic disease to the heart is the most common form of cardiac malignancy, and the pericardium is the most common site of cardiac involvement. The myocardium is less frequently involved and the endocardium least frequently involved. Except for pericardial malignancy manifesting as pain or effusion (with or without tamponade), cardiac metastases are frequently silent. Other signs of cardiac involvement include new heart murmurs, arrhythmias, heart failure, and embolization. Breast and lung carcinomas tend to spread to the pericardium

(55,56), whereas melanomas most often involve the myocardium (55,57). Overall, metastases to the heart occur in approximately 18% of patients who die of malignant tumors (58). This percentage is higher in specific subgroups, such as bronchogenic carcinoma patients, in whom a 31% incidence of cardiac involvement has been reported (59), and in melanoma patients, in whom over 50% of patients have myocardial involvement. In most autopsy series of soft tissue sarcoma patients, the incidence of cardiac metastases is approximately 25% (60). Lymphomas (61) and leukemias (62) frequently involve the heart (24 and 37%, respectively, in autopsy series).

Treatment depends on the type of malignancy and the nature of the cardiac problem. Management of pericardial effusion is discussed in Chapter 13. Radiation and chemotherapy may offer relief from symptoms secondary to myocardial involvement. Surgical removal of tumor may be helpful in relieving symptoms for patients with intracavitary obstructing tumors.

Primary tumors of the heart are far less common than metastatic tumors. Over 75% of primary tumors of the heart are benign. The malignant tumors are predominantly sarcomas and mesotheliomas. Treatment is problematical, but surgery appears to have a role in achieving local control of sarcomas. Surgical resection of mesothelioma is rarely possible.

B. Paraneoplastic Effects

Paraneoplastic cardiac problems include carcinoid heart disease, amyloid heart disease, and nonbacterial thrombotic endocarditis. Products of carcinoid tumors produce distinctive changes in the endocardium and (pulmonary and tricuspid) valves in some patients with the carcinoid syndrome. Carcinoid heart disease is not recognized clinically until cardiac murmurs or signs of right-sided heart failure develop, although echocardiographic findings may detect subclinical disease. Carcinoid heart failure may be a cause of disability or death in patients with carcinoid syndrome, and surgical relief of the cardiac problems may be indicated. Tricuspid valve replacement and pulmonary valvotomy (or valvectomy, or valve replacement) have been performed successfully in appropriate patients (63).

Amyloidosis occurs in approximately 10% of multiple myeloma patients. The median survival in the Kyle and Greipp series of 18 patients with amyloidosis and myeloma was 5 months (64). Cardiac involvement accounted for death in at least 40% of these cases. Cardiac involvement with amyloid is usually manifest as a restrictive cardiomyopathy with right-sided heart failure. The condition may simulate hypertrophic cardiomyopathy, constrictive pericardial disease, or even coronary artery disease (65). Patients are extremely sensitive to digitalis, and toxic deaths have occurred.

Nonbacterial thrombotic endocarditis (NBTE, marantic endocarditis) occurs in approximately 1.2% of autopsy patients and is most commonly found in patients with malignancy, especially adenocarcinomas (66). Cardiac failure is a possible complication of the coronary artery emboli and the myocardial infarction that may occur NBTE is most important as a cause of systemic emboli and distant organ toxicity. Cerebral, renal, and mesenteric circulations are frequently affected. Neurological events are the most common, ranging from focal deficits to general disorientation. (See Chap. 15.)

C. Drugs

Cardiac toxicity from drugs used in cancer patients is predominantly caused by chemotherapeutic agents. Allen recently reviewed this topic (67). Drug toxicity to the heart (outside the marrow transplant setting) is largely secondary to anthracyclines. Doxorubicin is the principal anthracycline used in oncology, and much of the literature deals specifically with this agent. Daunorubicin has similar toxicities, although at somewhat higher cumulative doses.

It is clear that when doxorubicin is given as intermittent bolus injections, the incidence of cardiotoxicity rises significantly at cumulative doses greater than 450 mg/m^2. Radiation therapy with cardiac exposure appears to enhance the risk of heart failure. Congestive heart failure may occur during therapy or after completing therapy, generally within 6–9 months. It has become apparent, with increasing clinical experience and increased numbers of patients who have lived many years following drug exposure, that cardiotoxicity may develop quite remote in time from initial drug exposure. Numerous patients have been reported who developed heart failure more than 5 years and as long as 14 years after completing chemotherapy (68–70).

An important point in clinical management is that many patients can be managed medically with excellent functional outcome despite very low cardiac ejection fractions. There are also data reporting recovery of cardiac function in some patients with severe heart failure (71). The prognosis for some of these patients may therefore be much better than once believed possible. If medical management fails to control the heart failure adequately and if the underlying cancer has been cured, cardiac transplantation is an option for some patients (72).

Various maneuvers have been used to try to minimize the risk of heart failure (73). These have included schedule modifications, such as continuous infusion of drug over 24–96 h, or the use of cardiac protectants. Use of a continuous infusion of drug allows greater total doses to be administered safely. The use of protective agents offers the possibility of reduced cardiac toxicity while maintaining antitumor efficacy.

Mitoxantrone (an anthraquinone and therefore structurally similar to the anthracyclines) appears to be less cardiotoxic than the anthracyclines (74). The risk of cardiotoxicity does not increase significantly until a cumulative dose of 160 mg/m^2 has been reached (equivalent to about 800 mg/m^2 of doxorubicin). Patients at the higher dose ranges should be monitored for left ventricular dysfunction, as are patients on doxorubicin.

Other drugs reported to have occasional cardiotoxicity (67) include bleomycin (pericarditis) and fluorouracil (5-FU) (angina and myocardial infarction). The cause of the 5-FU-induced cardiac symptoms and signs appears to be coronary spasm of the Prinzmetal type, and chest pain associated with 5-FU has responded to nitrates. The cardiotoxicity of cyclophosphamide generally occurs only at marrow transplant doses.

Interleukin-2 (IL-2) causes a broad range of cardiac toxicities that includes arrhythmias, ischemia, and hypocontractility (75). It has been postulated that cytokines, such as tumor necrosis factor, mediate the myocardiotoxic effects of IL-2. Interferon has been occasionally associated with cardiomyopathy (76).

V. LIVER FAILURE

A. Cancer

The liver has a large functional reserve capacity, and tumors involving the liver must replace approximately 65% of the liver before it begins to fail. Nonetheless, patients have presented with fulminant hepatic failure as the first manifestation of the cancer (77,78). These include cases of hemangioendothelioma, primary hepatocellular carcinoma, Hodgkin's disease, non-Hodgkin's lymphoma, acute leukemia, small cell lung carcinoma, breast carcinoma, bladder carcinoma, and pancreas as carcinoma. Other patients with a previous diagnosis of cancer developed fulminant hepatic failure later in the course of disease. Cases in the latter group include many of these diagnoses, but in addition may include melanoma, Merkel's cell tumor, and gastric carcinoma (77,79). In most of the patients with fulminant hepatic failure (regardless of the timing of presentation vis-à-vis the cancer diagnosis), imaging studies were not very helpful. In the Myszor and Record review (77), of 10 patients with ultrasound studies, 8 had a normal or large liver with homogeneous echo patterns and only 2 had studies suggesting metastatic disease. Liver scans in this review were equally disappointing. Although all 10 patients studied had abnormalities on liver scan indicating severe hepatocellular dysfunction, only 3 had filling defects. In 5 patients with computed tomographic scans of the liver, 3 were reported as normal. These data suggest that metastatic disease that involves the liver in such a way as to cause fulminant hepatic failure usually infiltrates diffusely and may therefore not be apparent on routine imaging studies. Because some of the neoplastic diseases noted earlier are responsive to therapy, the clinician must be alert to the possibility of cancer as a cause of fulminant hepatic failure. Recognition of a treatable cancer would at least allow the possibility of successful intervention.

B. Drugs

Chemotherapeutic drugs used for malignancy in the non–bone marrow transplant setting rarely cause severe hepatic complications. Perry has reviewed the topic

(80). One of the situations in which hepatic toxicity may occur and prove fatal is the use of floxuridine as an hepatic arterial infusion. Although floxuridine may be associated with a chemical hepatitis (in 50–100% of patients), with increases in transaminases, alkaline phosphatase, and bilirubin, this problem is almost invariably reversible. On the other hand, floxuridine may cause stricture of the intrahepatic and/or extrahepatic ducts (in 4–20% of patients), accompanied by an increase in alkaline phosphatase and bilirubin. This biliary sclerosis is irreversible. Attempts have been made to reduce the incidence of this problem by schedule alterations, such as limiting floxuridine infusion to the first week of a 5 week cycle followed by administration of bolus 5-FU via the implanted pump on days 15, 22, and 29 (81). Of 64 patients receiving this treatment approach, in none was treatment terminated because of toxicity, yet the response rate of 50% was in the range expected from studies using traditional 2 weeks on, 2 weeks off infusional schedules of floxuridine.

Hepatic venocclusive disease (VOD) has been reported for several chemotherapy drugs used at conventional doses. (See Chap. 21 for a discussion of VOD in the bone marrow transplant setting.) These include azathioprine, carboplatin, β-cytosine arabinoside (cytarabine), dacarbazine, dactinomycin, 6-mercaptopurine, and thioguanine (80). The clinical triad of jaundice, hepatomegaly, and ascites should lead one to suspect the diagnosis. Treatment is supportive after discontinuation of the offending drug.

Interferon-α frequently causes reversible increases in hepatic enzymes, but only one case of possible interferon-induced liver failure has been reported (82). IL-2 commonly causes reversible modest elevation of bilirubin and liver enzymes, but it has not been associated with severe hepatocellular damage (75).

There are two other drugs to be mentioned in regard to cancer patients and hepatic toxicity. The first is ketoconazole, which has been used in high doses as an antiandrogen for prostate cancer patients and in lower doses as an antifungal in cancer patients with mucosal candidiasis. This drug causes elevation of liver enzymes in some patients, and a few have died of hepatic toxicity. The other drug worthy of note is allopurinol, which is frequently used to reduce uric acid levels in patients treated for malignancy. Allopurinol has been linked to fulminant hepatic failure, presumably via a hypersensitivity reaction. There is also a report of tamoxifen exacerbating an allopurinol hepatotoxicity reaction (83).

VI. ADRENAL GLAND FAILURE

A. Cancer

The adrenal gland is a common site of metastatic disease, adrenal metastases occurring in 25% of autopsied cancer patients who had any evidence of metastatic disease (84). Lung, breast, kidney, and melanoma cancer patients with any evidence of metastatic disease have adrenal metastases approximately 50% of the time (84). Despite this high frequency of metastases to the adrenal gland, clinical adrenal insufficiency is quite uncommon. Nonetheless, Addison, in his original report of the syndrome bearing his name, included a patient with breast cancer who had bilateral adrenal metastases (85). Numerous patients in the literature have been reported to have adrenal insufficiency as a result of metastatic disease, but cases confirmed by appropriate hormonal evaluation are fewer in number (86,87). A patient reported in 1989 had adrenal failure caused by bilateral adrenal metastases as the sole manifestation of relapsing small cell lung cancer (88). One prospective evaluation of cancer patients with bilateral adrenal metastases revealed that 5 of 15 patients had adrenal insufficiency based on an abnormal cosyntropin stimulation test (87). The 5 patients had normal baseline cortisols but failed to exhibit a normal rise after stimulation. All these patients had resolution of nausea and anorexia after corticosteroid replacement, raising the possibility that their symptoms had been caused by compromised adrenal function.

B. Drugs

Adrenal insufficiency caused by drugs is an uncommon problem. The most frequent example in clinical oncology may be the patient on prolonged (>30 days) corticosteroid ("steroid") therapy, perhaps for brain metastases, who inadvertently has the steroids abruptly stopped. Several drugs in oncology are used specifically because they inhibit adrenal steroidogenesis. These include aminoglutethimide, mitotane (*o,p*′-DDD), and high-dose (400 mg every 8 h) ketoconazole. These agents all cause adrenal insufficiency and are routinely administered with replacement steroids. Patients frequently do not understand the rationale for use of certain drugs, however, and sometimes unilaterally discontinue medications. For this reason, physicians must carefully instruct patients in the importance of taking their steroids.

There is a report from the M. D. Anderson Cancer Center (89) of adrenal failure in several patients taking cyclic long-term alternating estrogen-progesterone for breast cancer. A total of 30 estrogen receptor-positive patients were treated with a physiological dose of estradiol (50 μg) by mouth for 7 days, followed by a pharmacological dose of medroxyprogesterone acetate (400 mg) by mouth daily for 21 days. Cycles were repeated after a 1 week rest period. Among the 17 responding patients, 3 developed clinical signs and symptoms of acute adrenal insufficiency toward the end of treatment or upon its withdrawal.

VII. SUMMARY

Organ failure, as discussed in this chapter, complicates the course of the disease of many patients with cancer. Organ failure as a result of cancer infiltration or paraneoplastic effects may be the presenting problem, or it may develop during the course of the disease when the patient is otherwise relatively asymptomatic. In these situations, the clinician must be alert to make the proper diagnosis. Early institution of therapy provides a chance to preserve organ function, improve or maintain performance status, and possibly improve survival. Drugs used in treating cancer patients frequently have major organ toxicities. Prevention or early detection of drug-induced toxicity optimizes organ function.

VIII. FUTURE RESEARCH AND PERSPECTIVES

Many lives are saved by the use of adjuvant chemotherapy. Patients with certain types of metastatic tumors can be cured with chemotherapy or multimodality treatment. Cure of cancer in a patient who develops fatal drug toxicity is a Pyrrhic victory. Sublethal toxicity that results in chronic organ dysfunction and reduces quality of life is less than a complete success. As more cancer patients are cured, reduction of drug toxicity will become an ever greater focus of clinical research.

SELECTED READING

Buxbaum JN, Chuba JV, Hellman JC, Solomon A, Gallo G. Monoclonal immunoglobulin deposition disease: light chain and light and heavy chain deposition diseases and their relation to light chain amyloidosis; clinical features, immunopathology, and molecular analysis. Ann Intern Med 1990; 112:455–464. The authors review the fibrillar (amyloidotic) and nonfibrillar forms of monoclonal immunoglobulin deposition that occur in overt myeloma or in the course of less aggressive plasmacytic dyscrasias.

Lopez JA, Ross RS, Fishbein MC, Siegel RJ. Nonbacterial thrombotic endocarditis: a review. Am Heart J 1987; 113(3):773–784. The entity of nonbacterial thrombotic endocarditis (NBTE) is reviewed. Although NBTE is most commonly found in patients with malignancy, the non-malignant etiologies are also discussed. Pathogenesis and clinicopathological findings are covered. Emphasis is placed on attempts at antemortem diagnosis because heparin treatment may be beneficial for patients with evidence of embolization.

Smolens P. The kidney in dysproteinemic states. AKF Nephrol Lett 1987; 4(4):27–42. Dr. Smolens presents an excellent, in-depth discussion of the renal syndromes caused by multiple myeloma, light-chain deposition disease, amyloidosis, and Waldenström's macroglobulinemia. He considers diagnosis, pathology, treatment, and prognosis for the various entities.

Weinman EJ, Patak RV. Acute renal failure is cancer patients. Oncology (Williston Park) 1992; 6(9):47–54. This is a concise overview of the topic of acute renal failure in cancer patients. Comments on the article by Dr. Thompson and further comments by Dr. Robeson provide additional perspectives on this complex problem.

REFERENCES

1. Garnick MB, Mayer RJ. Acute renal failure associated with neoplastic disease and its treatment. Semin Oncol 1978; 5(2):155–165.

42. Kane RD, Hawkins HK, Miller JA, Noce PS. Microscopic pulmonary tumor emboli associated with dyspnea. Cancer 1975; 36:1473–1482.
43. Logothetis CJ. Choriocarcinoma syndrome. Cancer Bull 1984; 36(2):118–120.
44. Benditt JO, Farber HW, Wright J, Karnad A. Pulmonary hemorrhage with diffuse alveolar infiltrates in men with high volume choriocarcinoma. Ann Intern Med 1988; 109:674–675.
45. Bagshawe KD, Noble MIM. Cardio-respiratory aspects of trophoblastic tumors. Q J Med 1966; 35(137):39–54.
46. Kelly MP, Rustin GJS, Ivory C, Phillips P, Bagshawe KD. Respiratory failure due to choriocarcinoma: a study of 103 dyspneic patients. Gynecol Oncol 1990; 38:149–154.
47. Baumann MH, Heffner JE. Bilateral vocal cord paralysis with respiratory failure; a presenting manifestation of bronchogenic carcinoma. Arch Intern Med 1989; 149:1453–1454.
48. Kreisman H, Wolkove N. Pulmonary toxicity of antineoplastic therapy. Semin Oncol 1992; 19(5):508–520.
49. Jules-Elysee K, White DA. Bleomycin-induced pulmonary toxicity. Clin Chest Med 1990; 11(1):1–20.
50. Twohig KJ, Matthay RA. Pulmonary effects of cytotoxic agents other than bleomycin. Clin Chest Med 1990; 11(1):31–54.
51. Comis RL. Detecting bleomycin pulmonary toxicity: a continued conundrum (editorial). J Clin Oncol 1990; 8(5):765–767.
52. Trump DL, Bartel E, Pozniak M. Nodular pneumonitis after chemotherapy for germ cell tumors. Ann Intern Med 1988; 109:431–432.
53. Goldiner PL, Carlon GC, Cvitkovic E, Schweizer O, Howland WS. Factors influencing postoperative morbidity and mortality in patients treated with bleomycin. BMJ 1978; 1:1664–1667.
54. Waid-Jones MI, Coursin DB. Perioperative considerations for patients treated with bleomycin. Chest 1991; 99:993–999.
55. MacGee W. Metastatic and invasive tumors involving the heart in a geriatric population: a necropsy study. Virchows Arch [A] 1991; 419:183–189.
56. Young JM, Goldman IR. Tumor metastasis to the heart. Circulation 1954; 9:220–229.
57. McAllister HA. Tumors of the cardiovascular system; atlas of tumor pathology (AFIP). Second series, fascicle 15, 1978.
58. Hanfling SM. Metastatic cancer to the heart; review of the literature and report of 127 cases. Circulation 1960; 22:474–483.
59. Goudie RB. Secondary tumours of the heart and pericardium. Br Heart J 1955; 17:183–188.
60. Hallahan DE, Vogelzang NJ, Borow KM, Bostwick DG, Simon MA. Cardiac metastases from soft-tissue sarcomas. J Clin Oncol 1986; 4:1662–1669.
61. Roberts WC, Glancy DL, DeVita VT. Heart in malignant lymphoma (Hodgkin's disease, lymphosarcoma, reticulum cell sarcoma and mycosis fungoides); a study of 196 autopsy cases. Am J Cardiol 1968; 22:85–107.
62. Roberts WC, Bodey GP, Wertlake PT. The heart in acute leukemia; a study of 420 autopsy cases. Am J Cardiol 1968; 21:388–412.

63. Lundin L, Hansson HE, Landelius J, Oberg K. Surgical treatment of carcinoid heart disease. J Thorac Cardiovasc Surg 1990; 100:552–561.
64. Kyle RA, Greipp PR. Amyloidosis (AL); clinical and laboratory features in 229 cases. Mayo Clin Proc 1983; 58:665–683.
65. Roberts WC, Waller BF. Cardiac amyloidosis causing cardiac dysfunction: analysis of 54 necropsy patients. Am J Cardiol 1983; 52:137–146.
66. Lopez JA, Ross RS, Fishbein MC, Siegel RJ. Nonbacterial thrombotic endocarditis: a review. Am Heart J 1987; 113(3):773–784.
67. Allen A. The cardiotoxicity of chemotherapeutic drugs. Semin Oncol 1992; 19(5):529–542.
68. Steinherz L, Steinherz P. Delayed cardiac toxicity from anthracycline therapy. Pediatrician 1991; 18:49–52.
69. Goorin AM, Chauvenet AR, Perez-Atayde AR, Cruz J, McKone R, Lipshultz SE. Initial congestive heart failure, six to ten years after doxorubicin chemotherapy for childhood cancer. J Pediatr 1990; 116(1):144–147.
70. Freter CF, Lee TC, Billingham ME, Chak L, Bristow MR. Doxorubicin cardiac toxicity manifesting seven years after treatment; case report and review. Am J Med 1986; 80:483–485.
71. Saini J, Rich MW, Lyss AP. Reversibility of severe left ventricular dysfunction due to doxorubicin cardiotoxicity; report of three cases. Ann Intern Med 1987; 106:814–816.
72. Hinkamp T, Sullivan H, Bakhos M, Grieco J, Pifarre R. Orthotopic cardiac transplantation in two patients with previous malignancy. Ann Thorac Surg 1991; 51:1004–1006.
73. Carlson RW. Reducing the cardiotoxicity of anthracyclines. Oncology (Williston Park) 1992; 6(6):95–108.
74. Weiss RB. Mitoxantrone: its development and role in clinical practice. Oncology (Williston Park) 1989; 3(6):135–147.
75. Siegel JP, Puri RK. Interleukin-2 toxicity. J Clin Oncol 1991; 9(4):694–704.
76. Sonnenblink M, Rosenmann D, Rosin A. Reversible cardiomyopathy induced by interferon. BMJ 1990; 300:1174–1175.
77. Myszor MF, Record CO. Primary and secondary malignant disease of the liver and fulminant hepatic failure. J Clin Gastroenterol 1990; 12(4):441–446.
78. Zafrani ES, Leclercq B, Vernant JP, Pinaudeau Y, Chomette G, Dhumeaux D. Massive blastic infiltration of the liver: a cause of fulminant hepatic failure. Hepatology 1983; 3(3):428–432.
79. Sawabe M, Kato Y, Ohashi I, Kitigawa T. Diffuse intrasinusoidal metastasis of gastric carcinoma to the liver leading to fulminant hepatic failure; a case report. Cancer 1990; 65:169–173.
80. Perry ML. Chemotherapeutic agents and hepatotoxicity. Semin Oncol 1992; 19(5):551–565.
81. Stagg RJ, Venook AP, Chase JL, et al. Alternating hepatic intra-arterial floxuridine and fluorouracil: a less toxic regimen for treatment of liver metastases from colorectal cancer. J Natl Cancer Inst 1991; 83:423–428.
82. Durand JM, Kaplanski G, Portal I, Scheiner L, Berland Y, Soubeyrand J. Liver failure due to recombinant alpha interferon (letter). Lancet 1991; 338:1268–1269.

83. Shah KA, Levin J, Rosen N, Greenwald H, Zumoff B. Allopurinol hepatotoxicity potentiated by tamoxifen. NY State J Med 1982; 82:1745–1746.
84. Glomset DA. The incidence of metastasis of malignant tumors to the adrenals. Am J Cancer 1938; 32:57–61.
85. Addison T. On the constitutional and local effects of disease of the suprarenal capsules, S. Highley, London, 1855; reprinted in Med Classics 1937; 2:244–280.
86. Sheeler LR, Myers JH, Eversman JJ, Taylor HC. Adrenal insufficiency secondary to carcinoma metastatic to the adrenal gland. Cancer 1983; 52:1312–1316.
87. Redman BG, Pazdur R, Zingas AP, Loredo R. Prospective evaluation of adrenal insufficiency in patients with adrenal metastasis. Cancer 1987; 60:103–107.
88. Guzzini F, Cozzi C, Cortese F, Gasparini P, Neri V, Pace L. Adrenal failure due to bilateral metastases as the sole manifestation of relapsing lung carcinoma; report of two cases. Tumori 1989; 75:634–636.
89. Hug V, Hortobagyi GN, Jones L. Adrenal failure in patients with breast carcinoma after long-term treatment of cyclic alternating oestrogen progesterone. Br J Cancer 1991; 63(3):454–456.

15

Neurological Complications

Jerzy G. Hildebrand
Hôpital Erasme, Université Libre de Bruxelles, Brussels, Belgium

I. INTRODUCTION

Neurological complications are common in cancer: approximately one of five patients, especially with generalized neoplasia, develop a major neurological insult most commonly caused by local extension or metastases of systemic cancer. A second group of neoplastic neurological lesions is caused by primary tumors of the nervous system.

The management of these complications includes in the first place specific antineoplastic therapies, for which the reader is refered to a recent monography (1). Quality of life however, especially in patients with neurological disorders, is also related to supportive care. The aim of this chapter is to consider the clinical presentation of the neurological complications of systemic cancer and the benefits and unwanted effects of the treatment of brain edema, metabolic encephalopathies, seizures, cerebrovascular diseases, peripheral pain, and weakness syndromes occurring in cancer patients.

II. BRAIN EDEMA

A. Physiopathogenesis and Clinical Presentation

Brain edema corresponds to an increase of brain volume as a result of an augmented water content. There are essentially three types of brain edema (2):

1. Vasogenic edema is caused by an increased permeability of brain capillaries and thus a disturbance of the blood-brain barrier. This edema involves primarily the white matter.

2. Cytotoxic edema is characterized by swelling of the cellular component and reduction in the brain's extracellular space.
3. The last variety, called interstitial edema, is seen in hydrocephalus, and the increase in water content predominates in the periventricular white matter.

Vasogenic edema is by far the most common type, especially in neurooncological pathologies. In tumor-related obstructive hydrocephalus, interstitial edema may also be present.

A variable degree of vasogenic edema surrounds almost every malignant primary or metastatic brain tumor. In many cases the symptoms and signs of the neoplasia may be hidden by the surrounding edema. As does brain tumor, brain edema may produce the following:

1. Generalized manifestations of increased intracranial pressure, such as headaches, somnolence, ataxic gait, and papilledema
2. Direct focal deficits
3. Remote focal signs resulting from displacement of intracranial structures, causing cingulate, uncal, or tonsillar herniations

In malignant tumors, the distinction between brain edema and neoplastic tissue may be extremely difficult. On computed tomographic (CT) scan, brain edema appears as an hypodense area surrounding the contrast-enchanced tumor tissue. However, in malignant tumor this area almost invariably contains neoplastic cells. Also, magnetic resonance imaging (MRI) does not permit an unequivocal distinction between tumor and peritumoral edema.

B. Treatment

Symptoms and signs of vasogenic brain edema are most effectively and most durably alleviated by glucocorticosteroids. The mode of action of corticosteroids on vasogenic brain edema is not fully elucidated, but they act, at least partially, by reducing capillary permeability and thus restoring the blood-brain barrier.

Corticosteroids also reduce the water content of the compressed spinal cord. However, the mechanism of the prompt pain relief observed in patients with epidural metastases remains unclear and is apparently independent of the effect on the edema. Dexamethasone and methylprednisolone are most commonly used to treat vasogenic edema. They differ mainly in their side effects. Their symptomatic effect is often dramatic and occurs within hours or few days. However, intermittent administration of even a very high dose of methylprednisolone does not prolong the survival of patients with malignant gliomas (3).

The cytolytic effect of glucocorticosteroids on brain tumor cells has not been unequivocally shown in clinical practice, except for non-Hodgkin's primary lymphomas of the brain (NHPL). NHPL may indeed disappear completely on CT scan within 24 h of glucocorticoid administration, and the remission, although usually short, occasionally lasts for years (4).

The usual daily dosage is 16 mg dexamethasone in four fractions or 80 mg methylprednisolone. Higher doses are occasionally necessary (5), but in our experiencc their benefit is often bland or transient. On the other hand, by not decreasing or discontinuing soon enough the administration of corticosteroids, one may be using unnecessarily high doses. In fact, Weissman et al. (6) showed in 20 patients with brain metastases that cerebral edema was efficiently controlled, even during radiation therapy, by decreasing the daily dose of dexamethasone from 8 to 2 mg and that corticosteroids could be discontinued at completion of the irradiation. From 14 of their patients who completed radiation therapy, only 1 needed to restart dexamethasone within 30 days.

Glucocorticosteroids also have salutary effects on nausea, vomiting, anorexia, and asthenia. However, the high frequency and severity of undesirable effects strongly limits their use in these circumstances.

In emergency cases, perfusions of 20% manitol are temporarily effective in reducing brain edema. In patients who do not tolerate glucocorticosteroids, glycerol given orally at an average daily dose of 1.5 g/kg body weight in four fractions is a safe alternative to corticosteroids.

C. Undesirable Effects of Glucocorticosteroids

Long-term administration of glucocorticosteroids is accompanied by a cohort of unwanted effects. The most important and the most common neurological manifestations are considered in this section. In one series these side effects were found in one of two patients (7). Their occurrence is largely unpredictable, because with the possible exception of hypoproteinemia, the risk factors for corticosteroid toxicity are unknown.

D. Psychiatric and Cognitive Disorders

Mental disturbances are less frequent with methylprednisolone or dexamethasone, the most communly used corticosteroids in neurooncology, than with natural corticosteroids or adrenocorticotropic hormone (ACTH).

Behavioral and personality changes, such as anxiety, nervousness, insomnia, and euphoria, are fairly common, but serious psychiatric manifestations, such as depression and acute psychotic and delirious reactions, occur in no more than 3% of cases. Depression may be seen in the early stages of corticosteroid therapy or during drug tapering. It usually vanishes after drug discontinuation. Acute psychotic and delirious reactions are characterized by paranoid behavior, often associated with visual or auditory hallucinations. In some patients these disorders rapidly respond to drug discontinuation; in others administration of major tranquilizers is necessary.

A decline in cognitive functions, possibly associated with cerebral atrophy, has been reported but is exceptional even in chronically treated patients.

E. Myopathy

So-called steroid myopathy corresponds to atrophy of type 2 muscle fibers. Clinically the syndrome is characterized by proximal weakness of the lower limbs and a variable degree of wasting of thigh muscles, producing difficulties in standing up or climbing steps. In very severe cases the neck and shoulder muscles are also involved. The most difficult differential diagnosis of steroid myopathy includes nutritional myopathies, in which, as in steroid myopathy, electromyography remains normal. Polymyositis and the Lambert-Eaton syndrome (LES) may also be clinically confused with steroid myopathy. However, the enzymatic and electromyographic changes found in polymyositis and the abnormalities on high-frequency stimulation test that characterize LES make the differential diagnosis much easier. Recently, Dropcho and Soong (8) reviewed 216 patients with primary brain tumors who received 2 weeks or more of continuous daily dexamethasone and found steroid-induced weakness in 23 (10.6%). In 15 (65%) the weakness developed between weeks 9 and 12 of treatment with a cumulative dose ranging from 580 to 1780 mg. These data suggest that treatment duration has a greater impact than the total dose of glucocorticosteroids. Another interesting finding of the study was the protective effect of antiepileptics, especially phenytoin.

F. Lipomatosis

Long-term steroid therapy leads to the redistribution of fat tissue, including its deposition in the epidural space. Often asymptomatic, epidural lipomatosis occasionally produces spinal cord compression and paraplegia. Epidural lipomatosis also favors paraplegia in patients with vertebral collapse, which is another complication of glucocorticoid therapy. Severe cases of spinal cord compression may require surgical decompression, but in milder cases discontinuation of steroids may restore the nerve function. Differential diagnosis from vertebral metastases may be difficult when vertebral fracture is present, whereas pure lipomatosis is easily differentiated from neoplastic tissue by MRI scan because of the typical density of the fat tissue.

G. Steroid Withdrawal Syndrome

Withdrawal of steroids mainly causes two neurological syndromes: steroid pseudorheumatism, characterized by acute, sometimes severe, myalgias and/or arthralgias, and pseudotumor cerebri syndrome, which manifest itself by headaches, papilledema, and sometimes impaired consciousness.

H. Nonneurological Complications

These side effects are not detailed here. They consist primarily of osteoporosis, avascular necrosis, mainly of the hip, hyperglycemia, gastrointestinal bleeding, and/or perforation and opportunistic infections.

III. METABOLIC AND TOXIC ENCEPHALOPATHIES

A. Physiopathogenesis and Clinical Presentation

An alteration in mental status, defined as a change in consciousness from mild confusion to coma, was, next to pain, the second most common symptom found by Clouston et al. (9) in patients referred to the Neurology Service of the Memorial Sloan-Kettering Cancer Center. Of 132 such patients, metabolic or drug-related encephalopathy was present in 80 (61%) and was the most common nonmetastatic neurological manifestation of symptomatic cancer. Focal neurological deficits, such as hemiparasis, aphasia, or focal seizures, may accompany diffuse encephalopathy but are not considered here if they occur in isolation.

Metabolic encephalopathies encountered in cancer patients are essentially of two kinds (Table 1). The largest group comprises metabolic encephalopathies mainly caused by dysfunction of vital organs, such as liver, lung, kidney and urinary tract, or mesenteric lymphatics, caused by metastatic spread or treatment toxicity. The second group represents truly paraneoplastic syndromes resulting from the production by the tumor cells, mainly small cell lung carcinoma (SCLC), of hormone or hormonelike substances.

The main cause of *toxic encephalopathies* in cancer patients is the administration of antineoplastic drugs (10,11), despite that most of them do not readily cross the blood-brain barrier.

1. Methotrexate (MTX) produces encephalopathy after either intrathecal or high-dose systemic administration. Signs of acute encephalopathy develop within hours of intrathecal administration, are often associated with a meningitic reaction, and resolve within 72 h. Acute encephalopathy also occurs in 1–2% of patients treated intravenously with high-dose MTX. Most patients recover spontaneously within 48 h. Concomitant radiation therapy increases the risk of MTX encephalopathy either by additive toxicity or by increasing the permeability of the blood-brain barrier to systemically administered drugs.
2. Encephalopathy is rare after methodichlorophen (DDMP) administration. It was observed only for doses of 3 mg/kg body weight or more.

Table 1 Acute Metabolic Encephalopathies in Cancer Patients

Metabolic disorder	Paraneoplastic production	Other causes related to cancer	Treatment
Hypercalcemia	Parathyroid hormone-related peptide, 1,25-hydroxy vitamin D	Bone metastases, multiple myeloma	Bisphosphonates, saline infusion, corticosteroids
Hypocalcemia		Malabsorption: postradiation lesions, mesenteric metastases, renal wasting of Mg and Ca caused by cisplatin	Intravenous or oral calcium
Hypophosphatemia	Deficit in 1,25-hydroxyvitamin D (?); other unknown factors	Cachexia, excessive glucose perfusion Respiratory alkalosis	K phosphate <60 mEq/24 h
Hypernatremia	ACTH (moderate)	Hemoconcentration, posterior pituitary metastases, cisplatin nephrotoxicity	Hydration, antidurietic hormone
Hyponatremia	Inappropriate secretion of antidiuretic hormone	Vincristine, cyclophosphamide Excessive hydration + chemotherapy	NaCl
Hypomagnesemia	—	Nephrotoxic chemotherapy (cisplatin)	
Hypoglycemia	Insulin, insulinelike products	Excessive consumption by tumor cells (?)	
Hyperglycemia	ACTH	Glucocorticosteroid therapy	
Uremia	—	Urinary tract obstruction Nephrotoxic chemotherapy	
Anoxia, anoxemia	—	Severe anemia, heart failure (doxorubicin) Primary or metastatic lung tumors, lung infections	
Hepatic failure	—	Liver primary or metastatic tumors *l*-Asparaginase	
Carcinoid syndrome	Serotonine ↑ in serum, ↓ in brain (?)	—	

3. Cortical disorders are also rare after systemic therapy using cisplatin. In addition, the possible neurotoxic effect of the drug must be differentiated from the ionic disturbances induced through renal toxicity or excessive hydration combined with chemotherapy.
4. Equally rare are cases of encephalopathy described in patients treated with vincristine (VCR). The physiopathogenesis of vincristine central nervous system (CNS) toxicity remains unclear. One mechanism is abnormal secretion of antidiuretic hormone as a result of the direct action of VCR on the hypothalamus or the peripheral volume receptors.
5. Two antipyrimidines, cytarabine and 5-fluorouracil, are primarily known to produce cerebellopathies. Occasionally, however, encephalopathy may develop.
6. Syndromes of usually mild encephalopathy, such as lassitude, sedation, or drowsiness, may be seen even when procarbazine, a monoamine oxidase inhibitor derivative, is given orally at daily doses of 150 mg or more. The drug also has a synergistic sedation effect when combined with barbiturates or phenothiazines. Severe encephalopathy is the main limiting factor to using procarbazine intravenously.
7. The administration of *l*-asparaginase may produce consciousness alteration ranging from confusion to coma, caused primarily by hepatic failure or, rarely, by thrombosis of an intracranial venous sinus. The latter complication is characterized by a clinical picture consisting of headaches, papilledema, seizures, and/or focal signs.
8. Very rare cases of encephalopathy have been reported with several alkylating agents, including nitrogen mustard, chlorambucil, cyclophosphamide, and, more recently, high-dose nitrosoureas and ifosfamide.
9. Interferons, whether administered intrathecally or systemically, commonly produce signs of acute encephalopathy. However, patients with nonneoplastic neurological diseases are not hindered by major CNS toxicity. Also, the administration of interleukin-2 with or without lyphokine activated killer (LAK) cells demands close surveillance for CNS toxicity, dose-related signs of encephalopathy being common.

In cancer patients, the differential diagnosis of metabolic or toxic encephalopathies includes the following:

First, multiple brain metastases, the most common CNS pathology in patients with systemic cancer. Mental changes are indeed seen in about 30% of patients, as the earliest clinical manifestation of cerebral or meningeal metastases.

Opportunistic CNS infections, among which *Listeria monocytogenes* and *Cryptococcus neoformans* figure prominently as causative agents, and progressive multifocal leukoencephalopathy caused by a papovavirus, should be ruled out next.

Finally, limbic encephalitis, a paraneoplastic disease usually associated with high titers of Hu antibody in the serum and cerebiospinal fluid (CSF) is a rare disease but should be taken into consideration especially in patients with SCLC.

B. Treatment

When facing recent mental disorders in a patient with generalized neoplasia, one must first rule out the possibility of multiple metastases (the most common etiology), then meningeal seedings, CNS infections, and finally paraneoplastic disorders. This may be achieved by performing brain CT scan with contrast enhancement, MRI scan with gadolinium of the brain and/or the spinal cord (very helpful to demonstrate meningeal metastases), and a lumbar puncture looking for evidence of leptomeningeal metastases or CNS infections. If these examinations are negative, metabolic or toxic encephalopathy becomes the most likely diagnosis. In making the diagnosis of metabolic encephalopathy, one must determine both the nature of the metabolic disorder and its physiopathogenesis (Table 1). Indeed, the management of these encephalopathies combines treatment of the underlying neoplasia and a rapid symptomatic correction of the metabolic abnormality. Both the dysfunction of vital organs as a result of metastases and the paraneoplastic endocrinopathies (production of hormones or hormonelike substances by the tumor cells) may respond to an appropriate antineoplastic therapy, whether surgery, radiation therapy, or chemotherapy. When the metabolic abnormality is attributed to chemotherapy, its administration must be discontinued. Sometimes, as in *l*-asparaginase-induced encephalopathy, dose reduction may suffice. Even if successful, however, these therapies do not usually produce immediate effects. Rapid symptomatic treatment is often necessary to correct the metabolic disorder.

The main treatments of metabolic encephalopathies are summarized in Table 1. Diphosphonates are the first-line therapy for hypercalcemia. In addition, hypercalcemia in myeloma or lymphoma patients responds, usually after a delay of 2–3 days, to corticosteroids. The reduction in hypernatremia must be progressive to avoid brain edema. It is recommended that the decrease in serum sodium should not exceed 15 mEq per 24 h and that of the osmotic pressure 20–30 mEq per 24 h. Hyponatremia lasting for less than 48 h may and should be corrected rapidly, but in chronic forms the increase in serum sodium should not exceed 15 mEq/liter per 24 h to avoid osmotic demyelinating syndrome.

The majority of drugs used in cancer chemotherapy do not cross the blood-brain barrier. Therefore, encephalopathies because of CNS toxicity are rate and are mainly seen after intrathecal and high-dose treatment. Their occurrence requires immediate discontinuation of drug administration; most drug-induced acute encephalopathies are reversible. In this chapter the CNS toxicity of intracarotid chemotherapy is not considered because the symptoms and signs are predominantly focal and the etiology is obvious.

IV. SEIZURES

A. Physiopathogenesis and Clinical Presentation

The main causes of acquired seizures in cancer patients are primary or metastatic supratentorial tumors, metabolic encephalopathies, toxicity of chemotherapeutic agents, and CNS infections. At least one-third of patients with supratentorial *primary tumors* suffer epileptic seizures. For similar pathologies seizure incidence tends to be higher in children than in adults. In some series the figures also tend to be higher in the more benign forms, such as low-grade astrocytomas or oligodendrogliomas. Patients bearing these tumors survive longer, however, and this factor by itself increases the risk of seizure. Seizures are often the presenting sign leading to earlier diagnosis of brain tumor, and this probably explains why in many studies the presence of seizures is a favorable prognostic factor for survival. Seizures caused by brain tumors are essentially focal, and a careful history may help to localize both the neoplastic and the epileptogenic focus. In some cases, however, seizures generalize so quickly that their focal nature may be overlooked. The incidence of seizures in brain *metastases* is about 20%. Although the figures vary greatly from one study to another, certain primaries—melanomas—and germ cell tumors appear more epileptogenic than other neoplasia.

The metabolic disorders most likely to cause epilepsy are hypoglycemia, hyponatremia, hypocalcemia, hypokalemia, uremia, and hepatic failure. Their physiopathogenic mechanisms are similar to those of the metabolic encephalopathies summarized in Table 1. Seizures are a frequent complication of intracarotid chemotherapy using nitrogen mustard and, more recently, nitrosourea derivatives (carmustine, BCNU, and HeCNU), cisplatin, or etoposide (VP-16-213), and in high-dose chemotherapy with methotrexate or carmustine. Beside these conditions, one must be very careful in attributing seizures to systemic chemotherapy despite that epileptic fits have been atttibuted to various agents, including VCR, decarbazine (DTIC), PALA, and others (10). In patients with generalized cancer treated by chemotherapy, brain or leptomeningeal metastases, metabolic disorders, or CNS infections are much more likely causes of epilepsy.

In the work-up of these patients, the epileptic nature of the "fit" is best established by a careful history, electroencephalographic recording, and determination of serum prolactin levels within 30 minutes following the seizure. Determination of the etiology requires a contrast-enhanced brain CT or MRI scan, a search for metabolic disorders, and possibly a lumbar puncture, mainly to rule out meningeal metastases or CNS infection.

B. Treatment

When seizures are caused by metabolic, toxic, or infectious disorders, prolonged administration of antiepileptic drugs is seldom required. On the contrary, patients with brain neoplasia suffering seizures will receive anticonvulsants. Yet, several factors complicate the use of antiepileptic drugs in cancer patients:

Epilepsy caused by brain tumors tends to be refractory to medical treatment.

Concomitant administration of chemotherapy (carmustine or cisplatin) or glucocorticosteroids makes it difficult to maintain stable blood therapeutic drug levels.

Anticonvulsants are neurotoxic and may produce, especially at high levels, neurological symptoms and signs.

We tend to follow the recommendation of Posner (12) by treating with antiepileptics only symptomatic patients, omitting prophylaxis in patients with primary or secondary brain tumors, except brain metastases in melanoma.

Carbamazepine and phenytoin appear today to be the most efficient drugs to control focal seizures, including these caused by cerebral neoplasia. There is a consensus to use these drugs as monotherapy at maximally tolerated doses rather than in combination. Phenytoin, which can be given intravenously, has the great advantage that it can be used, under electrocardiographic monitoring, to treat status epilepticus, a severe life-threatening condition that is not uncommon in patients with malignant brain tumors. In this condition phenytoin is given no faster than 50 mg per minute to a total dose of 18 mg/kg body weight. Thereafter the patients may be treated orally (13). The most troublesome neurological side effects of phenytoin are ataxia and nystagmus, which may mimic tumor progression. Phenytoin and also carbamazepinc have been reported to increase the risk of skin reaction to brain irradiation, which can lead occasionally to a fatal Stevens-Johnson syndrome (14).

The administration of carbamazepine may cause, especially in the elderly, drowsiness and intermittent diplopia. These side effects are minimized by increasing the daily dosage very slowly.

We tend to avoid the use of phenobarbital in patients with brain tumors because we believe it produces more sedation and more serious cognitive disorders than other anticonvulsivants and because 10–20% of patients with brain tumors develop pain and dysfunction of the shoulder or of the entire upper limb (shoulder-hand syndrome), usually contralateral to the tumor site (15). Nor do we consider valproate as the first-choice drug in patients with brain tumors because admittedly it is best indicated in generalized seizures. The drug is well tolerated, however, and hepatic failure has been observed only in children under 5 years old and when the drug was used in combination with other anticonvulsivants.

Diazepam (Valium), which is not used as chronic treatment for seizures, has two indications in neurooncology. Intravenous diazepam is recommended at a rate no faster than 2 mg/minute to stop seizures in status epilepticus, even before starting phenytoin. Its use has also been recommended to avoid seizures in patients with brain tumors when performing contrast-enhanced CT scan, 5–10 mg being given about half an hour before the procedure.

V. CEREBROVASCULAR DISEASE (CVD)

A. Physiopathogenesis and Clinical Presentation

Graus et al. (16) published in 1985 the most comprehensive study on cerebrovascular complications in patients with cancer based on a series of 3426 complete autopsies. CVD were found in 14.6% of patients, of which half were symptomatic. The frequency of hemorrhagic and ischemic lesions was about equal. CVD being, next to heart diseases and cancer, the third cause of mortality and morbidity in the West, their occurrence in cancer patients, especially in the elderly, is not necessarily related to the underlying neoplasia. We consider here the physiopathogenesis of CVD specifically related to cancer and review consecutively hemorrhagic and ischemic arterial lesions, then venous occlusions. This classification is of course arbitrary because in many patients different forms of CVD may coexist. For instance, the transformation of primary ischemic lesions into hemorrhagic lesions is common, especially in cancer patients, and in disseminated intravascular coagulation (DIC) both ischemic and hemorrhagic lesions may be found.

1. Hemorrhagic CVD

Intracerebral bleeding in cancer patients is caused primarily by coagulation abnormalities or intratumoral bleeding. The most commun source of intracranial hematomas in the Graus et al. (16) experience were *abnormalities of coagulation*, including hyperleukocytosis and probably thrombocytopenia. The underlying malignancy was acute leukemia in 69 of 88 patients; most of them had no signs of CNS leukemia. Of patients of this group 71% were symptomatic.

Intratumoral bleeding, the second cause of massive hemorrhage, may occur in primary (glioblastomas and oligodendrogliomas) or metastatic brain tumors. In the series of Graus et al., in which primary CNS tumors were not included, the metastases most frequently associated with intracerebral hemorrhage originated from germ cell tumors (hemorrhagic in 59.3%) or melanomas (30.9%), whereas brain metastases of lung cancer bleeded rarely (5%), and those of breast carcinoma exceptionally (0.9%). In 42.6% the intracerebral bleeding caused by metastases had an acute strokelike onset.

In *subarachnoid hemorrhage*, acute nonlymphoblastic leukemia was the most common underlying neoplasia. In these patients massive and symptomatic subarachnoid hemorrhage often leads to coma and rapid death.

Subdural hematomas were asymptomatic in three-quarters of 53 patients reported by Graus et al. Thrombocytopenia with or without DIC was present in all 25 patients with leukemia. All 27 patients with carcinoma had neoplastic infiltration of the dura. Another 10 patients had spinal subdural hematomas, all resulting from lumbar punctures; 8 of them were thrombocytopenic.

2. Ischemic CVD

Nonbacterial thrombotic endocarditis (NBTE), also called marantic endocarditis, occurs in 0.4–2.4% of cancer patients, primarily lung, gastrointestinal (pancreatic), prostate, or female genital tract carcinoma. NBTE is most likely to occur in cachetic, elderly patients with disseminated mucin-secreting cancer, but there are numerous exceptions (17). NBTE is a major cause of cerebral embolism in patients with carcinoma. General signs of NBTE include petechiae, leukocytosis, sometimes fever mimicking infectious endocarditis, and systemic embolisms. Neurological signs are the most prominent manifestations of NBTE, not only because emboli are located in the brain more often than in any other organ, but also because they are large and rarely remain asymptomatic. Neurological manifestations include focal deficits of abrupt onset and seizures, but not infrequently signs of diffuse encephalopathy are seen. DIC, present in about 25% of patients with NBTE, accounts for thrombocytopenia and independently produces cerebral arterial or venous occlusions and subdural and subarachnoid hemorrhages.

The etiopathogenesis of DIC may not differ fundamentally from that of NBTE, and as already mentioned, the two disorders can coexist. They differ statistically by the underlying neoplasia, however, and by the neurological presentation. Acute leukemia, lymphoma, and breast carcinoma are most commonly associated with intravascular coagulation. DIC is less often symptomatic than NBTE and thus less often diagnosed during life. Cerebral infarcts caused by DIC are multiple and small, and when symptomatic, they tend to produce more often a diffuse encephalopathy than focal deficits or seizures.

Less common causes of cerebral infarction or embolism in cancer patients include the following:

Septic infarction, which in the Graus et al. series was mainly associated with acute leukemia and was caused primarily by *Aspergillus*, *Candida*, or *Mucor*.

Tumor emboli primarily originate from cardiac tumors, such as myxomas or sarcomas. The majority of myxomas are diagnosed in adults aged 30–60 years. Cerebral emboli consisting of neoplastic cells occur rarely in carcinomas.

Postlymphographic embolization is a rare complication, especially because this examination procedure is now less frequently performed. The condition usually produces a diffuse self-limiting encephalopathy developing within a few hours following the diagnostic procedure (18).

Polycythemia, and to a much lesser extent *thrombocythemia* and *monoclonal gammapathies*, may lead to hyperviscosity and favor ischemic CVD.

Radiation-related lesions of large arteries may produce local thrombosis or distant emboli. These complications are seen after a delay ranging from months to over 20 years following irradiation. Postradiation lesions of the aortic arch may account for the pathogenesis of transient ischemic attacks, such as those observed in patients with Hodgkin's disease (19).

Clinically, CVD seen in cancer patients differ from these in the general population by a much higher frequency of diffuse encephalopathy (Table 2). Thus their differential diagnosis also includes toxic and metabolic encephalopathies and CNS infections.

The differential diagnosis of CVD presenting with acute focal deficits are brain metastases, which may mimic stroke even in absence of intratumoral bleeding, and brain abscesses. The most helpful diagnostic procedures to be performed in different forms of CVD in cancer patients are summarized in Table 2.

3. Venous Occlusions

A hypercoagulability state is common in malignant diseases and accounts for the high rate of thrombophlebitis with or without pulmonary emboli. In turn, thrombophlebitis may produce paradoxical brain emboli, but the incidence of this complication in cancer patients is unknown. In patients with brain tumors, and possibly other cerebral lesions, paresis through immobility and blood stagnation favors the occurrence of thrombophlebitis, which develops preferentially in the limb contralateral to the brain lesion.

Thrombosis of the cerebral veins and dural sinuses is a rare event even in patients with neoplasms. This complication results from metastatic infiltration or compression in most cases. The less common, nonmetastatic form may be caused by hypercoagulability or *l*-asparaginase treatment. Symptomatic patients present with signs of intracranial hypertension, headaches, seizures, and focal deficits.

B. Treatment

The management of CVD related to cancer first requires the identification of their etiopathogenesis. Table 2 indicates that the latter is often suggested by the

Table 2 Cerebrovascular Diseases in Cancer Patients[a]

Diagnosis	Main Pathogenesis	Main underlying neoplasia	Main clinical manifestation	Diagnostic procedures
Intracerebral hemorrhage	Coagulation abnormalities Hyperleukocytosis Thrombocytopenia Intratumoral bleeding Necrosis (?)	Acute leukemia (ANLL > ALL) Metastages Melanoma Germ cell tumor Lung carcinoma Glioblastoma Oligodendroglioma	Acute, strokelike in about 50%	CT, MRI scan Coagulation study Contrast-enhanced CT or MRI scan
Subdural hematoma Cerebral	Dural metastases Thrombocytopenia	Carcinoma Acute leukemia	Often asymptomatic	
Spinal	Thrombocytopenia plus LP	Acute leukemia Lymphoma	Asymptomatic or pain, paraparesis	CT, MRI scan
Subarachnoid hemorrhage	Meningeal metastases Thrombocytopenia	ANLL > ALL	↓ Consciousness Headache	CT, MRI scan LP, angiography
Nonbacterial thrombotic endocarditis	DIC Mucin secretion (?)	Lung carcinoma Gastrointestinal carcinoma Genital tract carcinoma Prostate carcinoma	Acute focal signs Seizures Sometimes diffuse encephalopathy	CT, MRI scan Cardiac echography Coagulation study

Intravascular coagulation		Acute leukemia Lymphoma Miscellaneous carcinoma	Diffuse encephalopathy Sometimes focal signs	Coagulation study
Septic emboli	*Aspergillus*, *Candida*, *Mucor*	Acute leukemia Lymphoma	Acute focal signs, diffuse encephalopathy	CT, MRI scan Chest, sinus x-ray Cultures
Tumor emboli	Neoplastic emboli Sometimes DIC, thoracotomy	Cardiac myxoma, sarcoma Lung carcinoma	Acute focal signs Sometimes diffuse encephalopathy	CT, MRI scans Chest x-ray
Postlymphography emboli	Lipid emboli	Lymphomas	Self-limiting encephalopathy	Chest x-ray Eyes, fundi
Postradiation vascular lesions	Arterial occlusion Emboli	Head and neck carcinoma	Stroke Transient ischemic attacks	Angiography
Hyperviscosity	Polycythemia Monogammopathy	Vaquez disease Myeloma, Waldeström's disease	Stroke	Blood examination Protein study
Cerebral venous and sinus occlusion	Dural metastases *l*-Asparaginase Hypercoagulability (?)	Miscellaneous carcinoma	Subacute intracranial hypertension, focal signs, seizures	MRI scan Angiography

[a]ANLL, acute nonlymphoblastic leukemia; ALL, acute lymphoblastic leukemia; LP, lumbar puncture; DIC, disseminated intravascular coagulation.

nature of the CNS lesion: hemorrhagic versus ischemic, the type of the underlying neoplasia (acute leukemia versus carcinoma), and the clinical presentation (focal deficits versus diffuse encephalopathy).

Evaluation of therapy of CVD in cancer patients is difficult because the outcome is related to many factors, including the spread of the underlying neoplasia, the patient's performance status, the sensitivity to antineoplastic treatment and the severity of its toxicity, and the importance of immunodepression. In the absence of adequate prospective trials, many treatment recommendations that follow may appear controversial.

Rapid correction of coagulation disorders, thrombocytopenia, or hyperviscosity probably represents useful prophylaxis of cancer-related CVD. The prognosis of patients presenting with massive acute cerebral hemorrhage is dismal, and neurosurgery is rarely indicated. Radiation therapy may help to stop bleeding caused by cerebral or dural metastases, however, especially those originating from radiosensitive neoplasia, such a germ cell tumors.

In symptomatic spinal subdural hematoma, decompressive surgery is indicated in patients with severe neurological deficit, but only after correction of the thrombocytopenia and if the general condition of the patient permits. The administration of heparin in NBTE seems useful to stop the occurrence of new neurological signs, and perhaps even to improve the patient's condition.

The occurrence of septic emboli may be prevented in leukemic patients by amphotericin B and is treated effectively by adequate antibiotics.

Postradiation vasculopathies are often segmental and amenable to surgical resection, which are recommended in symptomatic patients. Platelet antiaggregants should be used in inoperable patients. Because the effectiveness of heparin has been shown in cranial thrombophlebitis in a general population in a prospective and randomized study (20), we also recommend heparin in venous and sinus occlusion not caused by metastases in cancer patients.

VI. PERIPHERAL NEUROGENIC PAIN

The interest of early recognition and work-up of the peripheral neurogenic pain in cancer patients is of paramount importance for several reasons:

1. It may lead to an earlier diagnosis of a previously unknown neoplastic disease.
2. It points to new neoplastic locations in patients with an already known malignancy.
3. Finally, the success of its management is related to the precocity and the accuracy of the diagnosis.

The clinical presentation of the most common and most typical peripheral neurogenic pain syndromes is summarized in Table 3. This section emphasizes

Table 3 Main Peripheral Neurogenic Pain Syndromes Caused by Metastases

Pain location	Main associated signs	Most probable metastatic location	Structures involved
Unilateral frontal	Diplopia + exophthalmos	Orbital	Cranial nerves
Unilateral frontal	Diplopia + vein turgescence	Parasellar	
Facial (pain or numbness)	Nerve V Lesion	Middle fossa	
Glossopharyngeal neuralgia	Nerves IX, X, XI palsy	Jugular foramen	
Occipital	Nerve XII palsy, stiff neck	Occipital condyle	
Anterior aspect of chest and shoulder	Later, Horner's syndrome, eighth cervical and first and second thoracic root palsy	Lung apex (Pancoast's syndrome)	Eighth cervical segment First and second thoracic segments
Upper limb(s)	Signs of cervicobrachial plexopathy	Epidural, cervical, axillary	Cervicobrachial plexus and/or roots
Thoracic and upper lumbar root pain	Vertebral pain Later, signs of spinal cord compression	Epidural	Thoracic roots Upper lumbar roots
Lower limb(s)	Signs of lumbosacral plexopathy	Epidural, pelvic	Lumbosacral plexus and/or roots

the clinical presentation of these neurological abnormalities; pain aspects and their treatment are considered in Chapter 10.

1. Pain Related to Cranial Nerve Lesions

Five syndromes of cranial nerve lesions caused by metastases have been identified by Greenberg et al. (21). Unilateral frontal pain corresponds to two locations, orbital and parasellar; the three other pain locations are evocative of specific metastatic sites (Table 3). Although pain (sometimes numbness) may be the first manifestation, metastatic cranial nerve lesions are typically associated with other neurological deficits, summarized in Table 3. The identification of these different syndromes provides useful guidance for radiological investigations, although in many patients the syndromes may overlap.

Skull metastases are the most common cause of cranial nerve involvement in cancer patients, and the most useful complementary investigations include skull x-ray and isotopic and CT scans. If these examinations are negative, MRI scan with gadolinium and lumbar puncture is performed to rule out parenchymal or leptomeningeal lesions. It is only when all these investigations are negative that other etiologies, including the so-called idiopathic syndromes, may be considered, and even in these patients follow-up is required. Metastases may mimic other diseases, including Tolosa-Hunt syndrome, by both their clinical presentation and response to corticosteroids.

2. Pancoast's Syndrome

The first manifestation of this syndrome is an aching or burning pain caused by pleural involvement, reported to the anterior aspect of the chest and shoulder. Pancoast's syndrome points almost invariably to an apical pulmonary cancer. If the diagnosis is made at this early stage, an approximately 30% survival at 5 years may be expected (22). At later stages, when the eighth cervical and the first and second thoracic segments are involved, the chances for cure become dismal.

3. Plexopathies

Radicular pain is the initial manifestation of cancerous brachial or lumbosacral plexopathy in 80–90% of patients. The pain is rarely bilateral in the initial stages of this complication. The metastatic nature of plexus involvement is best confirmed by the evidence of neoplastic lesions on CT or MRI scan (23,24). These two procedures and myelography may also demonstrate epidural spread of the malignant tissue. If all these diagnostic procedures are negative and if a leptomeningeal carcinomatosis is ruled out by CSF analysis, the most likely, and also the most difficult, differential diagnosis becomes postradiation plexopathy in patients previously irradiated in this area. The clinical presentation of postradiation plexopathy differs from that of neoplastic lesions in that the first symptoms are numbness, paresthesia, or weakness rather than intense radicular pain. In addition, approximately 80% of lumbosacral plexopathies caused by radiation therapy are bilateral although asymmetrical. The presence of myokymia electromyography (EMG) favors a postradiation etiology (25).

Idiopathic plexopathies, such as the Parsonage-Turner (brachial plexus neuralgic amyotrophy) syndrome or its lumbosacral counterpart, occasionally occur in cancer patients, but their clinical presentation and course allow an easy differential diagnosis.

4. Thoracic and Upper Lumbar Radicular Pain

This symptom is the most common presentation of epidural metastases (26). It may be preceded or accompanied by vertebral ache. It is essential that epidural metastases be diagnosed at that early stage; before the development of signs of spinal cord compression. MRI scan and/or myelography best demonstrate epidural metastatic locations, which are multiple in about 17% of cases (27). Unless myelography is performed, lumbar puncture should be avoided in the work-up of epidural metastases: it may be hazardous and is rarely informative.

In cancer patients the differential diagnosis of epidural metastases includes abscesses, radiation-induced tumors, and epidural lipomatosis caused by corticosteroids.

5. Peripheral Neuropathies

Three types of clinically distinct peripheral neuropathies are seen with an increased frequency in cancer patients:

1. Sensory motor dying back polyneuropathy
2. Sensory neuropathy
3. Guillain-Barré-like polyneuritis

The two first varieties commonly manifest by burning and painful dysesthesia, whereas Guillain-Barré syndrome may be preceded by dorsal or lumbar pain. In addition to the differences in their clinical presentation, peripheral neuropathies are also diagnosed and differentiated from each other by electrophysiological features. Dying back neuropathy is characterized by a decreased amplitude of muscle and nerve potentials and/or slowing of motor and sensory nerve conduction velocities. Sensory neuronopathy is characterized by decreasing and eventually disappearance of sensory nerve potentials and Guillain-Barré syndrome by conduction blocks. The main causes of peripheral neuropathies specifically related to cancer are summarized in Table 4.

VII. FATIGUE AND WEAKNESS

According to Portenoy, quoted by Posner (12), fatigue is present in three-quarters of cancer patients and is the most frequent complaint. A specific mechanism,

Table 4 Cancer-Related Peripheral Neuropathies

Syndrome	Neoplastic compression or infiltration	Anticancer chemotherapy	Paraneoplasia
Dying back polyneuropathy	Very rare; seen in acute leukemias	*Vinca* alkaloids, procarbazine, Hexamethylamine	Common form of neurological paraneoplasia
Sensory neuronopathy	Posterior epidural matatases	Cisplatin, taxol	Denny-Brown sensory neuronopathy associated with SCLC
Guillain-Barré-like syndrome	Meningeal carcinomatosis	Suramin sodium	Associated with lymphomas, mainly Hodgkin's disease

similar to that of anorexia, that has been correlated with the production of tumor necrosis factor, has not been shown for fatigue. Many factors, however, including surgery, chemotherapy, radiation therapy, interferons, immunodepression, infections, anorexia and loss of weight, or feeling of sadness, may cause or at least aggravate the feeling of tiredness in cancer patients. Because fatigue is common in patients with generalized neoplastic diseases, several pathological conditions in which weakness is a prominant feature may be overlooked. These diseases include the Lambert-Eaton syndrome, hypokalemia and hypomagnesemia, polymyositis, and previously considered corticosteroid myopathy and predominantly motor neuropathies, including Guillain-Barré syndrome. These syndromes are compared in Table 5.

A. Lambert-Eaton Syndrome

1. Physiopathogenesis and Clinical Presentation

LES is an autoimmune diesease caused by antibodies directed against voltage-sensitive calcium channels. These channels are also expressed on the surface of the SCLC (but not other lung cancers), thus generating an autoimmune response that down-regulates the calcium channels of the presynaptic nerve terminals. Two-thirds of LES cases are associated with cancer, primarily SCLC. LES is a rare disease. Even in the selected group of SCLC patients its incidence is lower than 2%. In the majority of cases the diagnosis of LES precedes discovery of the underlying neoplasia.

LES is characterized by proximal weakness, which starts and predominates in the lower limbs, causing difficulty in climbing stairs or even standing up from a sitting position. Unlike in myasthenia gravis, the oculobulbar musculature is usually spared, but involvement of respiratory muscles is not rare and may account for respiratory distress, notably following general anesthesia. Signs of cholinergic dysautonomia, including dryness of mouth, skin, and eyes, impotence, obstipation, and urinary retention, are present in about 50% of cases. Tendon reflexes may be decreased or abolished. The diagnosis is confirmed by electrophysiological features that include (1) a low compound muscle action potential (CMAP); (2) a decrease in CMAP amplitude at low-frequency (<5 Hz) repetitive stimulation, and (3) an at least twofold increase in CMAP amplitude at high-frequency (20–50 Hz) stimulation. This typical pattern is not observed in all cases, however (28).

2. Treatment

Therapy of LES aims to (1) decrease the tumor volume, (2) increase the liberation of acetylcholine packets, and/or (3) inhibit the autoimmune reaction.

Table 5 Comparison of Selected Syndromes Causing Weakness in Cancer Patients

Syndrome	Relation to cancer	Main symptoms and signs	Main electrophysiological abnormalities	Laboratory examinations	Muscle biopsy	Treatment
Lambert-Easton symdrome	Paraneoplastic	Proximal weakness of lower limbs, cholinergic dysfunction	Low CMAP,[a] ↑ CMAP at high-frequency stimulation	Antibodies against Ca^{2+} channel	Not contributive	Tumor reduction, immunodepression, guanidine, diaminopyridine
Hypokalemia and hypomagnesemia	Toxic paraneoplastic	Widespread weakness	Usually not contributive	If severe, ↑ CK, myoglobinuria	Normal, vacuolar, or necrotizing myopathy	K^+ and Mg^+
Polymyositis	Paraneoplastic?	Proximal weakness dysphagia	Myopathic EMG, fibrillations	↑ Muscle enzymes, inflammatory changes	Necrotic and regenerative changes	Immunodepression
Corticoid myopathy	Prolonged treatment	Proximal lower limb weakness	Normal	Not contributive	Not contributive	Taper corticosteroids
Guillain-Barré syndrome	Paraneoplastic?	Weakness, tendon reflexes	Conduction blocks	↑ CSF protein	Not contributive	Plasmapheresis, immunoglobulins

[a]CMAP, compound muscle action potential.

1. Reduction in tumor volume by chemotherapy or radiation therapy has improved the clinical and electrophysiological signs, admittedly in a limited number of cases.
2. At least two drugs that increase the liberation of acetylcholine have been successfully used in LES therapy: guanidine chlorohydrate, 30 mg/kg in three to four daily fractions, and 3,4-diaminopyridine, 15–25 mg total dose given in four to five daily doses. The main side effects of these drugs are hematological, liver and/or renal toxicity for guanidine, and seizures for 3,4-diaminopyridine.
3. The benefit of immunodepressive treatments—corticosteroids or such drugs as azathioprine—may be delayed, thus limiting their use in cancer patients with a short life expectancy. The benefit of plasmapheresis has been established in LES treatment but is of short duration.

B. Hypokalemia and Hypomagnesemia

In cancer patients, paraneoplastic production of ACTH, malabsorption, incoercible diarrhea and vomiting, or administration of amphotericin B (through renal tubular damage) or cisplatin (through hypomagnesemia and renal toxicity) may cause potassium depletion. Chronic corticosteroid therapy may also cause hypokalemia, but corticosteroid myopathy is seldom related to ionic imbalance. Hypokalemic myopathy causes widespread weakness, which may or may not be painful, with depressed or absent tendon reflexes. Increased serum creatine kinase (CK) and myoglobinuria may be found. Pathological studies may be either normal or show vacuolar or, in most severe cases, necrotizing myopathy. Treatment consists of restoring serum potassium and magnesium levels and correcting the abnormality that led to the ionic imbalance.

C. Polymyositis and Motor Neuron Disease

Polymyositis is a diffuse inflamatory disease of predominantly proximal skeletal muscles. The majority of cases occur in patients without malignancy, and the association between polymyositis-dermatomyositis and cancer has been questioned (29). Recently, however, this association was reasonably established in a population-based study (30), which showed that patients with polymyositis have a moderately higher risk of cancer than the general population. Thus polymyositis may be regarded as a paraneoplastic disease, although the physiopathogenic relation to neoplasia has not been elucidated. When the characteristic skin rash is present (dermatomyositis), the diagnosis is usually made easily. In the absence of cutaneus lesions, however, the disease may be mistaken for metabolic or corticosteroid myopathy, or even LES, and possibly amyotrophic lateral sclerosis (ALS), low motor neuron disease (LMND), or Guillain-Barré syndrome.

The vast majority of ALS or LMND occurs in patients without neoplastic disease. However, an association was reported in the past mainly with lung and kidney carcinoma and, more recently, with Hodgkin's or non-Hodgkin's lymphoma (31). These, possibly paraneoplastic, forms of ALS are often accompanied by paraproteinemia, increased protein levels, and the presence of oligoclonal bands in the cerebrospinal fluid. The diganosis of polymyositis is based on the following:

1. Clinical features of progressive, predominantly proximal weakness combined in about 40% of cases with difficulty in swallowing or respiratory muscle weakness.
2. Myopathic changes on EMG with possible fibrillation potentials.
3. Increased levels of skeletal muscle enzymes.
4. Evidence of muscle fiber necrosis, inflammatory perivascular changes consisting predominantly of mononuclear cells, and signs of muscle fiber regeneration on biopsy.

Although treatment reports concerning paraneoplastic polymyositis are few and anecdotal, we use immunosuppressive therapy consisting of prednisolone (about 1 mg/kg body weight per day) given until significant clinical improvement and normalization of serum CK values. Azathioprine, cyclophosphamide, or methotrexate may be used either in combination with corticosteroids or if the latter fail.

REFERENCES

1. Hildebrand J, ed. Management in Neuro-Oncology, ESO Monographs, Berlin: Springer-Verlag, 1992.
2. Fishman RA. Brain edema. N Engl J Med 1975; 293:706–712.
3. Green SB, Byar DP, Walker MD. Comparisons of carmustine, procarbazine and high dose methylprednisolone as additions to surgery and radiation therapy for the treatment of malignant glioma. Cancer Treat Rep 1983; 67:121–132.
4. Van den Bent MJ, Vanneste JAL, Ansink BJJ. Prolonged remission of primary central nervous system lymphoma after discontinuation of steroid therapy. J Neurooncol 1992; 13:257–259.
5. Takakura K, Keiji S, Shuntaro H, Asao H. Glucocorticoid therapy. In: Takakura N, ed. Metastatic Tumors of the Central Nervous System. Tokyo: Igaku-Shoin, 1982:244–248.
6. Weissman DE, Janjan NA, Erickson B, et al. Twice daily tapering dexamethazone treatment during cranial radiation for newly diagnosed brain metastases. J Neurooncol 1991; 11:235–239.
7. Weissman DE, Dufer D, Vogel V, Abeloff MD. Corticosteroid toxicity in neuro-oncology patients. J Neurooncol 1987; 5:125–128.

8. Dropcho EJ, Soong SJ. Steroid-induced weakness in patients with primary brain tumors. Neurology 1991; 41:1235–1239.
9. Clouston PD, De Angelis LM, Posner JB. The spectrum of neurological disease in patients with systemic cancer. Ann Neurol 1992; 31:268–273.
10. Posner JB. Acute encephalopathy and seizures. In: Hildebrand J, ed. Neurological Adverse Reactions to Anticancer Drugs. Berlin: Springer-Verlag, 1990:55–65.
11. Graus F. Chronic encephalopathies. In: Hildebrand J, ed. Neurological Adverse Reactions to Anticancer Drugs. Berlin: Springer-Verlag, 1990:67–73.
12. Posner JB. Supportive care in the neuro-oncology patients. In: Hildebrand J, ed. Management in Neuro-Oncology. Berlin: Springer-Verlag, 1992:89–103.
13. Delgado-Escueta AV, Wasterlain C, Treiman DM, Porter RJ. Management of status epilepticus. N Engl J Med 1982; 306:1337–1340.
14. Delattre JY, Safai B, Posner JB. Erythema multiforme and Stevens-Johnson syndrome in patients receiving cranial irradiation and phenytoin. Neurology 1988; 38:194–198.
15. Taylor LP, Posner JB. Phenobarbital rheumatism in patients with brain tumor. Ann Neurol 1989; 25:92–94.
16. Graus F, Rogers LA, Posner JB. Cerebrovascular complications in patients with cancer. Medicine (Baltimore) 1985; 64:16–35.
17. Rosen P, Armstrong D. Non bacterial endocarditis in patients with malignant neoplastic diseases. Am J Med 1973; 54:23–29.
18. Andersen OF, Fogelberg MG, Rosencrantz NM, Weinfeld VA, Westin JE. Postlymphographic cerebral lipid embolization in vena cava superior syndrome. Cancer 1977; 39:79–84.
19. Feldman E, Posner JB. Episodic neurologic dysfunction in patients with Hodgkin's disease. Arch Neurol 1986; 43:1227–1233.
20. Einhaupl KM, Villringer A, Meister W, et al. Heparin treatment in sinus venous thrombosis. Lancet 1991; 338:597–600.
21. Greenberg HS, Deck MDF, Vikram B, Chu FCH, Posner JB. Metastasis to the base of the skull: clinical findings in 43 patients. Neurology 1981; 31:530–537.
22. Attar S, Miller JE, Satterfield J, et al. Pancoast's tumor: irradiation or surgery? Ann Thorac Surg 1979; 28:578–586.
23. Cascino TL, Kori S, Krol G, Foley KM. CT of the brachial plexus in patients with cancer. Neurology 1983; 33:1533–1557.
24. Thomas JE, Cascino TL, Earle JD. Differential diagnosis between radiation and tumor plexopathy of the pelvis. Neurology 1985; 35:1–7.
25. Aho I, Sainio K. Late irradiation-induced lesions of the lumbar plexus. Neurology 1983; 33:953–955.
26. Byrne TN. Spinal cord compression from epidural metastases. N Engl J Med 1992; 327:614–619.
27. Van der Sande JJ, Kroger R, Boogerd W. Multiple spinal epidural metastases; an unexpectedly frequent finding. J Neurol Neurosurg Psychiatry 1990; 53:1001–1003.
28. Oh SJ. Diverse electrophysiological spectrum of the Lambert-Eaton myasthenic syndrome. Muscle Nerve 1989; 12:464–469.
29. Lakhanpal S, Bunch TW, Ilstrup DM, Melton LJ. Polymyositis-dermatomyositis

and malignant lesions: Does an association exist? Mayo Clin Proc 1986; 61:645–653.

30. Sigurgeirsson B, Lindelof B, Edhag O, Allander E. Risk of cancer in patients with dermatomyositis or polymyositis. A population-based study. N Engl J Med 1992; 326:363–367.
31. Younger DS, Rowland LP, Latov N, et al. Lymphoma, motor neuron diseases, and amyotrophic lateral sclerosis. Ann Neurol 1991; 29:78–86.

16

Metabolic Complications of Cancer

William J. Slichenmyer and David S. Ettinger
Johns Hopkins Oncology Center, Baltimore, Maryland

I. INTRODUCTION

A variety of metabolic derangements can complicate the natural history of many types of cancer. This chapter describes some of the clinically important metabolic complications, with emphasis on the diagnosis and treatment of these often serious problems. Specifically addressed here are hyponatremia, hyperuricemia and tumor lysis syndrome, lactic acidosis, hypoglycemia, and hypomagnesemia. The clinical manifestations of hypercalcemia are also described here; the pathophysiology and treatment of this condition are described in Chapter 17.

II. CLINICAL MANIFESTATIONS OF HYPERCALCEMIA OF MALIGNANCY

Hypercalcemia can affect several target organs. These include the kidney, gastrointestinal tract, central nervous system, peripheral nerves and muscles, autonomic nervous system, and heart. Symptoms correlate better with the rate of rise of serum calcium levels than with the absolute level of the serum calcium (1). Other factors in the patient's clinical setting are important for the development of symptoms related to the hypercalcemia, such as the extent of underlying malignant disease, other comorbid states, or concomitant medications (1). The major manifestations in the central nervous system are depression, irritability, or disturbed sleep and can eventually lead to lethargy, confusion, stupor, or coma (1). Muscle weakness or hypotonia with absent deep tendon reflexes can also be seen in profound cases (1). Cardiovascular effects are shortening of the QT interval, broadening of the T wave, heart block with asystole, ventricular dysrhythmias, and increased sensitivity to digoxin (1). Gastointestinal manifestations include anorexia, vomiting, gastric atony, constipation, and possibly acute pancreatitis (1). The renal manifestations include polyuria, polydipsia, dehydration, acute renal insufficiency, and inability to concentrate the urine (nephrogenous diabetes insipidus) (1).

III. HYPONATREMIA

Hyponatremia, or low serum sodium concentration, is a potentially serious and relatively common disorder in cancer patients. Numerous factors can cause or contribute to hyponatremia, and most cases are mild and asymptomatic. Profound and symptomatic cases require prompt recognition and appropriate therapy.

A. Incidence

The prevalence of hyponatremia among hospitalized patients is 2.5% (2), and it is more frequent among cancer patients. It is the most common electrolyte disorder among cancer patients (3).

B. Pathophysiology

Factors that increase the ratio of water to sodium in the serum result in hyponatremia. The balance of sodium and water in the serum is regulated by vasopressin (also called antidiuretic hormone). Vasopressin is a small (nine amino acids) peptide hormone produced in the neurohypophysis. It is stored in the posterior pituitary bound to neurophysins within secretory granules. Release of these granules into the bloodstream is regulated by osmoreceptors located in the anterior hypothalamus (4). A steady, low level of release of the hormone normally maintains the plasma osmolarity in the normal range, usually very close to 290 mOsM. During times of increased osmotic pressure, the release of vasopressin is increased; during times of hypotonicity, release is inhibited.

Other secondary factors can regulate vasopressin secretion (4). Decreased extracellular fluid volume, sensed primarily via baroreceptors in the great veins and atria, increases vasopressin secretion. Other less important factors that stimulate secretion of vasopressin are low arterial blood pressure, high levels of angiotensin II, pain, and surgical stress. A number of drugs increase vasopressin secretion, including narcotics, nicotine, and barbiturates; alcohol and some narcotic antagonists can decrease the secretion of vasopressin.

Vasopressin acts in the collecting system of the kidney to inhibit the excretion of water (4). The hormone increases the permeability of the renal collecting ducts, thus permitting water to be reabsorbed into the hypertonic interstitium of the renal medulla. In the presence of vasopressin, over 99% of a load of filtered water can be reabsorbed. The result is hypertonic urine of low volume. Maximal urine concentration is approximately 1400 mOsM, approximately five times the osmolarity of plasma.

C. Etiology

A wide variety of diseases, conditions, drugs, and other factors can contribute to hyponatremia (Table 1). It is often useful to categorize these based upon various clinical parameters. One approach involves measurement of the serum osmolality as the initial step. If this is abnormally low, then clinical assessment of extracellular fluid volume further subdivides the categories into hypovolemic, euvolemic, or hypervolemic hyponatremia (5).

Somc other conditions, such as the infusion of hypertonic fluids (i.e., glucose and mannitol) and hyperglycemia as seen in nonketotic hyperosmolar hyperglycemia of non–insulin-dependent diabetes, induce an appropriate compensatory fall in the serum sodium (6). This is a physiological response to shifts of water from the intracellular compartment to the extracellular compartment. These states of low sodium concentration are important only in that they should be recognized as physiological adaptations to hypertonicity and do not require specific interventions.

Isotonic hyponatremia can also be caused by infusions of hypertonic mannitol or glucose. Moreover, "pseudohyponatremia" is a condition characterized by isotonic serum with a large portion of its volume replaced by nonaqueous substances, thereby lowering the measured sodium concentration. In particular, hypertriglyceridemia is associated with a decrease in the water compartment of the serum and an appropriate fall in the total quantity of sodium in that volume. The concentration of sodium in the water compartment remains normal, but in a given volume, less is measured. The same phenomenon occurs for patients with profound hyperproteinemia, such a Waldenström's macroglobulinemia. The true concentration of sodium can be obtained using an ion-specific electrode (6).

Hypotonic hyponatremia is much more common than the preceding conditions. This represents a truly low level of sodium relative to the amount of water in the serum. The classification further categorizes these heterogeneous disorders by the extracellular fluid volume (7). This requires the evaluation of many clinical factors, including obtaining a history of possible sources of sodium loss, such as vomiting, diarrhea, polyuria, output from a stoma, hemorrhage, or skin losses from burns, bullae, or other lesions. Any history to suggest increased fluid intake or retention, such as polydipsia, infusion of hypotonic fluids, congestive heart failure, liver disease, nephrotic syndrome, or renal failure, is also important. The physical examination should focus upon the presence or absence of tachycardia, postural hypotension, elevated jugular venous pressures, dependent

Table 1 Evaluation and Classification of Hyponatremia

- Hypertonic
  - Nonketotic hyperglycemia of diabetes mellitus
  - Infusions of mannitol or glucose
- Isotonic: infusions of mannitol or glucose
- Hypotonic
  - Hypervolemic
    - Congestive heart failure
    - Nephrotic syndrome
    - Cirrhosis
    - Renal failure
  - Euvolemic
    - SIADH
      - Tumor
        - Small cell lung carcinoma
        - Prostate carcinoma
        - Adrenal carcinoma
        - Hodgkin's lymphoma
        - Others
      - Antineoplastic therapy
        - Cyclophosphamide
        - *Vinca* alkaloids
        - Melphalan
        - Combined interleukin-1 and interleukin-4
      - Other drugs
        - Narcotics
        - Oral hypoglycemic agents
        - Phenothiazines
    - Renal failure
    - Hvpothyroidism
    - Adrenal insufficiency
    - Psychogenic polydipsia
  - Hypovolemic
    - Diarrhea (especially after cyclophosphamide with total-body irradiation for bone marrow transplant)
    - Vomiting
    - Draining fistulas
    - Cisplatin-associated salt-wasting nephropathy

rales, findings of pleural effusion or ascites, the third heart sound, skin turgor, and dependent edema. Use of an indwelling catheter for the measurement of central venous pressure is rarely required.

Hypovolemic hyponatremia is caused by loss of sodium, usually with a partial replacement by hypotonic fluids. A typical example is a patient with diarrhea who drinks water without sodium replacement. After a few days, hyponatremia with hypovolemia results. Vomiting or diuretics also commonly predispose an individual to this syndrome.

Two syndromes unique to the cancer patient population deserve mention. Cisplatin can induce a syndrome of salt-wasting nephropathy, such that large volumes of urine with a high sodium content are produced. In one series of 70 patients treated with cisplatin at doses of 100 mg/m^2 or higher, 8 developed this syndrome (8). All 8 had concomitant hypomagnesemia, with the syndrome arising 2–5 months after starting the cisplatin. The syndrome is distinguished from emesis-induced volume depletion by the inappropriately high urine sodium level (8). Another oncology-specific situation results from losses of sodium in the stool after total-body irradiation given in conjunction with high doses of cyclophosphamide. The effect seems to be related to the irradiation, because patients treated with high-dose etoposide plus high-dose cyclophosphamide do not have excessive fecal sodium output (9).

Euvolemic isotonic hyponatremia is most commonly related to the syndrome of inappropriate secretion of antidiuretic hormone (SIADH). This is discussed in greater detail in a subsequent section. Other etiologies in this category are psychogenic polydipsia, some cases of renal failure, and a condition known as the "reset osmostat." SIADH is distinguished from these conditions by the inability of the patient to excrete adequately a water load. Among cancer patients, a relatively frequent and usually mild iatrogenic cause is hyperalimentation fluid that supplies insufficient sodium.

Hypervolemic isotonic hyponatremia is usually associated with congestive heart failure, liver disease, or the nephrotic syndrome. These states share several common features, including increased total-body sodium and water, hypoalbuminemia, and peripheral edema. The other common feature is a reduced effective intravascular fluid volume, which in turn leads to elevated levels of vasopressin and diminished excretion of free water.

D. Syndrome of Inappropriate Secretion of Antidiuretic Hormone

This term is specifically applied to clinical situations with true hypotonic hyponatremia with isovolemia and no other identifiable etiology. It is characterized by inappropriate concentration of urine in the face of hypoosmolar serum. Many etiologies are known, including ectopic hormone production and secretion by tumors, increased pituitary release as a result of central nervous system (CNS) disease, pulmonary disorders, and the effects of many drugs. Among all patients with SIADH, the most common etiology is drug-induced, followed by tumor-associated SIADH (10).

Small cell lung cancer is the prototype tumor for ectopic production of vasopressin. Other tumors known to produce vasopressin and cause SIADH include some lymphomas and carcinomas of duodenum, pancreas, prostate, adrenal, esophagus, colon, head and neck, carcinoid tumor, thymoma, mesothelioma, esthesioneuroblastoma, and Ewing's sarcoma (11–13). Up to 40% of patients with small cell lung cancers have inappropriate vasopressin secretion, and approximately 10% of patients with small cell lung cancer have clinically apparent hyponatremia (14). The presence of SIADH does not correlate with the stage, sites of metastasis, or prognosis in patients with small cell lung cancer. The syndrome resolves as the tumor responds to chemotherapy or radiation (15). Relapses of the tumor are sometimes associated with return of the SIADH (15).

A variety of intracranial or intrathoracic processes are associated with SIADH (4). These include head trauma, brain tumors, meningitis, cerebrovascular accidents, pneumonia (fungal, bacterial, or viral), lung abscess, asthma, and mechanical ventilation. The vasopressin appears to be released from the posterior pituitary in these disorders. Increased, inappropriate vasopressin secretion is also noted, as mentioned, in hypothyroidism and adrenal insufficiency. Stress and pain, especially in the postoperative setting, can be associated with SIADH.

Many drugs can cause SIADH (4). The narcotic analgesics have been mentioned. Oral hypoglycemic agents, especially chlorpropamide and tolbutamide, are the most commonly cited examples. Phenothiazines, often used for their antiemetic properties in the oncology population, may be associated with SIADH. This may confound hypovolemic hyponatremia in the patient with poorly controlled chemotherapy-related emesis. At least three antineoplastic drugs are also associated with SIADH.

Cyclophosphamide is associated with hyponatremia and water intoxication, especially when large doses are administered as part of a bone marrow transplant regimen (16,17). This is particularly problematical because of the large volumes of intravenous fluids administered to these patients to prevent the development of hemorrhagic cystitis. The syndrome is relatively short-lived, and most patients have a spontaneous diuresis after a few hours. It is important to assess carefully the fluid status of such patients to prevent serious hyponatremia and volume overload. Aggressive use of diuretics can help to prevent dangerous sequelae (18). The syndrome can occur in the absence of elevated serum levels of vasopressin, suggesting that the cyclophosphamide or one of its metabolites acts in the collecting system of the kidney to mimic the effect of vasopressin (17).

Vinca alkaloids can also cause SIADH. A typical example is reported by Oldham and Pomeroy (19), who describe a 52-year-old female with a reticulum cell sarcoma of the neck. She presented 1 week after treatment with a vincristine-containing regimen (mechlorethamine + vincristine + procarbazine + prednisone) with disorientation and serum sodium level of 98 mM. Her symptoms diminished when she was treated with hypertonic saline, and her sodium level rose further with fluid restriction. Cases of accidental vincristine overdose have also been associated with SIADH (20). Recurrent and severe hyponatremia was observed in two of seven patients treated with combined vinblastine and interferon-γ, suggesting that this combination is particularly potent in inducing SIADH (21). In some cases of vincristine-related SIADH, serum vasopressin levels have been shown to be elevated (20), and a direct effect of vincristine in vitro upon rat neurohypophysis suggests that the SIADH results from release of hormone from the pituitary (22).

Other antineoplastic agents can cause hyponatremia. High doses of melphalan (>1 mg/kg) are associated with SIADH (23). Two patients treated with combined interleukin-2 and interleukin-4 developed hyponatremia probably caused by SIADH (24).

E. Diagnosis

The diagnosis of hyponatremia is usually made by obtaining an abnormally low sodium level as part of a multiassay panel of serum electrolyte determinations. Confirmation of the diagnosis requires exclusion of pseudohyponatremia or the uncommon hypertonic or isotonic hyponatremias by measurement of serum osmolarity. Any of the clinical manifestations of hyponatremia discussed here is an indication to measure the serum sodium level. Once the diagnosis is confirmed, a search for the underlying etiological factor(s) is required for appropriate therapy.

Identification of the etiology of hyponatremia begins with the history and physical examination. For patients with hypovolemic hyponatremia, if a cause for volume depletion is not obvious, consideration of surreptitious use of diuretics or laxatives may be important. Because adrenal insufficiency can result from metastatic disease or certain antineoplastic medications (aminoglutethemide and ketoconazole), exclusion of this disorder with an adrenocorticotropic hormone) (ACTH) stimulation test is also important in this situation. Thyroid function tests identify the rare patient with hypothyroidism presenting with hyponatremia. This may be particularly important for the patient with a history of radiotherapy to the neck.

In isovolemic hyponatremia, the comments regarding hypothyroidism and adrenal insufficiency also apply. Furthermore, if these disorders, renal insufficiency, and psychogenic polydipsia are excluded, then SIADH is likely. The presence of SIADH is confirmed by the finding of a urine sodium concentration greater than 20 mM and inappropriately concentrated urine (urine osmolality > 100 mOsMol/kg) in the setting of hypoosmolar serum (25). Levels of vasopressin are not required for this diagnosis. If not apparent, the cause of SIADH should be sought with emphasis on review of the patient's medications and evaluation of the thorax and brain.

In hypervolemic hyponatremia, a history of nephrosis, renal failure, congestive heart failure, or cirrhosis is usually obtained. The new onset of this clinical syndrome in the cancer patient should elicit a search for complications related to tumor progression, such as pericardial metastasis with tamponade physiology, extensive liver metastases with hepatic dysfunction, or portal or hepatic vein thrombosis. Nephrotic syndrome complicates several malignancies, including Hodgkin's lymphoma and a variety of carcinomas (25). Complications of cancer therapy should also be considered in this clinical setting, including anthracyclines, cyclophosphamide, and radiation-induced cardiac dysfunction. Echocardiogram or nuclear ventriculography (MUGA) may be very useful for evaluating ventricular function. If abnormal liver function tests are noted, then transfusion-associated viral hepatitis, hepatic venoocclusive disease, graft-versus-host disease of the liver, or hepatotoxic drugs should be considered.

F. Clinical Manifestations

The clinical manifestations of hyponatremia are related to the magnitude of and rate of change in the drop in sodium concentration (4). Most cases are mild and asymptomatic, requiring no intervention. Only when the sodium level falls below approximately 130 mM do symptoms arise. The usual early symptoms are nausea and malaise, typically occurring at levels below 125 mM. As levels fall to the range of 115–120 mM, headache, lethargy, or obtundation may occur. At sodium levels below 115 mM, seizures or coma may occur. Hyponatremia-induced brain edema and herniation can be fatal (26). Hyponatremia lowers the seizure threshold and may make manifest a previously undiagnosed brain metastasis. For the volume-depleted patient, diminished cardiac output and cerebral perfusion may also contribute to CNS symptoms.

G. Prevention

Because many cases of hyponatremia are iatrogenic, a high index of suspicion can allow early detection and appropriate intervention before symptoms arise. Intermittent monitoring of the serum sodium level is required for any cancer patient treated with diuretics, oral hypoglycemic agents, parenteral nutrition, intravenous fluids, narcotic analgesics, cyclophosphamide, or *Vinca* alkaloids. In patients with small cell lung cancer, CNS metastases, pulmonary tumors or infiltrates, renal insufficiency, or a history of fluid-retentive states the sodium level should be checked intermittently.

H. Treatment

The need for treatment depends on the severity of the hyponatremia and the presence or absence of symptoms (Table 2). Mild (serum sodium > 130 mM) and asymptomatic cases require no therapy; this is a transient phenomenon. The choice of therapy for more severe or symptomatic hyponatremia depends upon the etiology and the severity of the abnormality.

For mildly symptomatic hyponatremia in the patient with intravascular volume depletion, intravenous fluid replacement with normal saline is usually sufficient. The underlying causes of the volume depletion must be sought and corrected. Antiemetic or antidiarrheal therapy can usually prevent recurrence of the hyponatremia.

For moderate hyponatremia (serum sodium 120–130 mM) with only mild symptoms in the normovolemic or edematous patient, fluid restriction is the initial treatment of choice. Limiting the total daily fluid volume intake (including enteral and parenteral fluids) to 2 liters per day is adequate for most patients. More restrictive limitation of fluid intake may be required for some patients. Because many hyponatremic patients are thirsty (often despite total-body water excess), compliance with this degree of fluid restriction is difficult (4).

For patients with SIADH, other treatments are available if fluid restriction is unsuccessful. Demeclocycline has been used successfully in patients with small cell lung cancer (27,28). It is given orally in doses of 600 or 1200 mg per day in two to four divided doses. The higher dose is associated with better response of hyponatremia but also with greater toxicity, especially renal insufficiency in patients receiving other nephrotoxins. Because demeclocycline can induce a diuretic response, fluid restriction is not required when it is used. In one series

Table 2 Treatment of Hyponatremia

	Advantage	Disadvantage
Intravenous fluid replacement		Volume-depleted patients only
Fluid restriction	Safety	Slow Noncompliance
Demeclocycline	Efficacy Diuretic effect	Slow Nephrotoxic
Hypertonic saline	Rapid correction	Improper use can cause CNS damage Requires frequent monitoring of electrolytes Transient benefit

(27), a mean of 3.5 days was required for the serum sodium to rise above 130 mM, and the maximum response was reached at 9 days of therapy, with sodium levels over 140 mM.

Patients with profound hyponatremia require more aggressive therapy to prevent permanent neurological damage from the hyponatremia. These are patients with otherwise unexplained seizures or coma or with serum sodium levels below 115 mM. Caution is required because correcting the abnormality too quickly is also associated with permanent neurological sequelae, particularly the syndrome of central pontine myelinolysis (26,29). Cautious use of intravenous hypertonic (3%) saline or normal saline allows the sodium level to rise, but often only transiently, as the sodium load is excreted and the water retained under the influence of vasopressin. Addition of furosemide enhances the excretion of free water as these saline solutions are given (30). Although controversial, a useful guideline is to monitor frequently the serum sodium level during the first 24 h of treatment and to raise the sodium level no faster than an hourly rate of 2.5 mM, not more than 20 mM in any 24 h period (29) and to a level no higher than 135 mM (31). These emergency measures should prevent further serious neurological damage and allow institution of the more conservative treatments already mentioned.

I. Future Prospects

Antivasopressin drugs that bind to the vasopressin receptor are in development and may one day prove useful for patients with SIADH (4).

IV. HYPERURICEMIA AND THE TUMOR LYSIS SYNDROME

A. Definition

Hyperuricemia is a biochemical abnormality characterized by an elevated serum level of uric acid. In cancer patients this is associated with a variety of causes and diverse clinical syndromes. The most dramatic of these is the tumor lysis syndrome, a combination of biochemical abnormalities seen in some patients after rapid release into the blood of the contents of a large burden of malignant cells. Although relatively uncommon, the tumor lysis syndrome is important because of its potential for dangerous complications that can usually be minimized with proper management. Asymptomatic hyperuricemia is more common. Gout is a common medical disorder associated with chronic hyperuricemia that may coexist in patients with cancer and is not discussed further here.

B. Incidence and Etiology

The overall incidence of tumor lysis syndrome cannot be accurately estimated. One series of 37 patients with Burkitt's lymphoma found evidence of tumor lysis syndrome in 15 patients after chemotherapy (32). Tumor lysis causes renal failure in 10% of patients receiving induction chemotherapy for acute lymphoblastic leukemia (25). Patients with other types of high-grade non-Hodgkin's lymphoma or acute leukemia undergoing induction chemotherapy are also at relatively high risk. It is rare in solid tumors that are typically unresponsive to therapy, such as pancreatic, colorectal, and non–small cell lung cancer. The actual incidence of the syndrome has decreased dramatically in recent years because of the widespread adoption of prophylactic measures. The syndrome is occasionally seen in other chemosensitive solid tumors, such as small cell lung cancer and breast cancer (33). Patients with bulky tumor burden are at higher risk than patients with a smaller tumor load (32).

Hyperuricemia from other causes is much more common. If defined as a serum uric acid level greater than 7 mg/dl in men and greater than 6 mg/dl in women, this asymptomatic biochemical abnormality is found in 5–10% of adults in the United States. The incidence among cancer patients is probably somewhat higher, but reliable estimates are not available. In the majority of cases, hyperuricemia is asymptomatic and requires no specific intervention. Patients with tumor lysis syndrome, uric acid nephropathy, or gout are important exceptions who require treatment.

C. Pathophysiology

The tumor lysis syndrome occurs as a result of the disruption of a large number of tumor cell membranes, leading to the release into blood of intracellular constituents, including potassium, phosphate, and nucleic acids. Potassium is the principal intracellular cation, with a concentration within cells that is approximately 35-fold greater than in the extracellular fluid. Phosphate is the predominant intracellular anion. It, too, is approximately 30-fold increased in the intracellular space versus the extracellular space and may be especially concentrated in cells from rapidly proliferating tumors, such as acute lymphoblastic leukemia (34). The other important intracellular substances are nucleic acids. The purine nucleotides are biochemical precursors of xanthine, which is converted by the enzyme xanthine oxidase to uric acid. The tumor lysis syndrome is characterized by increases in the serum levels of potassium, phosphate, and uric acid.

Normally, the majority of a potassium load is excreted by the kidney. The proximal tubules reabsorb almost all the filtered potassium, and excretion is regulated by secretion in the distal tubules. When the filtered load of potassium is high, the amount secreted by the distal tubule rises, but this compensation is modest and is overcome during periods of tumor lysis syndrome. Patients with renal insufficiency have a markedly diminished capacity for potassium excretion and are at much higher risk for development of hyperkalemia.

Phosphate is normally reabsorbed in the proximal renal tubule. As serum phosphorus levels rise in the tumor lysis syndrome, some of the phosphate combines with calcium and deposits in bone. This leads to a fall in the ionized serum calcium level, which can be a clinically important manifestation of the tumor lysis syndrome. The hypocalcemia stimulates increased secretion of parathyroid hormone, which in turn reduces the renal tubular reabsorption of phosphate, with resultant increased phosphate excretion. Phosphate excretion capacity is diminished by renal insufficiency (35).

Like potassium and phosphate, uric acid is excreted by the kidney after tubular reabsorption and secretion. This excretion is decreased in states of renal insufficiency, in patients taking diuretics, aspirin, pyrazinamide, nicotinic acid, or ethanol, or in the presence of other organic anions, such as ketones or lactate. Uric acid can exist either as a sodium or potassium salt or in an acid form (36). The pK_a of this equilibrium is 5.75, so at physiological pH the salt form predominates. The salt is highly water soluble, but the acid is not. Therefore, in an acid environment, the equilibrium shifts to the less soluble acid form. This is important in the urinary tract, where pH may fall to below 5. In the tumor lysis syndrome, this can result in the deposition of uric acid crystals in the collecting tubules with resultant acute renal failure. This contrasts with the slowly progressive disorder of urate nephropathy, which is caused by the deposition of monosodium urate crystals in the renal interstitium, with a subsequent inflammatory response (36). The deposition of monosodium urate crystals in synovial tissues, if associated with an inflammatory response, results in an acute gouty arthritis (36).

D. Causes of Hyperuricemia and the Tumor Lysis Syndrome

The tumor lysis syndrome usually follows soon after initiation of cytotoxic therapy (32,34). The biochemical abnormalities are usually observed within 24 h of initiation of therapy, but some patients have onset delayed as much as 3 or 4 days or longer (37).

Hyperuricemia without tumor lysis syndrome may also arise in a setting of myeloproliferative disease, multiple myeloma, secondary polycythemia, thalassemia, pernicious anemia, or hemoglobinopathies (36). The feature common to all these disorders is rapid turnover of hematopoietic tissue with high rates of purine degradation.

E. Clinical Presentation and Natural History of the Tumor Lysis Syndrome

The initial manifestations of the tumor lysis syndrome are clinical biochemical abnormalities (Table 3). Typically, an increase in the serum potassium and

Table 3 Tumor Lysis products: Effects and Treatment

	Effect	Treatment
Potassium	Cardiac rhythm instability	Kayexalate (sodium polystyrene sulfonate) Insulin/glucose Forced diuresis Hemodialysis
Phosphate	Hypocalcemia	Calcium replacement (only if symptomatic)
	Obstructive uropathy ?	Forced diuresis Oral phosphate binding agents (prophylaxis)
Uric acid	Obstructive uropathy	Allopurinol (prophylaxis) Alkaline diuresis Hemodialysis

phosphorus levels is noted within 12 h of the initiation of chemotherapy in patients with acute leukemia, high-grade lymphoma, and other highly chemosensitive cancers. Elevations of the serum uric acid level are usually evident within 24 h with such tumors. Abnormalities in renal function follow 2 or 3 days later, corresponding to the time required for crystal deposition in the kidney (34).

Clinical signs and symptoms can arise in response to the hyperkalemia, hypocalcemia, or acute renal failure. Hyperkalemia is associated with abnormalities of cardiac conduction, especially at potassium concentrations greater than 6 mM (38). The earliest electrocardiographic manifestation is peaking and narrowing of the T wave. As the hyperkalemia becomes more severe, the QRS complex is widened and prolonged with decreasing amplitude of the R wave. Further worsening of hyperkalemia is associated with flattening and widening of the P wave, which can ultimately disappear. If treatment is inadequate, the wide QRS complex envelops the T wave, leading to a "sign wave" cardiogram. Unstable ventricular tachyarrhythmias soon follow.

The acute hypocalcemia associated with the tumor lysis syndrome may cause neuromuscular symptoms if it is sufficiently severe. Mild cases may be detected by Chvostek's sign, performed by tapping the seventh cranial nerve anterior and inferior to the external auditory meatus or at one of the branches located between the zygomatic arch and the corner of the mouth (39). Trousseau's sign is observed as tetany in the carpal muscles following the inflation of a blood pressure cuff to a pressure greater than the systolic for a duration of at least 3 minutes (39). More profound hypocalcemia may result in laryngospasm or lowering of the seizure threshold. Falling serum calcium is associated with prolongation of the electrocardiogram QT interval and may be associated with dysrhythmias. Severe hypocalcemia may rarely be associated with depression of myocardial contractility and heart failure (38).

The tumor lysis syndrome can cause acute renal failure (25,34,40,41). Oliguria (or even rarely anuria) with rising blood urea nitrogen and serum creatine levels and metabolic acidosis (in addition to the previously discussed hyperkalemia and hypocalcemia) are also present. Hypertension or congestive heart failure may result from fluid overload during acute renal failure. Uremic pericarditis, platelet aggregation dysfunction, nausea, anorexia, asterixis, and eventually seizures and coma are other possible manifestations of acute renal failure (42).

F. Prophylaxis and Treatment

The optimal management of tumor lysis syndrome begins well before the initiation of cytotoxic chemotherapy. The major prophylactic measures increase the urinary excretion of potassium and phosphorus and decrease the production of uric acid. This begins with vigorous hydration, usually without potassium replacement. The resulting increased urine volume decreases the urinary concentrations of phosphorus and uric acid, thus decreasing the likelihood of crystal deposition and renal damage. Vigorous hydration for at least 24 h before cytotoxic therapy and lasting until at least 48 h after the peak of biochemical abnormalities is recommended. Oral phosphorus-binding antacids help to minimize the absorption of dietary phosphorus and may even result in extraction of circulating phosphorus into the gut lumen and increase fecal phosphorus excretion. Antacids containing calcium should be avoided because of the possible systemic absorption of calcium, increasing the likelihood of ectopic deposition of calcium phosphate crystals. Aluminum hydroxide should be administered as 30 ml orally every 4 h for at least 3 days before initiation of chemotherapy. Allopurinol is crucial for the prevention of complications of hyperuricemia (32). Allopurinol inhibits the enzyme xanthine oxidase and prevents the formation of uric acid. Xanthine is excreted by the kidney and is less likely to cause renal damage than uric acid, although cases of xanthine crystals causing obstructive uropathy have been reported (43). For our patients at risk of tumor lysis syndrome, we prescribe allopurinol, 300 mg orally twice daily for at least 3 days, followed by 100 mg twice daily for 1 week starting 2 days before initiation of chemotherapy if possible.

When the initial doses of cytotoxic chemotherapy have been administered, frequent sampling of serum electrolytes is indicated. For patients with acute leukemia, monitoring the electrolytes every 4–6 h initially is recommended. For patients with lymphomas and chemosensitive solid tumors, monitoring two to four times daily for the first 48 h is recommended. If there are no abnormal electrolyte findings in the first 2 days, the frequency of these determinations can be decreased gradually over the next few days.

The electrolyte abnormalities are treated individually. For hyperkalemia, the first step in treatment is to eliminate any exogenous potassium from the diet or intravenous fluids (especially parenteral antibiotics and hyperalimentation). Urinary potassium excretion can be enhanced through the use of diuretics. The oral ingestion of sodium polystyrene sulfonate allows the exchange of cations in the intestine and enhances fecal potassium excretion. If the serum potassium level rises above 7 mM or there are electrocardiographic changes suggestive of hyperkalemia, more aggressive therapy may be indicated. Insulin stimulates the transport of potassium from the extracellular to the intracellular compartments, resulting in transient decreases in the serum potassium level. Regular insulin in doses of 5 units given intravenously every 15 minutes with 50 g glucose per hour can significantly decrease the serum potassium level. For refractory hyperkalemia, hemodialysis may be lifesaving.

Alkalinization of the urine enhances uric acid excretion. This is achieved with aggressive hydration and diuretics augmented by the addition of sodium bicarbonate to the intravenous fluids. Checking the urinary pH two to three times daily guides therapy. Because sodium bicarbonate therapy can provide large quantities of sodium, caution should be used to avoid iatrogenic hypernatremia.

For symptomatic hypocalcemia or cardiac arrhythmias associated with hyperkalemia, exogenous calcium may be lifesaving. Clinically observed levels of hypocalcemia may contribute to but do not cause dysrhythmias (38). Patients with asymptomatic hypocalcemia require no calcium replacement.

The renal insufficiency that develops during tumor lysis syndrome is usually transient and resolves spontaneously within a few days (32). Nonetheless, the temporary abnormalities may require institution of specific therapy. If oliguria or anuria arises, intravenous fluid flow rates must be significantly curtailed to prevent fluid overload and pulmonary edema. Extra vigilance for the development of hyperkalemia is required in the presence of renal insufficiency. Frequent cardiac auscultation and electrocardiography are also indicated. Early consultation with a nephrologist is beneficial for the management of fluid and electrolytes and the early initiation of hemodialysis, which is more effective than peritoneal dialysis in clearing uric acid (25).

In the management of the tumor lysis syndrome, the overriding concern is the ultimate outcome for the patient. Both patient and family should be reassured that, although potentially life threatening, with proper management the tumor lysis syndrome will resolve in a few days. Patient, family, and medical staff should be encouraged by the fact that lysis of tumor cells corresponds with a decreased tumor burden and hope for a significant antitumor response to therapy.

V. LACTIC ACIDOSIS

A. Definition

Lactic acidosis is defined as a constellation of clinical biochemical abnormalities of lactate metabolism and blood pH regulation. An elevation of the serum lactate level, depression of the serum bicarbonate level, and acidemia are required for the diagnosis (44). Although there is some discrepancy in the literature regarding the absolute levels of abnormality required, most authors agree that a venous blood lactate level above 5 mM and an arterial pH less than 7.35 are sufficient for the diagnosis of lactic acidosis.

This chapter focuses on only one of the two major categories of lactic acidosis. We do not consider further the type A lactic acidosis associated with hypoxemia or tissue hypoperfusion of various etiologies. Type B lactic acidosis is defined as that arising in the setting of adequate tissue perfusion and oxygen delivery. These have been further subdivided into type B_1, associated with various systemic diseases; type B_2, associated with drugs and toxins; and type B_3, associated with inborn errors of metabolism. This chapter addresses type B_1 lactic acidosis associated with various types of malignancy.

B. Incidence

This is an uncommon disorder. Fewer than 50 cases have been reported in the literature, although it may be underdiagnosed and infrequently reported. The majority of reported cases have arisen in the setting of newly diagnosed hematological malignancies, especially acute leukemias and high-grade lymphomas (45–47). A few cases have been recognized in patients with solid tumors. The majority of these cases have been associated with a very high tumor burden and involvement of the liver with extensive infiltrative or metastatic disease (32). Among the reported solid tumors, small cell lung cancer is the most frequently cited, followed by carcinoma of the breast, non–small cell lung cancer, and colon cancer (45,46,48,49).

Other settings for lactic acidosis have been described. Occasional cases secondary to profound thiamine deficiency have arisen in the setting of post–bone marrow transplantation or long-term total parenteral nutrition without adequate thiamine replacement (50,51). A few cases of severe lactic acidosis in patients with pheochromocytoma and elevated serum catecholamine levels have been described (52,53). In these patients, it is believed that vasoconstriction leads to a type A lactic acidosis.

C. Pathophysiology

Lactate exists in equilibrium with pyruvate, a product of glycolysis. Under normal circumstances, lactate is produced by many tissues, and the quantitatively most important are the brain, erythron, skin, and skeletal muscle (44). Leukocytes, platelets, and kidneys produce relatively smaller quantities of lactate. Under normal circumstances, the liver extracts lactate from the circulation and uses it as a substrate for gluconeogenesis. Skeletal muscle and kidney also contribute to extraction of circulating lactate, and the kidney can excrete lactate if the serum concentration rises above a threshold of 5–10 mM. Lactate levels in the serum rise to abnormal levels when the rate of production of lactate exceeds the capacity of these organs to clear it from the circulation. Lactic acidosis arises when lactate and hydrogen ion accumulate and exceed the capacity of the pH homeostatic mechanisms.

Patients with cancer-associated lactic acidosis probably have both increased lactate production and decreased clearance (45–47,49). Neoplastic cells are known to produce lactate in vitro, especially under conditions of reduced oxygen tension. Patients with leukemia and hyperleukocytosis can demonstrate artifactually low pO_2 and pH during the assessment of routine arterial blood gas studies if the specimen is given sufficient time for metabolism of the available oxygen and glucose (54). Clinical correlates of this phenomenon may occur in patients with leukemia who have sludging of circulating blasts in the peripheral circulation and decreased delivery of oxygen to the malignant cells. Rapidly growing solid tumors are known sometimes to "outgrow" their blood supplies, and the hypoxic zones can elaborate lactic acid (49).

Evidence of decreased clearance of lactate is indirect and is based upon the observation that the majority of reported cases involved patients with extensive hepatic infiltration or replacement by tumor (55). Some reported cases of cancer-associated lactic acidosis without hepatic involvement have been associated with profound hypoglycemia, which is an independent etiology of lactic acidosis more frequently seen in patients without cancer (55,56).

Lactic acidosis is clinically important because of the resulting acidemia. This can lead to hyperkalemia, reduction of the seizure threshold, systemic vasodilation, arterial hypotension, pulmonary vasoconstriction, decreased venous capacitance, myocardial depression, increased risk of ventricular dysrhythmias, or other cardiac conduction abnormalities. Furthermore, the use of pharmacological vasoconstrictors is impeded by an acidemic environment.

D. Diagnosis

Lactic acidosis typically arises in the setting of an advanced malignancy, especially acute leukemia, high-grade lymphoma, and small cell lung cancer. Tachypnea is a common symptom, resulting from stimulation of the respiratory center in the medulla oblongata in response to acidemia. A decreased serum bicarbonate level associated with an elevated anion gap is an indication to obtain arterial blood gas studies and measurement of arterial pH. Finding an elevated serum lactate level associated with acidemia is sufficient to make the diagnosis of lactic acidosis.

E. Natural History

The majority of patients reported in the literature died relatively soon after the diagnosis of cancer-associated lactic acidosis (44,49). This reflects the very poor prognosis of patients with acute leukemia or other tumors with very bulky disease and hepatic involvement. However, this grave prognosis is not uniform. Durable complete responses have been reported in patients with lactic acidosis and high-grade lymphoma (47,57), leukemia (45), and small cell lung cancer (58,59). The overall prognosis is determined by the chemosensitivity of the tumor, performance status of the patient, and other associated comorbid states, for example. Rather than being a contraindication to systemic antitumor therapy, for some patients lactic acidosis is an urgent indication for aggessive treatment.

F. Treatment

The mainstay of therapy is cytoreduction of the tumor, usually with combination chemotherapy. Specific management of the lactic acidosis may require invasive monitoring in the intensive care environment. Attempts to correct the arterial pH with bicarbonate have not been of proven benefit in other types of lactic acidosis (44), and there is some evidence that in malignancy-associated lactic acidosis, bicarbonate therapy may stimulate lactate production (55). Nonetheless, bicarbonate therapy is frequently provided to the patient with signs of impending fatal acidemia, such as cardiac rhythm instability or refractory hypotension. Hemodialysis and occasionally peritoneal dialysis with lactate-free dialysate may be of some benefit to patients with potentially life-threatening acidemia. Other supportive care should be provided as needed.

G. Future Consideration

Dichloroacetate (DCA) is an agent that may be of some clinical benefit to patients with malignancy-associated lactic acidosis. This agent acts to increase the activity of the enzyme complex pyruvate dehydrogenase, which in turn decreases pyruvate and lactate levels. A recently reported prospective randomized placebo-controlled clinical trial using DCA to treat patients with lactic acidosis and shock showed a decrease in lactate levels but no survival benefit from DCA (60). These results may not apply to patients with malignancy-induced type B lactic acidosis.

VI. HYPOGLYCEMIA

A. Definition and Incidence

Hypoglycemia, a decrease in the serum glucose concentration, is an uncommon complication of malignancy that can be dramatic and dangerous. Whipple's triad describes the diagnostic criteria: symptoms compatible with hypoglycemia, low serum glucose concentration, and resolution of symptoms with normalization of the serum glucose level (56). Although different authors and laboratories may disagree regarding the magnitude of the measured glucose concentration required for a diagnosis of hypoglycemia, most authors agree that an overnight fasting glucose level below 45 mg/dl (2.5 mM) is clearly abnormal, whereas those levels above 55 mg/dl (3.0 mM) are usually considered normal. Because the syndrome is so uncommon, incidence data are unknown.

B. Pathophysiology and Clinical Manifestation

Hypoglycemia occurs as a result of dysfunction of the normal homeostatic mechanisms that precisely regulate the blood glucose concentration. In the fasting state, hypoglycemia normally does not occur as a result of a fall in the serum insulin level from the postprandial peak elevations and a rise in glucagon levels. Glucagon stimulates hepatic glucose production and inhibits glucose utilization. Other glucose counterregulatory hormones, such as epinephrine, cortisol, and growth hormone, can also act during the fasting state to promote glucose production and limit glucose utilization. Maintenance of normoglycemia is a highly complex phenomenon, and for further information the reader is referred to specialized texts on carbohydrate metabolism (61,62).

The symptoms of hypoglycemia are related either to decreased delivery of glucose to the central nervous system (neuroglycopenia) or to release of epinephrine as a counter-regulatory response. Mild neuroglycopenia may be manifest as headache or hunger. More profound glucose deficits are associated with behavioral changes, confusion, vision problems, motor incoordination, seizures, and coma (63,64). In most cases of cancer-associated hypoglycemia, because the disorder is of slow and gradual onset, the brain has adapted to low glucose levels and symptoms arise only at profoundly low levels. Conversely, patients with a history of poorly controlled diabetes mellitus have hypoglycemic symptoms at relatively higher serum glucose levels (63). Symptoms related to epinephrine release include tachycardia, anxiety, diaphoresis, and palpitations. The symptoms usually abate quickly following return of the serum glucose level to normal (63). Severe and prolonged episodes of hypoglycemia may result in neuronal death or permanent neurological deficits (64).

C. Main Causes

The differential diagnosis of fasting hypoglycemia in the adult is given in Table 4 (65). As a memory aid, these are arranged in accordance with the acronym EXPLAIN. Exogenous causes include the administration of drugs, including insulin, oral hypoglycemic agents, sulfa antibiotics, ethanol, pentamidine (63), and the investigational anticancer drug chloroquinoxaline sulfonamide (66). Pituitary failure contributes to hypoglycemia through inadequate production of either growth hormone or cortisol (caused by the effects of deficient ACTH). Liver failure is associated with hypoglycemia in the end stages of the illness, probably because of inadequate gluconeogenesis (63). Adrenal insufficiency causes hypoglycemia as a result of insufficient production of cortisol or through destruction of the adrenal medulla and impaired epinephrine production (63). Insulinoma, typically a pancreatic islet cell tumor, secretes insulin independently of normal feedback inhibition mechanisms (67). Other neoplasms can be associated with hypoglycemia, especially large mesenchymal tumors. In an adult medical practice, exogenous agents account for the majority of cases of symptomatic hypoglycemia and are usually readily recognized (64). This is probably also true in the practice of general oncology, but hypoglycemia in the patient with insulinoma or non–islet cell tumors deserves special mention.

Approximately 66–80% of insulin-secreting tumors are benign adenomas of the pancreas (67,68). Malignant insulinoma accounts for approximately 10% of the cases, and the remaining 10% of patients with insulinoma have multiple islet cell tumors associated with the multiple endocrine neoplasia syndrome type I (68). Insulinomas cause hypoglycemia because the secretion of insulin fails to be suppressed normally when the serum glucose level is low (67).

Non–islet cell tumors associated with hypoglycemia are usually large masses of mesenchymal histology (i.e., sarcomas or mesotheliomas) and are usually found in the retroperitoneum or mediastinum (69). Although controversial for many years, accumulating data suggest that in many of these cases, the tumors produce and secrete a protein with insulinlike activity (70). The protein insulinlike growth factor II (IGF-II) has been implicated in many of these cases (71).

Table 4 Causes of Hypoglycemia In Cancer Patients

Exogenous agents: insulin, oral hypoglycemics, sulfonylureas, pentamidine, alcohol, salicylates, monoamine oxidase inhibitors, clofibrate
Pituitary insufficiency: inadequate growth hormone and ACTH
Liver failure
Addison's: autoimmune, infectious, or caused by metastatic disease
Insulinoma
Neoplasms: large mesenchymal tumors of abdomen or mediastinum

Although less potent than insulin, this peptide can bind to insulin receptors and mediate many of the effects of endogenous insulin. Not all tumors that produce IGF-II are associated with hypoglycemia; this may be because of the presence in some patients of a circulating protein that binds IGF-II and inhibits its activity (72–74). Other non–islet cell tumors associated with hypoglycemia are hepatocellular carcinoma and adrenal cortical carcinoma (69). The role of IGF-II in these tumors is unknown.

D. Diagnosis

As mentioned, fulfillment of Whipple's triad is required for the diagnosis of hypoglycemia. Identification of the specific etiology begins with a careful history and physical examination to rule out the use of exogenous hypoglycemic agents and a search for obvious signs of endocrine disorders or profound hepatic disease. When these have been excluded, the next step is an evaluation of nonsuppressible insulin secretion.

The determination of nonsuppressible insulin secretion is performed with a fasting test (75). Because this can induce potentially dangerous hypoglycemia and neuroglycopenia, the patient must be closely observed during this test. Supplies for the emergent administration of hypertonic glucose solutions must be on hand. The patient begins the test in the fed state with documentation of normoglycemia. The patient is then monitored throughout a period of fasting with periodic monitoring of the blood glucose level. This is initially performed on an hourly basis. The patient is observed closely for a fall in blood glucose and the onset of hypoglycemic symptoms. As the blood glucose is monitored hourly, simultaneous samples of blood are drawn for determination of serum insulin levels. When symptomatic hypoglycemia has been documented and the specimen for insulin level test is terminated. Some patients develop the hypoglycemia very slowly, and up to 72 h of fasting (with oral water intake permitted) may be required to reveal the metabolic abnormality.

The results of this test require careful evaluation (75,76). The absolute insulin concentration in the patient with an insulinoma may not exceed the normal range. In the patient with hypoglycemia, however, these values may be inappropriately high. Some authors have recommended calculation of the insulin-glucose ratio (mU/ml of immunoreactive insulin divided by mg/dl of glucose), a normal ratio being less than 0.3 (76). The finding of inappropriate insulin secretion should lead to a search for a pancreatic tumor.

For a patient who fulfills Whipple's triad in the absence of inappropriately secreted insulin, a search for other underlying tumors is indicated. Because these other lesions are usually quite large mesenchymal tumors, they are readily identified by computed tomographic scan of the chest, abdomen, or pelvis. Other imaging modalities may also be useful in individual cases. Measurement of serum

IGF-II levels is not considered routine practice and currently would add little to the plan for treatment of an individual patient.

E. Treatment

Optimal management of the hypoglycemia depends on the severity. For acute, profoundly symptomatic cases, after obtaining a specimen for determination of the blood glucose level, hypertonic glucose (50% dextrose) is administered intravenously. This may be followed by intravenous infusions of glucose-containing solutions. Milder cases can often be managed with frequent small meals. Such patients often learn to carry candy or other carbohydrate snacks with them and can ingest a little extra at the earliest onset of symptoms. More severe and prolonged cases may require the infusion of hypertonic glucose-containing fluids, but these are inconvenient for the patient and require frequent monitoring of serum electrolyte levels. For patients with insulinoma, oral diazoxide (200–600 mg daily) may suppress insulin release (67). A long-acting somatostatin analog may also be effective in controlling symptoms in patients with insulinoma (77).

The optimal management of patients with insulinoma or non–islet cell tumors requires antitumor therapy. Whenever possible, excision or surgical debulking should be performed (78). The majority of resected insulinomas do not recur. Resected sarcomas may recur, and if the primary tumor was associated with IGF-II and hypoglycemia, such symptoms may herald recurrence of tumor. If radiotherapy or chemotherapy can induce tumor regression, the hypoglycemia may be diminished in severity.

F. Future Considerations

The prognosis of patients with tumor-associated hypoglycemia depends upon eradication of the underlying tumor. We await the results of ongoing clinical trials in patients with islet cell tumors, sarcomas, and mesotheliomas. As our treatment of these underlying conditions improves, the management of hypoglycemia will be made easier.

VII. HYPOMAGNESEMIA

A. Definition and Incidence

Hypomagnesemia is defined as an abnormally low level of magnesium in the blood. The lower limit of normal varies among laboratories, but 1.3 mM (0.7 mM) is a typical threshold value. In cancer patients, mild, asymptomatic hypomagnesemia is relatively common, occurring in 17% of hospitalized cancer patients in one series (79). Symptomatic hypomagnesemia arises in 10% of patients treated with cisplatin (80). The prevalence of hypomagnesemia in other specific subpopulations of oncology patients remains undetermined.

B. Pathophysiology and Clinical Manifestations

Under normal circumstances, the dietary absorption and excretion of magnesium are well balanced. The average adult diet includes 20–30 mEq (10–20 mmol) per day, of which roughly one-third is absorbed, predominantly in the jejunum and ileum. Dietary absorption increases to 70% in magnesium deficiency states (81), although the mechanisms regulating this adaptation are unknown (82).

Excretion in the urine is regulated by tubular reabsorption. Approximately 30% of filtered magnesium is reabsorbed in the proximal convoluted tubule and 60% in the loop of Henle (81). Normally, about 5% of the filtered magnesium load is excreted in the urine. Magnesium infusions lead to increased urinary magnesium excretion, and decreased magnesium intake leads to diminished renal excretion (81).

Magnesium is an important intracellular cation (81). It is a cofactor required for the function of several enzyme systems and maintains the structural integrity of DNA, RNA, and ribosomes. The parathyroid gland requires magnesium for proper function, and magnesium depletion is association with decreased parathyroid hormone secretion and resistance of bone to parathyroid hormone action, leading to hypocalcemia (82). For incompletely understood reasons, hypomagnesemia often leads to renal potassium wasting and hypokalemia (81). This hypokalemia is usually refractory to therapy until the hypomagnesemia is corrected (82).

Hypomagnesemia can lead to neuromuscular irritability. This is clinically manifest as weakness, tremors, fasciculations, seizure, or coma. Trousseau's sign may be seen, but usually with coexistent hypocalcemia (81). Electrocardiographic abnormalities associated with hypomagnesemia include prolongation of PR and QT intervals and flattening of the T wave and are probably secondary to the associated hypocalcemia and hypokalemia (38). Dysrhythmias associated with hypomagnesemia include supraventricular and hypokalemia (38). Dysrhythmias associated with hypomagnesemia include supraventricular and ventricular tachycardias. Magnesium sulfate infusion is one of the treatments of choice for torsades de pointes (83). Cardiac toxicity from digitalis is exacerbated by magnesium deficiency (38,82).

C. Main Causes

In the general population, hypomagnesemia is associated with a variety of etiologies, outlined in Table 5, any of which can coexist in the patient with cancer. In the cancer population, the more common of these are related to alcoholism, decreased intake (because of anorexia or dysphagia), decreased gut

Table 5 Causes of Hypomagnesemia Among Cancer Patients

Diminished oral absorption
Alcoholism
Anorexis emesis
Nasogastric suction
Enteric fistula
Prior resection of small intestine
Inadequate parenteral nutrition formulation
Renal wasting
Cisplatin
Aminoglycosides
Amphotericin

absorption (short bowel syndrome, laxative abuse, biliary or enteric fistulas, or nasogastric suction), inadequate replacement in parenteral nutrition mixtures (84), or renal wasting (caused by diuretics, aminoglycosides, or cisplatin).

Cisplatin is well known to cause hypomagnesemia. In a study of 50 patients, 100% had an abnormally low magnesium level 3 months after starting cisplatin (80). In this study, the rate of onset of hypomagnesemia, but not the eventual severity of the abnormality, was related to the dose of platinum. This may be related to the vascular effects of platinum: modulation of intrarenal hemodynamics with a dopaminergic prodrug diminished renal wasting in one clinical study (85). Renal tubular necrosis or dysfunction is not required for the development of magnesium wasting after platinum (86). Magnesium is excreted despite a fall in the serum level to below normal. The effect can persist for many years after discontinuation of platinum therapy (87). Concomitant use of aminoglycosides or amphotericin with cisplatin may exacerbate the hypomagnesemia (88).

D. Diagnosis

The diagnosis of hypomagnesemia is readily made by determination of the serum magnesium level. Attribution of symptoms to hypomagnesemia is often more difficult, because patients typically have other electrolyte abnormalities and other clinical disorders that could contribute to the nonspecific signs and symptoms caused by hypomagnesemia. Resolution of clinical symptoms after replacement of magnesium provides additional indirect evidence of a causal role for hypomagnesemia in a given patient's symptom complex. Although the urinary magnesium output can be measured and may provide insight into the etiology of hypomagnesemia for a particular patient, this test seldom provides information useful in formulating a treatment plan.

E. Treatment

The mainstay of treatment of hypomagnesemia is increased intake, either oral or parenteral. For asymptomatic and mild cases, patients may require no therapy, and resumption of a normal diet may provide adequate replacement. For patients with platinum-associated or other renal wasting syndromes, chronic magnesium supplementation may be required. This may be given as magnesium sulfate at a rate of 1 g per hour. Seldom is more than 4 g required to reverse acute symptoms (83). Intramuscular magnesium sulfate may also be given in doses of 2–4 g but this is painful and should be avoided when possible. Oral magnesium replacement can be given to asymptomatic patients and is available in several preparations. One of these is magnesium oxide, which is available in 200 and 400 mg tablets that may be taken up to four times daily. Dose-related diarrhea may interfere with patient compliance with oral magnesium replacement (89).

The serum magnesium level may not rise immediately after initiation of replacement therapy. Several days of treatment may be required before the serum level rises into the normal range. Caution should be exercised when providing magnesium replacement to patients with renal insufficiency, because they may easily develop hypermagnesemia.

F. Prevention

Symptomatic hypomagnesemia can be prevented. Routine determination of the serum magnesium level in patients with poor dietary intake or absorption often finds asymptomatic patients with hypomagnesemia. Patients receiving cisplatin, aminoglycosides, or amphotericin should all have the magnesium level determined periodically. Some authors suggest that oral magnesium should be provided to all patients treated with cisplatin, and indeed this approach has been shown to be effective in preventing hypomagnesemia in this population (90). In patients with normal renal function, this strategy is safe, because any excess absorbed magnesium is quickly excreted into the urine. Finally, in patients receiving parenteral nutrition, the magnesium level must be periodically checked and replacement provided as needed.

REFERENCES

1. Bajorunas DR. Clinical manifestations of cancer-related hypercalcemia. Semin Oncol 1990; 17(2 suppl. 5):16–25.
2. Anderson RJ, Chung H-M, Kluge R, et al. Hyponatremia: a prospective analysis of its epidemiology and the pathogenetic role of vasopressin. Ann Intern Med 1985; 102:164–168.
3. Scheiner E, Isaacs M, Vanamee P. Water and electrolyte disturbances in cancer patients. Med Clin North Am 1976; 50:711–732.

4. Reeves WB, Andreoli TE. The posterior pituitary and water metabolism. In: Wilson JD, Foster DW, eds. Williams Textbook of Endocrinology. Philadelphia: W. B. Saunders, 1992:311–348.
5. Narins RG, Jones ER, Stom MC, et al. Diagnostic strategies in disorders of fluid, electrolyte and acid-base homeostasis. Am J Med 1982; 72:496–520.
6. Robertson GL, Berl T. Water metabolism. In: Brenner BM, Rector FC, eds. The Kidney. Philadelphia: W. B. Saunders, 1986:385–423.
7. Berl T, Anderson RJ, McDonald KM, et al. Clinical disorders of water metabolism. Kidney Int 1976; 10:117–132.
8. Perez E, Hutchison F, Gandara D, et al. Cisplatin-induced salt wasting nephropathy: clinical and laboratory parameters (meeting abstract). Proc Annu Meet Am Soc Clin Oncol 1987; 6:A1043.
9. Taveroff A, McArdle AH, Alton-Mackay M, et al. Hyponatremia associated with fecal sodium loss following intensive cytotoxic therapy (meeting abstract). Proc Annu Meet Am Soc Clin Oncol 1988; 7:A1096.
10. Verbalis JG. Tumoral hyponatremia (editorial). Arch Intern Med 1986; 146:1686–1687.
11. Waldman R, Narins RG. Hyponatremia: an approach to differential diagnosis and therapy. Del Med J 1982; 54:169–175.
12. Glover DJ, Glick JH. Metabolic oncologic emergencies. CA 1987; 37(5):302–320.
13. Osterman J, Calhoun A, Dunham M, et al. Chronic syndrome of inappropriate antidiuretic hormone secretion and hypertension in a patient with olfactory neuroblastoma. Arch Intern Med 1986; 146:1731–1735.
14. Odell WD, Appleton WS. Humoral manifestations of cancer. In: Wilson JD, Foster DW, eds. Williams Textbook of Endocrinology. Philadelphia: W. B. Saunders, 1992:1599–1624.
15. Greco FA, Richardson RL, Hande KR, et al. Treatment of inappropriate secretion of antidiuretic hormone in small cell lung cancer. Clin Res 1979; 27:385.
16. Defronzo RA, Braine H, Colvin M, et al. Water intoxication in man after cyclophosphamide therapy. Time course and relation to drug activation. Ann Intern Med 1973; 78:861–869.
17. Defronzo RA, Colvin OM, Braine H, et al. Cyclophosphamide and the kidney. Cancer 1974; 33:483–491.
18. Hantman D, Rossier B, Zohlman R, et al. Rapid correction of hyponatremia in the syndrome of inappropriate secretion of antidiuretic hormone. Ann Intern Med 1973; 78:870–875.
19. Oldham RK, Pomeroy TC. Vincristine-induced syndrome of inappropriate secretion of antidiuretic hormone. South Med J 1972; 65:1010–1012.
20. Wakem CJ, Bennett JM. Inappropriate antidiuretic hormone secretion associated with massive vincristine overdosage. Aust NZJ Med 1975; 5:266–269.
21. Bennett CL, Vogelzang NJ, Ratain MJ, et al. Hyponatremia and other toxic effects during a phase I trial of recombinant human gamma interferon and vinblastine. Cancer Treat Rep 1986; 70:1081–1084.
22. Rufener C, Nordman J, Rouiller C. Effet de la vincristine sur l'hypophyse pòsterieure de rat in vitro. Neurochirurgie 1972; 18:137–141.
23. Greenbaum-Lefkoe B, Rosenstock JG, Belasco JB, et al. Syndrome of inappropriate

antidiuretic hormone secretion. A complication of high-dose intravenous melphalan. Cancer 1985; 55:44–46.
24. Whitehead RP, Friedman KD, Clark DA. A phase I trial of sc interleukin-2 and interleukin-4 (meeting abstract). Proc Annu Meet Am Assoc Cancer Res 1992; 33:A1381.
25. Fer MF, McKinney TD, Richardson RL, et al. Cancer and the kidney: renal complications of neoplasms. Am J Med 1981; 71(4):704–718.
26. Sterns RH. Severe symptomatic hyponatremia: treatment and outcome. A study of 64 cases. Ann Intern Med 1987; 107:656–664.
27. Trump DL. Serious hyponatremia in patients with cancer: management with demeclocycline. Cancer 1981; 47:2908–2912.
28. Forrest JN, Cox M, Hong C, et al. Superiority of demeclocycline over lithium in the treatment of chronic syndrome of inappropriate secretion of antidiuretic hormone. N Engl J Med 1978; 298:173–177.
29. Berl T. Treating hyponatremia: what is all the controversy about? Ann Intern Med 1990; 113:417–419.
30. Hantman D, Rossier B, Zohlman R, et al. Rapid correction of hyponatremia in the syndrome of inappropriate secretion of antidiuretic hormone. An alternative treatment to hypertonic saline. Ann Intern Med 1973; 78:870–875.
31. Ayus JC, Krothapalli RK, Arieff AI. Changing concepts in treatment of severe symptomatic hyponatremia: rapid correction and possible relation to central pontine myelinolysis. Am J Med 1985; 78:897–902.
32. Cohen LF, Balow JE, Magrath IT, et al. Acute tumor lysis syndrome. A review of 37 patients with Burkitt's lymphoma. Am J Med 1980; 68:486–491.
33. Stark ME, Dyer MCD, Coonley CJ. Fatal acute tumor lysis syndrome with metastatic breast cancer. Cancer 1987; 60:762–764.
34. Ettinger DS, Harker WG, Gerry HW, et al. Hyperphosphatemia, hypocalcemia, and transient acute renal failure. Results of cytotoxic treatment of acute lymphoblastic leukemia. JAMA 1978; 239:2472–2474.
35. Monballyu J, Zachee P, Verberckmoes R, et al. Transient acute renal failure due to tumor-lysis-induced severe phosphate load in a patient with Burkitt's lymphoma. Clin Nephrol 1984; 22:47–50.
36. German DC, Holmes EW. Hyperuricemia and gout. Med Clin North Am 1986; 70:419–436.
37. Fer MF, Bottino GC, Sherwin SA, et al. Atypical tumor lysis syndrome in a patient with T-cell lymphoma treated with recombinant leukocyte interferon. Am J Med 1984; 77:953–956.
38. Rardon DP, Fisch C. Electrolytes and the heart. In: Hurst JW, Schlant RC, eds. The Heart Arteries and Veins. New York: McGraw-Hill, 1993:1557–1565.
39. Bates B. A Guide to Physical Examination, 3rd ed. Philadelphia: J. B. Lippincott, 1983.
40. Garnick MB, Mayer RJ. Acute renal failure associated with neoplastic disease and its treatment. Semin Oncol 1978; 5:155–164.
41. Monballyu J, Zachee P, Verberckmoes R, et al. Transient acute renal failure due to tumor-lysis-induced severe phosphate load in a patient with Burkitt's lymphoma. Clin Nephrol 1984; 22:47–50.

42. Brezis M, Rosen S, Epstein FH. Acute renal failure. In: Brenner BM, Rector FC, eds. The Kidney. Philadelphia: W. B. Saunders, 1986:735.
43. Band P. Xanthine nephropathy in a patient with lymphosarcoma treated with allopurinol. N Engl J Med 1970; 283:345.
44. Kreisberg RA. Lactate homeostasis and lactic acidosis. Ann Intern Med 1980; 92(part 1):227–237.
45. Sculier JP, Nicause C, Klastersky J. Lactic acidosis: a metabolic complication of extensive metastatic cancer. Eur J Cancer Clin Oncol 1983; 19:597–601.
46. Doolittle GC, Wurster MW, Rosenfeld CS, et al. Malignancy-induced lactic acidosis. South Med J 1988; 81:533–536.
47. Caspar CB, Oelz O. Lactic acidosis in malignant lymphoma (letter). Am J Med 1991; 91:197–198.
48. Evans TR, Stein RC, Ford HT, et al. Lactic acidosis. A presentation of metastatic breast cancer arising in pregnancy. Cancer 1992; 69:453–456.
49. Archer S, Bache-Wiig B. Lactic acidosis B associated with solid tumors. Minn Med 1986; 69:511–514.
50. Rovelli A, Bonomi M, Murano A, et al. Severe lactic acidosis due to thiamine deficiency after bone marrow transplantation in a child with acute monocytic leukemia (letter). Haematologica (Paris) 1990; 75:579–581.
51. Oriot D, Wood C, Gottesman R, et al. Severe lactic acidosis related to acute thiamine deficiency. J Parenter Enter Nutr 1991; 15:105–109.
52. Madias NE, Goorno WE, Herson S. Severe lactic acidosis as a presenting feature of pheochromocytoma. Am J Kidney Dis 1987; 10:250–253.
53. Bornemann M, Hill SC, Kidd GS. Lactic acidosis in pheochromocytoma. Ann Intern Med 1986; 105:880–882.
54. Chillar RK, Belman MJ. Pseudohypoxia due to leukemia and thrombocytosis. N Engl J Med 1980; 302:584.
55. Fraley DS, Adler S, Bruns FJ, et al. Stimulation of lactate production by administration of bicarbonate in a patient with a solid neoplasm and lactic acidosis. N Engl J Med 1980; 303:1100–1103.
56. Whipple AO, Frantz VK. Adenoma of islet cells with hyperinsulinism. Ann Surg 1935; 101:1299–1335.
57. Vandermolen LA, Swain S, Longo DL. Lactic acidosis in lymphoma: prompt resolution of acidosis with therapy directed at the lymphoma (letter). J Natl Cancer Inst 1988; 80:1077–1078.
58. Colman LK, Baker TM. Lactic acidosis with extensive oak cell carcinoma of lung—not necessarily a poor prognostic sign. Case report. Milit Med 1983; 148:440.
59. Rice K, Schwartz S. Lactic acidosis with small cell carcinoma, rapid response to chemotherapy. Am J Med 1985; 79:501–503.
60. Stacpoole PW, Wright EC, Baumgartner TG, et al. A controlled trial of dichloroacetate for treatment of lactic acidosis in adults. N Engl J Med 1992; 327:1564–1569.
61. Gerich JE, Campbell PJ. Overview of counterregulation and its abnormalities in diabetes mellitus and other conditions. Diabetes Metab Rev 1988; 4:93–111.
62. Defronzo RA. Lilly Lecture 1987. The triumvirate: B-cell, muscle, liver. Diabetes 1988; 37:667–687.

63. Cryer PE. Glucose homeostasis and hypoglycemia. In: Wilson JD, Foster DW, eds. Williams Textbook of Endocrinology. Philadelphia: W. B. Saunders, 1992:1223.
64. Malouf R, Brust JCM. Hypoglycemia: causes, neurological manifestations, and outcome. Ann Neurol 1985; 17:421–430.
65. Gale E. Causes of hypoglycaemia. Br J Hosp Med 1985; 33(3):159–162.
66. Rigas JR, Kris MG, Tong W, et al. Phase I trial of chloroquinoxaline sulfonamide (cqs): a unique agent selected for study based on activity in an in vitro stem cell assay (meeting abstract). Proc Annu Meet Am Assoc Cancer Res 1992; 33:A3160.
67. Boden G. Insulinoma and glucagonoma. Semin Oncol 1987; 14:253.
68. Fajans SS, Floyd JC. Diagnosis and medical management of insulinomas. Annu Rev Med 1979; 30:313–329.
69. Gorden P, Hendricks CM, Kahn CR, et al. Hypoglycemia associated with non-islet-cell tumor and insulin-like growth factors. A study of the tumor types. N Engl J Med 1981; 305:1452–1455.
70. Clark AJ. Glucose homeostasis. Jung RT, Sikora K, eds. Endocrine Problems in Cancer. Molecular Basis and Clinical Management. Heinemann Medical Books, 1984:71–88.
71. Daughaday WH, Emanuele MA, Brooks MH. Synthesis and secretion of insulin-like growth factor II by a leiomyosarcoma with associated hypoglycemia. N Engl J Med 1988; 319:1434–1440.
72. Zapf J, Schmid C, Guler HP, et al. Regulation of binding proteins for insulin-like growth factors (IGF) in humans. Increased expression of IGF binding protein 2 during IGF I treatment of healthy adults and in patients with extrapancreatic tumor hypoglycemia. J Clin Invest 1990; 86(3):952–961.
73. Baxter RC, Daughaday WH. Impaired formation of the ternary insulin-like growth factor-binding protein complex in patients with hypoglycemia due to nonislet cell tumors. J Clin Endocrinol Metab 1991; 73:696–702.
74. Zapf J, Kiefer M, Merryweather J, et al. Isolation from adult human serum of four insulin-like growth factor (IGF) binding proteins and molecular cloning of one of them that is increased by IGF I administration and in extrapancreatic tumor hypoglycemia. J Biol Chem 1990; 265:14892–14898.
75. Frerichs H, Creutzfeldt W. Hypoglycemia. 1. Insulin secreting tumors. Clin Endocrinol Metab 1976; 5:747.
76. Fajans SS, Floyd JC. Fasting hypoglycemia in adults. N Engl J Med 1976; 294:766–771.
77. Kvols LK, Buck M, Moertel LG. Treatment of metastatic islet cell carcinoma with somatostatin analogue (SMS-201-995). Ann Intern Med 1987; 107:162.
78. Doorneweerd DD, Nuttall FQ. Hypoglycemia in the adult: basic concepts and clinical disorders. Minn Med 1980; 63:513–517.
79. D'Erasmo E, Celi FS, Acca M, et al. Hypocalcemia and hypomagnesemia in cancer patients. Biomed Pharmacother 1991; 45:315–317.
80. Bell DR, Woods RL, Levi JA. Cis-diamminedichloroplatinum-induced hypomagnesemia and renal magnesium wasting. Eur J Cancer Clin Oncol 1985; 21:287–290.
81. Cronin RE, Knochel JP. Magnesium deficiency. Adv Intern Med 1983; 28:509–517.
82. Aurbach GD, Marx SJ, Spiegel, AM. Parathyroid hormone, calcitonin, and the

calciferols. In: Wilson JD, Foster DW, eds. Williams Textbook of Endocrinology. Philadelphia: W. B. Saunders, 1992:1397.
83. Tzivoni D, Banai S, Schuger C, et al. Treatment of torsade de pointes with magnesium sulfate. Circulation 1988; 77:392–397.
84. Frazier TG, Mucha ME, Rush IH, et al. Hypomagnesemia: higher risk using total parenteral nutrition in the treatment of patients with malignancies. J Surg Oncol 1980; 13:35–38.
85. Matheson L, Shearing C, Lee M, et al. Cisplatin nephrotoxicity: modulation by gamma-glutamyl L-dopa (meeting abstract). Proc Annu Meet Am Soc Clin Oncol 1989; 8:A275.
86. Teeling M, Pratt I, Casey B, et al. N-acetyl-beta-d-glucosaminidase (NAG) as an early predictor of renal tubular dysfunction on cisplatin nephrotoxicity (meeting abstract). Proc Annu Meet Am Soc Clin Oncol 1986; 5:52.
87. Schilsky RL, Anderson T. Hypomagnesemia and renal magnesium wasting in patients receiving cisplatin. Ann Intern Med 1979; 90:929–931.
88. Bar RS, Wilson HE, Mazzaferri EL. Hypomagnesemic hypocalcemia secondary to renal magnesium wasting: a possible consequence of high-dose gentamicin therapy. Ann Intern Med 1975; 82:646.
89. Strom M. Antacid side-effects on bowel habits. Scand J Gastroenterol 1982; 17(suppl 75):54–55.
90. Martin M, Diaz-Rubio E, Casado A, et al. Intravenous and oral magnesium supplementations in the prophylaxis of cisplatin-induced hypomagnesemia. Results of a controlled trial. Am J Clin Oncol 1992; 15:348–351.

17

Bone Metastases

Jean-Jacques Body
Institut Jules Bordet, Université Libre de Bruxelles, Brussels, Belgium

Bert Thürlimann
Kantonsspital, St. Gallen, Switzerland

I. MAGNITUDE OF THE PROBLEM

Single-lesion bone involvement in the absence of a known cancer may be caused by primary benign or malignant tumors. The relative frequency of primary bone tumors is listed in Table 1 (1). Metastatic spread is the most common presentation of neoplasm involving the skeleton, however, and multiple bone lesions are usually caused by metastatic dissemination of nonskeletal primary tumors. According to the series, 30–90% of patients with advanced cancer develop skeletal metastases (2). Patients with myeloma and patients with bone metastases caused by tumors with a high incidence, such as breast and prostate cancer, have a relatively long survival after the diagnosis of bone metastases compared with patients with extraosseous metastases only. The median survival is usually beyond 2 years, and about 10% of these patients are still alive 5–10 years after the first diagnosis of bone metastases. Osteolytic bone disease can thus be responsible for considerable morbidity and markedly decrease the quality of life. This must be kept in mind whenever planning the treatment of these patients.

The skeleton is the most common site of metastases in breast and prostate cancers. Breast cancer is the most common cancer in the Northern Hemisphere, and it is expected that 150,000 new cases per year of breast cancer will occur in the United States, in the 1990s (3). On the other hand, prostate cancer is currently the neoplastic disease with the highest number of estimated new cases in males in the United States. It is thus expected that 106,000 new cases per year will be diagnosed. About 30,000 deaths are estimated for 1990, making it

Table 1 Relative Frequency of Primary Bone Tumors

Primary benign bone tumors	%	Primary malignant bone tumors	%
Osteochondroma	12.0	Myeloma	30.0
Gigantocytoma	3.5	Osteogenic sarcoma	18.0
Osteoid-osteoma	3.0	Chondrosarcoma	10.0
Chondroma	2.5	Ewing's sarcoma	5.0
Fibroma	1.2	Malignant lymphoma	5.0
Hemangioma	1.0	(reticulum cell sarcoma)	
Benign osteoblastoma	0.6	Fibrosarcoma	2.5
Chondroblastoma	0.5	Malignant gigantocytoma	0.35
Chondromyxoid fibroma	0.5	Periosteal osteogenic sarcoma	0.30
Neurilemma	0.2	Mesenchymal chondrosarcoma	0.20
Hemangiopericytoma	0.1	Adamantinoma	0.20
Desmoplastic fibroma	0.1	Angiosarcoma	0.10
Lipoma	0.1		

Source: Adapted from Reference 1.

the second leading cause of cancer deaths in men (3). Of these cases 90% will have developed bone metastases during the clinical course. The overall incidence of bone metastases at autopsy of patients with a known primary tumor is shown in Table 2 (1). About 80% of all bone metastases have their origin from breast, lung, or prostate tumors, and more than 50% of these patients will develop bone metastases during the course of the disease. On the other hand, lung, breast, and prostate neoplasms are the most frequent causes of bone metastases in patients with an unknown primary tumor site, as can be seen in Table 3 (1).

II. PATHOPHYSIOLOGY

Although tumor-induced hypercalcemia (TIH) is often secondary to tumor-induced osteolysis (TIO), basic and clinical research has been primarily performed in the area of TIH, the findings of which are being secondarily applied to TIO.

A. Tumor-Induced Hypercalcemia

Increased calcium release from bone constitutes the main pathogenic factor leading to hypercalcemia in cancer patients. Tumor secretory products markedly stimulate osteoclast activity and proliferation, with a frequent inhibition of osteoblast activity, leading to a characteristic uncoupling between bone resorption and bone formation (4). This causes a rapid rise in serum calcium, which contrasts

Table 2 Frequency of Bone Metastases (%) According to Known Primary Tumor at Autopsy (n = 3317)

Breast, female	64.9
Prostate	58.8
Breast, male	50.0
Nasopharyngeal cancer	42.9
Kidney	38.6
Melanoma	35.5
Nasal sinus	33.2
Lung	32.1
Intestine + carcinoid	25.0
Liver	24.5
Cervix uteri	22.1
Bladder	18.1
Adrenal gland	16.7
Thyroid	15.2
Embryonal testis cancer	15.0
Pleural mesothelioma	14.3
Thymoma	14.3
Stomach	14.2
Esophagus	11.4
Larynx	11.1
Pancreas	10.3
Hypopharynx	9.1
Tongue	8.7
Malignant lymphoma	7.3
Ovary	6.2
Gallbladder	5.6
Corpus uteri	5.4
Colon	5.1
Rectum	3.2

Source: Adapted from Reference 1.

with relatively stable levels of serum calcium in primary hyperparathyroidism, in which bone formation is stimulated in parallel with bone resorption. The kidneys can also play a pathogenic role in the genesis and maintenance of TIH through a decrease in the glomerular filtration rate and an increase in the tubular reabsorption of calcium, itself a result of the decreased circulating volume and the specific renal effects of tumoral substances. However, the renal contribution relative to skeletal calcium release is still controversial.

When evaluating the interest in monitoring in TIH or TIO of the cross-linking

Table 3 Bone Metastases of Unknown Primary During Life: Frequency of Primary Tumor at Autopsy (%)

Lung	28.7
Breast, female	21.8
Prostate	11.4
Kidney	5.4
Malignant lymphoma	3.4
Cervix uteri	3.4
Stomach	3.4
Bladder	3.0
Liver	2.6
Colon	1.4
Pancreas	1.2
Melanoma	1.2
Ovary	1.0
Thyroid	1.0

Source: Adapted from Reference 1.

amino acids of collagen (pyridinoline, Pyr, and deoxypyridinoline, D-Pyr), we noted that these new markers of matrix bone resorption were less increased than the urinary excretion of calcium and that they also decreased less after bisphosphonate therapy (5). Coleman et al. similarly observed in patients with breast cancer and TIO that the decrease in Pyr and D-Pyr after oral bisphosphonate therapy was lower than the fall in urinary calcium excretion (6). These findings suggest a preferential removal of bone mineral compared with bone matrix during the process of malignant osteolysis and a similar preferential inhibitory activity of bisphosphonates, but these intriguing possibilities need further evaluation.

TIH is classically divided into three groups. Humoral hypercalcemia of malignancy (HHM) is defined as hypercalcemia occurring without evidence of bone metastases. Its frequency was previously estimated as less than 25%, but this figure is much higher when HHM is defined by biochemical parameters. Hypercalcemia apparently caused by bone metastatic involvement represents the largest group and typically complicates metastatic breast cancer. Hypercalcemia of hematological tumors constitutes a third and distinct group. Although this classification remains useful for teaching purposes, the boundaries between the three types progressively fade, notably because recent studies established the essential role of a parathormone-like substance, parathyroid hormone-related peptide (PTHrP), in all types of TIH.

The key role of PTHrP has been particularly well demonstrated in HHM. The findings of elevated urinary cyclic AMP with low PTH levels in a substantial proportion of hypercalcemic cancer patients provided the impetus for the isolation of a PTH-like factor in the 1980s. Purification of the PTH-like biological activity from tumors associated with HHM permitted the isolation of this new factor. The protein has been purified to homogeneity, sequenced, and cloned (7). PTHrP appears to have a crucial role in skeleton development, but also in the transport of calcium at the breast and placenta levels. Its effects are autocrine or paracrine in nature, and the only endocrine effect discovered so far concerns its pathogenic role in TIH. Several immunoassays have already been developed to measure circulating PTHrP. According to the published series, 46–90% of patients with TIH have increased circulating PTHrP levels (8). Virtually all hypercalcemic patients without bone metastases have elevated PTHrP levels, but with a sensitive assay, Grill et al. showed that this is also the case in two-thirds of patients with hypercalcemia and bone metastases (9). After reviewing all the assays described so far, Burtis concluded that two-site assays, including the measurement of large N-terminal regions, are optimal for TIH evaluation (10). Circulating PTHrP concentrations do not change after successful therapy of TIH with bisphosphonates, implying that elevated PTHrP levels indeed constitute a primary phenomenon and that PTHrP secretion does not appear to be regulated in vivo by serum calcium, at least in hypercalcemic subjects (8).

Cancer hypercalcemia, however, is a heterogeneous syndrome that cannot be fully explained by the ectopic secretion of a single osteolytic factor. As stated earlier, bone formation rate is often depressed in TIH, although PTHrP appears to act through PTH receptors. Also, in opposition to what is observed in primary hyperparathyroidism, circulating calcitriol levels are normal or reduced in patients with TIH, despite that PTHrP infusion in humans produces comparable effects to PTH. It is probable that other factors, such as transforming growth factors (TGFs) or cytokines, play at least a contributory role in many patients. For example, it was recently shown that inoculation into nude mice of Chinese hamster ovarian (CHO) cells transfected with the human TGF-α gene induced hypercalcemia and a marked increase in osteoclastic bone resorption, but no bone formation at sites of previous bone resportion could be observed (11). TGF-α could thus be involved in the inhibition of bone formation and in the uncoupling in bone turnover that are frequently observed in patients with TIH. Cytokines, such as interleukin-1 or tumor necrosis factor α, could also be responsible and could potentiate the hypercalcemic effects of PTHrP, as suggested by some in vitro data.

Cancer cells can thus make several hypercalcemic factors that probably work in concert, and a better delineation of the effects of PTHrP and of other osteotropic factors could come from studies of animals models of TIH in which CHO cells transfected with various peptides cDNAs are inoculated into nude mice (11).

B. Tumor-Induced Osteolysis

The tropism of certain cancers for the skeleton begins to be understood. The interactions between tumor cells and host stromal cells, the selective response of certain tumor cells to locally produced growth factors, and their attachment to basement membranes all play an essential role in this selective metastatic process. It has thus been shown that rat prostate cancer cells preferentially adhere to bone marrow-derived endothelial cells compared with endothelial cells of other organs or nonendothelial bone marrow cells (12). Moreover, in an animal model of lytic bone metastases, an antagonist to laminin, which is a basement membrane glycoprotein, inhibited the development of osteolytic lesions, whereas laminin had an opposite effect (13). The production of osteolytic substances by cancer cells, such as PTHrP, could also be important for the development of metastases in bone.

The pathogenesis of hypercalcemia of metastatic bone disease and of TIO itself have been less investigated than that of HHM, although it is now clear that bone destruction is essentially mediated by osteoclast activation rather than by the direct osteolytic effects of metastatic cancer cells, which would be important only in the late stages of TIO. For example, expression of collagenase by primary human tumors does not correlate with their metastatic potential (14). Moreover, microscopic studies have shown the existence of extensive osteoclastic activity adjacent to the tumor cells in animal models of bone metastases or in human bone invaded by cancer cells. The excellent response of hypercalcemia caused by bone metastases to antiosteoclastic drugs constitutes another important argument for an essential role of osteoclasts in neoplastic osteolysis compared with a directly mediated bone destruction by tumor cells.

The nature of the tumoral factor(s) responsible for osteoclastic activation remains unknown, but recent data indicate that PTHrP could play an essential role here, too. PTHrP-like substances are thus expressed by about 60% of human breast tumors, and circulating PTHrP levels can be elevated in up to two-thirds of patients with hypercalcemia associated with breast cancer and bone metastases (9). Breast tumors metastasizing to the skeleton produce PTHrP more frequently than the tumors metastasizing to nonosseous sites, suggesting a role for PTHrP in the genesis of TIO through stimulation of osteoclastic bone resorption (15). These data have already been confirmed by in situ hybridization techniques that can demonstrate the synthesis of PTHrP mRNA by primary breast tumors and by their metastatic cells. In a preliminary report, PTHrP mRNA was indeed expressed in 8 of 11 breast cancer metastases to bone but in only 3 of 15 metastases to nonbone sites (16).

Osteoclasts could be activated directly by tumor products or indirectly through an influence on other cells. Osteoblasts could well be important target cells for tumor secretory products and thus keep their central role in the control of normal bone metabolism. Evans et al. showed that myeloma cells secrete factor(s) that inhibit the proliferation of normal osteoblast-like cells and affect their differentiation (17). We also recently observed that breast cancer cells secrete factors that can inhibit the proliferation of osteoblastlike cells and apparently increase their sensitivity to osteolytic agents. The nature of the responsible factor(s) remains to be determined, but TGFs could play an important role. The following scheme can thus be tentatively proposed for the genesis of TIO following breast cancer invasion in bone. Local production of PTHrP and of other factors, such as TGFs, by cancer cells in bone would stimulate osteoclastic bone resorption through the osteoblasts, whose proliferation would also be inhibited, explaining the uncoupling in bone turnover. Increased osteoclast activity would cause local foci of osteolysis, which could further stimulate cancer cells proliferation because it is known that products of bone resorption can increase tumor cell growth (18). The reasoning remains speculative, but the data summarized here indicate that it is rational to target bone-resorbing cells for the treatment and prevention of TIO, even if much remains to be learned about the precise pathogenesis of TIO.

The pathogenesis of osteoblastic metastases, for example from prostate cancer, could be quite similar. PTHrP also appears to be produced by prostate cancer cells: recent immunohistochemical studies have found its presence in all 33 prostate tumors (19). Bone resorption is thus increased in patients with osteoblastic metastases from prostate cancer, as shown by biochemical markers. On the other hand, TGF-β probably has a crucial importance for the blastic reaction. It is produced in larger quantities by prostate cancer cells than by benign prostate cells, and the transition from benign prostate hyperplasia to cancer is associated with the induction of elevated TGF-β_1 production, which could be important in prostate cancer development and progression (20). The activation of TGF-β produced by the prostate or the bone tissue itself could be enhanced by prostate-specific antigen, which can also stimulate by itself the proliferation of osteoblastlike cells (21). Last, bone morphogenetic proteins (BMPs) could also play a role in the osteoinductive properties of prostate cancer cells. BMPs are expressed by several prostate cancer cell lines, and with the exception of BMP-5, they are more often expressed in patients with bone metastases than in patients without it (22).

III. CLINICAL PRESENTATION AND COMPLICATIONS

A. Symptomatic Patients

The hallmark of bone metastases is pain. Usually the pain is initially intermittent and related to activity but eventually becomes continuous and worsened by activity. Lumbovertebral metastases often present as low back pain that does not or only temporarily improves after symptomatic treatment. Vertebrae (69%), pelvis

(41%), femur (25%), and skull (14%) are the skeletal sites most commonly involved by metastatic cancer (23). The pattern of involvement is similar for most cancers, but prostate cancer shows predominant involvement of the pelvic bones. The most serious complication of vertebral metastases is epidural compression of the spinal cord. Patients usually complain of increasing back pain, but occasionally spinal cord compression can occur without pain. Any cancer patient with back pain and only the slightest signs of neurological impairment should have adequate radiological examinations to rule out spinal cord compression. Hypercalcemia and fractures constitute other classic complications of metastatic bone disease (see Selected Reading). The clinical presentation of hypercalcemia is reviewed in Chapter 16.

B. Asymptomatic Patients

The frequency of bone metastases depends on the intensity of the search, the primary cancer, and the stage or time within the course of the disease. For example, in breast cancer, bone metastases are detected in less than 1% of patients with T1 tumors, whereas the skeleton is the first site of relapse in almost one-third of cases after the primary treatment (Ref. 24 and Data on File, International Breast Cancer Study Group). At autopsy, bone metastases are discovered in the majority of patients with advanced cancer (Table 2).

Bone relapse as the first site of recurrence after primary treatment for cancer is especially frequent in breast, lung, and prostate cancers. It is thus useful to perform bone scintigraphy in conjunction with computed tomography or magnetic resonance imaging or, more rarely, sonography to allow the early detection and localization of bone lesions in patients with symptoms or signs suggesting metastatic disease. However, the role for these examinations in asymptomatic disease-free patients, for example in breast cancer, is much less clear. Regular bone scans in asymptomatic patients adds only minimal information in the follow-up of these patients. In our experience, such routinely performed bone scans detected only 4% of the relapses in asymptomatic breast cancer patients, whereas 88% of all relapses were discovered by taking the history and/or at the clinical examination. Because treatment of metastatic disease for neoplasms with high incidence, such as breast and prostate cancers, is still palliative, the knowledge about single or several bone lesions in asymptomatic patients is most probably of only marginal value for most clinicans. Even in the follow-up of clinical trials, regular bone scans are frequently no longer required for asymptomatic patients. There is thus no indication so far that early treatment of an asymptomatic systemic disease, beyond hope for cure, will change the course of the disease and/or maintain the quality of life.

C. Patients with Unknown Primary Cancer and Bone Metastases

Some patients present with bone metastases, alone or in conjunction with other metastatic sites, without evidence of a primary tumor. These patients usually present with pain in a bone site or with an unexplained fracture. Bone scans may be positive in 47% of asymptomatic and 88% of symptomatic patients (25). If a fracture is present, it must usually be stabilized by an orthopedic intervention, which will yield tissue that may give a clue to the tumor of origin. A serum protein electrophoresis and/or immunoelectrophoresis can suggest the diagnosis of multiple myeloma, and measurement of various serum tumor markers can also be useful in this situation. For example, elevated levels of prostate-specific antigen can point to a prostatic carcinoma. In this case, predominantly blastic bone lesions are usually seen. Blastic lesions, however, may also be seen in carcinoid tumors and thyroid, ovarian, and stomach cancer and very rarely in other tumors. A mixed blastic and lytic picture is more often seen in breast cancer. Special investigations in the search for the origin of bone metastases should concentrate on tumors that may have a specific therapy, such as prostate cancer, multiple myeloma, or breast or thyroid cancer. In the last case, even a curative approach is possible in some cases. Table 3 shows the frequency of the primary tumor at autopsy in patients presenting with cancer of unknown primary and bone metastases (1).

IV. DIAGNOSIS AND MONITORING OF BONE METASTASES

A. Bone Scintigraphy

Radionucleate imaging of the bone is a sensitive technique for the diagnosis of skeletal metastases. Whole-body imaging is performed with technetium 99m-labeled diphosphonate that is taken up preferentially at sites of increased osteoblastic activity. Osteolytic metastases are usually accompanied by increased osteoblastic repair. This seems especially true for tumors of the breast, prostate, lung, and kidney but is less frequent in myeloma and lymphoma. Therefore, bone scan is less accurate for the diagnosis of bone involvement in these last diseases, and a decreased uptake, called a photopenic lesion, is even frequently observed in multiple myeloma. Neither hot spots nor photopenic lesions are specific for skeletal involvement by cancer, however.

A single lesion of increased activity (hot spot) occurs in 6–8% of all patients with a known cancer. In a study of 273 such cases, 55% were found to represent metastatic disease; 25% were caused by trauma, 10% by infections, and 10% by various nonmalignant causes (26). Of the vertebral lesions, 80% proved to be metastatic compared with only 18% for rib lesions. The appearance of a new spot in a patient with a previously normal scintigraphy, however, is more specific for metastasis. When the bone scan shows a solitary lesion, additional investigations, such as computed tomographic (CT) scans, magnetic resonance imaging (MRI), or even biopsy, are necessary to establish the diagnosis. Figures 1 through 5 show

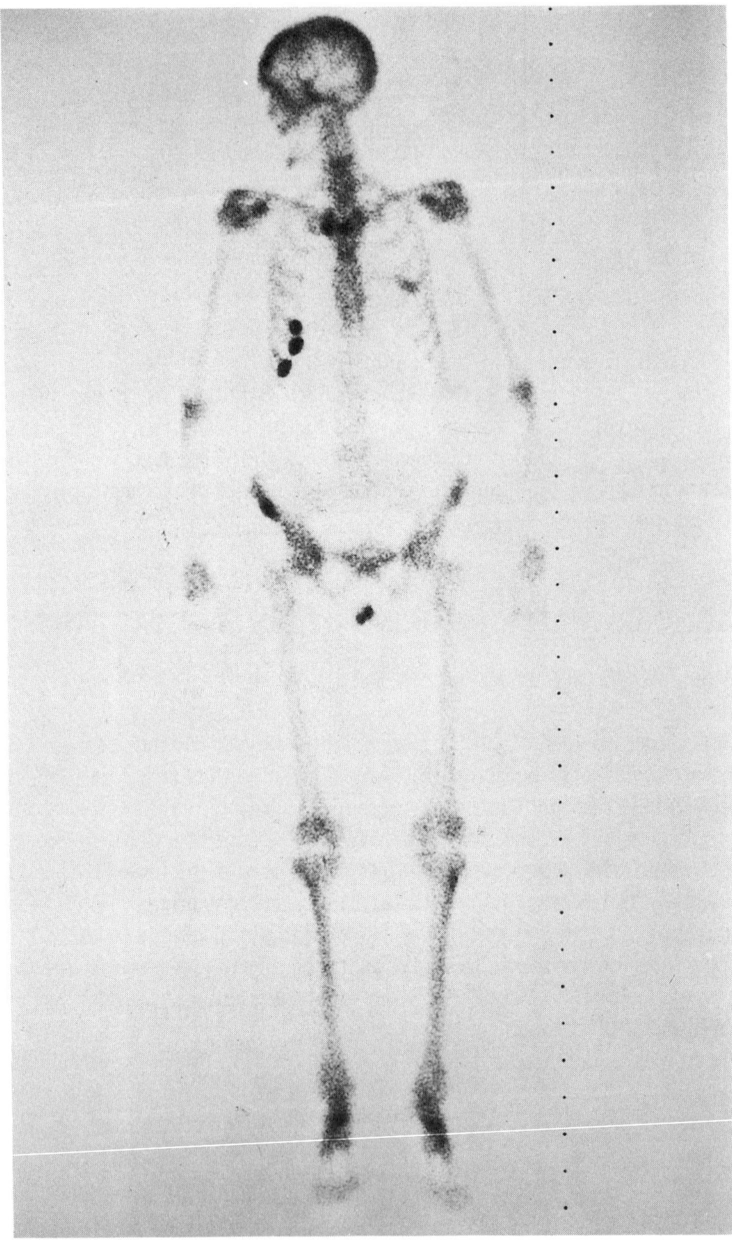

Figure 1 Pathological bone scan with hot spots on the right side in a line: right sternoclavicular joint, ventrolateral ribs, and spina iliaca anterior superior in a patient with breast cancer after she fell from a bicycle.

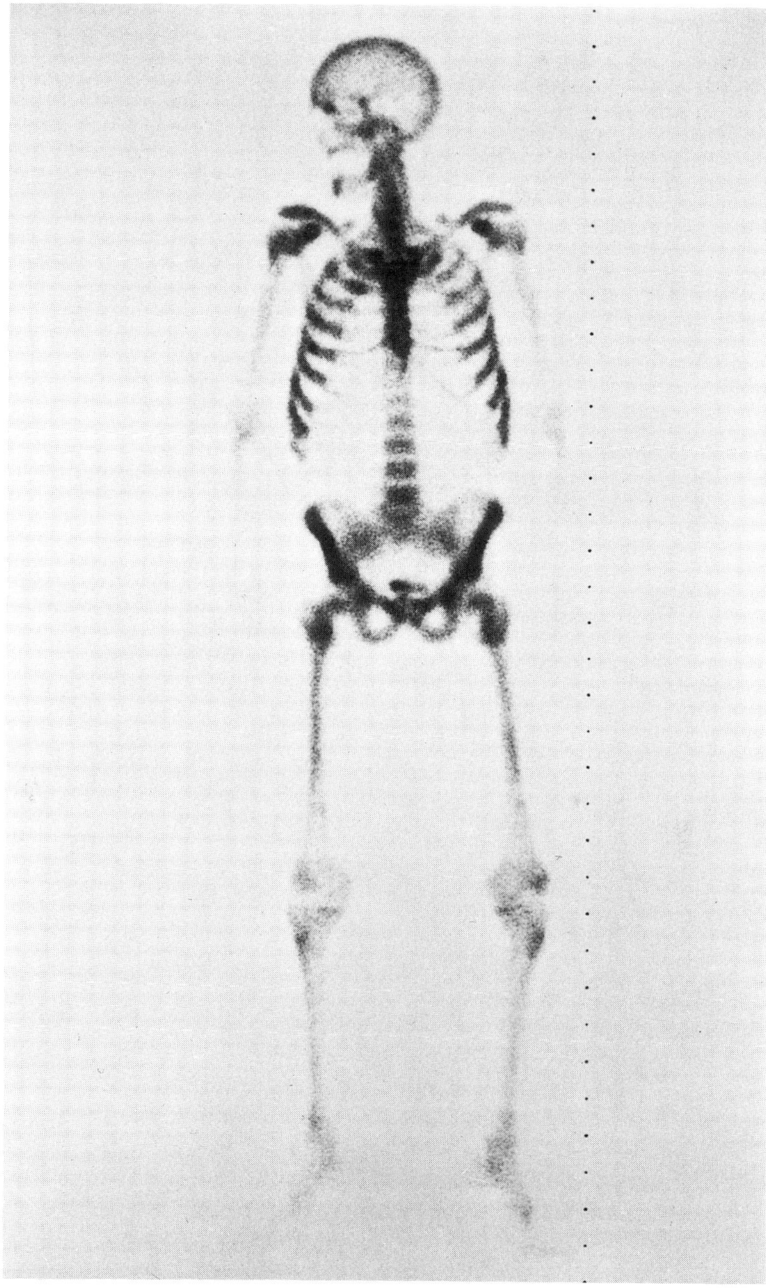

Figure 2 Metastatic prostate cancer with diffuse intense uptake of the radiopharmaceutical: only minor irregularities (left femur) and missing appearance of the kidneys.

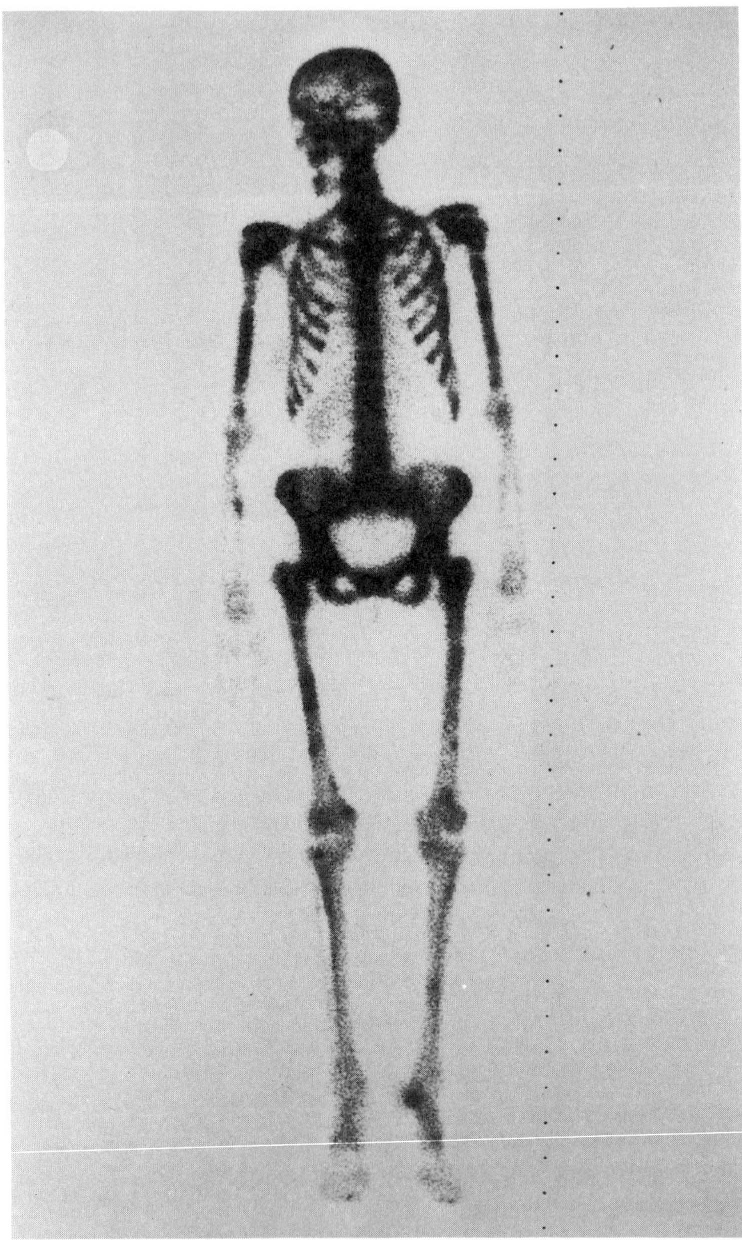

Figure 3 Bone scan of a patient with metastatic breast cancer and extensive diffuse bone and bone marrow involvement; the right kidney is not seen (and agenesis of the left kidney).

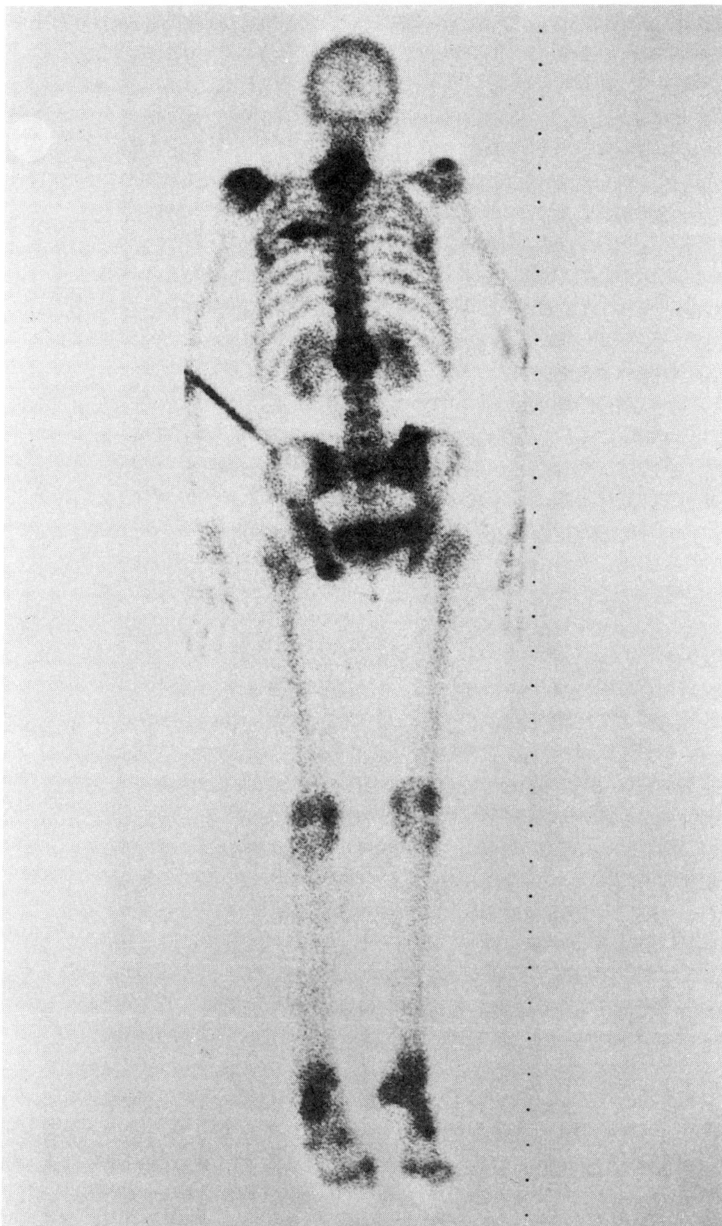

Figure 4 Bone scan of a patient with metastatic breast cancer and bone metastases with complete destruction of cervical and lower thoracic and lumbar vertebrae (seen on x-ray) and spinal cord compression. Note right urinary catheter.

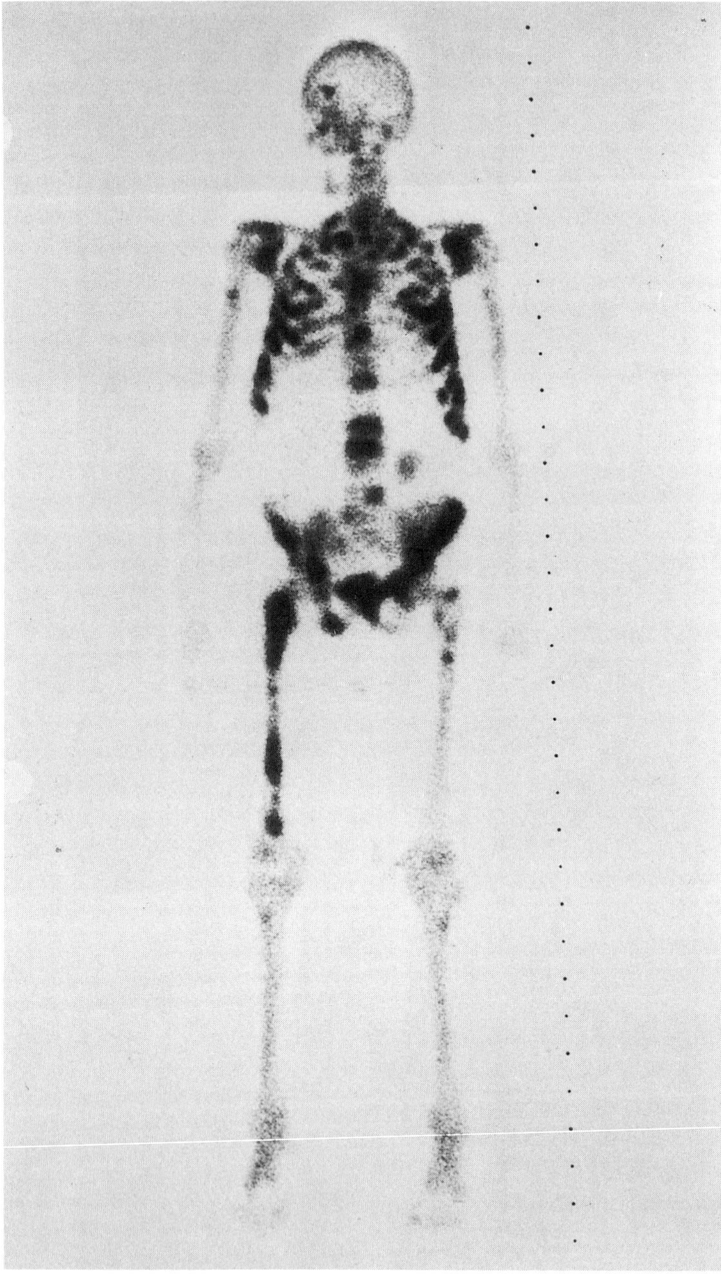

Figure 5 Bone scan of a patient with metastatic prostate cancer with extensive patchy but not diffuse metastatic disease.

examples of pathological bone scintigraphies (Institute of Nuclear Medicine, Kantonsspital, St. Gallen).

B. Radiography

Radiographs of hot spots or photopenic lesions detected by the bone scan facilitate differentiation of metastatic disease from other causes. In many instances no further tests may be required. As mentioned, the most common sites of metastases are the spine, pelvis, and femur. If the long bones are involved, the metaphyseal area is preferentially affected. Appreciation of the tumor size and shape and the possible multiplicity of the lesions enables the diagnosis of metastatic disease. Extraosseous extention rarely occurs in metastatic cancer but is characteristic of primary sarcomas of the bone. Primary multiple bony lesions may also be found, however, in histiocytosis, fibrous dysplasia, bone cysts, and compacta islands. At least 30% of the mineral bone must be replaced by soft tissue before an osteolytic lesion becomes apparent on plain x-rays, which explains the lack of sensitivity of the technique. The classic full bone survey is rarely necessary but remains valuable in myeloma patients, because bone scanning frequently does not give adequate information on the extent of bone involvement.

C. Computed Tomography

Computed tomography has been shown to be of value in confirming or excluding metastatic disease in the presence of hot spots on the bone scan. It is especially helpful if a single lesion is present (23) and/or plain radiographs are normal, particularly at the level of the spine. CT scans are also very useful to evaluate the extraskeletal manifestations of bone metastases, which is of special importance if other organs are affected. CT scans in these cases can detect early spinal cord compression or tumor involvement of neural structures (27). The treatment may be changed accordingly, by enlarging radiotherapy fields, for example.

D. Magnetic Resonance Imaging

Magnetic resonance imaging is of special value for evaluating the medullary component of bone. This is of special importance because most metastases start to grow in the spongiosa compartment. The infiltration leads to a higher cellularity and to a higher water content than in the normal marrow, which consists mainly of fat. Neoplastic tissue appears as a darker area on T1-related images. MRI is especially of value in diseases that involve the marrow compartment for a long time before invading the bone tissue itself. This is the case in myeloma, lymphoma, and leukemias (28,29). In a series of patients with multiple myeloma, MRI had a sensitivity of 100% (all cases confirmed by needle aspiration) compared with 20% for bone scan and 67% for radiographs (29).

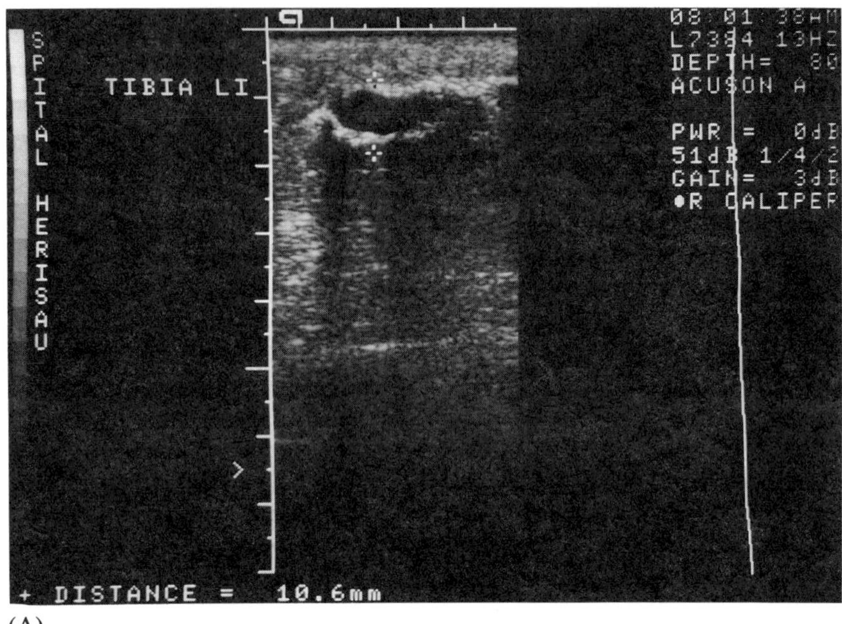

(A)

Figure 6 Ultrasound image (A) and corresponding x-ray (B) of a bone metastasis in the left tibia in a patient with brain and skeletal metastases of unknown primary. Cytological examination of fine-needle aspiration from the tibia showed oat cell carcinoma.

Compared with CT, MRI may be more sensitive in detecting bone involvement, especially in the spongiosa compartment, but extensive use of MRI investigations is restricted by its availability and cost and the necessity for the patient to stay in the machine without movement for a prolonged time. This can be difficult for many patients with bone metastases. Sonography can also sometimes be helpful to establish the diagnosis in certain locations (Fig. 6). The diagnosis of metastatic disease can be facilitated if a soft tissue structure can be identified within the bone picture.

E. Biochemical Markers

Traditionally, serum calcium and alkaline phosphatase have been used to monitor the skeleton as a possible site of relapse. However, serum calcium and alkaline phosphatase are frequently normal in patients with discrete bone metastatic involvement. Increased levels of alkaline phosphatase are found in patients with mixed or purely osteoblastic bone metastases. The differentiation between hepatic and bone sources can be made either by analysis of a second

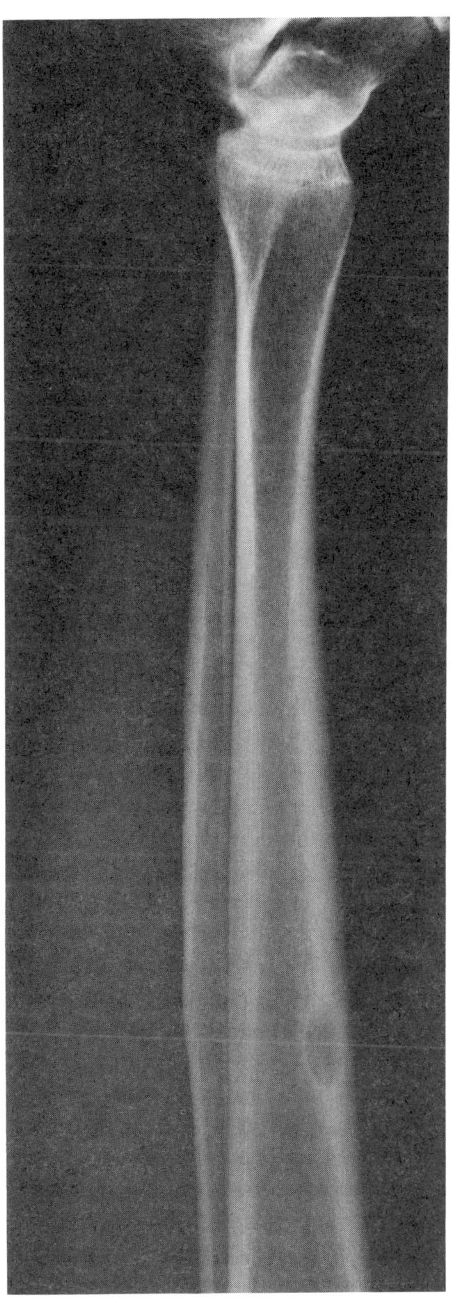

(B)

mainly cholestatic enzyme, such as gammaglutamyltransferase or leucinaminopeptidase. If both liver and bone are involved, isoenzyme electrophoresis can be performed to establish the relative contribution of hepatic and bone fractions of alkaline phosphatase. Classic biochemical parameters (with the exception of tumor markers) add actually very little to the diagnosis of a first relapse in the skeleton. The sensitivity of biochemical parameters has been shown to be inferior compared with that of bone scanning, so far, but sequential determinations of abnormal laboratory parameters, such as alkaline phosphatase, may be of value for monitoring disease activity and treatment efficacy. However, an initial rise in alkaline phosphatase levels after initiation or change of a systemic treatment does not mean by itself that the patient has progressive disease. A rise in alkaline phosphatase levels can as well indicate a higher activity of osteoblastic repair, which may be followed by clinically detectable tumor regression. The same is true for tumor markers but probably to a much lesser extent. A rise in tumor marker levels usually indicates progressive disease but, when occurring early, can also be the consequence of increased tumor lysis. On the other hand, rising levels of tumor markers often indicate disease progression or relapse weeks to months before becoming apparent clinically or by other investigations.

The utility of tumor markers for monitoring metastatic bone disease has been largely underevaluated so far. A simple and cheap method for monitoring bone metabolism, especially the balance between osteoblastic and osteoclastic activity, is the analysis of the calcium/creatine ratio in the second morning spot urine. Obviously this sample must be obtained without prior alimentary intake of calcium (overnight fast). Other parameters, such as alkaline phosphatase, osteocalcin, and hydroxyproline, are usually less reliable. Osteocalcin and alkaline phosphatase also represent mainly osteoblastic activity and may be used for monitoring patients with mainly osteoblastic bone metastases. Because most patients with exclusive osteoblastic activity do not develop clinically relevant bone-associated complications, monitoring of osteoblastic activity and bone metabolism is often not required.

The measurement of the pyridinoline crosslinks, pyridinoline and deoxypyridinoline, was recently introduced. Both are crosslinks of the fully built type I collagen and are eliminated unmetabolized by the kidney. They appear to have a higher sensitivity and specificity than hydroxyproline for osteoporosis, but their definite role for monitoring bone metabolism has yet to be determined. Recent studies in cancer patients did not establish the superiority of these new tests (5,6) compared with the calcium/creatinine ratio. Other markers of bone turnover are being developed, but more investigations are needed in cancer patients to know their value in monitoring bone metabolism, and urinary calcium and hydropyproline creatinine ratios in the second morning fasting urine remain the standard.

V. THERAPY

A. Treatment of Tumor-Induced Hypercalcemia

Cancer is the most frequent cause of hypercalcemia in hospitalized patients, whereas primary hyperparathyroidism is the leading cause in ambulatory patients. The differential diagnosis between TIH and primary hyperparathyroidism has been much simplified since the availability of assays specifically measuring intact parathyroid hormone. These assays permit a complete separation of PTH levels in the two conditions. Serum PTH concentrations are indeed elevated, or at least in the upper part of the normal range, in hyperparathyroid patients, whereas they are suppressed in patients with TIH. Primary hyperparathyroidism is not a rare disease, however, and both conditions can coexist, particularly in that an increased incidence of cancer has been previously reported in hyperparathyroid patients. On the other hand, as summarized earlier, commercial assays for PTHrP are now available and measurement of both PTH and PTHrP can be quite useful in a few patients for a correct differential diagnosis of hypercalcemia. The choice of the initial treatment for a hypercalcemic cancer patient is little influenced by this differential diagnosis, however.

1. Classic Therapeutic Means for TIH

An effective antineoplastic treatment remains the ideal means to obtain long-term control of serum calcium, but a marked reduction in the tumor burden is often not attainable, because hypercalcemia generally complicates advanced and refractory cancer. Forced saline diuresis with 6 liters or more per 24 h, combined with large doses of furosemide, must now be considered a risky and outdated procedure, but rehydration with intravenous saline should still be part of the initial therapeutic approach to the hypercalcemic cancer patient. Rehydration with saline infusions to restore the circulating volume only moderately reduces calcium levels, effecting a median decrease of only 1.0 mg/dl (30), but it interrupts the vicious circle of TIH by inhibiting the increased tubular reabsorption of calcium following hypovolemia. Moreover, rehydration improves the patient's clinical status, because several symptoms of hypercalcemia are caused or increased by the reduced circulating volume. Diuretics must only be administered after circulating volume has been restored if there are signs or risks of fluid overload.

Corticosteroids are still prescribed too often in TIH; their efficacy is actually limited to hematological malignancies. Intravenous administration of phosphate no longer has any place in the management of TIH because of the risks of extraskeletal calcium precipitation and renal insufficiency. Oral administration of phosphate (1–3 g elemental phosphorus) is certainly preferable, but its efficacy is limited by digestive secondary effects and is confined to hypophosphatemic patients with mild hypercalcemia.

The pathogenesis of TIH dictates that priority be given to agents that potently decrease bone resorption. Specific antiosteolytic therapy can be started simultaneously with rehydration (31). Calcitonin is a natural antiosteoclastic hormone, and its main advantages are a rapid onset of action and a negligible toxicity. It has, moreover, a calciuretic effect that contributes to its hypocalcemic activity (32). Recommended doses vary from 2 to 8 U/kg two to four times daily. However, the efficacy of calcitonin in TIH is variable, partial, and transient. Serum calcium usually starts to rise again after a few days, and there is no further response to an increase in the dose. Mithramycin (plicamycin) is another active antiosteoclastic agent, but its use is much limited by major potential toxicities, particularly when the administration is repeated. Plicamycin still has some defenders, but its use in TIH should progressively disappear. A recent randomized trial against the bisphosphonate pamidronate has demonstrated a poorer tolerance and a lesser efficacy of plicamycin compared with pamidronate (33).

Bisphosphonates are indeed very potent inhibitors of bone resorption that have dramatically changed the management of TIH.

2. Bisphosphonates for TIH

All bisphosphonates have a P-C-P bound in their structure, which is a prerequisite for their binding to the mineralized bone matrix and their inhibitory effects on bone resorption. The rest of the molecule differs among the various compounds and determines their relative potency and probably their precise mechanism of action. Clodronate directly acts on the mature osteoclasts and can have cytotoxic effects at the concentrations necessary to suppress bone resorption, whereas nitrogen-containing bisphosphonates are not toxic to the osteoclasts at therapeutic concentrations (34). Besides the still imprecisely understood effects of pamidronate on mature osteoclasts, the principal site of action of pamidronate is believed to reside in the terminal differentiation and final activation of osteoclasts. However, recent findings obtained with alendronate, a bisphosphonate quite similar to pamidronate, indicate that the drug preferentially goes to sites of active bone resorption and increases the permeability of the membrane of the osteoclasts to Ca^{2+} and to other ions, such as H^+ and NH_4^+, thereby making the osteoclast unable to resorb bone (34).

a. Etidronate. Etidronate (Didronel) is widely available, but it is the least potent of the clinically evaluated bisphosphonates. Prolonged treatment can inhibit bone mineralization and lead to osteomalacia, but this is not a concern in the acute treatment of TIH. Recommended doses for TIH are 7.5 mg/kg/day for 3 days, but some authors prolong the therapy for 7 days because the success rate seems to increase with treatment duration. In a double-blind multicenter trial including 202 patients treated for 3 days, 63% of the patients receiving etidronate became normocalcemic, against 33% in the control group receiving only saline infusions; when serum calcium was corrected for albumin levels, the response rates dropped, however, to 24 and 7%, respectively (30).

b. Clodronate. Clodronate (Ostac or Bonefos) has been given at doses varying between 300 and 1500 mg/day for 1–10 days. It is superior to placebo, and repeated administrations are well tolerated and have permitted a success rate of 80–90% (35). A single-day infusion is often poorly efficient in patients with markedly increased tubular reabsorption of calcium, and prolonged treatment appears to be superior to a 1 day administration.

c. Pamidronate. Pamidronate (Aredia) has been studied most often and is the most useful of the commercially available compounds. It was first administered as daily 15 mg 2 h infusions that were repeated for up to 10 days. In a multicenter trial, 90% of 132 patients with TIH treated in this manner became normocalcemic after a mean interval of 3–4 days (36). Such a therapeutic scheme is cumbersome, but particularly efficient, because serum calcium levels remain normal for a median of at least 3 weeks (37). Pamidronate can also be given as a single infusion over 4–24 h, and the efficacy of a single 24 h infusion is similar to a 3 day therapeutic scheme if the same total dose is administered (38). On the basis of a single dose-response study (39), the company marketing pamidronate recommends increasing the dose as a function of the pretreatment calcium levels, from 15–30 mg for calcium levels less than 12 mg/dl to 90 mg for calcium levels above 16 mg/dl. The existence of a dose-response relationship has actually been difficult to demonstrate and remains controversial. We could show it only when reviewing the therapeutic response to pamidronate in 160 patients with TIH. The success rate, considering Ca levels corrected for protein concentrations, was 80% for the groups that received a median dose of 0.5 or 1.0 mg/kg compared with 94% for the group that received 1.5 mg/kg ($p < 0.05$). As shown in Figure 7, the duration of normocalcemia was similarly more prolonged in the high-dose group (40). The dose-response relationship was significant only in patients with Ca levels above 12 mg/dl and in patients with an elevated index of tubular calcium reabsorption, which helps to resolve conflicting data in the literature, because after relatively low doses of pamidronate, the response is indeed less in patients with HHM than in patients with metastatic bone involvement. We suggest that a dose of 1.5 mg pamidronate/kg, around 90 mg for most individuals, is optimal for the treatment of TIH, except patients with mild hypercalcemia, for whom a dose of 1 mg/kg, around 60 mg, appears to be sufficient. At these dose levels, the efficacy of pamidronate is not significantly influenced by the tumor type or the degree of metastatic bone involvement. Elevated circulating PTHrP levels significantly influence the response to bisphosphonate therapy, and the few resistant patients often have markedly increased PTHrP levels (8).

Pamidronate is well tolerated, the only clinically detectable side effect being

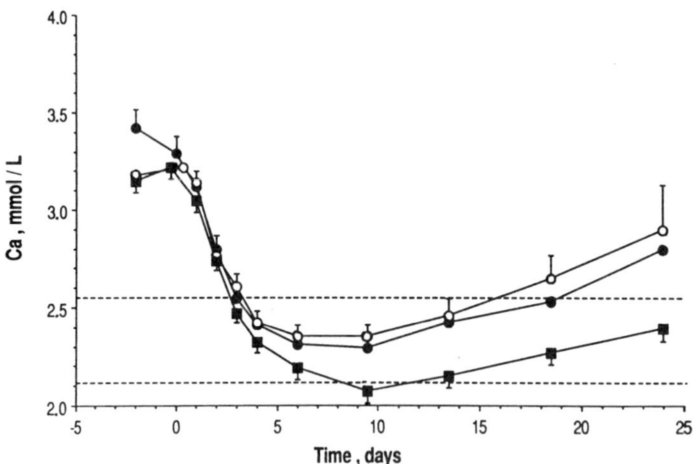

Figure 7 Effects of pamidronate on the decrease in serum calcium (Ca) in 160 hypercalcemic cancer patients divided according to the median dose received: (closed circles) 0.5 mg/kg, n = 35; (open circles) 1.0 mg/kg, n = 52; (squares) 1.5 mg/kg, n = 73. [Reproduced with permission from Body and Dumon (40).]

transient fever and a flulike syndrome in about one-fourth of the cases. Asymptomatic hypocalcemia and hypophosphatemia are often observed after therapy, and their incidence or severity is dose related (40). When hypercalcemia recurs, the efficacy of subsequent pamidronate infusions is progressively reduced. This is probably caused by an increased tumor mass and an enhanced release of osteolytic factors as the tumor progresses. Limited data indicate that higher doses of bisphosphonates can then be given successfully.

The superiority of pamidronate over etidronate, clodronate, plicamycin, and calcitonin has been demonstrated in prospective comparative trials (41). Besides saline infusions to restore circulating volume, there is no need to combine pamidronate with other hypocalcemic drugs, except in the few patients with severe, life-threatening hypercalcemia. In these patients, combining pamidronate with calcitonin is of particular value because of the rapid fall in serum calcium induced by calcitonin.

d. Alendronate and Newer Derivatives. Alendronate is a newer aminobisphosphonate that has been more often tested in nononcological patients. Its efficacy in TIH also appears to be dose related because the effects of a single 10 mg infusion are greater than the effects of a 2.5 or 5.0 mg infusion. After doses of 10–15 mg, at least 80% of the patients become normocalcemic, and alendronate superiority over clodronate and etidronate has already been demonstrated (42).

Newer and even more potent bisphosphonates are currently being studied, such as BM 21.0955 and CGP 42.446. Their increased potency compared with pamidronate and alendronate permits administering them at much lower doses and probably as short intravenous infusions. Other types of antiosteolytic compounds, such as gallium, are also under evaluation. The efficacy of gallium nitrate in TIH has already been shown to be superior to that of calcitonin and etidronate. Gallium is a potentially serious nephrotoxic agent, however, and it must be administered as a 5 day continuous infusion, which makes it unattractive for the management of TIH.

In summary, bisphosphonates have dramatically improved and simplified the management of TIH. Nowadays, the challenge for the clinician treating a hypercalcemic cancer patient is no longer to know how to treat but when not to treat. A single infusion of 60–90 mg pamidronate combined with saline infusions normalizes serum calcium in about 90% of hypercalcemic cancer patients. Alendronate, given at 10–15 mg, is probably as efficient, and newer bisphosphonates will probably not increase this response rate, but their ease of administration will make them particularly attractive for the management of normocalcemic cancer patients.

B. Treatment of Bone Metastases and Tumor-Induced Osteolysis

1. Traditional Antineoplastic Treatments

a. Systemic Treatment. The systemic treatment for bone metastases parallels usual therapies for other metastatic manifestations. These treatments are chosen according to the tumor type and to other factors influencing the probability of response. Furthermore, considerations must be made for the toxicity associated with these therapies. Chemotherapy, endocrine therapy, and bone-seeking isotopes contitute the various possibilities for antitumor treatment. Other agents, such as bisphosphonates and analgesics, are effective for the prevention and treatment of complications associated with osteolytic bone disease. Breast cancer and prostate cancer represent the majority of patients with bone metastases and are thus considered more specifically.

i. Breast Cancer. The skeleton is the most common site of distant recurrence after primary treatment of breast cancer. Most patients develop clinically relevant bone metastases during the course of the disease. It is also well known that patients with bone metastases as the first and exclusive site of relapse have a more favorable prognosis than patients with metastases at other sites. The more favorable prognosis of these patients may be related to the fact that receptor-positive breast cancers relapse more frequently in the skeleton than receptor-negative tumors.

Most patients with first relapse confined to the skeleton are treated with endocrine therapy because of their favorable prognosis. Tamoxifen is the treatment of choice for postmenopausal women in this group of patients. Response to treatment is variable and ranges from 4 to 40% (43). Such major differences in response rates might bc a result of different patient selection and because response assessment in the skeleton is a difficult task. In patients failing tamoxifen, aminogluthetimide is used frequently, and there is only little evidence of a dose-response effect to this drug. A frequently used regimen consists of 250 mg aminogluthetimide twice daily without hydrocortisone. Response rates to progestins when used as second-line therapy also appear to vary considerably, ranging from 0 to 50% in phase II studies (44). Second-line endocrine therapy with aminogluthetimide seems to have a slight advantage over other treatments at this stage of therapy (45). However, toxicities of second-line hormonal treatment after tamoxifen failure must be considered. Aminogluthetimide is associated with asthenia and skin rash in a substantial number of patients, and these effects are poorly related to the dose, whereas progestins, such as medroxyprogesterone acetate and megestrol acetate, are associated with an increased risk of thromboembolic complications and a marked weight gain in the majority of patients.

Chemotherapy is usually reserved for endocrine-resistant disease in breast cancer patients with bone metastases. A review of several chemotherapy studies showed response rates ranging from 0 to 30%. No evidence for the superiority of a single drug or a certain regimen has been found (46). However, the low response rate in the skeleton compared with other sites of disease does not reflect the whole palliative effect. Many patients achieving "no change" after systemic therapy actually benefit from excellent pain relief and an improvement in the quality of life. Along the same lines, survival of patients with no change for at least 6 months has been found to be comparable to that of patients with partial response (47). Comparisons of response rates in the skeleton are also biased by the inadequate reporting in older published trials. Strict criteria for response have not been applied and extramural or blinded reviews have only been rarely used to make the data more consistent. Furthermore, patients with bone involvement as the only site of metastases are frequently excluded from trials because of the difficulty in assessing response and time of disease progression.

ii. Prostate Cancer. The skeleton is the major and often exclusive site of metastatic disease in prostate cancer. Patients usually present with predominantly osteoblastic disease, making evaluation of treatment effects notoriously difficult. Specific tumor markers, such as prostate-specific antigen or acid phosphatase, can help to evaluate treatment response and treatment failure. Androgen deprivation leads to an improvement in symptoms in the majority of patients. The most commonly used form of therapy remains surgical castration, but it has been progressively susperceded by luteinizing hormone releasing hormone (LHRH) agonists. Responders to this procedure usually have a significant and early reduction in bone pain and an increased survival compared with nonresponders. Other means of endocrine treatment, such as LHRH agonists, flutamide, or combined treatment, did not show an improvement compared with surgical castration but are more acceptable to many patients. Estrogen therapy is assocated with considerable side effects and risks, especially if used at high doses (feminizing symptoms and cardiovascular events). Combined hormonal treatment of metastatic prostate cancer with so-called complete androgen blockade has not shown convincing superiority over androgen deprivation alone. The benefits of early initiation of androgen deprivation in asymptomatic patients with bone metastases compared with endocrine treatment delayed until complications or symptoms develop is currently under investigation. Second-line therapy after failure of androgen deprivation is not very successful in most cases. Many patients have a poor performance status and reduced hematological tolerance because of extensive bone involvement and prior radiotherapy. Relief from bone pain reportedly varies between 11% (48) and 54% (49), and duration of palliation is usually short.

b. Radiotherapy. Radiotherapy is often requested for patients with bone metastases and pain. The use of radiotherapy for the relief of metastatic bone pain indeed represents a large burden of work for radiotherapy departments. A review of the literature shows a large number of retrospective nonrandomized studies confirming the clinical usefulness of local radiation for bone pain. Data from retrospective studies show pain relief in up to 85% of the cases, but there is a considerable variation in the reported response rates (49). Traditional treatment consists of 30 Gy tumor dose in 10 daily fractions over 2 weeks. The histology of the primary tumor does not appear to have a major influence on the likelihood of pain relief. Early onset of pain relief, occasionally after one dose of radiotherapy, supports the hypothesis that tumor shrinkage caused by irradiation is not the only mechanism to achieve pain control in many patients.

The Radiation Therapy Oncology Group (RTOG) has conducted a prospective randomized trial for metastatic bone pain using several dose fraction schedules, ranging form 15 Gy over 1 week to 40.5 Gy in 15 fractions over 3 weeks. Excellent pain relief was reported in about half of the patients, and no difference between the various schedules could be found, except in patients with complete response in whom 40.5 Gy in 15 fractions was significantly more effective than 25 Gy in 5 daily fractions (50). Another prospective randomized trial compared 24 Gy in 6 fractions over 3 weeks with 20 Gy in 2 fractions over 1 week, and no difference in response could be found, 50% in each arm (51). A further prospective randomized trial compared 8 Gy as a single fraction to 30 Gy in 10 daily fractions, and again no difference could be seen between the two regimens, either for onset or for duration of pain relief (52). In conclusion, there is no evidence of a clear dose-response effect and no superiority of a particular therapeutic scheme, with the possible exception of more complete pain relief with total doses higher than 40 Gy in the RTOG study (50). However, pain and quality of life have generally been poorly evaluated in most radiotherapy studies. We need more prospective and well-conducted trials before being able to recommend one or the other therapeutic scheme.

Extensive bone involvement can be treated by hemibody irradiation using single fractions of 6–7 Gy, permitting an early onset of pain relief in a majority of patients. Hemibody irradiation is mainly used in patients with multiple myeloma and metastatic prostate cancer (53). Because of the greater irradiated body volume, toxicity is inevitably higher and, besides hematological toxicity, usually includes nausea and vomiting as well as diarrhea, especially if used in the lower hemibody. Upper hemibody irradiation can be associated with alopecia and pneumonitis. The greater toxicity and the small risk of life-threatening complications, such as pneumonitis, must be weighed against the frequently obtained pain relief, its early onset, and the prolonged effectiveness, as well as the convenience of a single radiation treatment for both patient and caregivers.

c. Radioactive Isotopes. An alternative to repeated irradiations in patients with extensive bone involvement by metastatic deposits is the use of radioisotopes for delivering radiation at the locations of multiple bone metastases. Differentiated carcinoma of the thyroid is the model for this kind of treatment, using a specific metabolic step in the cancer cell to allow transportation of radioisotopes (or possibly other agents) selectively to the tumor. Using this mechanism, differentiated thyroid carcinoma in advanced stages was the first cancer that could be cured with iodine 131.

Bone-seeking isotopes have also been used in other tumors. Radioactive phosphorus 32 and strontium 89 concentrate in areas with high bone formation and deliver radiation to the tissue within a range of a few millimeters. Strontium 89 has a long half-life of more than 50 days and a favorable energy range. It has been used for more than 50 years, but it was only recently tested in a placebo-controlled trial and was shown to be superior to placebo in pain relief (54). As expected, these agents can lead to bone marrow suppression, especially if given repeatedly (55). They must be reserved for osteoblastic metastases, typically from prostate cancer. Other isotopes, such as samarium 153-EDTMP and ^{117m}Sn (4+)DTPA (penteticacid) have a higher percentage of bone uptake and a better bone-blood ratio. It remains to be demonstrated whether these theoretical advantages will be confirmed in clinical trials.

2. Orthopedic Surgery

The strength of normal long bones is mainly determined by the cortical compartment, because cortical defects greatly reduce their resistance. A defect of a third of the diameter of a long bone decreases torsional strength by 70% (56). Destruction of less than 25% of the cortex is associated with minimal risk of fracture. A fracture rate of 3.7% has been reported when 25–50% of the cortex was destroyed, 61% for a destruction of 50–75%, and 79% when more than 75% of the cortex was involved by lytic lesions (57). Primary stabilization followed by irradiation is frequently used for impending fractures. It is easier to fix a bone with a lytic lesion while it is still intact, and better palliation is facilitated because of shorter and easier rehabilitation. Localized radiation could play an important role in preventing further osteolysis and loosening of implants in many patients, but the necessity for postoperative radiotherapy has not been demonstrated by prospective studies.

Pathological fractures requiring orthopedic surgery occur in about 9% of patients with malignant osteolytic bone disease (58). The evaluation of a patient with a pathological fracture or an impending fracture includes an assessment of many features, such as the general fitness for anesthesia and surgery, the diagnosis of the primary tumor, the dissemination of the disease, and the presence of other complications. During operation and especially in the postoperative period, additional complications can develop (infection, blood loss, and clotting disorders). Pathological transcervical femoral fractures are usually treated with arthroplasty. If the acetabulum is involved, total hip replacement is indicated. Femoral shaft fracture is usually treated with an intramedullary nail, whereas fractures in the metaphysis may require osteosynthesis with bone plates and screws. The majority of pathological fractures of the humerus and forearm are treated with intramedullary nailing, but fractures around the metaphysis may require plate fixation. Methyl methacrylate is often used in combination with metallic plates, rods, and implants. Its use also permits immediate filling and reconstruction of large defects. Postoperative irradiation is also frequently administered after orthopedic stabilization of pathological fractures. Radiotherapy does not appear to interfere with fracture healing (59). On the contrary, fractures of the humeral shaft treated by intramedullary nailing and postoperative radiation healed more rapidly than nonpathological fractures at the same site and with a greater amount of bone (60), but doses >30 Gy may be detrimental to bone consolidation.

Spinal instability presents with various degrees of back pain. Any movement can be associated with severe pain or might not be possible at all. Stabilization is usually achieved with implants fixed to the posterior spine. The implants must be fixed in at least two or preferably three vertebrae above and below the unstable segment. Additional anterior fixation may be necessary. Preoperative evaluation with radiographs, bone scans, and MRI are necessary to provide information on disease extent. A substantial proportion of these patients also have spinal cord or cauda equina compression. This information is necessary to allow optimal planning of both surgery and radiotherapy.

3. Inhibitors of Bone Resorption

The pathophysiology of metastatic bone destruction makes it logical to use inhibitors of osteoclast activity, which include plicamycin, the calcitonins, gallium nitrate, and the bisphosphonates. Plicamycin is a reasonably specific inhibitor of osteoclast activity, but long-term use is precluded by the toxicity of the compound. Calcitonin is widely prescribed for its analgesic activity, but its efficacy in this setting has been most often evaluated in uncontrolled trials. The results of two randomized double-blind trials are contradictory, even concerning the effects on bone pain. Studies of animal models of neoplastic bone involvement indicate that bisphosphonates are active in early and late stages of tumor bone destruction, whereas calcitonin appears to be able to inhibit TIO only in the early stages. The routine prescription of calcitonin for metastatic bone disease cannot thus be recommended, because recalcification of lytic bone metastases has not been demonstrated in a prospective trial and its possible analgesic activity in this setting compares unfavorably with that of classic major analgesics given the cost of the hormone. Gallium nitrate is a newly developed agent that is also able to inhibit bone resorption in cancer patients, but this compound needs further evaluation of its efficacy and toxicity.

Bisphosphonates are potent inhibitors of bone resorption that have opened the way for a noncytotoxic medical treatment of bone metastases. They have been used by the oral or intravenous route in patients with TIO.

a. Oral Bisphosphonates. The digestive absorption of bisphosphonates is generally less than 5% of the administered dose; it is variable and is dramatically inhibited by food intake. Combined with occasional poor tolerance and digestive side effects, this low and erratic absorption of oral bisphosphonates constitutes a major obstacle to their development as oral drugs. The absorption of newly developed aminobisphosphonates is similarly weak, from 0.3 to 2.0% according to the available studies. There are as yet few data in humans, but the mean bioavailability of a 300 mg oral dose of pamidronate has been estimated as around 0.3% (61). A similarly low figure of 0.5% has been reported for alendronate.

Etidronate is the least potent bisphosphonate, and its inefficacy in preventing the complications of metastatic bone disease was recently demonstrated in a double-blind trial involving 173 patients with multiple myeloma (62).

Most of the data have been obtained with clodronate or pamidronate. Two large-scale studies in patients with breast cancer metastatic to the skeleton, one with clodronate (63) and one with pamidronate (64), indicate that the prolonged administration of oral bisphosphonates can reduce the frequency of morbid skeletal events by 28 and 38%, respectively. A double-blind randomized trial of clodronate, 1600 mg/day, against placebo was performed in 173 patients with breast cancer metastatic to bone. In the clodronate-treated group, there was a significant reduction in the incidence of hypercalcemic episodes and vertebral fractures and in the rate of vertebral deformity. The combined rate of all morbid skeletal events was significantly reduced, but the survival of the two groups was similar (63). The tolerance of clodronate was excellent. On the other hand, a randomized placebo-controlled trial of 2.4 g clodronate daily for 2 years in 350 patients with newly diagnosed myeloma also showed a significant reduction in the proportion of patients presenting a progression of osteolytic bone lesions, 24 versus 12%, in an intention-to-treat analysis, although the progression rate of vertebral fractures was not significantly different between the two groups (65). Even more encouraging results were obtained with prolonged oral pamidronate therapy. The main study was performed by van Holten-Verzantvoort et al., who included 161 patients with breast cancer metastatic to bone in a prospective, but unblinded trial. The median follow-up was close to 2 years. The total number of complications was reduced by 38% in the pamidronate group. The incidence of hypercalcemia, bone pain, and symptomatic imminent fractures was reduced by 65, 30, and 50%, respectively. There was also a significant decrease in the need for systemic treatment changes and radiotherapy by 35 and 33%, respectively. However, there were no significant effects on the skeletal event-free period, on the survival, or on the radiological aspect of the lytic lesions. Dose-dependent efficacy was suggested by the authors, because greater effects were observed in the 29 patients who initially received 600 mg pamidronate daily than in the 52 patients who received 300 mg daily throughout the study. This high dose could not be maintained, however, because of gastrointestinal side effects, which demonstrates the need for more potent and less toxic compounds than pamidronate, at least for the oral route (64).

Despite these encouraging results, the place of oral bisphosphonates remains unclear in our opinion for the management of cancer patients. The poor and variable absorption of the existing compounds, the requirement to take the drug far from food intake, the occasional intolerance, superimposed on the frequent digestive complaints and lack of appetite of cancer patients, and the need for doses of bisphosphonates much higher in TIO than in benign conditions, all make the intravenous route more attractive than the oral route in cancer patients. However, this could change in the future with the newly developed compounds.

b. Intravenous Bisphosphonates. The introduction of biochemical assays for measuring pamidronate (66) has permitted physicians to begin to unravel its pharmacokinetics in patients. The distribution is rapid, with a mean apparent half-life ($T_{1/2}$) of less than 1 h (61). The skeleton acts as a sink, explaining why the apparent total plasma clearance is much higher than the renal clearance, which is similar to the creatinine clearance (61). Leyvraz et al. (67) reported that the mean body retention at 24 h was 60–70% for a 60 mg pamidronate infusion administered over a period of 1, 4, or 24 h. There was a considerable between-patient variability, from 42 to 91%, but the retention was not significantly influenced by the infusion rate. The bone retention of aminobisphosphonates seems to be definitely higher than that of clodronate, because figures of around 20% have been obtained in patients with metastatic breast cancer 3 days after drug administration (68). The lower bioavailability of clodronate could certainly contribute to its lower potency in vivo compared with aminobisphosphonates.

i. Pamidronate. Several phase II trials with intravenous pamidronate have already been performed in normocalcemic patients with lytic bone metastases. They are summarized in Table 4. In an open study of 28 patients with breast cancer metastatic to bone, Coleman et al. (69) showed that the fortnightly administration of 30 mg intravenous pamidronate as the only "antineoplastic" therapy induced a subjective improvement in about one-third of the cases and an objective sclerosis of osteolytic lesions in 4 patients. The median duration of this objective partial response was 10 months, and the disease was apparently stabilized in 11 other patients (69). Morton et al. (70) obtained apparently even better results in a small series of 16 patients treated with a similar therapeutic scheme but with an additional loading dose of pamidronate. In an early analysis of their dose-response trial, Lipton et al. reported that pain relief was more likely to occur when pamidronate was administered at doses of 60 and 90 mg every 2–4 weeks than at doses of 30 mg every 2 weeks (71). Similarly, in a review of 80 patients with breast cancer and painful bone metastases treated by pamidronate, Thürlimann et al. showed that the dose must be at least the equivalent of 20 mg weekly to obtain a significant analgesic effect (72). When pooling these data, a clear-cut relief of bone pain could apparently be obtained in more than one-third of the cases and an objective sclerosis of the lytic lesions in one-fourth (73). None of these studies were placebo controlled, however, and the evaluation was sometimes open to criticism. Moreover, the relatively high percentage of objective responses obtained by some authors (69,70) probably reflects a selection of patients with not very far advanced disease. These figures must thus be taken with caution, especially because, in each of these trials, the

Table 4 Intravenous Pamidronate in Breast Cancer-Induced Osteolysis

Author	Therapeutic scheme	Patients	Results	
			Recalcification	Analgesic effect
Coleman et al. (69)	30 mg every 2 weeks	28	4	9
Morton et al. (70)	30 mg every week × 4 then every 2 weeks	16	4	3
Thiébaud et al. (77)	60 mg every month × 4 then every 3 months	18	8	9
Lipton et al. (71)	30 mg every 2 weeks, 90 mg every 4 weeks	60	15	—[a]

[a]Not applicable.

investigators used different therapeutic schedules. On the basis of these limited pieces of information, it is tempting to conclude that a dose of 60–90 mg pamidronate administered every 3–4 weeks could constitute an adequate therapeutic scheme. Comparative and prospective trials in large series of patients, however, are needed before we can make strong recommendations concerning optimal therapeutic schemes in TIO.

Pharmacokinetic analyses could help in the selection of an adequate therapeutic regimen. Leyvraz et al. thus showed that the correlation between body retention and creatinine clearance is relatively weak ($r = 0.42$) but that there is a stronger association with the number of bone metastases. They thus found a mean ± standard deviation body retention of 51 ± 12% in patients with fewer than 5 metastatic bone sites compared with 76 ± 12% in patients with more than 15 bone metastases as evaluated by x-rays (67). These preliminary data suggest that the dose of bisphosphonates should perhaps be adapted to the degree of bone metastatic involvement. The bone compartment is not easily saturated, however, because pharmacokinetic parameters remained unchanged in four patients who received two to four infusions at monthly intervals. These data are actually not very surprising because they confirm the previous use of the "whole-body retention" of labeled bisphosphonates as an estimate of bone turnover. On the other hand, a single infusion of pamidronate has a prolonged efficacy on pain relief and on biochemical parameters of bone turnover, and for long-term treatment, it could be important to monitor the changes in biochemical parameters of bone turnover to avoid detrimental effects on bone formation (73).

Bisphosphonates are generally well tolerated, but prolonged therapy can cause hypocalcemia in patients with sclerotic metastases (74). Lytic bone metastases are evidently the main target of bisphosphonate therapy, and the only clinically detectable side effect of pamidronate that we have observed in breast cancer is a drug-related fever and a flulike syndrome that occur in about 20% of the cases, most often only after the first infusion.

ii. Perspectives. Several new bisphosphonates are under development, and the clinician will have an impressive and difficult choice within a few years. The new derivatives inhibit bone mineralization at the same or lower doses than etidronate, but their inhibitory potency on osteoclast activity is much more marked, implying that their therapeutic index becomes wider and wider. It has thus been shown in animal models of bone resorption that alendronate, risedronate, BM 21.0955, and CGP 42.446 are 5–10, almost 30, more than 50, and more than 500 times more potent than pamidronate, respectively, which is currently the most potent bisphosphonate commercially available (73,75). Human studies with BM 21.0955 and CGP 42.446 have been initiated, and it is hoped that the remarkable potency of these new compounds will permit us to administer them as a direct intravenous injection, maybe every 1–2 months, thus allowing very convenient therapeutic schemes. One can also speculate that it will be possible to administer such compounds orally at sufficiently low doses to reduce or possibly avoid digestive side effects and to have a marked and a prolonged inhibitory activity on bone resorption.

Existing bisphosphonates nevertheless already constitute a major therapeutic advance for patients with TIO. They successfully treat hypercalcemic episodes and exert significant analgesic and bone recalcification effects. Besides their favorable effects on the quality of life, bisphosphonates, if their price can be lowered, could also reduce the financial burden of metastatic breast cancer, because most of the time spent in the hospital and most of the financial costs are caused by complications of the disease rather than by the treatment itself (76). Pamidronate is also currently being tested as a preventive agent for prolonging the bone metastasis-free period in patients with extraosseous metastases but also in high-risk patients after mastectomy. There is currently no simple and reliable means to identify the patients who will later develop bone metastases and could thus benefit from preventive use of bisphosphonates, but the more frequent PTHrP expression by tumors that later invade the skeleton could help to select patients for trials aimed at preventing the development or the complications of TIO. The exact place of these compounds in our therapeutic armamentarium for the prevention and treatment of metastatic bone disease will appear more clearly within a few years. Finally, studies in cancer patients will also be of great benefit for the treatment and prevention of osteoporosis, for which bisphosphonates appear to be a very promising approach.

SELECTED READING

Body JJ. Bone metastases and tumor-induced hypercalcemia. Curr Opin Oncol 1992; 4:624–631.

Coleman RE, Rubens RD. The clinical course of bone metastases from breast cancer. Br J Cancer 1987; 55:61–66.

Lewington VJ. Targeted radionuclide therapy for bone metastases. Eur J Nucl Med 1993; 20:66–74.

Martin TJ, Grill V. Hypercalcemia in cancer. J Steroid Biochem Mol Biol 1992; 43:123–129.

Papapoulos SE, van Holten-Verzantvoort ATM. Modulation of tumour-induced bone resorption by bisphosphonates. J Steroid Biochem Mol Biol 1992; 43:131–136.

Poulsen HS, Nielsen OS, Klee M, Rorth M. Palliative irradiation of bone metastases. Cancer Treat Rev 1989; 16:41–48.

REFERENCES

1. Nolkins H. Tumorhandbuch: Pathologie und Klinik der menschlichen Tumoren. 2 Auflage, Band 3, Kapitel 22. Munich: Urban und Schwarzenberg, 1987.

2. Galasko CSB. Mechanisms of lytic and blastic metastatic disease of bone. Clin Orthop 1982; 169:20–27.
3. Garfunkel L. Statistics and trends. In: Holleb AI, Fink DJ, Murphy GP, eds. Textbook of Clinical Oncology. Atlanta: American Cancer Society, 1991:1–6.
4. Stewart AF, Vignery A, Silverglate A, et al. Quantitative bone histomorphometry in humoral hypercalcemia of malignancy: uncoupling of bone cell activity. J Clin Endocrinol Metab 1982; 55:219–227.
5. Body JJ, Delmas PD. Urinary pyridinium cross-links as markers of bone resorption in tumor-associated hypercalcemia. J Clin Endocrinol Metab 1992; 74:471–475.
6. Coleman RE, Houston S, James I, et al. Preliminary results of the use of urinary excretion of pyridinium crosslinks for monitoring metastatic bone disease. Br J Cancer 1992; 65:766–768.
7. Suva LJ, Winslow GA, Wettenhall REH, et al. A parathyroid hormone-related protein implicated in malignant hypercalcemia: cloning and expression. Science 1987; 237:893–896.
8. Body JJ, Dumon JC, Thirion M, Cleeren A. Circulating PTHrP concentrations in tumor-induced hypercalcemia: influence on the response to bisphosphonate and changes after therapy. J Bone Miner Res 1993; 8:701–706.
9. Grill V, Ho P, Body JJ, et al. Parathyroid hormone-related protein: elevated levels in both humoral hypercalcemia of malignancy and hypercalcemia complicating metastatic breast cancer. J Clin Endocrinol Metab 1991; 73:1309–1315.
10. Burtis WJ. Parathyroid hormone-related protein: structure, function and measurement. Clin Chem 1992; 38:2171–2183.
11. Yates AJ, Boyce BR, Favarato G, et al. Expression of human transforming growth factor α by Chinese hamster ovarian tumors in nude mice causes hypercalcemia and increased osteoclastic bone resorption. J Bone Miner Res 1992; 7:847–853.
12. Haq M, Goltzman D, Tremblay G, Brodt P. Rat prostate adenocarcinoma cells disseminate to bone and adhere preferentially to bone marrow-derived endothelial cells. Cancer Res 1992; 52:4613–4619.
13. Nakai M, Mundy GR, Williams PJ, Boyce B, Yoneda T. A synthetic antagonist to laminin inhibits the formation of osteolytic metastases by human melanoma cells in nude mice. Cancer Res 1992; 52:5395–5399.
14. Brown PD, Bloxidge RE, Anderson E, Howell A. Expression of activated gelatinase in human invasive breast carcinoma. Clin Exp Metastasis 1993; 11:183–189.
15. Powell GJ, Southby J, Danks JA, et al. Localization of parathyroid hormone-related protein in breast cancer metastases: increased incidence in bone compared with other sites. Cancer Res 1991; 51:3059–3061.
16. Vargas SJ, Gillespie MT, Powell GJ, et al. Localization of parathyroid hormone-related protein mRNA expression in breast cancer and metastatic lesions by in situ hybridation. J Bone Miner Res 1992; 7:971–979.
17. Evans CE, Ward C, Rathour L, Galasko CB. Myeloma affects both the growth and function of human osteoblast-like cells. Clin Exp Metastasis 1992; 10:33–38.
18. Kostenuik PJ, Singh G, Suyama KL, Orr FW. Stimulation of bone resorption results in a selective increase in the growth rate of spontaneously metastatic Walker 256 cancer cells in bone. Clin Exp Metastasis 1992; 10:411–418.

19. Iwamura M, di Sant'Agnese PA, Wu G, et al. Immunohistochemical localization of parathyroid hormone-related protein in human prostate cancer. Cancer Res 1993; 53:1724–1726.
20. Thompson TC, Truong LD, Timme TL, et al. Transforming growth factor β1 as a biomarker for prostate cancer. J Cell Biochem Suppl 1992; 16H:54–61.
21. Killian CS, Corral DA, Kawinski E, Constantine RI. Mitogenic response of osteoblast cells to prostate-specific antigen suggests an activation of latent TGF-β and a proteolytic modulation of cell adhesion receptors. Biochem Biophys Res Commun 1993; 192:940–947.
22. Bentley H, Hamdy FC, Hart KA, et al. Expression of bone morphogenetic proteins in human prostatic adenocarcinoma and benign prostatic hyperplasia. Br J Cancer 1992; 66:1159–1163.
23. Clain A. Secondary malignant disease of bone. Br J Cancer 1965; 19:15–29.
24. Coleman RE. Clinical aspects of metastatic bone disease In: Coleman R, Rubens RD, eds. Metastatic Bone Disease. Carnforth, Lancashire: Parthenon Publishing, 1992:11–26.
25. Gaber AO, Rice P, Eaton C, Pietrafitta JJ, Spatz E, Deckers PJ. Metastatic malignant disease of unknown origin. Am J Surg 1983; 145:493–497.
26. McNeil BJ. Value of bone scanning in neoplastic disease. Semin Nucl Med 1984; 14:277–286.
27. Weissmann DE, Gilbert M, Wang H, Grossmann SA. The use of computed tomography of the spine to identify patients at high risk for epidural metastases. J Clin Oncol 1985; 3:1541–1544.
28. Porter BA, Shields AF, Olson DO. Magnetic resonance imaging of bone marrow disorders. Radiol Clin North Am 1986; 24:269 288.
29. Daffner RH, Lupetin AR, Dash N, Sefczek RJ, Schapiro RL. MRI in the detection of malignant infiltration of bone marrow. Am J Roentgenol 1986; 146:353–358.
30. Singer FR, Ritch PS, Lad TE, et al., Hypercalcemia Study Group. Treatment of hypercalcemia of malignancy with intravenous etidronate. A controlled, multicenter study. Arch Intern Med 1991; 151:471–476.
31. Body JJ, Pot M, Borkowski A, Sculier JP, Klastersky J. Dose-response study of aminohydroxypropylidene bisphosphonate in tumor-associated hypercalcemia. Am J Med 1987; 82:957–963.
32. Hosking DJ, Gilson D. Comparison of the renal and skeletal actions of calcitonin in the treatment of severe hypercalcemia of malignancy. Q J Med 1984; 211:359–368.
33. Thürlimann B, Waldburger R, Senn HJ, Thiébaud D. Plicamycin and pamidronate in symptomatic tumor-related hypercalcemia: a prospective randomized crossover trial. Ann Oncol 1992; 3:619–623.
34. Sato M, Grasser W, Endo N, et al. Bisphosphonate action. Alendronate localization in rat bone and effects on osteoclast ultrastructure. J Clin Invest 1991; 88:2095–2105.
35. Rotstein S, Glas U, Eriksson M, et al. Intravenous clodronate for the treatment of hypercalcemia in breast cancer patients with bone metastases. A prospective randomised placebo-controlled multicenter study. Eur J Cancer 1992; 28A:890–893.
36. Harinck HIJ, Bijvoet OLM, Plantingh AST, et al. Role of bone and kidney in

tumor-induced hypercalcemia and its treatment with bisphosphonate and sodium chloride. Am J Med 1987; 82:1133–1142.
37. Body JJ, Borkowski A, Cleeren A, Bijvoet OLM. Treatment of malignancy-associated hypercalcemia with intravenous aminohydroxypropylidene diphosphonate (APD). J Clin Oncol 1986; 4:1177–1183.
38. Body JJ, Magritte A, Seraj F, Sculier JP, Borkowski A. Aminohydroxypropylidene bisphosphonate (APD) treatment for tumor-associated hypercalcemia: a randomized comparison between a 3-day treatment and single 24-hour infusions. J Bone Miner Res 1989; 4:923–928.
39. Thiébaud D, Jaeger J, Jacquet AF, Burckhardt P. Dose-response in the treatment of hypercalcemia of malignancy by a single infusion of the bisphosphonate AHPrPB. J Clin Oncol 1988; 6:762–768.
40. Body JJ, Dumon JC. Treatment of tumor-induced hypercalcemia with the bisphosphonate pamidronate: Dose-response relationship and influence of the tumor type. Ann Oncol 1994; 5:359–363.
41. Ralston SH, Gallacher SJ, Patel U, et al. Comparison of three intravenous bisphosphonates in cancer-associated hypercalcemia. Lancet 1989; 2:1180–1182.
42. Nussbaum SR, Warrell RP Jr, Rude R, et al. Dose-response study of alendronate sodium for the treatment of cancer-associated hypercalcemia. J Clin Oncol 1993; 11:1618–1623.
43. Lerner HI, Band PR, Isreal L, Leung PS. Phase II study of tamoxifen: 74 patients with stage 4 breast cancer. Cancer Treat Rep 1976; 60:1431–1435.
44. Hortobagyi GN, Buzdarr AU, Frye D, et al. Oral medroxyprogesterone acetate in the treatment of metastatic breast cancer. Breast Cancer Res Treat 1985; 5:321–326.
45. Harmsen HJ, Porsius HJ. Endocrine therapy of breast cancer. Eur J Cancer Clin Oncol 1988; 24:1099–1116.
46. Whitehouse JMA. Site-dependent response to chemotherapy for carcinoma of the breast. J R Soc Med 1985; 78(suppl 9):18–22.
47. Howell A, Mackintosh J, Jones M, Redford J, Wagstaff J, Sellwood RA. The definition of a no change category in patients treated with endocrine therapy for advanced carcinoma of the breast. Eur J Cancer Clin Oncol 1988; 24:1567–1572.
48. Scott WW, Jonson DE, Schmidt JE, et al. Chemotherapy of advanced prostatic carcinoma with cyclophosphamide of 5-fluorouracil: results of first regimen randomised study. J Urol 1987; 114:909–911.
49. Hoskin PJ. Scientific and clinical aspects of radiotherapy in the relief on bone pain. Cancer Surv 1988; 7:69–86.
50. Blitzer T. Reanalysis of the RTOG study of the palliation of symptomatic osseous metastases. Cancer 1985; 55:1468–1473.
51. Madsen EL. Painful bone metastases: efficacy of radiotherapy assessed by the patients: a randomized trial comparing 4 Gy × 6 vs 10 Gy × 2. Int J Radiat Oncol Biol Phys 1983; 9:1775–1779.
52. Price P, Hoskins PH, Eaton D, Austin D, Palmer SG, Yarnold JR. Prospective randomized trial of single and multifraction radiotherapy schedules in the treatment of painful bone metastases. Radiother Oncol 1986; 6:247–255.
53. Hoskin PJ, Ford HT, Harmer CL. Hemibody irradiation for metastatic bone pain. Clin Oncol 1989; 1:41–42.

54. Lewington VJ, McEwan AJ, Ackery DM, et al. A prospective randomized double-blind crossover study to examine the efficacy of strontium-89 in pain palliation in patients with advanced prostate cancer metastatic to bone. Eur J Cancer 1991; 27:954–958.
55. Robinson RG. Radionuclides for the alleviation of bone pain in advanced malignancy. Clin Oncol 1986; 5:39–49.
56. Pugh J, Sherry H, Futterman B, Frankel VH. Biomechanics of pathological fractures. Clin Orthop 1982; 169:109–114.
57. Fidler M. Incidence of fracture of bone metastases in long bones. Acta Orthop Scand 1981; 52:623–627.
58. Higinbotham NL, Marcove RC. The management of pathological fractures. J Trauma 1965; 5:792–798.
59. Gainor WJ, Buchert P. Fracture healing in metastatic bone disease. Clin Orthop 1983; 178:297–302.
60. Galasko CSB. The management of the skeletal metastases. J R Coll Surg Edinb 1980; 25:143–161.
61. Daley-Yates PT, Dodwell DJ, Pongchaidecha M, Coleman RE. Howell A. The clearance and bioavailability of pamidronate in patients with breast cancer and bone metastases. Calcif Tissue Int 1991; 49:433–435.
62. Belch AR, Bergsagel DE, Wilson K, et al. Effect of daily etidronate on the osteolysis of multiple myeloma. J Clin Oncol 1991; 9:1397–1402.
63. Paterson AHG, Powles TJ, Kanis JA, McCloskey E, Hanson J, Ashley S. Double-blind controlled trial of oral clodronate in patients with bone metastases from breast cancer. J Clin Oncol 1993; 11:59–65.
64. Van Holten-Verzantvoort ATM. Kroon HM, Bijvoet OLM, et al. Palliative pamidronate treatment in patients with bone metastases from breast cancer. J Clin Oncol 1993; 11:491–498.
65. Lahtinen R, Laakso M, Palva I, Virkkunen P, Elomaa I, Finnish Leukaemia Group. Randomized placebo-controlled multicentre trial of clodronate in multiple myeloma. Lancet 1992; 340:1049–1052.
66. Flesch G, Hauffe SA. Determination of the bisphosphonate pamidronate disodium in urine, by pre-column derivatization with fluorescamine, high-performance liquid chromatography and fluorescence detection. J Chromatogr 1989; 489:446–451.
67. Leyvraz S, Hess U, Flesch G, et al. Pharmacokinetics of pamidronate in patients with bone metastases. J Natl Cancer Inst 1992; 84:788–792.
68. Pentikäinen PJ, Elomaa I, Nurmi AK, Kärkkäinen S. Pharmacokinetics of clodronate in patients with metastatic breast cancer. Int J Clin Pharmacol Ther Toxicol 1989; 27:222–228.
69. Coleman RE, Woll PJ, Miles M, Scrivener W, Rubens RD. Treatment of bone metastases from breast cancer with (3-amino-1-hydroxypropylidene)-1,1-bisphosphonate (APD). Br J Cancer 1988; 58:621–625.
70. Morton AR, Cantrill JA, Pillai GV, McMahon A, Anderson DC, Howell A. Sclerosis of lytic bone metastases after disodium aminohydroxypropylidene bisphosphonate (APD) in patients with breast carcinoma. BMJ 1988; 297:772–773.
71. Lipton A, Glover D, Harvey H, et al. Disodium pamidronate (APD)—a dose-seeking study in patients with breast and prostate cancer: preliminary report. In: Bijvoet

OLM, Lipton A, eds. Osteoclast Inhibition in the Management of Malignancy-Related Bone Disorders. Lewinston, NY: Hogrefe & Huber, 1991:33–44.
72. Thürlimann B, Morant R, Jungi WF, Radziwill A. Pamidronate for pain control in patients with malignant osteolytic bone disease: a prospective dose-effect study. Support Care Cancer 1994; 2:61–65.
73. Body JJ. Medical treatment of tumor-induced hypercalcemia and tumor-induced osteolysis: challenges for future research. Support Care Cancer 1993; 1:26–33.
74. Francini G, Gonnelli S, Petrioli R, Conti F, Paffetti P, Gennari C. Treatment of bone metastases with dichloromethylene bisphosphonate. J Clin Oncol 1992; 10:591–598.
75. Mühlbauer RC, Bauss F, Schenk R, et al. BM 21.0955, a potent new bisphosphonate to inhibit bone resorption. J Bone Miner Res 1991; 6:1003–1011.
76. Richards MA, Braysher S, Gregory WM, Rubens RD. Advanced breast cancer: use of resources and cost implications. Br J Cancer 1993; 67:856–860.
77. Thiébaud D, Leyvraz S, von Fliedner V, et al. Treatment of bone metastases from breast cancer and myeloma with pamidronate. Eur J Cancer 1991; 27:37–41.

18

Ostomy Care

Debra Broadwell Jackson
Clemson University College of Nursing, Clemson, South Carolina

I. INTRODUCTION

As the success rate because of earlier diagnosis and more effective cancer therapy increases, more individuals are finding that they live with a cancer diagnosis. Cancer as a chronic illness requires that health care professionals view the patient from the perspective of functional abilities rather than as a disease process. Patients and families may not realize that the impact of cancer requires coping with changes over an extended period and that cure may be possible for some types of cancer.

A discussion of ostomy care as related to supportive cancer care should be placed in an appropriate context. An *ostomy* is a surgical procedure that may be indicated when a person has colon, bladder, or gynecological cancer that cannot be managed by less body altering surgeries. The surgery results in the creation of a stoma and is performed for curative reasons, although occasionally a stoma is constructed for palliative treatment. Adjuvant therapy may precede or follow surgery.

A common public myth is that cancer of the colon or bladder automatically results in an ostomy. The fear of ostomy often delays diagnosis and/or treatment for people who fear having diversional procedures. The number of ostomies performed each year have decreased as new, sphincter-sparing surgeries are developed, but each person undergoing ostomy surgery deserves a comprehensive and caring approach to learning self-care. This chapter focuses on the care of patients who have had cancer of the bowel, bladder, or gynecological systems that necessitates the surgical creation of a permanent stoma or ostomy. Although recognizing that stomas for feeding (esophagostomy) and drainage (gastrostomy) are used for supportive care, this chapter is limited to the care of the person with a colostomy, ileostomy, or ileal conduit (urinary diversion or urostomy). However, the pouching and skin care techniques discussed may be applied to all stomas.

II. SIGNIFICANCE OF THE PROBLEM

Cancer is second to heart disease as the leading cause of death in the United States. The number of new cases of cancer involving the colon and rectum, urinary bladder, and female genital organs has not shown signs of decreasing. More than 120,000 new cases of colorectal cancer are diagnosed each year in the United States (1).

The public is becoming more aware of the signs and symptoms of cancer and carcinogens associated with the development of certain cancers, and health screenings are publicized widely to encourage early diagnosis. (2).

A major concern for health professionals is the delay between symptoms and diagnosis. Hurney and Holland (3) report that early symptoms of bladder and colon cancers may be present for months before a person seeks medical help. The vague signs and symptoms often associated with cancer may delay the diagnosis even more. An average lag time from appearance of symptoms to the diagnosis of colorectal cancer was 8.25 months in a study of 200 patients conducted in England (4). Ignorance, denial, fear of mutilation, and excessive modesty were associated with delays in seeking diagnosis. Holland reports that fear of having an ostomy may also cause a delay in diagnosis (5).

A. Colon Cancer

Several strategies identified for the management of colon cancer include identification of carcinogens and protection of the bowel from these substances, screening of the general population over 50 years of age, follow-up of high-risk individuals, adequate primary surgical management in conjunction with adjuvant therapy, and aggressive therapy for localized recurrence (6). The risk factors for colorectal cancer are found in Table 1. Colon cancer has received increased publicity recently as new research has suggested a DNA defect associated with familial cancer of the colon (7). More importantly, recent studies indicate that stool for occult blood may be an important screening tool despite the number of false positives. The American Cancer Society and the National Cancer Institute recommend that men and women over the age of 50 be screened by fecal occult blood tests to detect early colorectal cancers (8). Positive screening results

Table 1 Risk Factors: Colorectal Cancer

Over 40
Low-fiber and high-fat diets
Family history of colon cancer
Previous colorectal cancer
Adenomatous polyps
Family history of familial polyposis coli
Ulcerative colitis
Crohn's disease
Previous pelvic radiation

indicate the need for a complete diagnostic evaluation, including colonoscopy or barium enema x-ray plus flexible sigmoidoscopy.

Unfortunately, the literature shows that community-based patients may not receive a complete evaluation of abnormal test results (8–10). The low rate of complete evaluations following screening reduces the potential benefits of performing community screening programs. Morbidity and mortality levels are not reduced through early identification of colorectal lesions if follow-up is inadequate or missing (8).

Colon and rectal cancers are categorized as *primary* if they develop from the bowel and *metastatic* when the cancer spreads from adjacent or distant sites. Metastatic colorectal cancers can develop from lymphoma, leiomyoscaroma, malignant melanoma, and cancer of the breast, ovary, prostate, and lung (11).

The primary treatment for adenocarcinoma of the colon and rectum is surgical resection, with the approach determined by the site of the lesion and the presence or absence of adjacent organ involvement.

B. Bladder Cancer

Bladder cancers are more common in men than women, and although bladder cancers may occur at any time, the tumors are more common after 60 years of age. The incidence of bladder cancer is lower than that of colorectal cancer, with approximately 45,000 new cases in the United States each year (11). The cause of bladder cancers remains unknown, although several environmental agents have been implicated (see Table 2). Repeated exposure to risk factors increases the incidence of bladder cancer. Occupational exposure often leads to bladder cancer 40–50 years after exposure to chemicals and aniline dyes, but toxins from cigarette smoking may be a greater risk. Approximately half of bladder cancers are in smokers (12). The more a person smokes increases the risk significantly.

Transitional cell carcinomas account for 95% of bladder cancers, followed by

Table 2 Risk Factors: Bladder Cancer

Category	Specific agent
Occupational toxins	
Aromatic amines	Dyes, leather tanning
Organic chemicals	
Cigarette smoking	2-Naphthylamine and nitrosamine
Artificial sweeteners	Cyclamates
Foods	Coffee
Infectious agents	Schistosomiasis
Drugs	Phenacetin, cyclophosphamide

squamous cell (3%) and adenocarcinoma (2%) (13). The majority of bladder tumors originate from epithelial cells. The exposure to toxic substances over time is associated with these lesions. Chronic irritation of the bladder seems associated with squamous cell cancers of the bladder. In Egypt, approximately 70% of bladder cancers are squamous cell carcinomas and are secondary to schistosomiasis infections. These organisms may be found in contaminated water. When a person becomes infected, the eggs are laid in the muscle wall of the bladder and intestine. The irritation of the ova in the bladder wall progresses to squamous cell carcinoma (12).

Bladder tumors recur more frequently when they invade the layers of the bladder wall. This predictable pattern influences the treatment programs provided to patients. The tumors recur in the same stage and grade as the original tumor (12). Solid tumors are more likely to invade the muscle wall of the bladder and to metastasize early.

The key to diagnosis is painless hematuria, gross or microscopic. Additionally, patients may complain of altered patterns of elimination, with increased urinary frequency and flank pain associated with ureteral obstruction or metastasis.

Noninvasive bladder tumors are treated with transurethral resections, laser fulguration, and intravesicular chemotherapy. Surgery is limited to invasive tumors and may include partial or radical cystectomy or cystoprostatectomy, urinary diversion, adjunct chemotherapy, and adjunct radiation therapy (13). The urinary diversion may be incontinent or continent (Kock, Indiana, Mainz, or University of California, Los Angeles pouch).

C. Pelvic Malignancy

Pelvic exenteration is performed in both sexes for a variety of pelvic malignancies, including colorectal carcinoma and, occasionally, radiation necrosis. The most frequent indication for this procedure is radioresistant, recurrent, or advanced cervical cancer. Anterior pelvic exenteration involves removal of the urinary bladder and the distal segments of the ureters with a resultant urinary diversion. In women, the female reproductive organs are removed, including all or part of the anterior vagina. Posterior pelvic exenteration includes the removal of the colon, rectum, uterus, vagina, and adnexa. A colostomy is required, but the bladder is intact. A total pelvic exenteration includes the removal of all reproductive organs, bladder, colon, and rectum with resultant colostomy and urinary diversion (14). The indications for this high-risk surgery are weighed carefully by the physician and family. The inclusion in this chapter is related to the care and management of the diversions.

III. SURGICAL PROCEDURES

A. Colostomy

Colostomy means an opening into the colon and can be surgically created anywhere along the length of the large intestine (*ileostomy* refers to small intestinal ileum). Three types of primary colostomies are the end, the loop, and the double barrel and refer to the general surgery required (Fig. 1).

An end colostomy is the most common procedure for colorectal cancer involving the low rectum and anus. The surgeon brings the bowel through a small opening in the abdominal wall and cuffs the lumen back upon itself and sutures to the skin at the base, to create the stoma, the externalized bowel that remains (15). The innermost muscosal layer of the bowel wall is exposed when the stoma is created. The distal diseased colon, rectum, and anus are removed in a procedure called abdominoperineal resection or the Miles resection. The abdominoperineal resection involves an abdominal incision used to free part of the bowel and create the stoma and the perineal incision through which the distal portion, rectum, and anus are removed. A large defect is left during the surgery. Three types of closures may be used for the perineal area: primary closure, partial closure, or open and packed. A primary closure, which heals much faster, is indicated if there is adequate hemostasis, no infection, and no fecal contamination. A partially closed wound includes the use of a Penrose drain in the midline perineal incision, facilitating drainage. The open and packed management is used when necessary to control bleeding (16).

When the distal colon or rectum is not removed, two procedures may be selected. The rectal stump is oversewn and left in situ, called a Hartmann's pouch. The patient has an end colostomy and the rectum and anus are intact. Mucus drainage from the rectum is expected and included in the patient's education (Fig. 2). Hartmann's pouch is indicated when the surgeon does not want to do an anastomosis and the patient is unable to tolerate the larger, more traumatic perineal resection (15).

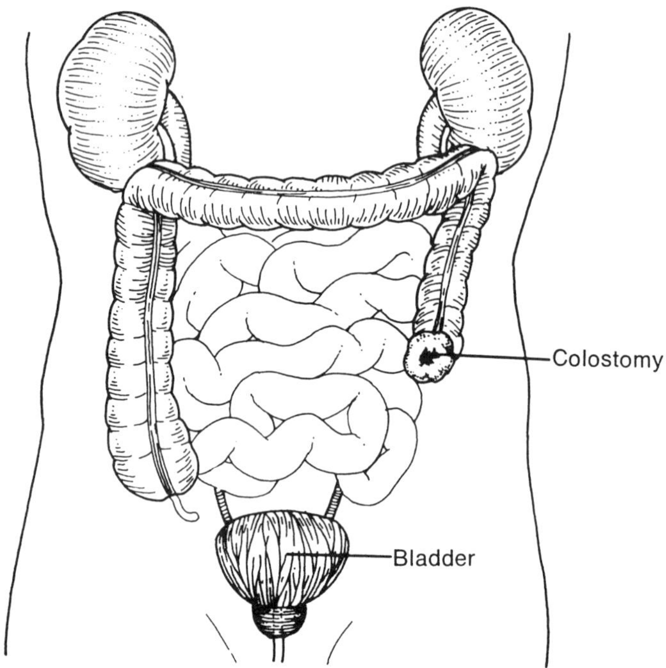

Figure 1 Resection of the rectosigmoid colon with construction of a sigmoid colostomy. (From Broadwell DC, Jackson BS. Principles of ostomy care. St. Louis: C. V. Mosby, 1982.)

The distal bowel may be brought through the abdominal wall and a second stoma created. This procedure is called a double-barrel stoma. The stoma leading to the functional bowel is the functioning, colostomy stoma. The stoma leading to the distal bowel is nonfunctioning, except for mucus drainage. Mucus may drain from the rectum as well. This surgery is most effective from the patient's point of view when the stomas are separated so that the functioning stoma can be pouched, and the nonfunctioning stoma is covered with a nonsterile dressing or pad (17).

A loop stoma is performed by bringing a loop of bowel through an abdominal incision; the posterior wall of the bowel is supported for 5–7 days by a rod or bridge. The anterior wall of the loop is opened transversely and forms one stoma with two distinct openings. The surgery results in a larger, oval stoma. The loop stoma is indicated in emergency or palliative surgery. Most loop colostomies are performed for blunt trauma and perforating injuries than for cancer (15).

Many surgeons have developed techniques to be used to save the sphincter

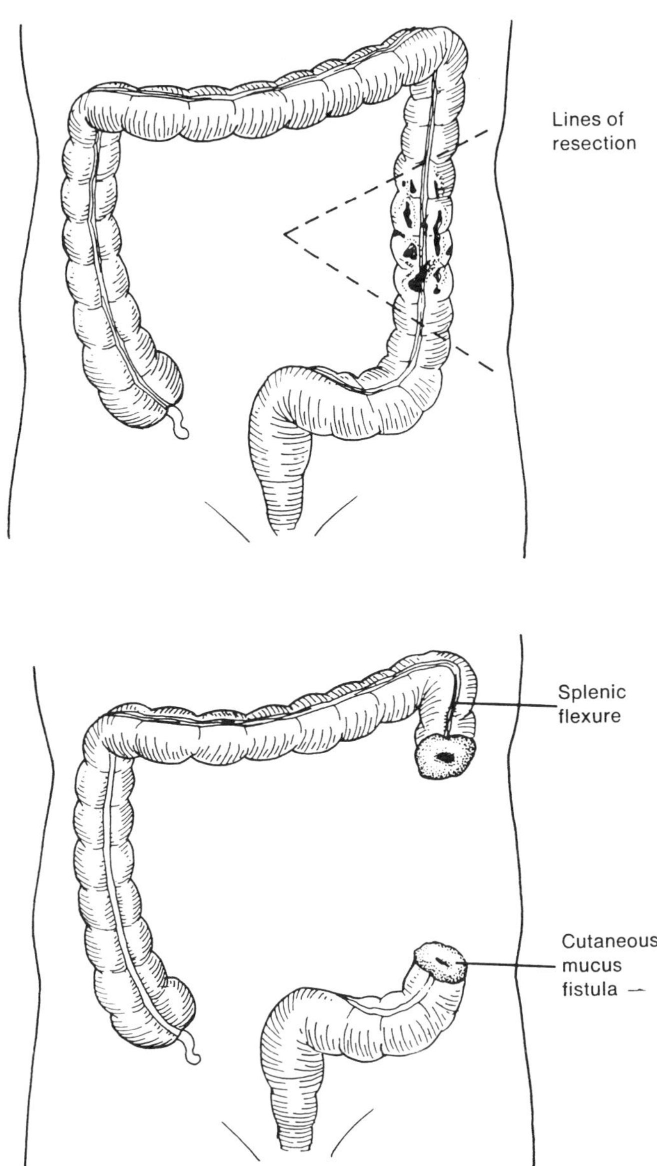

Figure 2 Disease or injury to a colon segment requires resection of the segment and may result in a double-barrel colostomy. (From Broadwell DC, Jackson BS. Principles of ostomy care. St. Louis: C. V. Mosby, 1982.)

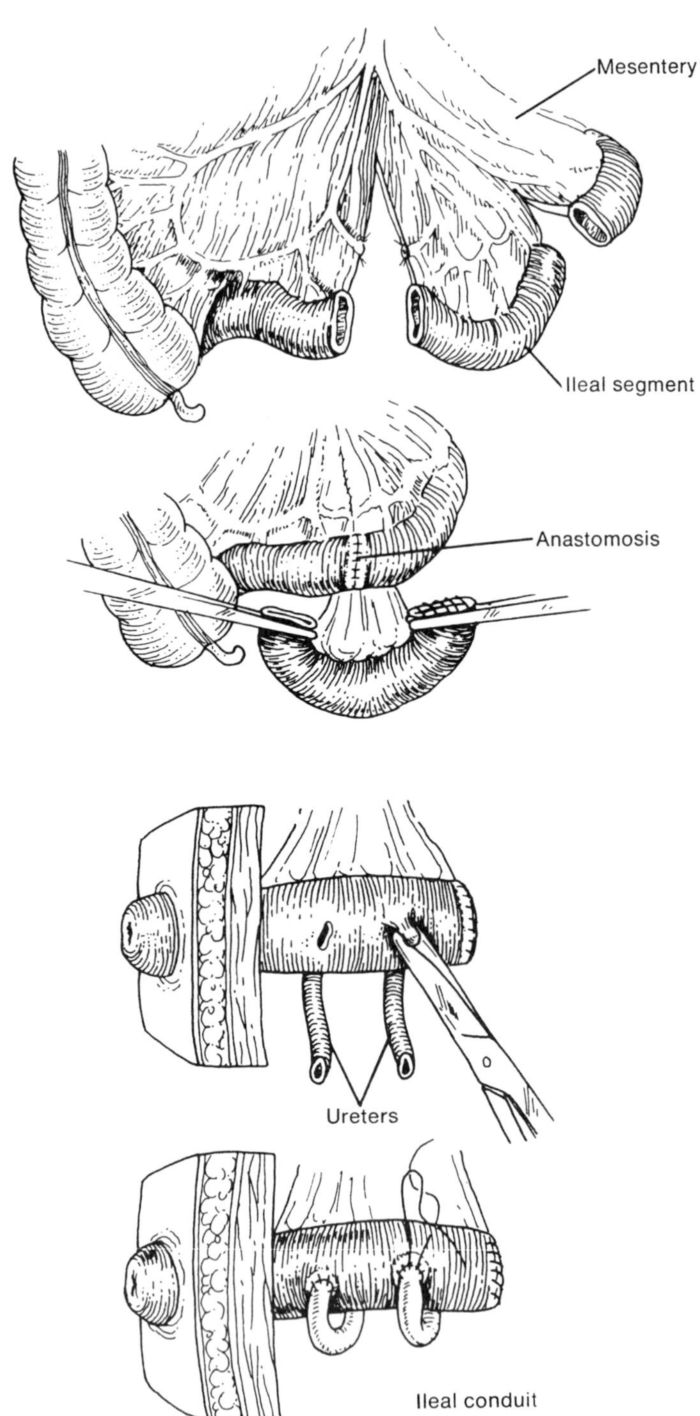

Mesentery
Ileal segment
Anastomosis
Ureters
Ileal conduit

mechanism and normal bowel elimination whenever possible. Colon resections are much more common than colostomies, particularly permanent colostomies with abdominoperineal resections. Continent procedures for persons requiring total colectomy, decreasing the number of permanent ileostomies, are available, including the Kock pouch and ileoanal reservoirs that preserve the anal sphincter.

B. Urinary Diversion

A "urinary diversion" is a general term that refers to the diversion of urine away from the urethra and/or bladder. A urinary diversion may be necessary for many clinical reasons. When the bladder is removed for cancer, the most common type of diversion is the ileal conduit. A ureterostomy can be performed and is described here briefly. The ileal conduit was first described by Bricker in the early 1950s (18). Until the refinement of the continent urinary diversion in the late 1980s, the Bricker procedure was the standard diversion for bladder cancer that did not respond to other nonsurgical methods of treatment. A 6 inch segment of ileum is removed from the small intestine with its mesentery intact. The intestinal tract is reanatomosed. One end of the segment is closed, and the other end is brought through the abdominal wall to form the stoma. The ureters are implanted into the ileal segment, which is now a conduit for the passage of urine. (Fig. 3). The conduit should empty freely and easily without residual urine remaining in the segment. An excessively long conduit may result in urinary stasis associated with increased urinary tract infections and electrolyte imbalance caused by urine reabsorption by the ileum. (Fig. 4).

Continent urinary diversions are gaining favor over the traditional ileal conduit in many major medical centers. The continent procedures lower the long-term negative consequences associated with ileal conduits. Pernet and Jonas (19) report a high rate of renal deterioration following ileal conduit as survival rates increase. In addition, continent procedures eliminate the need for an external collecting device or pouch, which may leak unexpectedly and requires regular maintenance and care. The major reason that continent procedures have increased is the research on clean intermittent catheterization, which allows a clean procedure be used for emptying the internal reservoir rather than a sterile procedure (20).

Several types of urinary continent procedures are being performed, and two are discussed in this chapter: the Kock pouch and the Indiana pouch. The Kock urinary

---

Figure 3 Construction of ileal conduit. (A) Segment of ileum is isolated from the gastrointestinal (GI) tract with its mesenteric blood flow. (B) GI tract is reanastomosed. (C) Ureters, which are located retroperitoneally, are brought into the abdominal cavity. Incisions are made in the conduit for ureteral implantation. (D) Abdominal stoma is mature, and the ureters are anastomosed to the ileum segment in an end-to-side fashion. (From Broadwell DC, Jackson BS. Principles of ostomy care. St. Louis: St. Louis, 1982.)

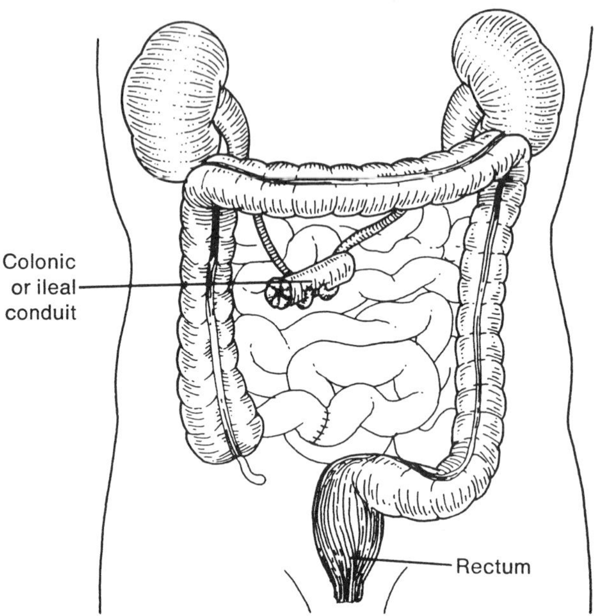

Figure 4 Completed ileal conduit. Note reanastomosed ileum. (From Broadwell DC, Jackson BS. Principles of ostomy care. St. Louis: C. V. Mosby, 1982.)

reservoir is a variation of the Kock continent ileostomy. Approximately 60–80 cm ileum is used to create an internal pouch with two intussuscepted nipple valves. The afferent limb prevents reflux of urine from the internal pouch back toward the ureters, which are anastomosed to the distal portion of the limb. The efferent limb is brought out through the abdominal wall to form a stoma, and the nipple valve prevents leakage from the Kock pouch. The surgery is lengthier, by 1–2 h. The most serious complication of this surgery is the loss of continence.

The Indiana or ileocecal pouch uses 20 cm cecum and 15 cm terminal ileum, and an additional segment of ileum or colon is used as a patch to complete the pouch construction. The distal portion of the ileum is anastomosed to the colon to reestablish bowel continuity. The cecum and the patch segment are opened and connected to form a pouch. The ureters are tunneled into the taeniae of the colonic segment, creating an antireflux mechanism. The ileal segment is brought through the abdominal wall to form a stoma. Continence is achieved by the ileocecal valve and plication of the ileum to form a long outflow tract (20). Several surgical variations have been reported in the literature and address different methods of providing continence. The care and management of the continent urinary diversions are similar.

IV. REHABILITATION AND TRAJECTORY OF PATIENT OUTCOME

Rehabilitation is a dynamic, goal-directed process designed to help individuals to function at their maximum level within the limitations and constraints of the disease and treatment protocols (21). The physical, mental, emotional, social, sexual, and economic potential of the individual is used to design a comprehensive rehabilitation program.

The success of the rehabilitation following ostomy procedures depends on four major factors: the commitment of the health care team to provide ongoing evaluation and planning for changes as the person lives with cancer and a stoma; the identification of a planned rehabilitation program with a key individual to coordinate the activities within and among team members; the involvement of patient and family in the process from the initial screening; and the effectiveness of communications between team members, which directly impacts the success of the rehabilitation program in general and for individual patients.

Throughout the phases of the disease—treatment, remission, cure, and death—cancer rehabilitation must be individualized. Whereas certain responses and coping behaviors are seen in persons faced with life-threatening illness, each individual has a unique response and personal interpretation of the meaning of illness and its treatment (18). Patient and family education is essential. The patient and family need to have an understanding of the trajectory of the disease, treatment, and outcome. The doctor and nurse have many opportunities to explain to the patient and family what will happen. Health care professionals who have worked with many people undergoing diversions for cancer have a knowledge of the stages families can expect.

A person with an ostomy will experience many changes in functional ability. Teaching the patient and family about the disease, the treatment and side effects, and the procedures to improve, maintain, or support changes in functions is integral to successful rehabilitation (22).

A. Ostomy Adjustment

The adjustment to ostomy surgery requires time: time to grieve for the loss and changes resulting from surgery; time to adapt to a new method of elimination; time to learn that others are accepting of you, the individual; and time to have new experiences and successes. Patients often discuss retirement at the time of diagnosis. The health care team can help people to wait to make major life decisions until the treatment is completed. Ambulatory patients diagnosed and undergoing treatment for cancer identified three physical parameters that changed during the treatment: level of physical activity, sleeping habits, and weight. Body image, a psychosocial dimension, and economic status also changed over time

(23). The research by Frank-Stromborg and Wright (23) did not support the assumption that a diagnosis of cancer produces a marked change in lifestyle. Interestly, the author found in a study of 289 individuals with colostomies, ileostomies, and urinary diversions that 75% of colostomy subjects and 80% of urinary diversion subjects were not employed or retired, compared with 50% of ileostomy subjects. The average age of patients receiving both the colostomy and urinary diversions was 17 years older than the ileostomy patients, which probably accounted for the difference in employment (24).

B. Diagnosis and Decision for Surgery

Cancer of the colon and rectum has often been called the cancer no one talks about (17). Societal impression related to living with a colostomy or a urinary diversion are a major consideration in educating the public and play an important role in the preoperative education of persons diagnosed with bladder or rectal cancer. An ostomy creates a physical change in the body, alters normal elimination patterns, and affects sexual functioning. The quality of life is of considerable importance to everyone. However, quality of life is a daily question for a person with an abdominal stoma who is confronted with bowel and bladder function daily (2). To a considerable extent, the quality of life following ostomy surgery is dependent upon the surgeon to create a stoma that is well-placed, of proper length, and pouchable. Druckerman (25) reviewed six key areas in the management of permanent colostomies: diet, medication, irrigation and training, use of appliances and dressings, care of the skin, and general measures. This classic study, conducted in 1938, is still relevant. Current research (24) suggests that these areas continue to be of importance and have refined general measures to include sexual functioning, emotional adaptation and adjustment, management of complications, and living with an ostomy issues.

C. Preoperative Teaching

People who need to have ostomy surgery benefit from an enterostomal therapy (ET) nurse, ostomy nurse, or oncology nursing specialist visit when the decision is reached that an ostomy is necessary. The nurse can augment what the physician has explained. Some patients and families are in shock and hear little if anything the physician has so carefully said. Patients and families need to know that their feelings and reactions are normal and expected (17).

The patient wants to know everything and nothing. For the most part, patients' questions can guide the discussion and the depth of the answers provided. A quiet, unhurried environment is necessary. The language should be down-to-earth, lay language. Handouts and patients materials are helpful, but only if the material is related to the patient and the institution. Written material does not substitute for the nurse's time in answering questions and concerns. Topics that should be included in the preoperative discussions are found in Table 3.

Questions at this time can be managed in general rather than specific terms. A person may want to know how they will go the bathroom, but the answer does not have to include every step in emptying a pouch. The answer is simply, "While sitting on the toilet, you can open the bottom of pouch and empty the stool or urine into the toilet."

Patients are interested in the sensations that they can expect before, during, and after surgery. A trajectory of the surgical process is helpful: what will happen when and how will this influence me, will it hurt and for how long, and when will I go home? A person following colostomy surgery can expect to have a nasogastric tube until bowel sounds return and will be on intravenous fluids until tolerating food.

Table 3 Preoperative Teaching Guidelines

Common questions	Suggested methods
What is an ostomy?	Define in lay terms the type of ostomy. Drawings are helpful.
What will the stoma look like?	Describe the stoma, its normal red color, peristaltic motion, lack of sensory nerve endings.
Will the ostomy be hard to take care of?	Discuss in general terms the management for the appropriate stoma.
What does a pouch or bag look like?	Show a pouch that is likely to be used at discharge as well as the pouch applied in surgery, if different.
How do I go to the bathroom after this surgery?	Discuss methods for emptying the pouch.
Will my diet change?	Discuss the return to normal diet.
Will I be able to manage at work	Identify current employment activities, and explore with the patient any anticipated management issues.
Can I bathe or shower?	Discuss general activities of daily living and how having an ostomy does not necessarily lead to change.
Will I be sick or disabled?	Explore the patient's fears or concerns about the outcome of surgery and the diagnosis. Be as supportive and encouraging as possible.
What else should I know?	Some patients are hesitant to ask relationship and sexual questions. Initiate the discussion.

The preoperative teaching session is the time to define terms for use, for example, stool, feces, and bowel movements are options for discussing colostomy output. Colostomy output may be appropriate for nurses or doctors, but patients need a more comfortable, familiar term. People also have trouble with urinary output. The health care provider can help by providing patients with acceptable words.

The preoperative visit provides an opportunity for patient and family assessments that can guide the health team in planning a comprehensive teaching and rehabilitation program. The patient and family level of understanding of the disease and treatment protocol can be evaluated. Any preconceived ideas or misunderstandings can be clarified immediately. It is always helpful to ask whether the patient and family know anyone with an ostomy and decide whether the experience was positive or negative. Physical limitations that may interfere with a person's ability to manage the ostomy may be identified, and methods for adaptation can be initiated. Social and family networks are essential to successful rehabilitation, and assessments of support groups should be included. Personal concerns include sexual functioning, and these should be addressed openly and honestly. The nurse needs to know what the physician has said regarding potential nerve damage and build on this information as she or he discusses alternatives.

In summary, people with ostomies eat normal diets, wear the clothes they wish to wear, and resume all the presurgical activities they enjoy.

V. STOMAL PLACEMENT

The most important predictor of successful rehabilitation is a well-constructed stoma, properly located on the abdomen (26). The quality of life following ostomy surgery is link directly with the person's ability to maintain a pouch seal, avoiding unplanned leakage of stool or urine and odors, despite his or her physical activities. A stoma that is retracted below the skin level or at the skin level is difficult to pouch; leakage of stool or urine and skin irritation are common. Stomas located in folds or dimples, near scars or bony prominences, or too low for patient to see create difficult pouching situations.

The doctor or ET nurse trained in stoma marking should decide before surgery the appropriate placement for the stoma (see Table 4). Stoma marking is not difficult in ambulatory adults of normal weight and good abdominal musculature. The patient is observed in standing, sitting, and bending positions, as well as supine (Figs. 5 and 6). Bending at the waist and hips shifts the abdomen and should be observed carefully. Flexing the legs at the hips while standing is also observed. The patient should sit in a chair and slowly bend forward as if to touch the floor. Careful observation of the abdomen during this step of stoma marking

Table 4 Criteria for Stoma Site Selection

1. The patient is able to see the stoma when sitting or standing.
2. The stoma avoids abdominal scars, folds, and creases when the patient is sitting, standing, or supine.
3. The site allows a 2 inch diameter of smooth skin surrounding the stoma.
4. The stoma avoids the costal margins, superior iliac crest, and symphysis pubis.
5. The stoma is located over the rectus abdominis.

detects troublesome folds or creases. Running your finger along a fold may lengthen the crease and bring attention to a potentially difficult area.

The method for marking the stoma varies and bears some consideration. The use of methylene blue injections (0.01 ml) forms a permanent tattoo, and if for some unforeseen reason the marked stoma site is not used during surgery, the patient retains a tattoo. The scratching of the skin with a sterile needle to mark the location is uncomfortable for the patient and can lead to a localized infection. A black waterproof felt marker is neither permanent nor painful but may fade during the surgical preparation. A compromise used by many physicians and ET nurses is to mark the site preoperatively with a waterproof marker. The patient

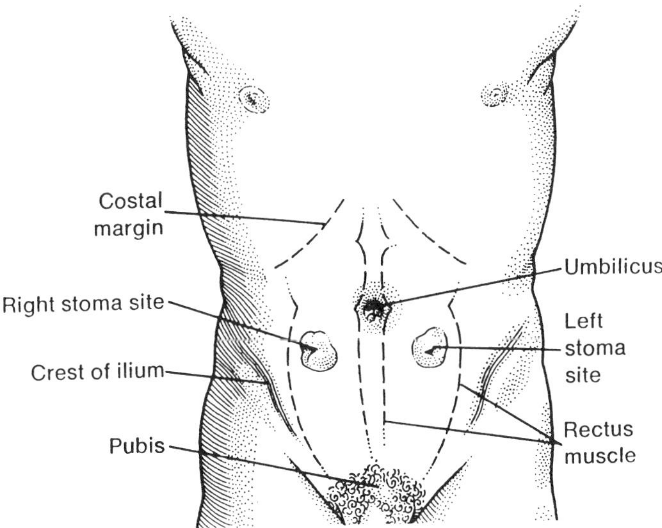

Figure 5 Right and left lower quadrant abdominal stoma sites for an ambulatory adult of normal weight. (From Broadwell DC, Jackson BS. Principles of ostomy care. St. Louis: C. V. Mosby, 1982.)

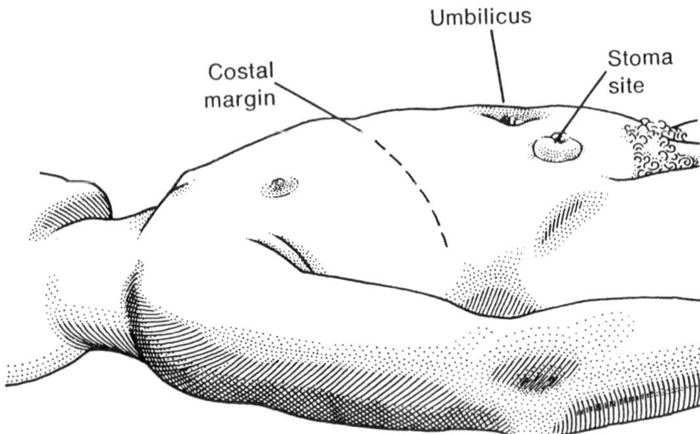

Figure 6 Lower quadrant stoma sites for a supine adult of normal weight. (From Broadwell DC, Jackson BS. Principles of ostomy care. St. Louis: C. V. Mosby; 1982.)

can darken the spot before and after presurgical scrubs or showers the night before surgery. Once the patient is in the operative suite, and asleep, the doctor scratches the marked skin with a needle.

Special considerations for marking the stoma are discussed in the remainder of this section.

1. Obesity

If the patient is obese, the stoma may be sited in the upper quadrant or level with the umbilicus to allow adequate visualization after surgery. Otherwise, the patient will have great difficulty in changing the pouch without assistance. The locations of the inferior coastal margin and the iliac crest are carefully noted while the person is sitting. The stoma site should be at least 2 inches below the inferior costal margin, above and lateral to the umbilicus (Figs. 7 and 8).

2. Two Stomas

When a patient requires two stomas, such as a double-barrel colostomy, the functioning stoma is position for pouching and should be in an ideal location. The nonfunctioning mucus fistula is placed approximately 3 inches away from the functioning stoma to prevent interference with the pouch.

If a person will have two functioning stomas, they should be on opposite sides of the abdomen. The criteria for locating each stoma should be used in determining location (Fig. 9).

3. Nonambulatory Patients

The patient must be observed using all prosthetic devices, such as corsets or braces. If the patient uses a wheelchair, observe the patient in the chair and in

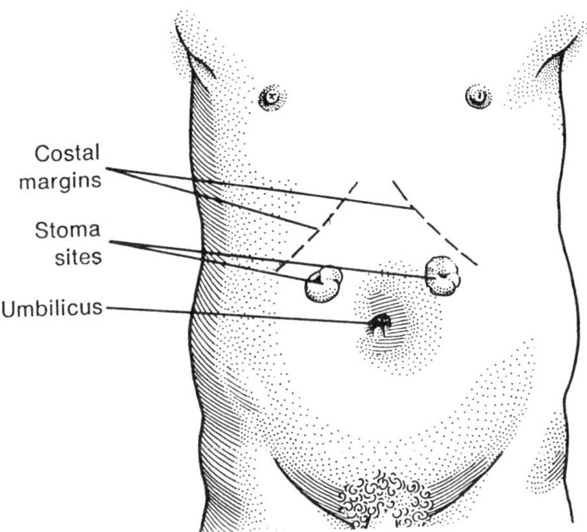

Figure 7 Right and left upper quadrant abdominal stoma sites for an ambulatory adult with an obese or enlarged abdomen. (From Broadwell DC, Jackson BS. Principles of ostomy care. St. Louis: C. V. Mosby, 1982.)

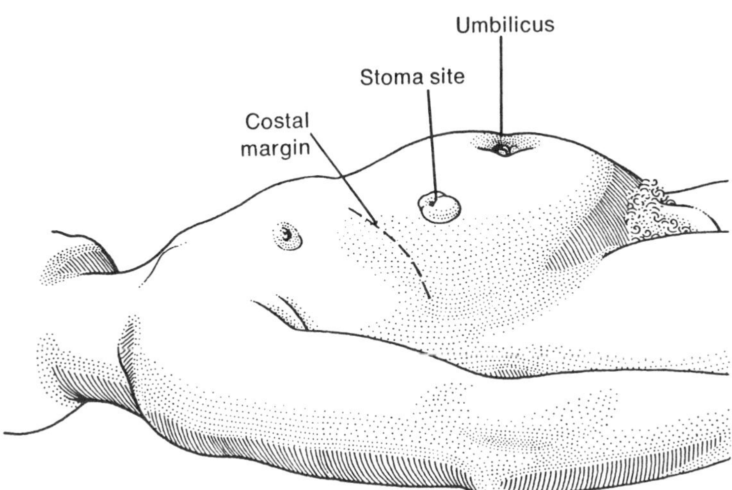

Figure 8 Upper quadrant stoma sites for a supine adult with an obese or enlarged abdomen. (From Broadwell DC, Jackson BS. Principles of ostomy care. St. Louis: C. V. Mosby, 1982.)

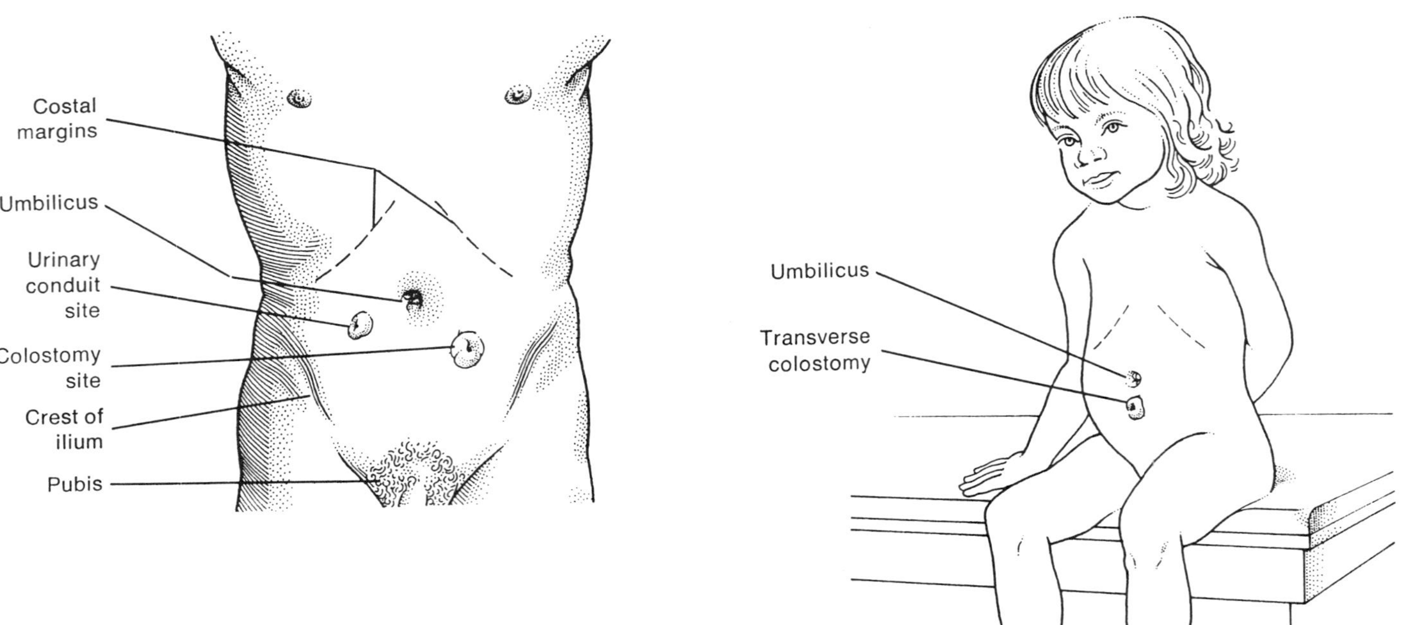

Figure 9 Two abdominal stomas: urinary diversion, right lower quadrant, and fecal diversion, left lower quadrant. (From Broadwell DC, Jackson BS. Principles of ostomy care. St. Louis: C. V. Mosby, 1982.)

transferring from bed to chair. In most situations, the stoma is placed above or level with the umbilicus (Fig. 10). Weight gain is common in nonambulatory patients as they age, and often the person gains the weight in the abdomen (Fig. 11). Folds are common when the thighs are flexed while sitting in a wheelchair.

The nonambulatory patient with an extremely difficult abdomen for stoma site selection may benefit from wearing a pouch containing warm water placed at the proposed site for 1–2 days. This technique is not recommended for all patients, but the importance of the appropriate stoma location is generally understood, and most patients are cooperative and interested.

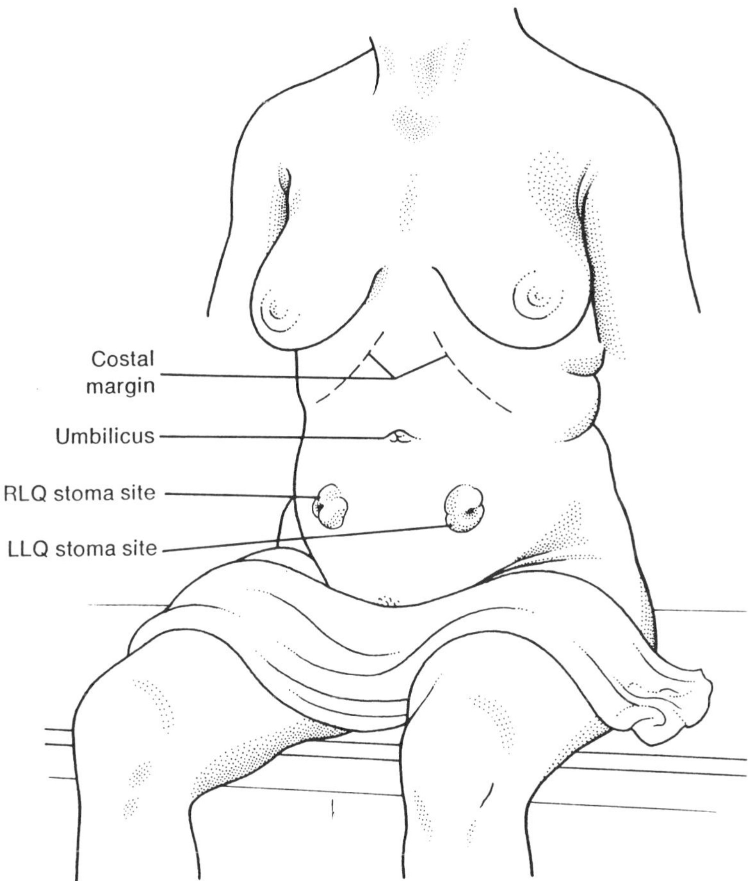

Figure 10 Right and left lower quadrant abdominal stoma sites for a nonambulatory female adult of normal weight. (From Broadwell DC, Jackson BS. Principles of ostomy care. St. Louis: C. V. Mosby, 1982.)

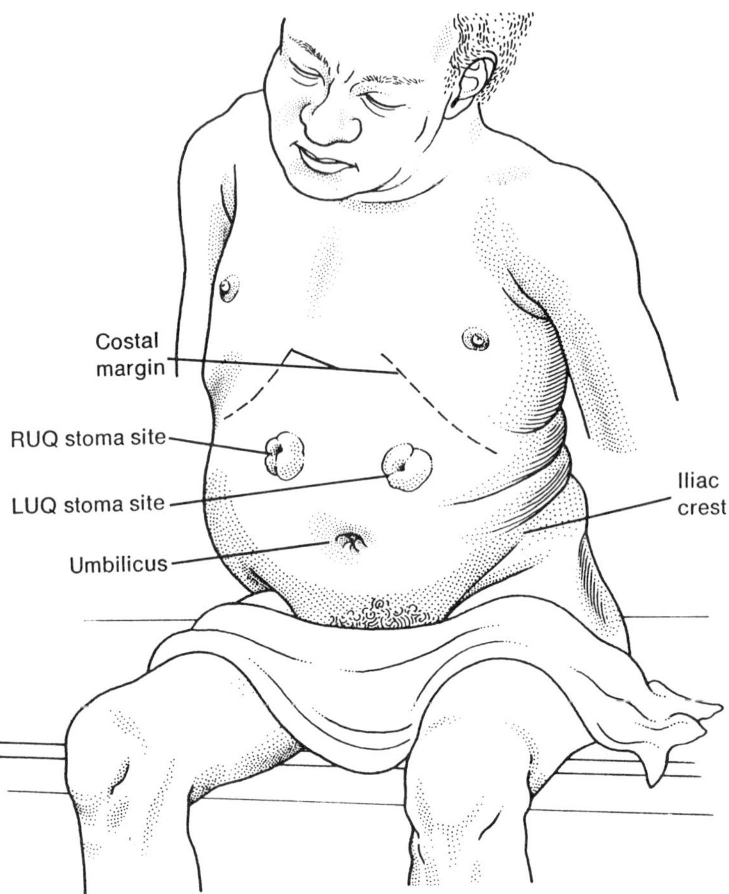

Figure 11 Upper quadrant abdominal stoma sites for a nonambulatory patient with spinal deformity and asymmetrical abdomen. (From Broadwell DC, Jackson BS. Principles of ostomy care. St. Louis: C. V. Mosby, 1982.)

4. Thinness

Slender men and women may have a different set of considerations. Men tend to have a narrow pelvis, and if they wear their belts below the umbilicus, stoma location may be a problem. Movement and bony prominences may compromise the pouch seal integrity when the stoma placement is in the lower abdominal quadrant. Placement of the stoma higher on the abdomen necessitates clothing changes or the pouch may be visible. Women tend to have an easier time adapting to a higher belt line than men. The broader pelvis also makes placement slightly easier.

5. Summary

When a patient has a particularly difficult abdomen for stoma site selection, the surgeon and ET nurse should discuss the situation together. In these individuals, moving a stoma even a fraction of an inch may make a major difference in ostomy management.

VI. POSTOPERATIVE TEACHING AND CARE

The care of all diversions begins with the application of a postoperative pouch and skin barrier in the operating room. In most situations, a transparent pouch is used in the hospital to allow ease of visualization of the stoma for color and edema and of the stomal (mucocutaneous) suture line. In colostomies and ileostomies, normal bowel function may not return for several days, but the pouching system protects the skin from mucous drainage and unexpected fecal output. With an ileal conduit, the urine drainage from the stoma begins during surgery (27,28).

A pouching system includes a pouch and some form of skin protection, from solid barrier to paste to liquids. The pouch itself has a faceplate, which attaches the pouch to the skin or to the skin barrier. The faceplate may be adhesive or may have a Tupperware type of connection. The pouch system should be changed regularly in the postoperative period, primarily for teaching the patient and family. Early discharge from the hospital has created a need for family involvement to begin immediately and for the patient to participate in his or her care when feasible. Table 5 provides an outline for changing a pouching system. (Universal precautions must be followed when changing a pouch.) A variety of one- and two-piece drainable pouching systems is available.

A. Selection of Equipment

The steps in selecting appropriate pouching systems are of utmost importance. No single pouch or skin barrier works on everyone. An effective pouching system is one that contains the effluent and protects the skin in a comfortable, cost-effective manner. This implies a "good seal" (18). A good seal is present when the skin protector and pouch adhere to the skin from the base of the stoma to the outer edge of the faceplate. This is differentiated from a seal that does not allow effluent to escape from the outer edge of the seal and drainage collects between the stoma and outer edge, called a "hidden leak" (18). The following assessments are needed to select the appropriate equipment for a person with an ostomy:

Table 5 Principles of Changing a Pouch

I. Assemble all equipment.
   A. To cleanse the skin, used cotton balls, Kleenex, toilet paper, washcloths, towels, premoistened towelettes.
   B. Pouch.
   C. Skin barriers.
   D. Pouch closure (rubber band, clip).
   E. Tape and/or belt.
   F. Equipment for cleansing or disposing of used pouches.

II. Assemble pattern.
   A. A paper towel may be used to trace a pattern.
   B. The pattern should hug the stoma but not ride up on it.
   C. Always label the pattern for top or skin side.
   D. Not only is the stomal opening important in making a pattern, the outer dimensions of the pattern must also be considered. The pattern should avoid hip bone, pubic area, ribs, and folds at waist or navel.

III. Use a Skin barrier (if applicable).
   A. Use half, quarter, or full wafer (4 × 4), depending on the size of the stoma and abdomen.
   B. Round the corners, or conform the wafer to the shape of the adhesive on the pouch.
   C. Trace the stomal pattern on the paper side.
   D. Cut hole on pattern line: line is not visible when the opening is cut.
   E. Smooth sides of the opening with finger.

IV. Apply the pouch.
   A. Pouch opening should be *slightly larger* (1/8–1/4 inch) than the opening of the skin barrier (paper can cut the stoma).
   B. Trace pattern on the paper side of the pouch (use the opening from the skin barrier that has already been cut).
   C. Cut the hole larger than the line of the pattern (cut outside the line).
   D. The edges around the opening should be smooth.
   E. Remove paper backing from the pouch, center the openings, and apply the shiny side of the skin barrier to the pouch if you want to apply as a one piece.
   F. If using a two-piece system, assemble system before applying to abdomen in the early postoperative period to prevent discomfort.

V. Empty the pouch. (Remember to use the universal precautions during the change procedure.)

VI. Remove pouch (if disposable, place in Baggie).

VII. Cleanse skin.
   A. Use warm water: soaps are not necessary and leave a film residue.
   B. It is not necessary to remove all barrier left on the skin: abrasions may be caused by rough cleansing, and other barriers tend to "burn" for a few minutes when applied.

VIII. Dry well.
IX. Note any changes in the skin or stoma (color, size, ulcerations).
X. Remove backing, and apply skin barrier (if not attached to pouch in step 4).
XI. Center and apply clean pouch.
XII. Close end.
XIII. Tape and/or belt.
XIV. Check supplies, and reorder as necessary.

Source: Adapted from Jackson D B, Sorrells S. Colostomy care. Plainsfield, NJ: Patient Education Press, 1988.

Type of ostomy
Size and contour of the abdomen
Condition of the peristomal skin
Physical and mental status of patient
Physical activities of patient
Financial situation of patient and family
Personal preference of patient

The type of ostomy suggests the consistency and content of the drainage from the stoma. This should indicate the need for and type of skin protection, the type of pouch closure, the appropriate pouch material, the need for preventive measures, and potential problems. A urinary diversion pouch should contain an antireflux valve and a spout closure. Colostomy pouches should be odor proof and drainable.

The size and contour of the abdomen and the presence of folds, creases, scars, and bony prominences determine the shape and size of the faceplate of the pouch. The pouch length and width are determined by the patient's torso and clothing. The extralong postoperative pouches that are used commonly in hospitals are not appropriate for discharge and are questionable for hospital use.

The condition of the peristomal skin influences the selection of skin protective products and skin care treatments. An effective pouching system should prevent skin breakdown, and once the skin is irritated, the length of time a pouching system stays on is limited. Skin turgor, texture, moisture, and secretions also influence the length of time a pouching system remains intact. Patients who perspire heavily in the summer may need an alternative system during these months.

Physical and mental status assessment of the patient is essential for determining whether the patient is capable of self-care, a family member will help or provide the care at home, or a home nurse referral is necessary. The patient and family are the best resource for planning care and teaching programs. The techniques required in applying, emptying, and caring for a pouching system should be considered by working closely with the patient. One pouch closure may work better for the patient than a second closure.

Physical activities affect the abdomen. Children are more active, in different ways than adults. Adults who are active sports enthusiasts may experience less success with the length of time a pouch seal remains intact. The hospitalized and recently discharged patient is less active than a person 3 or 6 months following surgery. The pouching system may need adjustment or changing as the person with an ostomy regains his or her presurgical activity level. This is one major reason that posthospital follow-up is so important.

The financial situation is of major concern to the patient and family. The nurse should work with the patient and family to select a cost-effective pouching system. Cost is only one factor to be considered. The other variables to be evaluated include the length of time a pouch can be worn, the prevention of skin problems, the ease of application, and patient comfort and confidence with the system.

Personal preference is a consideration in the selection of a pouch and skin barrier. The color, opaque to clear, precut to starter openings, two versus one piece, the length, and the shape may vary from person to person. The nurse's role in pouch selection is to provide the best possible system to prevent unnecessary leakage, odor escape, and skin breakdown. As the patient gains experiences, he or she may experiment with systems, but during the initial postoperative period, the patient may not have the knowledge to make informed choices unless educated to do so.

B. Peristomal Skin Integrity

The loss of skin integrity in the peristomal area may be related to several variables: the composition, consistency, and quantity of the effluent; the underlying disease process; treatments and medications; surgical construction and location of the stoma; skill of the care givers; skill and interest of patient in self-care; and the availability of proper supplies. In addition, nutrition, age, general health status, personal hygiene, activity, and rest patterns affect the body's ability to maintain skin integrity (29).

The person with an ostomy is at risk for damage to the epidermis around the stoma. Peristomal irritation that may be observed includes primary lesions (papules, vesicles, abscesses, and nodules) and secondary lesions (crusts, scales, erosions, ulcerations, and atrophy). Full-thickness wounds involve both the epidermis and the dermis, whereas partial-thickness lesions involve the epidermis.

Skin breakdown associated with ostomies may originate from four primary etiologies: allergies, mechanical trauma, chemical reactions, and infections. Although less common, peristomal skin breakdown may be associated with the primary disease of the patient, such as Crohn's disease, or with treatment protocols, such as chemotherapy and radiation therapy.

1. Allergies

Sensitivities have been reported to skin barriers, powders, pouches, clamps, belts, and adhesives. The skin may appear erythematous, edematous, eroded, weeping, or bleeding (30). Patients may report initial symptoms of itching, stinging, and/or burning. The skin irritation is limited to the area in contact with allergen.

Systemic allergic responses to products in contact with the stoma mucosa have been reported (29). If a person has a history of allergies, the nurse should observe the patient for 30 minutes after applying any new product, pouch, solid barriers, pastes, or powders. This is not difficult to do, and patient teaching can continue while the nurse is with the patient and family. Localized reactions (skin) take longer to appear but are not life threatening.

Many sensitivities are associated with the misuse of products. Skin barriers applied to wet rather than dry skin, moisture under a plastic pouch, and thick applications of bonding agents are frequent causes of skin problems. Many patients report sensitivity to paper or microporous tapes. These sensitivities are often tape burns associated with the misuse application of tape. When tape is applied to skin and stretched tightly across a dressing, tension is placed on the skin and "tape burns" or vesicles appear. A patient may associate this with an allergic reaction. Because many ostomy products are available with a similar tape, the use of these products depends on patient sensitivities versus misuse.

2. Mechanical Trauma

Pressure, friction, or stripping of adhesives or skin barriers may result in mechanical trauma to the skin. Repeated, frequent removal of pouching systems is the most common cause (29). The first sign is erythema or redness that does not disappear when the pouching system has been removed for several minutes. Prolonged and continued irritation results in loss of epidermis, with denudation and erosions of the skin followed by scales, patches, and crusts.

Prevention of mechanical trauma may be accomplished by regular changes of the pouching system every 4–7 days or whenever leakage occurs. If the pouching system is leaking frequently, then reevaluate the system and select a system that works better before the skin is irritated.

3. Chemical Irritants

The most common chemical irritants are stool and urine. Any drainage left in continuous contact with the skin results ultimately in irritation. Skin barriers appropriately sized to fit the stoma and protect the skin prevent problems by eliminating exposure of the skin to stool and/or urine. The skin barrier can hug the stoma, but the pouch opening should be 1/8 inch larger than thc stoma.

Although not common in hospitals, accumulation of amorphous ammonium phosphates (urine crystals) may appear on the stoma or skin of a person with an ileal conduit. Urine crystals are more common with alkaline urine. The salts appear as white, gritty particles (31). The prevention of urine crystals includes appropriate cleansing of all equipment, maintenance of an acid urine, and carefully calibrated stomal openings (31).

Certain chemicals in glues, solvents, soaps, and detergents may irritate the peristomal skin. If burning or stinging sensations are reported by the patient, remove the system and cleanse the skin carefully. Soaps are avoided in the peristomal area, because many leave a residue on the skin. This is not to imply that people never wash the peristomal skin with soap, but it is important to provide a thorough rinsing. When patients return home, recommend a shower, if possible, during the pouch change. The running water helps remove any soap residue (29).

4. *Infections*

The most common infection is caused by *Candida albicans (Monilia)*. The skin appears brightly erythematous, with papulular and vesicular lesions. Satellite vesicles are common. As the infection progresses, serous weeping is followed by scaling and crusting (29). *Candida* infections are more common in urinary diversions and are related to the extensive bowel preparation before surgery and the moist environment of the peristomal area. Diagnosis of *C. albicans* infection can be made by visual inspection and by skin scrapings prepared with potassium hydroxide. The treatment is nystatin (Mycostatin) powder (29). Steroid sprays are not recommended unless severe inflammation is present and extends beyond the peristomal area.

Bacterial infections are less common. *Staphylococcus aureus* may present as a large patchy, erythematous, crusty area with plaques (30). Organisms should be identified by culture of the affected area. The appropriate topical or systemic antibiotic is then ordered. Skin barriers do not adhere to an ointment initially after applied. Apply the ointment, and expose the skin to air, light, and heat. As the ointment begins to be absorbed, the skin barrier can be applied.

5. *Chemotherapy*

The basal cells in the epidermis rapidly divide and, therefore, are more susceptible to the effects of chemotherapy. Skin reactions can be minimized or prevented by adding solid skin barriers to the pouching system, if these are not routinely used, changing pouches when a leak occurs, and early recognition of bacterial or fungal infections. A discoloration, deep red and purple, may be caused by 5-fluorouracil and bleomycin (32). A generalized skin breakdown may occur with methotrexate, bleomycin, and adrenocorticoids that does not subside until the causative agent is discontinued (32).

6. Radiation Therapy

Skin reactions with radiation therapy may vary from a mild loss of hair to a deep, purplish erythema with blistering. Prevention includes minimizing trauma and irritation; reducing friction; avoiding solvents, soaps, ointments, and lotions; avoiding direct sunshine and heat; and keeping the area dry (29). The skin should be gently cleansed with warm water and patted dry, not rubbed. If the stoma is in the direct field of radiation, remove the pouching system during the treatment if possible. If the pouch or a segment of faceplate is in the radiation field, move or remove the pouch during treatment. The faceplate or skin barrier can often be adjusted or trimmed to remove it from the field of radiation.

The treatment of peristomal skin is more difficult than the prevention. Table 6 provides a summary of common types of peristomal skin problems and steps for treatment.

VII. DIAGNOSTIC PROCEDURES FOLLOWING DIVERSIONAL SURGERIES

A. Colostomy

The most common diagnostic procedures following colostomy are diagnostic radiology studies or further intestinal surgery that requires bowel preparation. The first questions to be answered should include the reason for the bowel preparation, the usual consistency and volume of the patient's stool, and the length and function of the proximal bowel (33). If the patient has an end-sigmoid colostomy, the bowel preparation cleanses the proximal colon, and a combination of liquid diets, oral laxatives, and colostomy irrigations may be used. Suppositories are not used because they are expelled from the stoma before being absorbed. If repeated colostomy irrigations are required, saline rather than tap water is recommended for the procedure to reduce any fluid and electrolyte imbalance (33).

If the distal bowel is intact, the nurse should clarify whether both segments of colon are to be cleansed or the distal (nonfunctioning) or the proximal bowel. When irrigating a distal bowel segment, the returns are expected through the rectum unless a blockage is present in the segment of distal bowel. When Hartmann's pouch is to be cleansed for surgery, the volume of solution is determined by the length of retained distal colon. A low-volume enema is suggested when the rectosigmoid colon has been left (33).

B. Urinary Diversion

The most important test done following urinary diversion that is most often performed incorrectly is obtaining a urine specimen for culture and sensitivity

Table 6 Peristomal Skin Management

- I. Rash
  - A. Location can be under the tape, under the faceplate, and on any part of the skin where the pouch comes in contact with the skin. A generalized reddish appearance that covers an entire area, similar to a diaper rash, is seen.
  - B. Cause
    1. Leaking appliance
    2. Perspiration
    3. Allergies to tape
  - C. Treatment
    1. Use heat lamp and/or hair drier to dry the skin.
    2. Sprinkle a small amount of powder (karaya, stomahesive) on the skin, wipe off the excess, then blot with a skin sealant to seal the powder to the skin.
    3. Powder the skin on which the pouch lies (not under the faceplate).
    4. Make or buy a pouch cover.
    5. Wearing a pouch belt too tight may break the seal.
- II. Erythematous skin
  - A. Location may be under the tape, under the faceplate, and on any part of the skin in contact with the pouch.
  - B. Cause
    1. Allergic response
    2. Mechanical trauma
  - C. Treatment
    1. Remove pouch every 48–72 h or more often if patient complains of pain.
    2. Cleanse the skin with warm water, and pat dry.
    3. Expose skin to light, air, and heat for 20 minutes.
    4. Use a solid skin barrier covering all erythematous skin.
    5. Use a different pouching system if erythremia is related to an allergic response.
- III. Eroded or denuded skin
  - A. Location is under faceplate or tape.
  - B. Cause
    1. Mechanical trauma
    2. Chemical irritant
  - C. Treatment
    1. Change system every 24–48 h to treat the skin.
    2. Cleanse with warm water, and pat dry.
    3. Apply Burow's solution (aluminum acetate) compresses for 20 minutes (Optional step).
    4. Expose skin to air, heat, and light.
    5. Apply powder or paste (not containing alcohol).
    6. Apply solid skin barrier.

IV. Ulcerated area on stoma.
  A. Location is anywhere on stoma.
  B. Cause: Stomal opening of the pouch was too small and/or activities caused the faceplate to rub or cut into stoma.
  C. Treatment
    1. Enlarge the size of the pouch opening (opening should be at least 1/8 inch larger than stoma).
    2. Evaluate patient activities; may need a different size or shape of faceplate.
    3. Loosen the belt; if too tight, it may cause the faceplate to ride into stoma.

V. Infected or irritated hair follicles
  A. Location is under the faceplate, raised red areas (similar to acne) at the shaft of the hair follicle.
  B. Cause: Not keeping the area under the faceplate shaved.
  C. Treatment
    1. Must allow the irritation to improve before removing any more hair by shaving or cutting.
    2. Use hair drier and/or heat lamp to dry the skin, if oozing is present.
    3. Use a skin barrier between the skin and faceplate until irritation improves. Try to leave on 24–48 h.

VI. Water-logged skin (urinary diversion)
  A. Location is between opening of the faceplate and the stoma.
  B. Cause is too much skin exposed between the stoma and the faceplate and the urine pools on the skin.
  C. Treatment
    1. Use heat lamp and/or hair drier in area.
    2. Cover area with a pectin-based skin barrier, hugging the stoma.
    3. Decrease the size of stomal opening in faceplate.

VII. *Candida albicans* infection
  A. Location is on skin surrounding the stoma. May extend beyond the faceplate: reddened skin with raised lesions.
  B. Cause is fungal infection of the skin.
  C. Treatment
    1. Use heat lamp and/or hair drier on the area.
    2. Apply Mycostatin powder to the area, blow off the excess powder, and seal this in with a thin coat of a skin sealant. Apply pouch in the usual manner. (You need a prescription for Mycostatin.)
    3. Drink lots of fluids. Add buttermilk or yogurt to your diet.

VIII. Alkaline urine crystals
  A. Location is on the stoma and/or around the stoma base.
  B. Cause is alkaline urine and a predisposition for stone formation.
  C. Treatment
    1. Swab vinegar solution (1 part vinegar and 1 part water) on the stoma when changing the pouch.

Table 6 (*Continued*)

2. Insert vinegar solution into the pouch while it is being worn. For a minor formation, insert four times a day. (Remove antireflux valve from the pouch.
   a. Empty the pouch.
   b. Instill 1–2 ounces of vinegar solution into the pouch.
   c. Encourage patient to lay down so the solution bathes the inside of the pouch and the stoma for approximately 20 minutes.
   d. Empty the pouch, and rinse with cool water.

Note: The vinegar solution may discolor the stoma, making it appear "blanched" or "white." It will return to its normal red color in a few minutes.

3. Use vinyl or plastic pouches until the condition clears, or use new rubber pouches. Rubber pouches tend to precipitate crystals inside the pouch, which may cause bleeding and irritation to the stoma.

Source: Adapted from Jackson DB, Sorrells S. Urinary diversion care. Plainfield, NJ: Patient Education Press, 1988.

from an ileal conduit or other form of urinary diversion. The urine should be obtained from the conduit by introducing a catheter through the stoma using sterile techniques. Often a specimen is taken from the pouch in the doctor's office, resulting in a positive culture, regardless of whether a urinary infection is present.

After hand washing and donning sterile gloves, the nurse or doctor should establish a sterile field. The stoma is cleansed or "prepped" with three swabs soaked in an antiseptic solution. The stoma is cleansed with each swab once. A fourth, sterile swab is used to remove any remaining cleansing solution from the stoma. A lubricated catheter is introduced through the stoma opening into the conduit. The drainage end of the catheter is placed in a sterile container and held below the level of the abdomen to facilitate drainage from the conduit. It is necessary to wait for urine to drain into the container because the conduit is not a reservoir and does not hold urine.

VIII. COMPLICATIONS ASSOCIATED WITH DIVERSIONAL PROCEDURES

A. Stomal Complications

In the early postoperative period, the stomal complications that may occur include bleeding, ischemia and necrosis, and skin-mucosa separation. Stomal complications that may occur in the late postoperative period (months to years following surgery) include melanosis coli, prolapse, hernia, retraction, stenosis, and laceration. Careful observation of the stoma during each pouch change provides for early diagnosis of any complication.

B. Alterations in Sexual Function

Ostomy surgery and adjuvant therapy may directly or indirectly alter the sexual function of the patient. Surgery for low-lying rectal cancers and bladder cancer damages the nerves and structures essential for penile and vaginal intercourse. Men experience erectile and ejaculatory problems. The degree of impotence is related to the amount of tissue resected (34). For women, the changes are not as apparent. Women may experience decreased lubrication and coital pain. Gynecological cancers may result in the loss or shortening of the vagina.

Radiation therapy may result in nerve damage, alteration in vascular flow, and tissue changes that affect sexual function. Chemotherapy may cause impotence, sterility, depressed libido, and the appearance of secondary sex characteristics. Indirectly, both radiation and chemotherapy result in side effects that negatively impact on sexual functioning, including depression, nausea, vomiting, and general malaise.

Patients and their partners benefit from open and honest discussions about sexual functioning and alternatives that are available following surgery and recuperation. Referral to a counselor for assistance should be considered for each patient and partner.

IX. RESOURCES FOR FAMILIES

A major resource for persons having ostomy surgery is a person who has undergone similar surgery. The United Ostomy Association (2001 West Beverly Boulevard, Los Angeles, CA 90057) and the International Ostomy Association (15 Station Road, Reding, Berkshire RG1 1LG, UK) are self-help groups designed to help people who have had surgery. The organizations are operated by volunteers who have stomas and who demonstrate for others that people with stomas can rehabilitate and live successful and productive lives, marry and have children, work, and play and grow. The group meetings allow members to share experiences and to share solutions. Visitors are available for hospital or home visits as well as phone calls.

The American Cancer Society (1599 Clifton Road NE, Atlanta, GA 30329) also serves as a major resource for persons undergoing ostomy surgery. The society provides education for lay public and the medical profession. The American Cancer Society has played an instrumental role in developing screening programs for detecting colorectal cancers.

X. FUTURE PERSPECTIVES

The future of ostomies will be in the new surgeries being developed and refined that will eliminate the need for external devices and stomas. Fewer and fewer stomas will be created that are permanent. The advantages for future patients include no fears of odor or embarrassing leakages. For some, no pouch will be required, although other procedures will be needed, such as intermittent catheterization. As more people live with cancer as a chronic illness, the future for all will brighten.

SELECTED READING

Hampton BG, Bryant RA. Ostomies and continent diversions. Nursing management. St. Louis: C. V. Mosby, 1992. This book is an in-depth coverage of ostomies. The authors have assembled a wealth of information on the indications for surgeries, the surgical techniques, and all aspects of the physical and emotional care needed for patients and families. An excellent resource.

Doughty DB, Jackson DB. Gastrointestinal disorders. St. Louis: C. V. Mosby, 1993. This text examines the gastrointestinal diseases, their treatment, and nursing implications in detail. The sections on ostomy include patient education materials and highlights for question and answer sections with patients and families. The complication and management of ostomies are detailed.

REFERENCES

1. Fry RD, Fleshman JW, Kodner IJ. Cancer of the colon and rectum. Clin Symp 1989; 41(5):2.
2. Jackson BS, Broadwell DC. Ostomy surgery: an overview of historical, current, and future perspectives. Semin Oncol Nurs 1986; 2(4): 227–234.
3. Hurney C, Holland J. Psychological sequelae of ostomies in cancer patients. CA 1986; 36:26–41.
4. Perez CA, Knapp RC, DiSaia PJ, et al. Gynecologic tumors. In: DeVita VT, Hellman S, Rosenberg SA, eds. Cancer: principles and practice, 2nd ed. Philadelphia: Lippincott, 1985: 1013–82.
5. Holland J. Psychological aspects of cancer. In: Holland JF, Frei E, eds. Cancer medicine, 2nd ed. Philadelphia: Lea and Febiger, 1982.
6. Sugarbaker PH, Gunderson LL, Wittes RE. Colorectal cancer. In: DeVita VT, Hellman S, Rosenberg SA, eds. Cancer: principles and practice, 2nd ed. Philadelphia: Lippincott, 1985: 795–884.
7. Ezzell C. Colon cancer's newly mapped gene puts it all in the family. J NIH Res 1993; 5(6):38–39.
8. Myers RE, Balshem AM, Wolf TA, Ross EA, Millner L. Screening for colorectal neoplasia: physicans' adherence to complete diagnostic evaluation. Am J Public Health 1993; 83(11):1620–1622.

9. Khubchandani IT, Karamchandani M, Kleckner F, et al. Mass screening for colorectal cancer. Dis Colon Rectum 1989; 32:754–758.
10. Simon J. Occult blood screening for colorectal carcinoma: a critical review. Gastroenterology 1985; 88:820.
11. Bryant RA, Buls JG. Pathophysiology and diagnostic studies of gastriointestinal tract disorders. In: Hampton BG, Bryant RA, eds. Ostomies and continent diversions: nursing management. St. Louis: C. V. Mosby, 1992; 299–348.
12. Droller MJ. Transitional cell cancer: upper tracks and bladder. In: Walsh PC, Gittes, RF, Perlmutter, AD, and Stamey, TA, ed., Campbell's urology, 5th ed. Philadelphia: W. B. Saunders, 1986.
13. Gray M. Genitourinary disorders. St. Louis: C. V. Mosby, 1992.
14. Hampton BG. Nursing management of a patient following pelvic exenteration. Semin Oncol Nurs 1986; 2(4):281–286.
15. Fazio VW. Cancer of the colon and rectum. In: Broadwell DC, Jackson BS, eds. Principles of ostomy care. St. Louis: C. V. Mosby, 1982: 148–166.
16. Atkinson KG. Abdominoperineal resection of the rectum. In: Broadwell DC, Jackson BS, eds. Principles of ostomy care. St. Louis: C. V. Mosby, 1982:186–205.
17. Dobkin KA, Broadwell DC. Nursing considerations for the patient undergoing colostomy surgery. Semin Oncol Nurs 1986; 2(4):249–255.
18. Broadwell DC, Jackson BS. Principles of ostomy care. St. Louis: C. V. Mosby, 1982.
19. Pernet FPPM, Jonas U. Ileal conduit urinary diversion: early and late results of 132 cases in a 25 year period. World J Urol 1985; 3:140.
20. Rolstad BS, Hoyman K. Continent diversions and reservoirs. In: Hampton BG, Bryant RA, eds. Ostomies and continent diversions. Nursing management. St. Louis: C. V. Mosby, 1992:129–162.
21. Dudas S. Rehabilitation concepts of nursing. J Enterostomal Ther 1984; 11:6–15.
22. Broadwell DC. Rehabilitation needs of the patient with cancer. Cancer (August 1 Suppl) 1987; 60:563–568.
23. Frank-Stromborg M, Wright P. Ambulatory cancer patients' perception of the physical and psychosocial changes in their lives since the diagnosis of surgery. Cancer Nurs 1984; 7:117–130.
24. Jackson DB. Variables affecting ostomy patient outcomes. NIH grant number 1 R15 NRO2929-01, research study in process.
25. Druckerman LJ. The management of a permanent colostomy. Am J Dig Dis 1938; 5:382–385.
26. Watt R. Stoma placement. In: Broadwell DC, Jackson BS, eds. Principles of ostomy care. St. Louis: C. V. Mosby, 1982: 329–339.
27. Alterescu KB. Colostomy. Nurs Clin North Am 1987; 22(2):281–289.
28. Erickson PJ. Otomies: the art of pouching. Nurs Clin North Am 1987; 22(2):311–320.
29. Broadwell DC. Peristomal skin integrity. Nurs Clin North Am 1987; 22(2):321–332.
30. Watt RC. Pathophysiology of peristomal skin. In: Broadwell DC, Jackson BS, eds. Principles of ostomy care. St. Louis: C. V. Mosby, 1982:241–256.
31. Watt RC. Nursing management of a patient with a urinary diversion. Semin Oncol Nurs, 1986; 2:265–269.
32. Rodriques DB. Special considerations: care of the ostomy patient receiving cancer

therapy. In: Broadwell DC, Jackson BS, eds. Principles of ostomy care. St. Louis: C. V. Mosby, 1982:381–389.
33. Erwin-Toth P, Doughty DB. Principles and procedures of stoma management. In: Hampton BG, Bryant RA, eds. Ostomies and continent diversions: nursing management. St. Louis: C. V. Mosby, 1992:29–103.
34. Shipes E. Sexual function following ostomy surgery. Nurs Clin North Am 1987; 22(2):303–310.

19

Information, Education, and Counseling: Essentials of Supportive Cancer Care

Agnes Glaus
Kantonsspital, St. Gallen, Switzerland

Gertrude Grahn
Lund University, Lund, Sweden

I. INTRODUCTION

Supportive care in cancer patients is a concept that has evolved in the last two decades. The struggle against cancer as a life-threatening disease was primarily understood in terms of the destruction of cancer cells, the stopping of tumor growth, and the increase in survival time. The progress of medical science in the twentieth century allowed many patients to understand that even cancer could be cured, or at least controlled, over years. Thus success has inspired hope and improved quantity and quality of life for many patients. Once it became possible to increase survival time, the quality of life debate became more relevant. Death was no longer seen as the greatest and sole enemy of quality of life.

Quality of life is of concern for cancer patients in all stages of the disease. Supportive care therefore deals with patients from the time of diagnosis to the time of cure, relapse, or death. Palliative care can be seen as part of supportive care, which deals especially with the suffering of patients with incurable disease during the terminal phase of their lives. Supportive care bridges so-called curative care wih palliative care, because its activities, feelings, and attitudes pay regard to physical, psychological, and social coping with progressive illness and survival (1).

Supportive care also bridges the efforts of different health care professionals; it is an interdisciplinary endeavor. To be supportive means to care for patients from different viewpoints, accepting other professionals as specialists and patients as competent claimants (2). Information, education, and counseling are one part of supportive care, which needs a strong link between professions and patient to be effective and complementary. It has been said that the ability to care for oneself and to exercise control over daily activities may improve psychological as well as moral well-being, which again is considered the most significant dimension of quality of life (3). This implies that information, education, and counseling are major concerns for patients and, from their viewpoint, probably the most relevant aspects of supportive care.

II. THE CONCEPT OF SUPPORTIVE CARE AND ITS RELATION TO INFORMATIONAL NEEDS

Providing support for others is considered a key aspect of nursing. However, definitions about the nature and behaviors of support are vague. A supportive care model was developed by O'Berle to articulate a specific palliative nursing role. This model includes six interwoven dimensions: valuing, connecting, empowering, doing for, finding meaning, and preserving one's own integrity (4). This model raises the question of whether being supportive is different from caring and whether it is representative of a specific role. Support is cited as an integral component of care, which is defined by Leininger as "those assistive, supportive or facilitative acts towards or for an individual or group, intended to ameliorate or improve a human condition or life way" (5). Similarly, Paternoster defines caring as "warmth, compassion, support and concern" (6). The supportive care model by O'Berle seems to be highly compatible with the holistic view of caring as described by the experts Benner and Wrubel (7).

In this sense, support for cancer patients seems to be an integral component of nursing, medical, and psychosocial care. This support could be explained as helping methods to deal with specific physical and psychological problems, but also as attitudes and feelings that mediate the supporter to act. In cancer care, this refers, apart from any tumor therapy, to assisting in adjustment to new circumstances (physical and psychological), to understanding treatments, to combating the side effects of therapy, to relieving symptoms, and to helping the patient cope. Orem describes support as encouragement, assurance, communication, and physical help with the aim of enabling the patient to control and direct action in the situation, once support has been received (8). However, some cancer patients cannot, or can no longer, control and direct actions. For those who are able to do so, information, education, and counseling become crucial prerequisites to gaining control and directing action.

III. INFORMATION

A. Definition and Aim

Information giving is described as an important element of teaching. It may not be the same as teaching, the latter inferring an interactive process whereby learning takes place, which may subsequently be used to influence behavior. From research conducted in patients who were due for tests or surgery, clues emerge to explain the mechanism of how information giving or patient teaching helps individuals (9):

1. Anxiety is alleviated by reducing the area of "unknown" experiences, fears and fantasies being corrected by providing a realistic account of what will happen.
2. The role of instruction helps patients to know what is expected of them and how to do things, which will improve their experiences and recovery. Through this confidence they can behave in a useful way and feel less dependent and helpless.

Information giving is described as a process in which there is only one-way exchange. Topics may be limited and unquestioned, data factual only, and the relationship neutral but authoritative (10). Information giving in itself provides only a small amount of interaction or assessment of individual needs. The level of negotiation on content is usually low. Goals may not be discussed, and continuing sessions may be lacking. This kind of information can easily be obtained but not easily retained. A bad example of one-way information is the misuse of written, informed consent, in which patients sign a paper with information on procedures and possible outcome. In practice, patients badly understand the text and unfortunately often cannot discuss it with anyone.

It becomes evident that the underlying ethical attitudes of the health care professionals may play a major role in how information is given. On one side, these professionals, especially doctors and nurses, mostly lack education concerning communication skills. Nursing and medical education in Europe usually does not include teaching principles. On the other side, the relationship between patient and caregiver plays a crucial role. Whenever a paternalistic attitude prevails, patients are not involved in the information process. What can they be told about, if they are not allowed even to know the diagnosis? Patients are coming to understand that knowledge about illness and medical care is not the exclusive property of health professionals (11). Information is essential if respect for the autonomy of the patient is to be considered.

Sound knowledge, communication, and teaching skills, as well as a partnershiplike relation between caregiver and patient, allow mere information to become a process with a two-way exchange. They build the framework for the actual impartation of information (Fig. 1).

B. Imparting Information

Clear guidelines have become commonly accepted for the actual imparting of information (12). New, oral information must have the following characteristics:

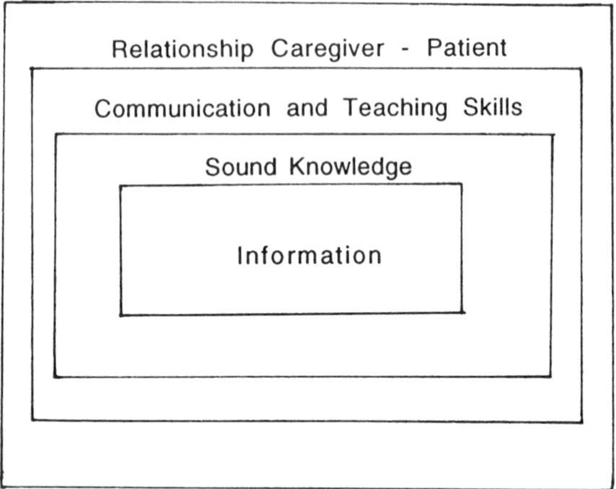

Figure 1 Framework for imparting the cancer diagnosis.

Carefully planned, sequential, and logical
Covers the most important points first
Related to the next event
Limited amount of information
Includes questions to elicit patient's understanding
Complemented by written or audiovisual material if possible

Informal patient information may represent the most common type of information and refers to all unplanned patient-staff communication. Even though this may be effective, it can scarcely be pursued or measured by outcome. Essential information must be given in a methodological and timely planned intervention.

Formal, planned information giving has a specific content, for example information about the diagnosis. Questions related to the person of the informer, to the receiver of the information, and to the how and where of information giving, are described later in the specific context of cancer care.

IV. INFORMATION ABOUT CANCER: STILL A QUESTION?

Paterson found in 1954 that cancer was regarded as the most alarming disease a person could contract, and 50% of the sample believed that it was incurable (13). Today there is still something about cancer that causes more fear and anxiety in individuals than any other disease, even though one-third to half of these patients are treated successfully and can be cured (14). There is still no worldwide agreement about whether to inform the patient about cancer. In 1979, however,

Novack and Plumer suggested that 95% of patients in the United States were told the diagnosis when cancer was discovered (15). In some other countries, a consensus has emerged that it is best to tell the "truth." This does not seem to be the case in Latin countries, where cancer is still treated as a taboo and the sociocultural background stipulates withholding the diagnosis cancer. A study from Spain shows that establishing a "conspiracy of silence" around the patient is the usual manner of "communicating." A survey of 167 cancer patients reveals that only 15% of them are aware of their diagnosis (16). In view of the imminent unification of Europe and inevitable intermigration of populations, disclosure of a cancer diagnosis to patients of different cultural origins becomes an important issue.

A. Aim of Communicating the Diagnosis of Cancer

In countries where patients are told about the disease, health care professionals and patients believe in the right to know. From the ethical point of view, this refers to the principle of respect for autonomy. Who, if not the patient, can decide which course of action maximizes his or her welfare? The information allows the patient to gain knowledge about illness and treatment and helps to decide further steps. It gives the opportunity to set priorities in life, to set realistic goals, to understand treatments, and to comply with or refuse them. If the patient is kept in ignorance, he or she cannot know how to cope with the situation.

B. Who Communicates the Diagnosis?

There is no question about the fact that the truth is communicated by more than merely words. Professionals and relatives or friends may express their knowledge in nonverbal signs. The expression on the physician's face, silence, increased attention, and avoidance strategies, as well as signals from the own body, may promptly inform the patient. Everyone around the patient is communicating in some way.

1. Role of the Physician

If the information about cancer is a formal, planned intervention, the responsibility is likely to be the doctor's. Because today many doctors are involved in the diagnostic procedure, the questions evolves on which doctor is meant to be the informer. Many primary care physicians initially convey warnings or suspicions to patients and schedule them for consultation with surgeons or oncologists. Lind documented that the majority of patients first learned the diagnosis of cancer from a surgeon who performed a biopsy and only a minority were told by their primary care physicians (17). Today, advances in radiological imaging complicate the question of who should do the telling. Experience suggests that the doctors who are involved only at the diagnostic stage should pass the results to the primary physician or to the oncologist, who will also discuss treatment options. Further research is needed to identify whether the person telling the diagnosis is of importance to patients or if this concern is overridden by the diagnosis itself.

2. Role of Nurses and Other Health Care Professionals

It has been said that hospital staff can be divided into announcers and nonannouncers. Doctors are the primary announcers. When it comes to information about the patient's condition, nurses are nonannouncers (18). There seems to be a gap between the primary announcers and the nonannouncers. The primary announcement, in everyday practice, very soon becomes a message that must be repeated. This repetition can be classified as an announcement, and at that time, the telling person is often likely to be the experienced nurse. Translation into the patient's own vocabulary, in which hiding behind medical terms is no longer possible, can be very painful. At this stage, information is transformed into counseling.

There are few official instructions about the type of information nurses are allowed to release. There is anecdotal evidence that nurses sometimes cannot or do not want to escape from breaking the rule of withholding information. Their closeness to patients makes it difficult to hide anything. Experience shows that nurses push withholding doctors to tell the truth because they, like the patient, suffer from the "silent conspiracy." It has been suggested that the greater the power of a nurse and the lesser the social distance between the doctor and nurse, the less the nurse feels bound to hospital rules (18). Here, power is not defined; it can be interpreted as knowledge, experience, position, and communication skills. It becomes evident that the degree of collaboration between doctor and nurse and the expert role of nurses, as well as their ideological perspective, have immediate influence on truth telling.

Tilley found that patients acknowledged nurses as sources of certain information. They preferred to receive information from the nurse concerning the event of illness and about what to expect in the future. However, patients preferred to receive medically oriented information from doctors (19). These findings suggest that nurses and doctors can and must have different emphases in information giving.

Little research has been done on the role of auxiliary staff, physiotherapists, social workers, cleaners, or the clergy in the informal communication. It is not known how much information, if any, these individuals pass on to patients and relatives.

C. When and Where Should the Diagnosis Be Told?

Patients relate that the time of uncertainty is very difficult. The period between suspicion and the results of a biopsy or radiologic procedure seems endless to patients. They may push doctors to rapid conveyance of information, immediately after biopsy or radiography. Because the revision of an initially benign diagnosis is an unlikely but potentially traumatic consequence, many institutions respect the following rule:

> Never inform a patient about the cancer diagnosis before the final proving report is available (biopsy or cytology).

This rule prevents unnecessarily burdening patients with a cancer diagnosis that might turn out to be only a suspicion or later, false.

However, delaying until the biopsy report is available lengthens the time of uncertainty. To overcome this problem, physicians may relate the diagnosis over the telephone. Lind and Delvecchio found that 42% of a studied patient population in the United States was told either in the recovery room or over the telephone. A significantly greater percentage of the patients told over the telephone expressed negative feelings about the timing of information, compared with those told in a hospital room or doctor's office (17). Negative feelings were related to being upset when caught off-guard or in a nonprivate setting. To overcome this problem, the following rule might be helpful:

> Making an office appointment to tell the patient the diagnosis is preferable to telling the patient the diagnosis over the telephone. If an office appointment is not possible, the phone call should be scheduled to give the patient the opportunity to prepare psychologically and choose an adequate locality.

In the same study, patients indicated that learning the diagnosis of cancer sooner is not necessarily better. The circumstances and mode of telling bad news seem to be crucial. If the diagnostic results are negative, telling the good news over the telephone has not been received negatively (17). As outpatient diagnosis of cancer becomes more common, the question of how to tell patients who are not hospitalized will be increasingly relevant, not only in American but also in European countries, from where we have little knowledge concerning information via telephone calls.

Another important point is the readiness of the patient to be informed. Patients distressed about being told in the recovery room believed that they had not fully recovered from anesthesia and did not have sufficient mental clarity to cope effectively with learning the diagnosis at that time (17).

> Psychoactive medication, inability to concentrate, discomfort (e.g., pain), or anxiety interferes with the patient's readiness to receive information.

It is not evident from research whether the presence of a spouse, relative, or close friend is important to patients when receiving bad news. Experience shows that many patients come to the office together with a significant person. If the principle of respect for autonomy is to be regarded and if it is not allowed by law to inform someone other than the patient, the patient must agree with the involvement of another person.

It remains the patient's choice to share the truth with someone else.

Experience shows that patients find it helpful if they are offered to learn the diagnosis together with a significant other person.

If the information is given in a patient's room, care should be given that no other patients are in the room. Never inform patients "en passant" in a corridor. Ensure that everyone is seated comfortably. As an informer, never remain standing in front of patients who are seated or in bed.

D. How to Inform Patients About Cancer

Many questions concerning the "how" of truth telling are still unexplored. What do patients understand by the terms used by doctors and nurses? What does "tumor" or "malignancy" mean to them? If doctors use terms other than cancer, do they want to leave the patient with more hope? Another reason that has been suggested is that it is a reflection of the fears and anxiety of the doctor (18). Bearing in mind how difficult it is to disclose such a diagnosis, this reason is very understandable. Caregivers are vulnerable people, too.

To care for someone means to respond to a person who matters. It means to feel an interest in, to feel concern for. Caring in this sense is the essence of a helping relationship (20). If this concept of care underlies medical, nursing, or social care, how a life-threatening diagnosis is told cannot be cold, neutral, or without sympathy. This is the opposite of paternalistic withholding of the truth. Physicians who comfortably and confidently convey clear information and who can ask sensitively about the patient's reaction are usually perceived as more empathic, concerned, and trustworthy (21).

The Swiss Working Group for Clinical Cancer Research (SAKK) developed a method for assessment of the efficiency of the first interview between an oncologist and a cancer patient (22). Videotaped interviews were analyzed. Three dimensions formed the basis for assessment of the first information concerning cancer diagnosis.

1. Dimension: Content of Information (Cognitive Aspects)

This dimension deals with the cognitive aspects of the information. It refers to diagnostic, therapeutic, and prognostic information. Ideally, the language of the informer is clear and well understood by the patient.

Information is understandable to the patient (words and content): no unexplained medical terms and diagnosis clear and unequivocal.

Style and structure of talk are not rigid, allowing patient to interrupt.
Informer realizes that questions may already contain information.
Informer listens to already available knowledge and builds on it or corrects misunderstanding.
Don't talk down to the patient.
Use the word *I*, not *we* or *one*.
Pay attention to the equal contribution of speaking time between informer and patient.
Content of information is not too dense; informer does not speak too fast and asks questions to elicit understanding.
Listen and respond to the patient's comments.
Information is topic centered: no mention of minor things or unlikely events.
Relationship to patient is more important than completeness of information.
Avoid cross-examination style or induction of guilt.

2. Dimension: Emotional Warmth (Affective Aspects)

In oncology there remains this unresolvable conflict between the emotional involvement and the distance needed to be able to help. This closeness-distance problem is determined by the personality of the informer and by the patient. Emotional warmth manifests itself by the degree of attachment, positively but also negatively. An informer who takes over the depressed feelings of the patient and thus also becomes depressed is a negative example.

The informer shows respect and esteem for the individual's reaction and experience.
Remain friendly and considerate.
Encourage patient.
Show interest, and remain natural.
Verbal and nonverbal expressions remain congruent (e.g., friendly words are not accompanied by hostility).
Informer must realize that the information is more constructive and supportive with some patients and more defensive and distant with others, depending on the relationship to the patient.

3. Dimension: Patient Centeredness (Interactive Aspect)

This dimension allows the patient to feel personally understood. It refers to taking up all direct (verbal) and indirect patient information (affect, facial expression, and gestures). Critiques or doubts can be verbalized. It also refers to the need to explain the personal meaning or cause of the disease or to the expression of anxiety concerning death.

Anxiety concerning death and suffering can be verbalized.
Do not trivialize or console without objective facts.
Be reassuring and calming on the basis of objective facts.
Patient can express his or her reactions.
Do not blame anyone involved in treatment and care.
Listen and respond to individual interpretations of causes and meaning of disease; be ready to keep the talk flexible.

High patient centeredness may lead to "overidentification" by the informer. This overidentification can go along with fear and anxiety and can make it difficult for physicians and nurses to carry on with aggressive treatments, for example in research protocols.

Ideal information giving involves all three dimensions equally (Fig. 2). The information is clear and understandable; the informer shows emotional warmth and pays attention to the patient's personal way of reacting. Practice shows that this balance is often difficult to achieve because individual factors of both parties are involved; circumstances also play a crucial role. Videotaping of such important talks and subsequent analysis with regard to the three dimensions together with peers and psychooncologists could be a good learning method for nurses and doctors to prevent routinized and poor information giving. Routinized health care professionals are in danger of forgetting that their information might change everything in the life of the person concerned.

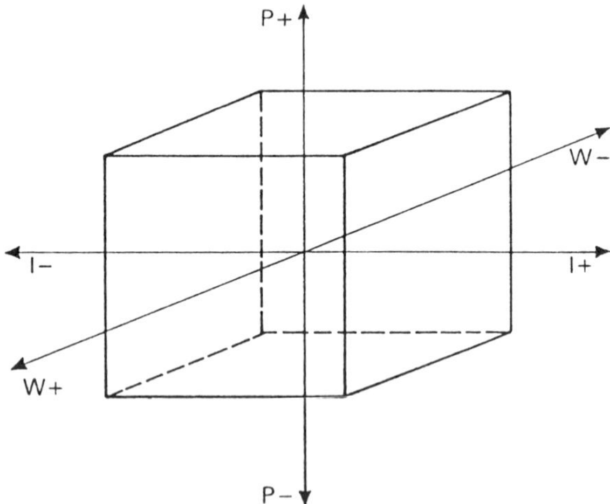

Figure 2 The balance of the three dimensions in truth telling: I, information, P, patient centeredness, and W, emotional warmth.

V. INFORMATION: AN ONGOING PROCESS IN CANCER CARE

Information is much more than disclosure of the diagnosis of cancer; it remains essential throughout the course of the illness. It is a continuing need when patients must cope with the disease and also with treatments or symptom control and when they have to live with a limited life expectancy.

Helpful information enables the patient to have control over side effects or symptoms, such as pain, and it enables them to live with obstacles. It helps them to understand why specific reactions happen and why specific measures are being taken. Some patients say that they do not want to know about every detail because it would scare them. Others want to know and document all analyses, including leukocyte counts and drug doses. "Good news," such as indications of tumor regression or of recovery from such side effects as leukopenia, are helpful to inspire hope and to encourage the patient.

During the course of illness and treatment, complications unrelated to tumor progression may arise. Such events must be explained to patients carefully because they observe changes very precisely and interpret them as tumor progression and are unnecessarily scared. This refers, for example, to prolonged therapy-induced leukopenia, to thrombosis or pulmonary embolism, or to unrelated infection.

Some other information seems to be harmful to patients. This especially relates to blunt information concerning the prognosis. Even though it may be realistic from statistical evidence that some patients have a short and determined life expectancy, it remains questionable when doctors speak of a "specific" survival time, because this is never known for an individual patient. Experience shows that patients being told a specific survival time (in weeks or months), but who then live longer, additionally suffer because they feel they are "over their time," which makes living difficult. Modern diagnostic procedures, such as relevant tumor markers, may enable patients and caregivers to follow the course of illness much more precisely. However, relating such fluctuations may be absolutely irrelevant for advanced cancer patients, because they in turn may induce additional anxiety. The following German proverb might be a helpful guide in many situations:

> Everything you say should be true, but not everything that is true needs to be told.

VI. EDUCATION: A BASIS FOR COPING WITH CANCER

Interest in the psychosocial aspects of being a cancer-diagnosed patient has grown considerably during the last decade. Supporting patients by means of education to achieve an *understanding* of occurrences in their efforts to cope with the cancer experience has become acknowledged within cancer care but more seldom given the attention it deserves.

A. Understanding the Cancer Experience

Research studies have shown that many cancer patients and their significant others want to understand better the events to which they are exposed and experience throughout the course of cancer. They seek information regarding the disease and treatment. They want support in passing through and making sense of the situational demands, which they perceive to exceed their personal resources. They want to be actively involved during the period of treatment as well as during the rehabilitation phase and/or the terminal phase (23–26).

For health care professionals, supportive care in this respect means to describe and explain for the patient what can be expected or to provide the patient with a means of coming to grips with what has been experienced. It entails outlining and organizing core features of the unfamiliar situation in a meaningful way and do so in light of recognizing and respecting the patient as a person with an unique history, with unique expectations and an unique meaning attached to the experience of illness. Patients seeking an understanding, an ability to infer from the information they have received, might have their coping efforts facilitated by learning more about the disease and their own reactions to it, as expressed by Marie Curie: "Nothing in life is to be feared; it is to be understood." Thus, providing a means to understand the cancer experience merges into the field of education (27).

B. Theoretical Frame for Learning and Coping

Everyone agrees that health care professionals must describe and explain many things for the patient, who wants to learn about and understand the current situation. Informing patients is generally oriented toward explaining the diagnosis, describing the treatment modalities and their side effects, and so on, in a one-way communication. For skill acquisition, demonstrations are commonly used.

Education, because it is an interactive process, moves beyond imparting information to increase the knowledge base and beyond demonstrations for skill acquisition. Education aims at growth and changes in the way a person thinks, feels, and acts in a holistic sense. For an understanding of events to occur, the cognitive and affective domains concurrently are influenced to increase, modify, or bring about changes in knowledge, attitudes, values, and skills to direct actions. In the teaching-learning process information, demonstration and emotional support are interwoven strands.

Growth and *change* are two dynamic words to describe learning and advancement in an educational endeavor. Varying learning theories have made attempts to capture the phenomena of growth and change related to core features in the current context, social structures and individual differences. The perception of education and its pedagogical consequences has varied from ancient to modern times (28). Fundamental conditions for learning and understanding to take place have been investigated and described in classic pedagogical learning models (e.g., Refs. 29–31). To apply knowledge of human learning processes is judicious in supporting patients and their significant others to achieve understanding.

The process of teaching and learning consists of educational experiences planned to meet individual learning needs, readiness, interests, and capabilities. Providing concrete experiences within the learner's world and allowing the learner to take on an active role give rise to increased ability and readiness for actions. Patient education is a valuable tool in empowering patients to make informed choices, which have an impact on their maintenance of and/or improvement in well-being and quality of life. It is a powerful device in building up confidence for living with cancer also when approaching death (32).

People use different strategies to give the events of daily life a decent order and to achieve understanding of unfamiliar events. When an event is perceived as a threat to well-being or touches the very core of life, as does a cancer diagnosis, the situational demands could, according to Lazarus and Folkman, be appraised as exceeding personal resources. Common strategies of daily life become insufficient or inappropriate. In attempts to manage a situation that thus is changed beyond control, the person constantly tries to modify cognitive, emotional, and behavioral efforts to solve the problem and/or reappraise the current situation in a process of coping (33–35). Changes in thoughts, feelings, and actions are interwined and interdependent strands in the process of coping. This is parallel to the process of learning, in which cognitive and affective domains are influenced to bring about changes in knowledge, attitudes, values, and skills to direct actions. This is why education is a valuable tool in developing and supporting coping strategies.

Education as a base for coping with events throughout the course of cancer is very much a question of finding congruence between what the patient expects, is exposed to, and experiences. When patients and their significant others struggle with demands they consider to exceed their personal resources, support in learning and becoming familiar with facts and feelings related to the cancer experience will influence their coping ability (32).

The essence and aim of patient education within the frame of psychosocial interventions in cancer care are to provide for intellectual and emotional growth and change. This aim is accomplished by giving patients opportunities and tools that are supportive of coping with the cancer experience and supportive also of living with cancer when life expectancy is limited.

C. Assessing Learning Needs

The first step in the interactive process of education is to identify the need or request a person has for knowing something or for gaining an ability to do something. Before staff members enter an educative process, it is important to establish the patient's own needs in terms of information and support. Assessing learning needs comprises an assessment of the content to be taught as well as the method to be used in accordance with assessed learning capacity and motivation. An accurate assessment results in mutually agreed goals for the teaching-learning endeavor. Learning occurs over time, and assessment of learning needs is an ongoing activity.

Because the need for information about the disease and treatment and the request for support in efforts to cope with the cancer experience are well documented within cancer care, the assessment area is mostly easy to review. However, even if items are well known, it is important in needs assessment to notice obstacles, if any, and to notice patients who are unable to identify and/or express their learning needs.

Learning requires emotional readiness or motivation. Needs identified by the learner will promote learning efforts and stimulate the learning process. Most important in assessing learning needs is thus to help patients and their significant others in identifying their learning needs. Not seldom are a patient's learning needs defined from the staff members' viewpoint. In a paternalistic way, staff members tend to "know best" the learning needs of their patients; they decide what their patients ought to know about procedures before and after surgery, about chemotherapy-induced side effects, and so on. The patients' perceptions of what is essential for them to know about in their coping efforts and their expectations, their experiences, and the meaning they attach to the situation, as well as their learning capacity, may not be congruent with what caregivers perceive.

The predominantly identified learning needs of cancer patients are cognitive and connected to the disease, treatment and side effects, and procedures. Assessments tend to ignore emotional dimensions, which are profound determinants of the coping capacity. The emotional detatchment of health care professionals is mainly a result of lack of training in communication and counseling (36).

A complete and accurate assessment provides a base that in a holistic sense has the potential to meet individual learning needs to provide comprehensive information and sufficient support. For the beginner, a checklist with itemized learning needs complemented by items suggested by the patient can sometimes be useful when teaching individuals as well as groups (37).

1. Adult Learners

Within the theory of adult learning it is emphasized that the adult learner has a desire to articulate his or her own needs and to make choices in moving from dependence toward self-direction when the climate communicates acceptance and support. Much of adult learning entails relearning. Adult learners are highly motivated to learn when their past experiences are considered and later used as a resource for further learning. Successful adult learning is also based on recognizing and respecting the learner's efforts, competence, and progress when reassessing learning needs. A "learning by doing" style is a challenge for adult learners, and their desire for active participation should be noted when needs are assessed (38).

Because adult learners may be of advanced age, impairment of vision or hearing may militate against proper understanding. Assessment of such age-related factors is crucial.

2. Learners with Low Literacy Skills

To assess the learning needs of patients with low literacy skills is not easy. It takes specialized knowledge to estimate their literacy and comprehension. To reach them in patient education sessions and to find the level at which communication is possible is a challenge for staff members. Efforts to simplify language in verbal communication and written materials, for example, are not always successful, because persons with low literacy skills process information differently from other persons. It is important to work with special sensitivity in assessing the needs of these patients; despite the intellectual handicap, their need for information and emotional support are equal to that other patients (38).

3. Learners with Different Cultural Backgrounds

A diversity of cultural beliefs and values may complicate educational ventures if not assessed properly. Some issues are of special importance to consider, and staff members involved in patient education must learn about salient cultural features. Religious beliefs or cultural traditions may determine what can be communicated and disclosed. Such concepts as the human body, health, disease, and illness are perceived in different ways and have different meanings in different cultures, and nonverbal signals can be interpreted in many ways.

D. Planning and Implementing

Patient education is a psychosocial intervention aiming at supporting the patient in coping with the cancer experience. As such, patient education should become an integral part of cancer care, planned for, accomplished, and evaluated, as is the rule for other interventions. Although there are many similarities between providing supportive education to reduce confusion regarding the cancer experience and, for example, giving antiemetics to reduce nausea and vomiting, one is mandatory, whereas the other is incidental. Based on the needs assessment and the mutually agreed goals for teaching and learning, a structured plan must be outlined. In planning for patient education the guiding principles should be as follows (when the patients' significant others participate, the same principles are applicable):

Confirm and respect the patient as a person with individual expectations, experiences, and reactions.
Consider the contextual influence on distress and coping.
Adopt the patient's perspective, and structure the content to allow reflections.
Focus information vividly and consistently on core features in a comprehensive and applicable way.
Use pedagogical principles for adult learning, modified to accommodate assessed learning needs, capability, readiness, motivation, and attentional fatigue.
Take correct timing into consideration.

It is crucial to adjust the amount of information to assessed learning capacity; otherwise the educational intervention will be overwhelming and confusing. As a consequence of predominantly assessed cognitive learning needs, the main learning activities used in patient education are lectures, group discussions, and demonstrations. Cognitive learning is thus emphasized. The emotional dimension is more seldom addressed. Thus the patient's experiences and reflections are not used to develop values compatible with his or her quality of life and supportive of self-esteem and confidence, for example.

For each topic staff members must select the activities that are most conductive to the intended change. It is important that topics be presented in sequence, interspersed with pauses to give opportunities for repetition, feedback, and questions. Videotapes, slides, and printed material, for example, are useful complements. If produced locally, the written material should reflect the guiding principles earlier mentioned. When elderly patients participate, it is especially important that the letters in printed material be large enough. For participants to be comfortable, it is a good rule to start with simple concepts slowly presented. Consistency as to content and method should be considered when planning as well as when accomplishing educational sessions. Because patient education is often a team effort, the members of the team should reach a consensus in answering the following questions: What content? For what purpose? With what method? Before staff members take on responsibility for patient education, a training course for "patient educators" is mandatory.

Learning requires directed attention. Concentration difficulty is occasionally a problem even for healthy adult learners. When illness and treatment are added, the difficulties may be more manifest and reduce the patient's attentional capacity. Attentional fatigue must be considered in the education of patients (39). Readability-tested printed material used in combination with pictures facilitates attention.

Patient education should start as soon as patients and their significant others want. For some patients the optimal time is directly after the diagnosis; for others it is weeks or months later. The plans developed for education at these different stages of the cancer experience will have very different structures based on the needs assessment.

Careful planning considers timing as a very important factor, but it can sometimes be difficult to squeeze in educational interventions at the time most appropriate from the patient's point of view. It should be remembered, however, that poor timing has caused much unneccessary anxiety and confusion. When patient education is placed within the frame of cancer rehabilitation, there is a risk that education is considered first when discharge from the hospital is discussed.

What best serves the aim of an educational venture determines the choice of teaching format. Group teaching has been reported as just as effective as individual teaching (40). Both strategies have their advantages and disadvantages. The main advantages to group education are similar to the disadvantages to individual teaching: opportunities of sharing with and gaining support from other patients with similar experiences, amount of time available, and cost of staff time. Increased consistency and congruence between assessed needs and planned interventions, together with flexibility and opportunities to facilitate patients to play an active role, despite depression, anxiety, or impairment, are some of the advantages of individual teaching.

E. Evaluation

Evaluation aims to investigate whether the participants have attained the mutually agreed goal. When patient education is evaluated, it is with almost no exception a question of measuring to what extent behavioral objectives used to define expected outcome have been achieved. Evaluation is straightforward: what is expected can be measured. Several methods are used to evaluate goal achievement. Self-care activities, such as the performance of breast self-examination, can be evaluated by direct observation. Tests are used before and after a teaching session to measure progress in learning. Sometimes patients, family members, or staff members are asked to answer questions in structured interviews and questionnaires. All these forms of evaluation focus explicitly on learning outcomes that are defined in detail (38).

When facilitating coping efforts, the desired outcome to be evaluated is the process, not the product. The process of coping, with its intertwined and interdependent strands of changes in thoughts, feelings, and actions, can hardly be fragmented into measurable variables, however. Unstructered interviews in terms of narrative is one approach in which information about increased ability to cope with the cancer experience can be systematically collected.

F. Educational Programs for Coping with Cancer

In the United States, Johnson developed in 1979 an educational program for cancer patients and their family members called I Can Cope and showed that the program improved the patients' ability to adapt to living with cancer (41). Today almost half a million people in the United States have participated in the program. During the last decade, similar programs have been developed in Australia, entitled Living with Cancer, and in Sweden, entitled Learning to Cope and Living with Cancer.

The Swedish program has been adapted to the learning needs of Swedish cancer patients and their significant others. The program provides a framework for individual needs to be met and individual resources to be cultivated. To make the program also an opportunity for the patient's significant others has been much appreciated. The educational intervention has been evaluated, showing that familiarity with facts and feelings throughout the course of cancer influenced the coping capacity by increasing self-esteem and confidence in living with cancer. The program Learning to Cope and Living with Cancer is unique in the education of patients; patients and their significant others have been actively involved in developing and evaluating not only the program but also the learning material (32).

Educational programs have been shown to have an impact on patients' ability to cope with cancer experiences. A successful educational intervention to support coping efforts is characterized by the following:

Pay due respect to the patient's expectations and experiences.
Base the intervention on assessed learning needs.
Anchor it in pedagogical principles regarding the learning process.

Although patient education has been shown to be a powerful intervention, it is still in many health care settings a new concept and a new way of thinking, slowly recognized. Patient education is an appealing concept, however, and interest in using education as an intervention to support patients and their significant others to cope with the cancer experience is growing.

VII. COUNSELING: PART OF INFORMATION AND EDUCATION

In this chapter, counseling refers only to information and education of patients with cancer. The following definition is used by the British Association for Counselling: "The task of counselling is to give the client an opportunity to explore, discover and clarify ways of living more satisfyingly and resourcefully" (42). This definition indeed shows that counseling is part of the information and education process. It goes a step further than informing and educating: it supports people in finding individual ways of living and coping with their disease or in mobilizing for recovery. Counseling in this sense can be seen as coaching. The coaching function in nursing has been described as follows: nurses who have come to grips with the culturally avoided or uncharted and can open ways of being and coping for the patient and the family (43).

Nurses and doctors usually are not counselors but health care professionals who can have counseling skills. To "do" counseling has also been described as "giving personalised care" (44). It usually does not have to do with sessions on a formal basis but rather with situations within everyday care. The effectiveness of counseling might be related to the relationship between patient and caregiver. Those caring for patients understand as a result of their own experience, awareness, and vulnerability (45).

Counseling in cancer patients can therefore be seen as an individual two-way exchange, loosely structured, with the aim to learn and to cope. Topics are agreed but not limited, and there is an emphasis on feelings with reference to facts and action (10).

Counseling can allow people to interpret the illness and work from their own perspective. This includes the meaning of the disease, the cause, or the treatment. It gives those concerned an opportunity to inform nurses and doctors about their beliefs. This does not exclude the possibility of offering a different interpretation or eliciting harmful fantasies. Realistic facts may help the patient to reduce guilt feelings or anxiety or prevent them from harmful alternative therapeutic strategies.

Counseling also comprises the interpretation of the patient's condition. Experience shows that talking about deterioration of the disease is very difficult if the destruction of realistic hope is to be prevented. Realistic hope here refers to living without physical, spiritual, and psychological distress and to the support offered to achieve this aim. Here, discussing goals and negotiation, as well as finding new perspectives, becomes crucial. What can the perspectives be, when death is impending or when physical or psychological limitations cannot be overcome? A deep connection between patient and doctor, based on thorough information, described as "connexional dimension," has the attribute of a relationship and may be much more supportive and helpful than mere information giving (46).

Interpretation of the side effects of therapy or complications not related to tumor progression is another part of counseling. In curative situations, it also can mean convincing patients overwhelmed by the cancer diagnosis that there is hope of successful treatment and cure. Many patients still believe that there is no chance to survive such a disease. Many also need to be reassured that cancer is a noncontagious illness. Questions on family planning or sexual problems are important points of counseling when helping to cope with disease and treatment.

Apart from information giving and education through doctors and nurses, specific counseling may be the professional counselor's task. The role of the psychologist, psychiatrist, clergy, or art therapist in cancer care is not described in this chapter.

VIII. CONCLUSIONS AND PERSPECTIVES

Although in some parts of the world it is the right of patients to be informed about cancer, in others it is still use and tradition to withhold the truth. Whether the "silent conspiracy" is part of culture and whether this needs to be changed need further, thorough research projects. This becomes especially true when facing the inevitable intermigration of populations in Europe. Apart from the "whether or not" question, there are many details to be explored when telling the truth. Changing medical technology and methods create new situations, and research will also have to focus on very old topics concerning communication, relationship, and given circumstances that are essential to caring information giving, education, and counseling.

Professional information and education through nursing and medical personnel is part of effective counseling. To communicate effectively, nurses and doctors need to develop their communication skills. Unfortunately, medical and nursing education, at least in Europe, usually does not include sufficient time in teaching and communication principles, which explains the often experienced lack of such skills. Health care professionals obviously need different teaching strategies, which again need to be underpinned by future research.

REFERENCES

1. Senn HJ, Glaus A. Supportive Care in Cancer, Vol. II. Recent Results in Cancer, Vol. 121. Heidelberg: Springer, 1991.
2. Gaut D. Development of theoretically adequate description of caring. West J Nurs Res 1983; 5(4):313–324.
3. Padilla G, Grant M. Quality of life as a cancer nursing outcome variable. Adv Nurs Sci 1985; 8:45–60.
4. O'Berle K, Davies B. Support and caring: exploring the concepts. Oncol Nurs Forum, 1992; 19(5):763–767.
5. Leininger M. The phenomenon of caring. In: Leininger M, ed. Caring: An Essential Human Need. Proceeding of the Three National Caring Conferences. Thorofare, N.J.: C. B. Slack, 1981:3–15.
6. Paternoster J. How patients know that nurses care about them. J NY State Nurs Assoc 1988; 19(4):17–21.
7. Benner P, Wrubel J. The primacy of caring. Stress and coping in health and illness. Menlo Park, CA: Addison-Wesley, 1988.
8. Orem D. Nursing Concepts of Practice. New York: McGraw-Hill, 1985.

9. Wilson-Barnett J, Osborne J. Studies evaluating patient teaching: implications for practice. Int J Nurs Stud 1983; 20(1):33–44.
10. Wheeler D. Counselling collegues—the role of the staff counseller. Counselling 1984; 47:17–19.
11. Parker M. A nursing inservice curriculum for patient education. Nurs Health Care 1983; 4(3):142–146.
12. Wepp P. Teaching patients and relatives. In: Tiffany R, ed. Oncology for Nurses and Health Care Professionals. London: Harper and Row, 1988.
13. Paterson R, Aitken J. Public opinion on cancer. Lancet 1954; 857.
14. Pitot H. Fundamentals of Oncology. New York: Marcel Dekker, 1986.
15. Novack D, Plumer R. Changes in physicians attitudes toward telling the cancer patient. JAMA 1979; 241:897–900.
16. Estapé J, Palombo E. Cancer diagnosis disclosure in a Spanish hospital. Ann Oncol 1992; 3:451–454.
17. Lind S, Delvecchio M. Telling the diagnosis of cancer. J Clin Oncol 1989; 7(5):583–589.
18. McIntosh J. Processes of communication, information seeking and control associated with cancer. Soc Sci Med 1974; 8:167–187.
19. Tilley J. The nurses role in patient education: incongruent perceptions among nurses and patients. J Adv Nurs 1987; 12:291–301.
20. Travelbee J. Interpersonal Aspects of Nursing. Philadelphia: F. A. Davis, 1966.
21. Holland J. Now we tell—but how well? (Editorial). J Clin Oncol 1989; 7(5):557–559.
22. Meerwein F. Das Erstgespräch auf der Abteilung für Medizinische Onkologie. Bern: SAKK Publication, 1985.
23. Grahn G, Johnson J. Learning to cope and living with cancer. Learning needs assessment in cancer patient education. Scand J Caring Sci 1990; 4:173–181.
24. Houts et al. Information needs of families of cancer patients: a literature review and recommendations. J Cancer Ed 1991; 6(4):255–261.
25. Derdiarian A. Informational needs of recently diagnosed cancer patients. Cancer Nurs 1987; 10(2):107–115.
26. Hinds C. Suffering: a relatively unexplored phenomenon among family caregivers of non-institutionalized patients with cancer. J Adv Nurs 1992; 17:918–925.
27. Grahn G. Coping with the cancer experience. Part I. Developing and implementing an education and support program. Submitted.
28. Grahn G. Educational situations in clinical settings. A process analysis. Acta Univ Upsaliensis. Ph.D. dissertation. Uppsala Studies in Education, Vol. 27. Stockholm: A & W International, 1987.
29. Piaget J. Psychologie et pédagogie. Paris: Editions Denoël, 1969.
30. Dewey J. Experience and Education. New York: Collier Books, 1980 (1963).
31. Montessori M. From Childhood to Adolescence. New York: Schocken Books, 1973 (1948).
32. Grahn G, Danielsson M. Coping with the cancer experience. Part II. Evaluating an education and support program. Submitted.
33. Lazarus R, Folkman S. Stress, Appraisal and Coping. New York: Springer, 1984.
34. McHaffie HE. Coping: an essential element of nursing. J Adv Nurs 1992; 17:933–40.

35. White N, Richter J, Fry C. Coping, social support and adaptation to chronic illness. West J Nurs Res 1992; 14:211–224.
36. Fallowfield L. Problems in communication to cancer patients. In Glaxo Symposium: Progress in Supportive Care. Wien, 1992.
37. Wilson E, Desruisseux B. Stoma care in patient teaching. In: Wilson-Barnett J, ed. Patient Teaching. London: Livingstone, 1983:95–118.
38. Rankin S, Stallings K. Patient Education. New York: Lippincott, 1990.
39. Cimprich B. A theoretical perspective on attention and patient education. Adv Nurs Sci 1992; 14(3):39–51.
40. Lindeman C. Patient education. Annu Rev Nurs Res 1988; 6:29–60.
41. Johnson J. The effects of a patient-centered educational program on persons' adaptability to live with a chronic disease. University of Minnesota, Ph.D. dissertation, 1979.
42. Godden M, Charles D. What is counselling? BAC Newslett 1984; 27:14.
43. Benner P. From Novice to Expert. Menlo Park, CA: Addison-Wesley, 1984.
44. Jourard SM. The Transparent Self. New York: Van Nostrand-Reinhold, 1971.
45. Tschudin V. Counselling Skills for Nurses. London: Baillière Tindall, 1987.
46. Surbone A. The information to the cancer patient: psychosocial and spiritual implications. Support Care Cancer 1993; 1:89–91.

20

Drug Delivery Systems: Infusion and Access Devices

Rebecca S. Finley
University of Maryland School of Pharmacy, and University of Maryland Cancer Center, Baltimore, Maryland

David A. Van Echo
University of Maryland Cancer Center, and University of Maryland, Baltimore, Maryland

I. INTRODUCTION

In the United States it is estimated that 25–50% of all patients receive some form of intravenous therapy (drugs or fluids) during their hospitalization. Although much intravenous therapy is accomplished by simple gravity administration, the steadily increasing use of potent medications and advances in critical care medicine and other specialty areas has led to an increase in the use of electronic infusion devices to ensure safe and accurate drug delivery. Research in intravenous drug delivery technology has demonstrated that the method of delivery strongly influences the resulting serum concentrations of medications (1–3). When medications have a narrow therapeutic index (e.g., cytotoxics) or must be carefully titrated to achieve a specific physiological response (e.g., cardioactive drugs), accurate drug delivery may have a profound influence on patient outcome, both therapeutic and toxic.

During the past decade, major advances in mechanical drug delivery systems have enabled clinicians to administer diverse therapeutic regimens safely and efficiently in a variety of settings (4). These advances in mechanical drug delivery technology have impacted both vascular access and infusion devices. Although infusion systems are widely used in almost every health care setting in which parenteral drugs are administered, the use of "high-tech" devices is most widespread in settings in which either patients are receiving multiple drugs or the drugs are given via innovative infusion schedules (e.g., circadian timing or alternating infusions); in addition, these high-technology devices are also used in alternative settings (e.g., home care) in which health care professionals are not immediately available to supervise and manage drug administration. The increased use of continuous subcutaneous infusions and regional (e.g., epidural, intraarterial, or intraperitoneal) drug delivery has also diversified the need for infusion and access devices. Other catalysts that have stimulated advancements in infusion technology are listed in Table 1.

II. INFUSION DEVICES IN ONCOLOGY

The comprehensive and optimum management of patients with malignant diseases often includes a wide spectrum of parenteral drugs, intravenous fluids, and blood products. The collective administration of all these therapies may involve the use of a multitude of infusion rates and schedules, ranging from intermittent bolus injections to continuous infusions to patient-controlled administration. Thus, it is not surprising that the variety of infusion devices available today is quite extensive and diverse. Table 2 summarizes some of the basic and optional features of infusion devices.

Historically, most devices have been designed for in-hospital use and for a single, continuous flow rate of an infusion. The expanding use of multiple-drug regimens and more innovative infusion techniques (e.g., on-demand therapy) and the desire to make the drug delivery process more efficient (e.g., preprogrammed administration of intermittent doses or tapering an infusion rate), as well as the use of more infusions outside the hospital or clinic setting, mandated the development of technology that can safely, accurately, and efficiently deliver such infusions. Examples of these technologies are the patient-controlled analgesia, multichannel, and parenteral nutrition devices.

Table 1 Trends in Infusion Therapy That Stimulated Advancement in Infusion Device Technology

Use of prolonged continuous infusions (e.g., chemotherapy)
Innovative infusion patterns (e.g., circadian timed, alternating, or sequential infusions)
Administration of potent drugs when a precise infusion rate is critical to the efficacy and/or safety
Administration of cancer chemotherapy, antibiotics, total parenteral nutrition via ambulatory infusions
Anatomically targeted regional drug delivery (e.g., intraarterial, hepatic arterial, intraperitoneal, epidural)

Table 2 General Assessment of Infusion Device Needs[a]

Criteria	Alternatives
Setting related	Circle most applicable choices:
Setting in which infusion devices will be used	Hospital-inpatient Clinic-outpatient Home care
Patient population	Adult Pediatric Neonatal
Persons responsible for	
Programming	Nurse, pharmacist, patient
Drug preparation	Nurse, pharmacist, patient
Administration	Nurse, pharmacist, patient
Troubleshooting	Nurse, pharmacist, patient
Therapy related	
Range of infusion rates	
Range of infusion durations	
Types of infusion schedules or patterns	Intermittent Continuous On-demand
Range of infusate volumes	10–100 ml/day 50–3000 ml/day
Red blood cell transfusions	Yes No
Arterial infusions	Yes No Hepatic arterial
Multiple drugs simultaneously	Yes, two to four No If yes, drugs likely to be physically and chemically compatible: yes or no
Alarms and safety features	
Low battery	Yes or no
Occlusion	Yes or no
Air in line	Yes or no
Low volume	Yes or no
System malfunction	Yes or no
Cost related	Enter approximate amounts
Pump	
Drug reservoirs	
Tubings	
Power source	
Ancillary needs: computer or programming unit	

[a]Identification of this information assists in determining specifications for infusion device selection.

A. Special Features of Infusion Devices and Applications in Oncology

1. On-Demand or Patient-Controlled Dosing

Many infusion devices are capable of delivering a fixed dose of a medication when a demand button is depressed. This feature has been most widely used in the delivery of patient-controlled analgesia (PCA) (5); however, it may also be used in the administration of "as-needed" antiemetics or other medications for symptom management. PCA is widely accepted by both patients and health care providers as a method for managing postoperative pain (5,6). Many of the PCA devices can administer continuous (basal rate) infusions in addition to delivering bolus doses when needed (7). The combination of continuous infusion opioids with patient-controlled bolus doses during acute exacerbations of pain provides greater pain control and patient satisfaction. This application of PCA for "breakthrough" pain during continuous infusion of an opioid is often used to provide optimal pain control in patients with cancer-related pain requiring parenteral therapy (8).

PCA devices are used for intravenous, subcutaneous, and epidural analgesia (8–13). Most PCA devices enable the health care provider to program both the dose to be administered (both basal infusion rate and bolus dose) and the lockout interval. The use of a lockout feature disables the demand button for a predetermined length of time and prevents the patient from receiving repeated bolus injections in rapid succession. A lockout interval of 5–30 minutes is generally recommended. Many of the PCA devices record the number of times the patient attempts to deliver a dose (even during lockout periods), so the clinician can adjust or titrate dosages and lockout intervals more appropriately, if necessary. Some devices also allow the programmer to set a maximum number of doses to be delivered in a specified time period, and others have a default setting that determines the maximum number of doses. PCA pumps also have security features that prevent tampering with the program, and most feature a locking system to prevent tampering with the drug reservoir. A useful feature, especially when analgesia is being titrated, is the ability to display or print out a detailed record of the analgesic use. This feature generally provides data regarding the total cumulative dose delivered in a specified interval, the number of attempts or demands, and a summary of the programmed regimen.

Electronic PCA devices designed for in-hospital use must be placed near the patient's bedside, either on a stand or attached to an intravenous (IV) pole. Hospital PCA pumps utilize either syringe or collapsible IV bag drug reservoirs. These devices feature a remote dosing button that can be attached to the bed railing or patient's bed clothing for easy access. Examples of PCA devices for use in the hospital include the Harvard Bard PCA pump, the Abbott LifeCare PCA Classic and PCA Plus, the Becton Dickinson PCA, and the Strato PCA infuser.

Ambulatory PCA devices can be carried by the patient in a pouch or holster and most have a dosing button on the pump; some also have a remote button. Although ambulatory PCA devices have many of the same safety and security features of the hospital models, many of these devices allow access to some programming functions by the patient or family to facilitate titration of analgesics at home. When ambulatory PCA is used, it is imperative that patients and their families or caregivers demonstrate the ability to understand the principles of PCA and general pump management. Examples of ambulatory PCA devices include the CADD-PCA by Pharmacia Deltec, the Bard Ambulatory PCA, and the Provider One by Abbott. Although most PCA pumps have been designed specifically for either hospital or ambulatory use, some have been marketed for either. For example, the Bard Ambulatory PCA and the CADD-PCA are both available with an optional pole-mounting device and a remote demand button.

The Baxter PCA Infusor system is a nonelectronic, lightweight, disposable device consisting of two components. The Infusor is an elastomeric infusion device with an attached microbore tubing. The Patient Control Module, attached to the tubing, resembles a wristwatch with a demand button on the top. When the button is depressed, a 0.5 ml dose is administered. No doses are delivered between depressions of the demand button. This nonelectronic device has a relative delay or "lockout" period of about 6 minutes, which is the time required to refill the 0.5 ml bladder of the unit. The dose administered to the patient can be varied only by changing the concentration of the infusate within the Infusor. Clinical evaluation of this device has demonstrated safety, effectiveness, and patient satisfaction (14).

2. *Programmable Capabilities*

In addition to long- or short-term continuous infusions, many newer infusion devices can also be programmed to deliver innovative or complicated infusion schedules without human intervention each time a rate or dose change is made. Examples of some programmable capabilities of infusion devices include (1) delivery of intermittent doses at preset intervals, (2) administration of cycled parenteral nutrition solutions that taper the flow rate at the start and end of infusions, and (3) delivery of chronotherapeutic regimens that administer varying rates of infusion depending on the time of day. Some newer devices also allow reprogramming (and troubleshooting) at a distant site and transfer of the new program via modem. In this case, a home care patient's infusion may be titrated and changed without a visit from a health care professional or the patient returning to the clinic.

3. *Multichannel Devices*

In response to the increasing number of parenteral drugs individual patients must receive concurrently, several manufacturers have developed devices capable of facilitating the delivery of drugs from multiple (two to four) reservoirs. Examples of multichannel devices are the IMED Gemini PC-4, Omni-Flow Therapist, and the VIVUS 4000 by I-Flow. Each channel of these devices is programmed independently, and some are designed to accommodate syringes in addition to collapsible bags or glass bottles. The multichannel devices may either deliver drugs through a single IV line via a manifold system or administer each channel through a separate tubing or catheter.

4. Future Applications

Research and development of closed-loop mechanisms are now underway that will be able to adjust infusion pump delivery rates in response to physiological (or other measurable) responses using some type of sensor. Currently, such technological applications are being investigated in anesthesia, in which delivery of anesthetics may be automatically titrated in response to the patient's vital signs and indicators of level of consciousness. An example of a closed-loop technology, under development, that has application in oncology consists of a PCA device for opioid administration connected to a pulse oximetry monitor. If the patient becomes hypoxic (presumably because of opioid-induced respiratory depression), the device may alarm, turn off, or decrease the dosage.

B. Ambulatory Infusion Devices

Ambulatory infusion devices may include any of the features detailed in Table 2; however, these devices are also small enough to allow the patient to remain active. The ambulatory devices may be divided into categories on the basis of their pumping mechanism, type of reservoir, reusability, rate and duration of infusion capabilities, programming capacity, number of infusion channels, and cost. Table 3 describes the specifications and features of a few representative ambulatory infusion devices available in the United States.

The use of an ambulatory device should provide both the patient and the clinicians caring for them a safe, practical, and relatively uncomplicated method of administering parenteral therapy. The selection of an ambulatory device is dependent on factors related to the patient, the therapy (e.g., the drug, volume to be administered, and rate of infusion), and the infusion service (nursing and pharmacy) that will be coordinating the patient's care. Patients who are being evaluated for an ambulatory infusion must either be capable of learning necessary procedures for managing their therapy (such as changing drug reservoirs or batteries and responding to alarms) or have a caregiver who will assume this responsibility. The more the patient (or caregiver) can master such responsibilities, the more independent they can become from the institution or infusion service. Conversely, the more complex the infusion system, the more likely it is that the patient will continue to be dependent on the institution or infusion service.

Table 3 Examples of Infusion Devices Currently Marketed in the United States: Manufacturers' Specifications

Name/model (manufacturer)	Pumping mechanism	Drug reservoir, accessories	Battery, power source	Range of infusion rates (ml/h)	Alarms and safety features	Keep open rate (ml/h)	Program modes	Weight	Size
Hospital, single channel									
Gemini PC-1 (IMED)	Linear persistaltic (both pump and controller modes)	Any standard IV container Dedicated tubing	Electrical with rechargeable battery (approximately 5 h)	0.1–999 ml/h in pump mode 0.1–500 ml/h in controller mode	Occluded Check IV set Close door Air in line Occluded, patient side Occluded, fluid side Partial occlusion, fluid side Malfunction Infusion complete, KVO Low battery	1 ml/h or set rate if <1 ml/h	Continuous Volume to be infused Auto taper		27.5 × 20.6 × 16.5 cm
EZ-1 volumetric infusion pump (Ivion)		Any standard IV container	Electrical with rechargeable battery (6 h life)	0.1–999.9 ml/h	Pump not infusing Cassette, door open Patient occlusion Bottle occlusion Air in cassette System check KVO ≤ 1 ml/h Infuse all Low battery	≤ 1 ml/h	Continuous	5 kg	26.7 × 17.1 × 18 cm
PCA Infuser Model 310 (1VAC)	Syringe	Standard syringes	Size D alkaline disposable batteries	Continuous 1–60 ml/h PCA, 0.1–99.9 mg	Low volume Low battery Programming error Syringe not primed No syringe Access code error Tampering Empty syringe Occlusion		Continuous PCA	6.6 kg	6.3 × 12.5 × 2.9 inches

Table 3 (*Continued*)

Name/model (manufacturer)	Pumping mechanism	Drug reservoir, accessories	Battery, power source	Range of infusion rates (ml/h)	Alarms and safety features	Keep open rate (ml/h)	Program modes	Weight	Size
Model 570, variable pressure, volumetric pump (1VAC)		Any standard IV container Dedicated tubing	Electrical with rechargeable battery (approximately 5 h)	1–999 ml/h in 1 or 0.1 ml/h increments	Empty container Closed clamp Low battery Occlusion Open door Air in line Malfunction	Yes	Continuous		
Quest 521 Intelligent Pump (Kendall McGraw)	Volumetric positive-pressure displacement reservoir	Any standard IV container Syringe Dedicated tubing	Electric with rechargeable battery (approximately 8 h)	1–999 ml/h	Occlusion Close/open Door Low battery Low volume Raise bag		1–999 ml/h Programmable up to nine rates per time period	5.45 kg	24.8 × 24.1 × 13.3 cm
Hospital, multichannel									
Gemini PC-2 (1MED) Two channels	Linear peristaltic (has both pump and controller modes)	Any standard IV container Dedicated tubing	Electrical with rechargeable battery (4–5 h life)	0.1–999 ml/h in pump mode 0.1–500 ml/h in controller mode	Check IV set Close door Air in line Occluded, patient side Occluded, fluid side Partial occlusion, fluid side Check ECD malfunction Low battery Infusion complete, KVO	1 ml/h, or set rate if < 1 ml/h	Continuous infusion	8.4 kg	26.9 × 30.2 × 18.3 cm
Omni-Flow 4000 (Abbott) Four channels	Piston diaphragm	Bag, bottle, syringe Dedicated tubing	Electrical with rechargeable battery (approximately 5 h)	1.4–800 ml/h	Automatic air elimination		Continuous	6.0 kg	28.58 × 23.16 × 17.8 cm

Horizon (McGraw) Modular system, up to six on standard IV pole, more on critical care pole	Volumetric, positive-pressure displacement reservoir	Any standard IV container	Electrical with rechargeable battery	Standard mode: 0.1 – 999.9 ml/h Micromode 0.1 – 99.9 ml/h	Air in line Door open Downstream occlusion Hold time exceeded Container empty Low battery Set loaded improperly Upstream occlusion	0.1 – 3 ml/h	Continuous Sequential delivery of up to nine different rates and volumes	5.3 kg	31.5 × 12.2 × 31 cm
Ambulatory, single channel									
WalkMed 440 PIC (Medex division of Ivion)	Linear peristaltic	Disposable 65, 150, and 250 ml bags Dedicated pump sets	9 V disposable (450 – 650 ml per battery)	1 – 30 ml/h (can also be programmed as mg/h)	Near end of program Volume limit Occlusion System malfunction Low battery Depleted battery End of infusion Door open Programming error Lockout levels	0 – 9.9 ml/h	PCA Intermittent Continuous	360 g	4.6 × 11.2 × 10.2 cm
WalkMed 350 (Medex Ambulatory Infusion Systems, division of Ivion)	Linear peristaltic	Disposable 65, 150, and 250 ml bags Dedicated pump sets	9 V alkaline battery (3 – 21 days)	0.1 – 19.99 ml/h (increments of 0.01 ml)	Occlusion System malfunction Low battery Depleted battery Prime Door open		Continuous	360 g	4.6 × 11.2 × 10.2 cm
WalkMed PCA (Medex Ambulatory Infusion Systems)	Linear peristaltic	Disposable 65, 150, and 250 ml bags Dedicated pump sets	9 V alkaline battery (1 – 21 days depending on infusion rate)	0.1 – 19.99 ml/h (increments of 0.01) or 0.1 – 30 ml/h (increments of 0.1 ml)	Near end Volume limit Occlusion System malfunction Low battery Depleted battery End of infusion Total volume delivered Programming error		Continuous Continuous with patient-activated bolus Bolus only	360 g	4.6 × 11.2 × 10.2 cm

Table 3 *(Continued)*

Name/model (manufacturer)	Pumping mechanism	Drug reservoir, accessories	Battery, power source	Range of infusion rates (ml/h)	Alarms and safety features	Keep open rate (ml/h)	Program modes	Weight	Size
Provider One (Abbott)	Rotary peristaltic	Any collapsible IV bag Dedicated tubing	Two disposable 9 V lithium batteries (4800 ml) or 12 V rechargeable (4000 ml)	1–400 ml/h	Occlusion Cartridge improperly inserted Programming error Computer error Air in line Low battery Low reservoir End of infusion	1 ml/h	Continuous Tapering	400 g	132 × 86 × 33 cm
Provider 5500 (Pancretec/ Abbott)	Rotary peristaltic	Any collapsible IV bag Dedicated tubing					Continuous PCA		
Pain Management Provider (Abbott)	Rotary peristaltic	Any collapsible IV bag Dedicated tubing		0.1–25 ml/h in 0.1 ml increments	Security lockbox available		Continuous Loading Dose PCA (suitable for epidural injection)		
CADD-Plus (Pharmacia Deltec)	Linear peristaltic	50, 100, 250 ml custom cassettes or any collapsible IV bag with custom adapter	9 V disposable alkaline or lithium battery	0.1–75 ml/h	High pressure Low reservoir Low battery Power-up failure Pump in stop mode Programmed volume depleted High pressure System error	0–10 ml/h	Continuous Intermittent	425 g	2.8 × 8.9 × 16 cm

CADD-1 (Pharmacia Deltec)	Linear peristaltic	50, 100, 250 ml custom cassettes or any collapsible IV bag with custom adapter	9 V disposable alkaline or lithium battery	0–2999 ml/24 h or 90 ml/h in fixed high-flow mode	Power-up fault Pump in stop mode Low battery Low reservoir volume Programmed volume depleted High pressure System error		Continuous	425 g	2.8 × 8.9 × 16 cm
CADD-PCA ambulatory infusion pump Model 5800	Linear peristaltic	50, 100, 250 ml custom reservoir or any IV bag with remote adaptor	9 V alkaline or lithium battery	0–20 ml/h (may also be programmed in mg/h)	Power-up failure Low battery Depleted battery Low reservoir Programmed volume depleted High pressure System error		Continuous Patient-activated bolus Continuous plus patient-activated bolus	425 g	2.8 × 3.5 × 6.4 cm
CADD-TPN ambulatory infusion system Model 5700 (Pharmacia Deltec)	Linear peristaltic	Collapsible IV bag with dedicated adaptor tubing	9 V alkalkine (6 h) or lithium (18 h) battery or rechargeable battery pack (11 h) or a.c. adaptor	10–400 ml/h	Low reservoir Programmed volume depleted Infusion period completed Low battery Depleted battery Invalid rate High pressure Power-up fault System error	5 ml/h	Continuous Continuous with tapering	369 g	2.8 × 8.9 × 13.3 cm
SideKick (I-Flow)	Spring-driven infusion	50 and 100 ml minibags Custom IV sets that determine flow rate	Self-contained spring	50, 100, or 200 ml/h	None		Continuous		
Intermate LV system (Baxter)	Elastomeric	Unit is a disposable balloon reservoir	None	50–100 ml/h	None	NA	Continuous		

Table 3 (*Continued*)

Name/model (manufacturer)	Pumping mechanism	Drug reservoir, accessories	Battery, power source	Range of infusion rates (ml/h)	Alarms and safety features	Keep open rate (ml/h)	Program modes	Weight	Size
Infusor (Baxter)	Elastomeric	Unit is a disposable balloon reservoir	None	0.5 – 5 ml/h	With patient control module attachment lockout of 15 or 60 minutes		Continuous PCA		
Ambulatory, multichannel									
The VIVUS 4000 infuser (I-Flow Corporation) Four channel	Positive displacement	Any IV bag Dedicated tubing Manifold line to connect up to four tubings to single IV line Programmer required for operation Communicator unit for remote programming	5 (5000 ml delivery) or 10 (10,000 ml delivery) AA disposable alkaline batteries, 1.5 V d.c. or external 110/120 V a.c. adaptor	0.1 – 200 ml/h	Low battery Dead battery Occlusion Empty reservoir Internal malfunction Runaway Open door	0.1 – 200 ml/h	Continuous Sequential Continuous/ bolus Intermittent	1.05 kg	19.7 × 11.43 × 5.1 cm
Intelliject (Ivion) Four channel	Rack-and-pinion drive (syringe driver)	Dedicated 30 ml syringes and manifold	Two 9 V disposable batteries	5.4 – 40 ml/h per channel	Occlusion Low battery Low reservoir Program error Electronic fault	Any preset rate	Continuous Bolus Continuous plus bolus Sequential Alternating	1.54 kg	25.4 × 16.5 × 7.1 cm

Therapy-related factors that influence the selection of an ambulatory device include the number of drugs to be administered and their physical and chemical stability and compatibility, the duration of the infusion, the schedule or pattern of infusion, and the volume of infusate. If a drug is not stable in the drug reservoir for at least 24 h, it may be very difficult to design an acceptable ambulatory routine. Obviously, the size and type of the drug reservoir are critical factors in selecting the most appropriate device.

Although many of the early-generation infusion devices used syringes as the reservoir (e.g., Autosyringe and Graseby), today's ambulatory devices use a variety of reservoirs that include syringes, varying sizes of collapsible bags contained within plastic cassettes, elastomeric balloons, and standard collapsible IV containers (e.g., Viaflex bags). Such devices as the Abbott Provider series can use any IV bag along with the dedicated Provider tubing. If the 24 h volume of infusate is large, a device that can accommodate a large-volume infusion (e.g., parenteral nutrition or hydration fluids) must be used. The more frequently that the drug reservoir must be exchanged, the greater is the risk of complications, including infection and air embolism. In addition, frequent reservoir exchanges are more inconvenient for the patient.

The range of infusion rates a pump may provide is also critical when selecting a device. Several of the ambulatory devices, such as the WalkMed 350, were designed for the administration of small-volume chemotherapy (e.g., fluorouracil and floxuridine) and have infusion rates ranging from 0.1 to 10 ml per 24 h, whereas such devices as the CADD-TPN (Pharmacia Deltec) and the Abbott Provider One are capable of infusing at rates necessary for parenteral nutrition or hydration.

Disposable batteries are the most common type of power source used by the ambulatory devices. Most devices operate at maximum capacity (i.e., infusion rate) for at least 2–4 days on a single 9-V alkaline or lithium battery. Some devices use rechargeable batteries. Even though this may appear economical, patients must be supplied with an adapter for recharging and either must schedule times when mobility is limited for recharging or be given extra rechargeable batteries. This may add to patient confusion and inconvenience. Some devices, such as the Abbott Provider One, may also be plugged directly into an electrical outlet as an alternative to a disposable battery as a power source. If devices are selected that use disposable batteries, patients should be given extra batteries. Another practical feature of many devices is the ability to maintain memory protection for the operating program during battery exchange.

The ambulatory devices have a variety of safety features or alarms, which may include low battery, system malfunction, line occlusion, air in the line, and low volume remaining in the reservoir. In addition, many devices decrease the flow rate to a "keep-open" rate if the reservoir is not changed by the time the volume is at a critically low level to prevent clotting and line occlusion. On most devices the alarms are both audible and visible (liquid crystal display screen or warning lights).

Several elastomeric devices are also currently marketed in the United States and are most widely used for home or ambulatory therapy. These disposable pumping devices are lightweight and deliver the infusate at a constant rate determined by the lumen of the tubing or outflow valve from the balloon-like reservoir. Devices are available that infuse at rates ranging from 0.5 to 200 ml/h. The devices that administer at low rates are designed for prolonged continuous infusion, whereas the devices that flow at high rates are used for intermittent administration (e.g., antibiotics) or bolus doses (e.g., chemotherapy). These devices do not have the alarms and safety features found on most mechanical devices, however; therefore they may not be appropriate for medications that require a critical infusion rate to sustain vital functions (e.g., dobutamine) or that may be associated with toxicity if extravasation occurs. For patients requiring long-term therapy, they may also be relatively expensive compared with reusable mechanical devices.

If the patient is to receive multiple drugs that are not compatible, either a multichannel device or multiple single-channel devices must be used and a regimen must be designed to assure that incompatible drugs do not interact in the infusion system (including the vascular access device).

Some ambulatory infusion devices have advanced technology programming and drug delivery capabilities that facilitate administration of novel or complicated infusion profiles (e.g., circadian-timed, alternating, or sequential regimens). Other devices may be monitored and programmed using a modem and telephone lines (i.e., VIVUS 4000 by I-Flow), which allow closer patient follow-up and rapid response to acute needs for changes in drug delivery. This type of device may be utilized to provide improved supportive or palliative care in the home for patients with advanced disease. The use of these high-technology devices can improve overall patient care; however, the cost of these devices and their accessories is usually greater than that of more traditional ambulatory devices. They also require more programming time on the part of the clinician and may require extensive education of the patient or caregiver. Therefore, the need for a high-technology device must be carefully scrutinized before its selection.

C. Implantable Infusion Devices

The implanted infusion devices were developed for the long-term administration of medications either systemically or regionally. They are generally placed subcutaneously in either the lower abdomen or subclavicular region. The implantable infusion systems have been used primarily for administration of hepatic arterial infusions (15–17). In addition, they may be used for intravenous, other arterial, intraperitoneal, and epidural infusions of medications, including chemotherapy, analgesics, anticoagulants, and antispasmodics (e.g., baclofen) (18,19). The device consists of a pumping mechanism, the drug reservoir, and a catheter inserted into the artery, vein, or anatomical space in which the drug is to be administered. Several types of power sources or pumping mechanisms have been used for implantable devices. Infusaid first introduced a system that consisted of an inner drug reservoir and an outer charging fluid chamber separated by flexible bellows. The two-phase charging fluid is condensed into a vapor when compressed (i.e., the drug reservoir is filled). The vapor exerts a constant pressure on the bellows, resulting in a constant flow of the contents of the drug reservoir through an outlet capillary and into the catheter. As the pressure in the charging chamber decreases during flow, the vapor gradually changes to a fluid once again. The infusion rate of this type of device is preset during the manufacturing process and is determined by the outflow capillary diameter. The Medtronics implantable device uses a lithium battery as a power source. In addition, the infusion rate may be adjusted by use of an external programming unit and a wand placed over the pump.

The drug reservoir of the implantable devices is contained within the unit, and models are available with volume capacities ranging from about 20 to 50 ml. The drug is added to the device by palpating the pump to locate the injection port and inserting a needle through the skin and diaphragm of the port. Some models are available that also have a second port that can be used for bolus injections (the port bypasses the reservoir and delivers the drug directly into the catheter).

These devices are costly (approximately \$3000–5000, depending on the brand and model selected), and initial costs of implantation are also high because a surgical procedure is required. If the devices are used long term in a patient, they have been reported to be less costly overall than an external system because disposable tubings and reservoirs are not necessary (except for the syringe and needle used to fill the device) and the care and maintenance are less than that necessary for external or percutaneous systems (20).

The incidence, type, and severity of complications related to the use of the implantable systems may be somewhat dependent on the experience of the surgeon with the implantation of the particular device, as well as that of the clinicians providing follow-up care and refilling of the reservoir. Reported complications include arterial thrombosis, catheter occlusion secondary to blood clotting or precipitation of the drug, pocket infections, and catheter dislodgement from the pump (21). In addition, specific regional therapies (e.g., intraarterial or intraperitoneal chemotherapy) may cause toxicities that are quite different from their systemic effects (e.g., biliary sclerosis secondary to hepatic arterial floxuridine). Like the elastomeric devices, the implantable devices also do not have alarms, so complications or interruptions in drug delivery may not be realized immediately.

D. Nonintravenous Applications of Infusion Devices

Besides intravenous drug delivery, infusion devices are commonly used for the administration of drugs subcutaneously, intraarterially, and epidurally (8,10–13,15). Central venous lines generally have pressures of 15–20 mm Hg; however, intraarterial pressures range from 150 to 250 mm Hg. Solutions flow from an area of higher pressure to one of lower pressure; therefore, devices to be used for intraarterial drug delivery must provide a significantly higher pumping pressure to overcome intraarterial pressure. The use of microbore tubing or an in-line filter raises the "downstream" pressure even more, necessitating a higher pumping pressure in such situations. The implantable infusion devices have been the most widely used devices for intraarterial infusions of hepatic arterial chemotherapy (15–17), as well as carotid artery drug delivery in the treatment of brain tumors (18).

Devices designed for the administration of intravenous drugs are not necessarily suited to administering solutions through an epidural catheter. The combination of the high back-pressure created by the epidural space and the in-line filter recommended for epidural injections is frequently enough to activate the high-pressure occlusion alarms on many devices. Although some devices may be able to deliver very low infusion rates (e.g., those used for continuous epidural infusions), the high pressure generated by a rapid injection (e.g., bolus injection during PCA) often triggers the occlusion alarm. The desirable characteristics of a device for epidural PCA therefore include accuracy of infusion against the back-pressure of the epidural space and the ability to deliver a bolus dose without activation of the occlusion alarm while retaining the ability to detect an occlusion (22). An occlusion pressure of approximately 1200 mm Hg is recommended. Although relatively high occlusion pressures are desirable for epidural administration, they delay detection of an occluded catheter or cannula, which may result in poor-quality analgesia or a dangerously high bolus dose when the occlusion is cleared (as a result of the rapid administration of the stored volume or the fluid that collects behind an occlusion).

E. Summary: Selection of Infusion Devices for Oncology Settings

Because of the diverse infusion device market and the variety of infusion needs, it is common for clinical services to need more than one type or model of a device. However, it is impractical and potentially dangerous (because of staff confusion or unfamiliarity with multiple devices) and may be excessively expensive (as a result of costs of devices and the dedicated disposable tubings for each) to have more than a few types of devices, and therefore an objective assessment process must be applied to determine the specific needs of the setting.

Selection of the most appropriate infusion devices for any clinical setting should be based on an assessment of the infusion requirements of the patients.

This assessment must include information regarding the number and types of therapies being administered simultaneously, the range of infusion rates and volumes of infusate, and whether the patients are institutionalized or ambulatory, as well as other factors listed in Table 4. Compatibility of the infusion system with drug products in clinical use must also be considered (see Sec. IV). Finally, such issues as the cost of the device and necessary disposables (e.g., tubing and drug reservoirs), flexibility of leasing and purchase contracts, and available technical support and service must also be considered when selecting infusion devices. Many institutions and clinical services use predetermined evaluation tools for device selection. Once devices are selected for evaluation or use in a clinical setting, a qualified biomedical engineer should evaluate the technical performance and projected service and maintenance requirements.

III. VASCULAR ACCESS DEVICES

Throughout the late 1970s and early 1980s, the expanding use of more complex chemotherapy regimens using more irritating, sclerosing, and vesicant drugs, as well as the use of prolonged continuous infusion regimens, posed considerable dilemmas for drug delivery via peripheral venous access. The increasing use of intravenous supportive care medications, including total parenteral nutrition, antiemetics, antimicrobials, and analgesics, further compounded the need for safe and dependable venous access. Because of the need for prolonged or long-term intermittent cycles of therapy and supportive medications, a wide variety of vascular access devices suitable for long-term placement and ambulatory use have been developed. These devices provide extended venous access for patients requiring frequent venipunctures (drug and blood product administration and blood sampling) and for patients with less than optimal peripheral venous access secondary to obesity, prior therapy with irritating drugs, or advanced age.

A. Tunneled Central Venous Catheters

The development of the Silastic Broviac and Hickman catheters in the 1970s permitted long-term vascular access with few complications (23,24). Once placed, this type of catheter is tunneled subcutaneously for a short distance to provide a barrier between the skin exit site and the vascular entrance site. The catheter is usually placed in the cephalic vein and passed into the superior vena cava with the catheter tip at the entrance of the right atrium. A Dacron cuff around the catheter (under the skin) just below the exit site promotes the ingrowth of fibrous tissue, which creates an additional barrier to microorganisms and helps to hold the device in place.

Since the development of the Broviac and Hickman catheters, a wide variety

Table 4 Features of Infusion Devices

Feature	Explanation and significance	Application
Types of infusion devices		
Controllers	Regulate flow rate with gravity pressure; can only utilize pressure available from height difference of IV container and patient IV site; unable to deliver fluid when resistance overcomes gravity pressure; most are nonvolumetric and only estimate volume delivered from number of drops	Administration via peripheral venous access
Pumps	Generate positive pressure needed to infuse fluid at set rate up to a preset occlusion pressure; most are volumetric	Administration via peripheral or central venous access, epidural, subcutaneous; delivery of viscous infusates; administration of drugs or fluids requiring in-line filter
Syringe pumps	Deliver contents of a syringe over a set period of time	Same as above; commonly used to administer small volumes (e.g., neonatal administration)
Volumetric devices	Regulation of infusion according to a specific volume of fluid (e.g., ml/h)	Most mechanical IV pumps currently available are volumetric devices
Nonvolumetric devices	Regulation of fluid delivery by counting of drops delivered; drop rate must then be converted to an approximate fluid rate; less accurate than volumetric devices because drop size may differ depending on viscosity of fluid and type of tubing	Most available controllers are nonvolumetric devices
Pumping mechanisms		
Peristaltic	Peristaltic pumps achieve their pumping action by progressively squeezing the flexible tubing to force the fluid along the tube lumen from the reservoir toward the infusion site	

Linear	Series of adjacent pressure points or valves progressively squeeze the tubing along a length of tubing in a wave-like motion; variation uses valves at each end of the length of tubing that passes through the pump; piston located between these valves, and when it is depressed, the exhaust valve opens and the contents of the tubing are forced out; when the piston moves up, the exhaust valve closes and the intake valve opens, allowing the tubing to fill	Many of the ambulatory devices, including the CADD and WalkMed series, apply this type of pumping mechanism
Rotary	Tubing is wound around a shaft that rotates around one or more rollers to squeeze the tubing closed	Provider series uses this type of technology
Positive-pressure displacement	Fluid from the reservoir enters a volumetric cassette or chamber that is part of the tubing set; mechanically, the pump displaces the volume from the chamber and toward the distal (patient) end of the tubing	Many of the pumps designed for in-hospital use this type of pumping mechanism
Screw	Motor-driven screw progressively forces plunger into syringe barrel	Syringe pumps use this type of pumping mechanism
Drug reservoir		
Standard IV container, glass or plastic	Standard IV container can be used as the drug reservoir rather than purchasing a dedicated reservoir	In-hospital devices, Provider series (collapsible bags only), CADD-TPN
Manufacturer-specific cassettes	Disposable drug reservoirs must be used in conjunction with a particular device, many of these reservoir requiring more pharmacist time in filling than conventional drug reservoirs (e.g., bags, bottles, syringes)	Custom cassettes used with the CADD series are examples

Table 4 *(Continued)*

Feature	Explanation and significance	Application
Syringes	Pumps use syringes as the drug reservoir, generally limited to specific brands and sizes of syringes	Intelliject device uses only custom syringes available from the manufacturer
Alarms (may be audible and/or visible) and safety features		
Low battery	Power is low or depleted; most devices signal before power is completely depleted to allow time for battery replacement or recharging	Necessary on all in-hospital and ambulatory devices that use rechargeable or disposable batteries to alert staff, patient, or caregiver of impending power loss
Occlusion	Devices have a preset maximum occlusion pressure they can generate in an attempt to overcome resistance to flow; alarm sounds when the pump reaches this point, and it indicates that the fluid cannot overcome the resistance and drug delivery has stopped	Detect occlusions within the lumen of the vascular access device (e.g., drug precipitate or kinking) or at the tip (e.g., blood clot)
Air in line	Detects air bubbles in the line; in some cases, the device is able to dispel air from the tubing; other devices alarm and stop the pump	Important with ambulatory devices that use conventional collapsible IV bags (air should be removed from bags before connection; however, this safety feature prevents unremoved air bubbles from reaching the patient)
Low volume	Reservoir fluid is almost depleted; most devices determine this by subtracting the amount infused from the amount programmed to be infused; many devices alarm intermittently after the volume reaches a critically low amount (e.g., 5–10% of total) and begin to alarm continuously once the reservoir is depleted	Alerts staff or patients so that reservoir can be changed to avoid clotting and retain patency at end of the IV tubing

Program end	Programmed infusion duration or volume is completed; most devices either stop or convert to a KVO rate	Notify staff or patient that infusion is complete
System malfunction	Electronic malfunction	
Infusion pattern capabilities		
Continuous	Device delivers fluid at a set rate until the rate is changed or discontinued	Most widely used type of infusion pattern; many intermittent medications are also given by a series of short infusions using the continuous mode
Intermittent	Pump turns on and off at specified intervals to deliver preprogrammed amounts of fluid	Frequently used for antibiotic administration
On-demand	Button on the pump or a remote device is depressed to deliver a specific, preprogrammed amount of fluid	Most widely used for patient-controlled analgesia; however, has also been used for administration of antiemetics and anxiolytics
Tapering	Device is capable of gradually increasing and/or decreasing infusion rate, usually at the beginning and end of a continuous infusion	Cyclic total parenteral nutrition
Sequential	Multichannel devices can administer drugs in a preprogrammed succession	Chemotherapy regimens, incompatible combinations of antibiotics or antiemetics
Keep open	When the reservoir volume becomes low or the desired bolus dose is administered, the pump automatically converts to a low (predetermined) infusion rate to maintain venous access patency	Usual keep vein open rates are 1.0 ml/h

of similar devices have been marketed for both pediatric and adult use. Brands and models of catheters may differ in (1) the number of lumens, (2) the catheter material, (3) the diameter of the catheter and that of each lumen(s), and (4) the type of catheter tip. Representative types of catheters marketed in the United States are described in Table 5. Tunneled catheters are usually made of either silicone or polyurethane. The size of the catheters range from a French size 3 (pediatric) to 12.5–13.0 (double or triple lumen), with lumens ranging from 0.5 to 2.0 mm in diameter. Single-, double-, and triple-lumen catheters are available. Each lumen is distinct within the catheter, and thus incompatible drug-containing solutions may be infused simultaneously through separate lumens. As the fluids exit from the lumens into the vessel, central venous blood flow is rapid and solutions are rapidly diluted and dispersed. Consequently, there does not appear to be any significant risk of incompatibility at the exit sites of the lumen tips. Such catheters as the Hickman and Broviac are hollow tubes with openings on both the proximal and distal tips. The Groshong differs because it is designed with a pressure-sensitive distal tip valve and a "slit" valve on the side of the catheter. Pressure from fluids being infused through or withdrawn from the Groshong cause the valve to open inward or outward. When the valve is closed blood does not flow back into the catheter, thus eliminating the need for heparin locking of the catheter and decreasing the risk of air embolism (25). The most common complications reported with these devices are infections (exit site, tunnel, or systemic); other complications include venous thrombosis, catheter occlusion, and incorrect positioning of the catheter (26–28).

B. Subcutaneous Vascular Access Ports

The vascular access ports consist of a small-volume reservoir with a Silastic (self-sealing) septum connected to a central venous catheter. The port is made of plastic, stainless steel, or titanium. The entire system is placed subcutaneously, usually in the anterior chest wall. Once implanted, the port is only slightly noticeable. Access to the device is obtained with a specially designed noncoring needle (e.g., Huberpoint) placed through the skin and septum of the port. The septum is designed to withstand 1000–2000 punctures, depending on the gauge of the needle. These devices are widely used for intermittent and prolonged continuous infusions. Between infusions, the system is generally flushed and locked with heparinized saline at monthly intervals. Single- and double-lumen devices are available. One design of the subcutaneous port is attached to a Groshong catheter. In addition to complications similar to those associated with the tunneled catheters, pocket infections and needle dislodgement from the septum have also been reported with the ports. Rarely the port can flip sideways or upside down in the pocket, thereby preventing needle access. This is caused by disconnection of the fixation sutures from the underlying structure (29).

C. Peripherally Inserted Central Venous Catheters (PICC)

These devices are made of flexible polyurethane or silicone and have also been called long-arm or long-line catheters. PICCs are inserted via the antecubital fossa and threaded into the basilic, median antecubital basilic, or cephalic vein through the subclavian vein, with the tip resting in the superior vena cava. They can be placed at the bedside by specially trained nurses and have remained in place for several weeks to several months (30). Like the tunneled catheters, the PICCs are also available in single- and multilumen designs. Major complications associated with PICCs include phlebitis at the insertion site or along the vein, infection at the insertion site, sepsis, cellulitis, withdrawal occlusion, thrombosis, catheter occlusion secondary to obstruction or kinking, and catheter tip migration (31,32).

The P.A.S. PORT (Pharmacia Deltec) differs from other available PICCs because it has a small titanium port with a silicone septum attached to the polyurethane catheter. It is used in conjunction with the CATH-FINDER catheter tracking system. This catheter tracking system uses a locator wand (with audible and visual signals) in conjunction with anatomical landmarks (e.g., third rib and sternum) for guidance to determine the catheter tip location. Noncoring needles (e.g., Huber needle) of 20 gauge or less are necessary for access.

D. Nonvenous Access Devices

A wide variety of access devices are also available for the regional administration of chemotherapy or other drugs. These include arterial and intraperitoneal ports, intraperitoneal catheters, and intraventricular reservoirs. Arterial ports and catheters have been developed primarily for the administration of hepatic arterial chemotherapy; however, they have also been used for administration of regional therapy for head and neck tumors and sarcomas (32,33). The arterial catheters have a smaller lumen than central intravenous catheters because of the small size of the arteries (e.g., hepatic) that are cannulated. Because of the small lumen, these devices are not generally used for blood drawing because of a high risk of clot formation (33).

Intraperitoneal catheters (e.g., Tenckhoff peritoneal dialysis catheter) and implanted ports (similar to the venous ports) connected to an intraperitoneal catheter are widely used for the administration of chemotherapy into the peritoneal cavity for the management of ovarian cancer, mesotheliomas, melanomas, and colorectal cancer with peritoneal metastases. Examples of intraperitoneal ports include the Port-A-Cath intraperitoneal access system by Pharmacia Deltec and the Macroport intraperitoneal port by Strato Medical Corporation. The lumens of the catheters are much larger than the venous catheters. The catheter tip has many small holes that facilitate drainage of peritoneal fluid after treatment (or dialysis) is completed (34,35). The tip is placed in the abdominal cavity, and the port is placed subcutaneously in a pocket beneath the skin. It is affixed to the fascia of the muscles overlying an anatomical area that provides support and stability (36–38). Complications associated with these devices include infections (catheter track, pocket, and peritonitis), development of a fibrin sheath on the catheter tip that prevents outflow (drainage), abdominal pain, bowel perforation, and paralytic ileus (38).

Direct intraventricular administration of drugs can be accomplished with a small, subcutaneously placed reservoir connected to a small catheter leading to the lateral ventricle of the brain (39). These ventricular access devices are commonly referred to as Ommaya reservoirs, after the innovator. The 0.3–1.0 ml silicone or polypropylene reservoir is dome shaped (1.5–2.7 cm in diameter) and self-sealing, and the catheter is about 18 cm in length. A polypropylene needle guard at the base of the reservoir prevents needle puncture (40,41). Examples include the standard Ommaya reservoir (V. Mueller Baxter/Meyer Schulte) and the Accu-Flo cerebrospinal fluid (CSF) reservoir (Codman Shurt Leff, Inc.) The drug solution is injected into the reservoir, and then the reservoir is gently pumped. Shapiro et al. demonstrated that methotrexate administered through such a device is distributed rapidly and evenly in patients with meningeal leukemia and meningeal carcinomatosis (42). The reservoir also makes it possible to withdraw samples of CSF for cytological, biochemical, or bacteriological testing.

E. Summary: Selection of Vascular Access Devices

Tables 5, 6, and 7 describe only a representative fraction of the vascular access devices available in the United States today. Selection of the most appropriate type and model of device for a particular patient is based on factors that include the number of concomitant therapies the patient will need (to determine the number of lumens desirable), the anticipated duration of therapy (i.e., how long the device will be required), whether placement of a particular device would place the patient at increased risk of bleeding or infection, the ability of the patient or caregivers to participate in the maintenance of catheter care, and the need for the device to be frequently used for blood drawing.

For such devices as the tunneled catheters or implanted ports, the patient must be involved in the decision to place the device and must be made aware of the potential advantages of the device as well as its risks. To minimize risk, it is strongly recommended that institutions or alternative clinical settings that utilize these devices develop explicit policies and procedures regarding their placement and care. Such policies and procedures should include information regarding patients who are considered high risk for device-related complications, patient education materials, and detailed information regarding the care of the access device, including maintenance of patency, care of the exit site, and use of thrombolytics for occlusion.

Table 5 Tunneled Central Venous Catheters: Some Devices Currently Marketed in the United States

Model/material (manufacturer)	French size of catheter	Inner diameter catheter (mm)	Total lumen volume (priming volume, ml)
Single-lumen devices			
Hickman single-lumen catheter/silicone (Bard)	9	1.6	1.8
Groshong single-lumen catheter/silicone (Bard)	7 and 8	1.3 –1.5	0.7–1.2 ml
Quinton single-lumen central venous access catheter/silicone (Quinton)	3.9–9.7[a]	0.75–1.5	0.9–2.0 ml
Harborin single-lumen central venous catheter/polyurethane (Harbor Medical Devices)	7	1.5	0.9
Double-lumen devices			
Hickman dual-lumen catheter/silicone (Bard)	7	0.8/1.0	0.6/0.8
	9	0.7/1.3	0.6/1.3
	12	1.6/lumen	1.8 each lumen
Leonard dual-lumen catheter/silicone (Bard)	10	1.3/lumen	1.3/lumen
Groshong dual-lumen catheter/silicone (Bard)	9.5	1.1/1.33	0.5/0.8
Cook TPN double-lumen central venous catheters/silicone (Cook Critical Care)	5	0.5/lumen	0.2/lumen
	7	0.7/1.0	0.4/0.6
	9	1.0/1.3	0.6/1.0
	12	1.0/1.6	1.6/2.3
Quinton RAAF dual-lumen central venous catheters/silicone	9	1.1/lumen	1.2/lumen
	12	1.5/lumen	2.2/lumen
	13.5	2.0/lumen	2.5/lumen
Triple-lumen catheters			
National Support Catheter/polyurethane (Arrow International, Inc.)	7		0.7/0.5/0.5
Hickman triple-lumen catheter/silicone (Bard)	12.5	1.0/1.0/1.5	0.7/0.7/1.6
Quinton triple-lumen central venous access catheter/silicone	11.7	1.0/1.0/1.25	1.0/1.1/1.2

[a]Depending on model.

Table 6 Peripherally Inserted Central Venous Catheters (PICC): Some Devices Currently Marketed in the United States

Model or trade name/material (manufacturer)	French size	Lumen diameter (mm)	Length (cm)	Priming volume (ml)
Single-lumen catheters				
Groshong PICC/silicone (Bard)	4	0.8	56	0.3
C-PICS/silicone (Cook Critical Care)	5	0.91	60	0.6
V-Cath/silicone (HDC Corporation)	2	0.3	40	0.1
	4	0.9	60	0.4
L-Cath PICC/polyurethane	5	1.2	56	0.9
(Luther Medical Products, Inc.)	3.5	0.7	56	0.4
	2.6	0.5	56	0.2
Double-lumen catheters				
D/L PICC/silicone (Bard)	5	0.8/0.6	55.9	0.4/0.3
Double-lumen Per-q-cath/silicone (Bard)	4	0.5/0.3	60	0.1/0.6
	5	0.8/0.4	60	0.3/0.1

IV. PHARMACEUTICAL CONSIDERATIONS IN THE SELECTION AND USE OF DRUG DELIVERY SYSTEMS

The safe and effective delivery of any drug or fluid is dependent not only on the accuracy of the delivery system but also on the physical and chemical compatibility of the infusate with all components of the system with which it comes in contact. Factors that must be evaluated include the drug reservoir materials, diluents, resultant pH, temperature at which the drug (in the system) will be stored and infused, exposure to light, and duration of time from drug preparation until completed administration. It is important to emphasize that compatibility of the drug with the infusion system applies not only to the drug reservoir (e.g., syringe, bag, or cassette) but also to the tubing, in-line filters, access devices, or other apparatus through which the infusate solution passes during drug delivery.

If multiple drugs are to be administered simultaneously, the physical and chemical compatibility of the admixture must be assured in the specific type of delivery system under simulated conditions of use (e.g., temperature, concentrations, diluents, and drug reservoir). This is particularly important when nontraditional (i.e., not glass or polyvinyl chloride, PVC) drug reservoirs are used. The increased availability of ambulatory and implanted infusion devices has led to the use of many innovative drug reservoirs. Most drug compatibility studies have been performed in either glass or PVC containers, and it should not

Table 7 Venous Access Implanted Ports[a]

Model or trade name/materials [base diameter/height/septum diameter, mm] (manufacturer)	Inner diameter of catheter (mm)	Port volume (ml)	Catheter volume (ml)	Total priming volume (ml)
Single-lumen ports				
Hickman titanium port/titanium port, silicone catheter [31.7/14/12.7] (Bard)	1.6	0.6	1.5	2.1
Hickman titanium port and Groshong catheter/titanium port, silicone catheter [31.7/14/12.7] (Bard)	1.5	0.6	0.6	1.2
MRI plastic port/plastic port, silicone catheter [31.7/15/12.7] (Bard)	1.6	0.6	1.5	2.1
Celsite venous drug delivery system/epoxy-coated titanium port, silastic catheter [26 × 32/12/12] (Burron Medical, Inc.)	1.1	0.6	0.76	1.4
Vital Port single-lumen/titanium port, silicone catheter [30/12.7/12.7] (Cook Pacemaker Corp.)	1.4	0.5	1.1	1.6
Vital Port MRI/plastic polysulfone port, silicone catheter [30/12.7/12.7] (Cook Pacemaker Corp.)	1.6	0.5	1.4	1.9
Port-A-Cath/titanium or stainless steel port, silicone catheter [25.4/13.5/11.4] (Pharmacia Deltec)	1.0	0.49	0.3	0.8
Port-A-Cath low profile/titanium port, silicone catheter [25.4/10.1/9.5] (Pharmacia Deltec)	1.0	0.28	0.39	0.7
P.A.S. PORT venous system/titanium port, polyurethane catheter [26.7/10/6.6] (Pharmacia Deltec)	1.0	0.13	0.6	0.7
LifePort venous system/titanium or delrin (plastic) port, silicone catheter [31.8/12.4/12.7] (Strato Medical Corporation)	1.5	0.6	1.3	1.9

Table 7 *(Continued)*

Model or trade name/materials [base diameter/height/septum diameter, mm] (manufacturer)	Inner diameter of catheter (mm)	Port volume (ml)	Catheter volume (ml)	Total priming volume (ml)
LifePort low profile/titanium port, silicone catheter [24.1/9.7/10.2] (Strato Medical Corporation)	1.0	0.4	0.6	1.0
Infuse-A-Port/plastic, polysulfone port, silicone catheter [30–38/11–14/8–13] (Strato Medical Corporation) Available port styles: Microport, Macroport, SnapLock Macroport	1.0	0.3 MicroPort 0.7 MacroPort 0.8 SnapLock	0.4 0.4 0.4	0.9 1.1 1.2
Double-lument ports				
MRI dual plastic port with Septum Finder, Ridge and Groshong Catheter/plastic port, silicone catheter [45.1/14.6/12.7] (Bard)	1.0/1.3 lumen	0.8/lumen	0.6/lumen	1.4/lumen
Vital Port dual lumen/titanium port, silicone catheter [29/12.7/12.7] (Cook Pacemaker Corporation)	1.2/lumen	0.5/lumen	0.8/lumen	1.3/lumen
S.E.A. Port dual lumen/titanium port, polyurethane catheter [32 × 40/12/0.21 inches^2 (Harbor Medical Devices)	1.4/lumen	0.8/lumen	0.7/lumen	1.5/lumen
Port-A-Cath dual lumen/titanium port, silicone catheter [45.6/13.5/11.4] (Pharmacia Deltec)	1.4/lumen	0.97/lumen	0.1/lumen	1.0/lumen
LifePort dual lumen/Delrin (plastic) port, polyurethane catheter [46.1 × 28.7/13.3/12.7/septum] (Strato Medical Corporation)	1.4/lumen	0.5/lumen	1.1/lumen	1.6/lumen

[a]Examples of devices available in the United States. Most of these devices are available in various catheter sizes and lengths. Some ports are available in both titanium and plastic. Some are also available in a low-profile design for patients with smaller body mass.

be assumed that an admixture would have the same final stability if placed in a different type of reservoir. Potential compatibility problems associated with changing drug delivery systems include leaching of plasticizer from the drug reservoir or administration tubing, adsorption to the reservoir or tubing, and change in particle size that may not be compatible with the pore size of an in-line filter. The use of such drug products as paclitaxel, which contain solubilizers that leach plasticizers from PVC, and recombinant DNA products, which may adsorb to delivery systems, emphasize the need for careful pharmaceutical evaluation of the entire drug delivery process.

When reviewing compatibility studies, it is also very important to assess whether the new drug delivery system will alter the final drug concentrations of any drugs in the admixture. Many drug admixture compatibility or stability studies have been performed in conditions simulating large-volume parenterals and "traditional" (e.g., 1 liter containers) drug delivery systems. In clinical practice, however, the emphasis on home administration of chemotherapy and other pharmaceuticals has shifted drug delivery toward the use of small, ambulatory devices. These devices often necessitate highly concentrated infusates in comparison to the more traditional large-volume admixtures.

REFERENCES

1. Nahata MC, Powell DA, Durrell D, et al. Delivery of tobramycin by three infusion systems. Chemotherapy 1984; 30:84–87.
2. Nahata MC, Durrell DE, Miller MA. Accuracy of tobramycin piggyback delivery using gravity flow versus controller. Am J Hosp Pharm 1986; 43:947–949.
3. Pleasants RA, Sawyer WT, Williams DM. Effect of four intravenous infusion methods on tobramycin pharmacokinetics. Clin Pharm 1988; 7:374–379.
4. Kwan JW. High-technology i.v. infusion devices. Am J Hosp Pharm 1991; 48(suppl 1):S36–51.
5. Graves DA, Foster TS, Batenhorst RL, et al. Patient-controlled analgesia. Ann Intern Med 1983; 99:360–366.
6. White PF. Patient-controlled analgesia: a new approach to the management of postoperative pain. Semin Anesth 1985; 4:255–266.
7. Barkas G, Duafala ME. Advances in cancer pain management: a review of patient-controlled analgesia. J Pain Sympt Management 1988; 3:150–160.
8. Swanson G, Smith J, Bulich R, New P, Shiffman R. Patient-controlled analgesia for chronic cancer pain in the ambulatory setting: a report of 117 patients. J Clin Oncol 1989; 7:1903–1908.
9. Bauman TJ, Batenhorst RL, Graves DA, Foster TS, Bennett RL. Patient-controlled analgesia in the terminally ill cancer patient. Drug Intell Clin Pharm 1986; 20:297–301.
10. White PF. Patient-controlled analgesia. II. Comparative studies and alternative routes of administration. In: Stanley TH, ed. Anesthesiology and Pain Management. Amsterdam: Kluwer, 1991:245–248.

11. Urquhart ML, Klapp K, White PF. Patient-controlled analgesia: a comparison of intravenous versus subcutaneous hydromorphone. Anesthesiology 1988; 69:428–432.
12. Chrubasik J, Wiemers K. Continuous-plus-on-demand epidural infusion of morphine for postoperative pain relief by means of a small, externally worn infusion device. Anesthesiology 1985; 62:263–267.
13. Sjostrom S, Hartvig D, Tamsen A. Patient-controlled analgesia with extradural morphine or pethidine. Br J Anaesth 1988; 60:358–366.
14. Wermeling DP, Foster TS, Rapp RP, Kenady DE. Evaluation of a disposable, nonelectric, patient-controlled-analgesia device for postoperative pain. Clin Pharm 1987; 6:307–14.
15. Balch CM, Urist MM, Soong S, et al. A prospective phase 2 clinical trial of continuous FUDR regional chemotherapy for colorectal metastases to the liver using a totally implantable drug infusion pump. Ann Surg 1983; 198:567–573.
16. Niederhuber JE, Ensminger W, Gyves J. Regional chemotherapy of colorectal cancer metastatic to the liver. Cancer 1984; 53:1336–1343.
17. Barone RM, Byfield JE, Goldfarb PB, et al. Intra-arterial chemotherapy using an implantable infusion pump and liver irradiation for the treatment of hepatic metastases. Cancer 1982; 50:850–862.
18. Phillips TW, Chandler WF, Kindt GW, et al. New implantable continuous administration and bolus dose intracarotid drug delivery system for the treatment of malignant gliomas. Neurosurgery 1981; 11:213–218.
19. Penn RD. Drug pumps for treatment of neurologic diseases and pain. Neurol Clin 1985; 3:439–451.
20. Lanning RM, Hrushesky WJM. Cost comparison of wearable and implantable drug delivery systems. Proc ASCO 1990; 9:322.
21. Hohn D, Rayner AA, Economou JS, et al. Toxicities and complications of implanted pump hepatic arterial and intravenous floxuridine infusion. Cancer 1986; 57:465–470.
22. Baldwin AM, Ilsley AH, Kluger MT, Owen H. Assessment of a new infusion pump for epidural PCA. Anaesth Intensive Care 1991; 19:246–250.
23. Broviac JW, Cole JJ, Schribner BH. A silicone rubber atrial catheter for prolonged parenteral alimentation. Surg Gynecol Obstet 1973; 136:602–606.
24. Hickman RO, Buckner CD, Clift RA, et al. A modified right atrial catheter for access to the venous system in marrow transplant recipients. Surg Gynecol Obstet 1979; 148:871–875.
25. Hadaway LC. Evaluation and use of advanced I.V. technology. Part I. Central venous access devices. J IV Nurs 1989; 12:73–82.
26. Hiemenz J, Skelton J, Pizzo PA. Perspectives on the management of catheter-related infections in cancer patients. Pediatric Infect Dis J 1986; 5:6–11.
27. Lazarus HM, Lowder JN, Herzig RH. Occlusion and infections in Broviac catheters during intensive cancer therapy. Cancer 1983; 52:2342–2348.
28. Reed WP, Newman KA, DeJongh CA, et al. Prolonged venous access for chemotherapy by means of the Hickman catheter. Cancer 1983; 52:185–192.
29. Bothe A, Daly J. Technical aspects of vascular access for infusional chemotherapy. In: Lokich JJ, ed. Cancer Chemotherapy by Infusion. Chicago: Precept Press, 1987:59–73.

30. Masoorii S, Angeles T. PICC lines: the latest home care challenge. RN 1990; 44–51.
31. Rutherford C. A study of single lumen peripherally inserted central line catheter dwelling time and complications. J IV Nurs 1988; 11:169–173.
32. Winters V, Peters B, Coila S, et al. A trial with a new peripheral implanted vascular access device. Oncol Nurs Forum 1990; 17:891–896.
32. Johnson S, Patt YZ. Caring for the patient on intraarterial chemotherapy. Are you ready? Nursing 1981; 81:108–112.
33. Winters V. Implantable vascular access devices. Oncol Nurs Forum 1984; 11:25–30.
34. Swenson KK, Erikson JH. Nursing management of intraperitoneal chemotherapy. Oncol Nurs Forum 1986; 13:33–39.
35. DeGraff PW, Mellema MM, ten Bokkel Huinink WW, et al. Complications of Tenckhoff catheter implantation in patients with multiple intraabdominal procedures for ovarian carcinoma. Gynecol Oncol 1988; 29:43–49.
36. Hoff ST. Concepts in intraperitoneal chemotherapy. Semin Oncol Nurs 1987; 3:112–117.
37. Almadrones L, Yerys C. Problems associated with the administration of intraperitoneal therapy using the Port-A-Cath system. Oncol Nurs Forum 1990; 17:75–80.
38. Howell SB. Intraperitoneal catheters for chemotherapy. J Vasc Access Nurs 1990; 1:8–10.
39. Ratcheson RA, Ommaya AK. Experience with the use of the subcutaneous cerebrospinal-fluid reservoir: preliminary report of 60 cases. N Engl J Med 1968: 279:1025–1031.
40. Esparza DM, Weyland JB. Nursing care for the patients with an Ommaya reservoir. Oncol Nurs Forum 1982; 9:17–20.
41. Hagle ME. Implantable devices for chemotherapy: access and delivery. Semin Oncol Nurs 1987; 3:96–105.
42. Shapiro WR, Young DF, Mehta BM. Methotrexate distribution in cerebrospinal fluid after intravenous ventricular and lumbar injections. N Engl J Med 1975; 293:161–166.

21

Bone Marrow Transplantation

D. Bron
Institut Jules Bordet, Université Libre de Bruxelles, Brussels, Belgium

I. INTRODUCTION

Bone marrow transplantation (BMT) is now an accepted form of therapy with increasing indications in a variety of malignant diseases, genetic disorders, and aplastic anaemia.

Morbidity and mortality within the first 100 days is substantial, particularly following allogeneic BMT. The possibility that this therapeutic procedure might induce toxic death is of particular concern when survival of the patients without BMT may be considerably longer (i.e., chronic myeloid leukemia in first year of chronic phase). Patients undergoing such treatment suffer prolonged marrow aplasia, significant nonmarrow toxicities, profound immunosuppression, and unique complications, such as graft-versus-host disease (GVHD). This requires maximum supportive care, including close monitoring of clinical and laboratory parameters to anticipate or detect as early as possible complications. In addition, the dedication and expertise of the medical and nursing team is required.

This chapter focuses on the prevention, treatment, and follow-up of early and late complications in patients undergoing BMT. Topics such as prevention of bacterial and fungal infections, transfusions, antiemetics and oral care are discussed in other chapters of this handbook.

II. SIDE EFFECTS OF CONDITIONING

Despite its increasing success, bone marrow transplantation remains limited by toxicities occurring in both the early and the late posttransplantation periods.

A. Cytotoxic Drug Toxicity

High-dose cyclophosphamide (CY) chemotherapy is used for its antineoplastic and immunosuppressive effects in preparation for BMT. A unique cardiotoxicity is associated with high-dose CY. Manifestations of CY cardiotoxicity range from an asymptomatic pericardial effusion with reduction in electrocardiographic voltage to myopericarditis and congestive heart failure (CHF), which may be fatal. Braverman et al. prospectively studied the incidence, risk factors, and course of cardiotoxicity following high-dose CY administration (1). CY toxicity is thought to be caused by toxic endothelial damage followed by extravasation of toxic metabolites with resultant myocyte damage and interstitial hemorrhage and edema. Microthrombosis leading to further ischemic damage may be responsible for more serious cardiotoxicity leading to death. Braverman et al. report 35% of baseline fractional shortening (by M-mode echocardiogram). The risk of cardiotoxicity is directly related to the dose, and the authors suggest fractionating high doses of CY to reduce cardiotoxicity, as reported in animal models, without losing the therapeutic efficacy. Prior radiation therapy was not found to predispose to cardiotoxicity in at least three studies. Increased toxicity related to prior administration of anthracyclines remains questionable. Only a history of clinical CHF or a baseline ejection fraction less than 50% was an independent predictor of cardiotoxicity.

The administration of high-dose CY is also associated with hemorrhagic cystitis. This complication is uncommon, but its treatment is difficult. A recent randomized study suggested that bladder irrigation does not prevent hemorrhagic cystitis, but mesna administration is mandatory (2).

Busulfan has been associated with seizures during its administration or shortly thereafter. Because it is known that high blood levels of busulfan can persist for 24–48 h after the end of oral busulfan administration, antiseizure prophylaxis should include phenytoin for at least 48 h after the last dose (3).

B. Mucositis

Mucositis is a frequent complication of BMT conditioning, but the severity of mucositis may be reduced by the administration of acyclovir, suggesting an important role of herpes simplex virus in the development of oral mucositis. The pathogenesis of this mucositis could be related to the increased tumor necrosis factor α (TNF-α) serum levels observed after BMT. TNF-α being involved in the pathogenesis of mucositis, graft-versus-host disease, and venoocclusive disease, a phase I study using pentoxifylline (2 g/day p.o.), which interferes with TNF-α transcription, was conducted in high-risk allogeneic transplanted patients. In this series of 30 patients, the incidence of mucositis, liver dysfunction, renal insufficiency, and GVHD was significantly reduced compared with historical controls (4). The hospitalization duration and survival seemed to be improved.

Ciprofloxacin, another drug that interferes with TNF-α transcription, has been reported to enhance hematopoietic recovery and improve survival in a murine model (5). Addition of ciprofloxacin to pentoxifylline could be even more beneficial to the transplant patients. Randomized studies are now ongoing and will gather more convincing data.

C. Hemolytic-Uremic Syndrome

Recently, renal dysfunction and hemolytic-uremic syndrome have come to be recognized as late complications after marrow transplantation. Hemolytic-uremic syndrome occurs as early as 30 days and as late as 2 years after BMT. It may be benign, with complete resolution of symptoms, but patients in whom the hemolytic-uremic syndrome develops early after transplantation are more likely to die (6). Risk factors and preventive measures to avoid this complication require further investigation.

III. GRAFT-VERSUS-HOST DISEASE

Graft-versus-host disease remains a significant problem following allogeneic BMT. The risk of significant grade II–IV GVHD is associated with increasing age and any combination other than a female-to-female donor-recipient pair. Other but less important risks are associated with female donors who are immunized and donors who are cytomegalovirus (CMV) positive (7). The essential requirements for the development of GVHD have been summarized by Billigham et al.:

1. The graft must contain immunologically competent cells.
2. The recipient must express relevant transplantation antigens that are capable of immunologically stimulating donor cells.
3. The recipient must be immunologically deficient, that is, incapable of mounting an immune response.

These requirements are present not only after allogeneic transplantation but also after transplantation of solid organs containing lymphoid tissue and after transfusion of nonirradiated blood products, particularly in immunocompromised patients. Under certain circumstances, GVHD has been demonstrated after autologous or syngeneic BMT.

The pathogenesis of this reaction is currently understood as a two-step process with, first, an activation of donor T cells by recipient tissue antigens and, second, secretion of cytokines, such as TNF-α, interferon-γ (IFN-γ), interleukin-1 (IL-1), and IL-2, by activated donor T lymphocytes, which attack recipient skin, liver, and intestinal tract (8).

Acute GVHD generally develops within 2–8 weeks of marrow transplantation. Clinical manifestations include fever, skin rash, jaundice, diarrhea, and vomiting, and in some hyperacute cases, capillary damage and fluid retention are observed. Patients may present with mild bilirubin abnormalities but marked transaminase elevations. Although not universally accepted, the Seattle classification is the most common grading system (Table 1).

The clinical picture may suggest the diagnosis of GVHD, but only skin or rectal biopsies can assess the diagnosis; liver biopsy is also needed to differentiate GVHD from venoocclusive disease and toxic or viral hepatitis.

A. Prevention of Acute GVHD

Methotrexate with cyclosporine has been shown to be the most effective combination in decreasing the incidence of GVHD. There is a concern because of the higher relapse rate after methotrexate and cyclosporine compared with cyclosporine alone (9). However, actuarial relapse-free survival is not different. Low trough levels of cyclosporine A 2 weeks after BMT, usually caused by adapted doses to nephrotoxicity, are associated with a high risk of GVHD (10). Cyclosporine A and methotrexate combination was compared to T cell depletion of the marrow using CD6 and CD8, acute and chronic GVHD were higher in the T cell-depleted group (11).

Anti-IL-2 receptor monoclonal antibodies have also been tested in the prevention of GVHD with promising results, but further studies are clearly warranted (12).

B. Treatment of Acute GVHD

Steroids are the classic treatment for acute GVHD. Generally methylprednisolone is given intravenously (IV) at 2 mg/kg/day, and 30–50% respond to this treatment.

Table 1 Grading of GVHD

Skin desquamation (%)	Gastrointestinal tract	Liver	Grade
<50	—	—	I
<50	Diarrhea (<500 ml)	↗ Bilirubin (<20 μM)	II
>50	Diarrhea (<1.5 liters)	↗ Bilirubin (>20 μM)	III
>50	Diarrhea (>1 liter) Ileus	↗ Bilirubin (>20 μM) ↗ AST, ALT[a]	IV

[a]AST, aspartate aminotransferase; ALT, alanine aminotransferase.

It is important to note that a response to GVHD therapy does not mean a loss of graft-versus-leukemia effect. When clinicians are faced with a steroid-resistant GVHD, several alternatives are now available, such as antithymocyte globulins (ATG), anti-IL-2 receptor antibodies, azathiopine, and anti-TNF antibodies (13).

Patients who may benefit from anti-IL-2 receptor antibodies seem to be those who have low levels of soluble CD8 receptor, IL-2 receptor and TNF-α in the serum (14).

C. Treatment of Chronic GVHD

Chronic GVHD occurs to some extent in approximately 40% of recipients in allogeneic BMT. Chronic GVHD differs from acute GVHD in its pathogenesis, target organs, and clinical presentations, which are summarized in Table 2. T cells in chronic GVHD react in an autoimmune fashion against histocompatibility alloantigens of the host. These T cells release cytokines and stimulate collagen production. Although this may be associated with a beneficial graft-versus-leukemia effect under certain circumstances, it generally leads to significant morbidity and mortality. Much of the management of these patients resolves around symptomatic therapy of the associated skin disease, Sjögren's syndrome, and severe immunosuppression with infectious complications (Table 3) (15).

It is generally recommended that chronic GVHD be treated with steroïds, but in case of thrombocytopenia, a poor prognostic factor, cyclosporine, should be added (16). In severe chronic GVHD resistant to steroïds and cyclosporine, azathiopine should be tried. Recent papers reported successful preliminary results with thalidomide (17,18). For the treatment of drug-resistant cutaneous GVHD, a combination of 8-methoxypsoralen (methoxsalen) and ultraviolet A was tested in 11 patients: 6 complete and 5 partial responses were observed (19).

IV. LIVER DYSFUNCTION

Hepatic dysfunction frequently occurs after BMT, and various etiologies, such as venoocclusive disease, graft-versus-host-disease, infections, drug injury, or

Table 2 Clinical Features of Chronic GVHD

Skin muscle	Sclerosis, depigmentation, alopecia, contractures with restriction of movement
Liver	Jaundice caused by biliary obstruction, liver failure, cirrhosis
Exocrine glands	Sicca syndrome, ocular damage, anhydrya
Gastrointestinal tract	Ulceration, malabsorption, weight loss, pancreatic insufficiency
Lungs	Bronchiolitis, recurrent chest infections, pneumothorax
Blood cell count	Cytopenia by decreased marrow production or autoimmune destruction

Table 3 Management of GVHD

Prevention	
In vitro	T cell depletion of donor marrow
	Irradiation of blood products
In vivo	Cyclosporine (12 mg/kg/day)
	Methotrexate (10 mg/m^2 days 1, 3, 6)
	Steroids (prednisone, 2 mg/kg/day)
	Anitlymphocyte globulins (0.15 g/kg × 5 days)
	Pentoxifylline (2 g/day)
Treatment	
Acute	Steroids
	Antilymphocyte globulins
	Anti-CD2, anti-CD5
	Anti-IL-2
	Anti-TNF
Chronic	Steroids
	Cyclosporines
	Antilymphocyte globulins
	Thalidomide

parenteral nutrition, must be distinguished. Time of onset, duration, treatment, and prognosis are different for each diagnosis.

A. Venoocclusive Disease (VOD)

VOD is a consequence of toxic injury to the liver resulting from the high-dose chemo- and radiotherapy used to condition the patient. It is the most common life-threatening complication of conditioning regimen-related toxicity, and it is clinically suspected if jaundice, weight gain, and painful hepatomegaly develop in the first 2 weeks after BMT (20). The incidence of VOD is lower in autologous BMT than allogeneic BMT, and this led to speculation about the immunological mechanisms involved in the pathogenesis of VOD.

The pathogenesis is not fully understood, but the toxic concentration of active metabolites of antineoplastic agents in the centrolobular zone of the liver sinusoids may lead to the obstruction of small intrahepatic venules by edematous, injured, and necrotic hepatocytes. It is believed that the release of TNF-α potentiates cytotoxicity and activates coagulation, leading to more severe obstruction of hepatic sinusoids and venules. This can cause a shift of fluid containing sodium and albumin from the intravascular to the extravascular space; the clinical picture then consists of edema, ascites, abdominal pain, hepatomegaly, and impaired liver function with icterus. In severe cases with prolonged liver dysfunction, renal insufficiency may develop secondary to prerenal failure. In patients treated with cyclosporine, prostacylin release from endothelial cells is reduced, and this may facilitate capillary thrombosis.

A number of contraindications exist between published risk factors from different institutions. McDonald et al. stratified the potential risk factors for developing VOD into three areas: (1) pretransplant factors, (2) marrow conditioning and type of transplant, and (3) clinical course factors.

Among pretransplant factors, elevated SGOT above the upper normal limit is one of the strongest risk factors for VOD, and the increased risk is proportional to the degree of SGOT elevation. In most series, the causes of pretransplant hepatitis are primarily non-A, non-B hepatitis, more likely hepatitis C. In the multivariate analysis by McDonald and colleagues, an additional risk is related to septicemia and/or the use of broad-spectrum antibiotics (including vancomycin and amphotericin B). It could be that persistent fever requiring the use of these drugs reflects increased levels of TNF-α involved in the pathogenesis of VOD. Other pretransplant risk factors include disease states, positive CMV serology, patients heavily pretreated with chemotherapy, and older age. However, some of these factors were not confirmed in recent studies (21).

The conditioning regimen is the major risk for VOD when more intensive cytoreductive regimens are administered. The administration of high-dose busulfan is often incriminated in the increased risk of VOD (22). However, the rate of VOD varies greatly after conditioning with busulfan and cyclophosphamide. This marked variability is now better understood by pharmacological data: the apparent volume of distribution and clearance rate were twice as high in children, and this could explain the higher risk in adult patients who received doses calculated per body weight (16 mg/kg). The hepatotoxicity of total-body irradiation (TBI) is sharply increased as the total TBI dose is increased despite the use of fractionated schedules.

Jaundice, hepatomegaly, fluid retention, and ascites may be nonspecific findings, and a liver biopsy can be useful to distinguish VOD from acute GVHD and infection of the liver. Because patients are generally severely thrombocytopenic, a transvenous liver biopsy should be used instead of percutaneous liver biopsy, which carries an increased risk of hemorrhage. However, these clinical manifestations early after transplantation are highly suggestive of VOD, ascites or significant weight gain usually not being seen in drug-induced hepatotoxicity. Acute GVHD usually appears after the first 2 weeks and without ascites.

Of patients presenting with VOD, 30% ultimately die from hepatorenal failure. Therefore, several prophylactic options have been proposed (Table 4). The most spectacular results have been observed with pentoxifylline (2 g/day), a TNF-α blocker that lowers the TNF-α level in the serum of treated patients (4). Another option was reported by Attal and colleagues in a randomized study comparing the continuous infusion of low-dose heparin (100 U/kg/day) and no prophylactic

Table 4 Management of Venoocclusive Disease

Prevention
Pentoxifylline
Heparin
Prostacyclin
Treatment
Electrolyte balance surveillance
Fluid restriction with preservation of renal perfusion
Maintenance of osmotic pressure (albumin)

treatment. The heparin-treated group was significantly superior ($p < 0.01$) to the control group. The effect was achieved without an increased risk of bleeding (23). Prophylactic infusion of prostacyclin may also be effective, but side effects, such as fluid retention and painful extremities, are limiting toxicities.

The treatment of VOD is limited to symptomatic measures: a restriction of sodium intake to achieve a negative sodium balance. The total volume of perfusion should be reduced, but renal perfusion must be maintained. Albumin (up to four times 25 g IV/day) is useful to maintain the osmotic pressure. Hemoglobin should be maintained at a level of $\geq$ 10 g/dl to provide sufficient oxygen to hepatocytes and renal tubular cells. Spironolactone is recommended if serum creatinine is normal. Administration of tissue plasminogen activator can reverse bilirubin elevation in some patients, but experience with this approach is limited. Drugs, such as cyclosporine, methotrexate, sedatives, and analgesics, need dose adjustment or discontinuation.

B. Acute and Chronic GVHD

The hepatotoxicity of acute GVHD is probably the result of both cellular attack (by T lymphocytes) and cytokines, such as TNF and IFN. In the majority of patients, some degree of skin or intestinal involvement in acute GVHD is present concurrently. Usually, transaminases and serum bilirubin are moderately increased. Acute liver failure with ascites, coagulation disorders, and encephalopathy is uncommon. In some cases, liver biopsy is required to make the diagnosis. The treatment of GVHD was described earlier.

The majority of patients with chronic GVHD show some degree of hepatic involvement: the main targets of chronic GVHD of the liver are the small interlobular bile ducts. A biopsy is often needed to exclude other pathologies. Rarely, hepatic failure and cirrhosis are observed.

The treatment was detailed earlier. About half of these patients remain free of chronic GVHD after immunosuppressive drug withdrawal.

C. Infections

The most common infections of the liver in BMT recipients are of viral origin: hepatitis B or C, cytomegalovirus, varicella-zoster (VZV), and herpes simplex (HSV).

V. PREVENTION OF VIRAL INFECTIONS

Viral opportunistic infections, primarily CMV infections, represent a major infectious problem in transplant patients. However, significant progress has been made in identifying risk factors for the prevention and treatment of CMV infection (24). In addition to pneumonitis, retinitis, and hepatitis, CMV has been associated with a delay in the recovery of platelets after allogeneic and autologous BMT (25,26). However, CMV is rarely a life-threatening complication in autologous BMT, and in this setting, CMV prophylaxis is not recommended (27).

Several centers have reported that screened (CMV-negative) blood products can prevent CMV infection in seronegative recipients with seronegative donors, and this aspect will be discussed in Chapter (28). Four recent studies have also demonstrated that leukocyte-depleted blood products can prevent CMV infection in CMV-negative patients (29). Even in patients receiving marrow from a CMV-positive donor, leukocyte-depleted blood products could reduce the incidence of CMV infection (30).

For CMV-positive recipients, two approaches have been widely studied: (1) immunoprophylaxis with high doses of intravenous immunoglobulins (IVIG) and (2) antiviral drug prophylaxis using acyclovir or ganciclovir.

A. High-Dose IgG Immunoglobulins

There are several reasons to support immunoprophylaxis in the prevention of CMV infection: hyperimmune immunoglobulins have proven useful in the prevention of various viral infections, such as hepatitis, varicella, and rubella. Other rational bases derive from animal data showing that hyperimmune immunoglobulins are able to protect immunosuppressed or newborn mice against CMV-induced interstitial pneumonia. Also, after allogeneic BMT, patients with a higher antibody response to CMV antigens have been reported to have a better outcome (31).

At least five controlled studies have shown a decrease in the incidence of interstitial pneumonia, whereas the incidence of CMV infection is not always significantly reduced. In addition, in a large comparative study reported by the Seattle group, several other advantages to the treatment with IVIG have been pointed out: a reduced risk of GVHD, a reduced incidence of bacterial septicemia, and a reduced number of pneumonitis. The mechanism of action of these IVIG is not fully elucidated. IVIG increase the circulating level of specific anti-CMV (and anti-bacteria) immunoglobulins with cytotoxic and neutralizing activities. It is also likely that the increase in the IgG level in the serum and respiratory tract decreases the risk of infectious problems, including CMV. The reduced incidence of GVHD could be related to antilymphocyte antibodies or to a blockade of Fc receptor on CD8 lymphocytes, which are involved in the GVHD process. A relationship exists between CMV infection and acute GVHD, and a reduced incidence of GVHD could probably have an indirect effect in the prevention of CMV infection (32).

Two new promising immunological approaches are currently being investigated in phase I trials: the first is the administration of human monoclonal anti-CMV antibodies, which should have more consistent anti-CMV activity from lot to lot (33,34), and the second is adoptive immunotherapy using T cell clones obtained from serpositive donors. Actually, it has been shown that transplant patients with a specific anti-CMV T cell response have a better outcome than patients unable to have such a cytolytic T cell response (35).

Although the role of IVIG in CMV prophylaxis is still debated, the other beneficial effects of IVIG have led many centers to adopt this immunoprophylaxis using 500 mg/kg weekly for the first 100 days and monthly up to 12 months.

B. Antiviral Drug Prophylaxis

The first convincing study was reported by Meyers in 1990 using acyclovir at the dose of 500 mg/m^2 every 8 h from day 7 to day 30 in allogeneic transplanted patients. In this series, the incidence of both CMV infections and interstitial pneumonia was reduced (36). However, acyclovir is not the optimal antiviral drug, and ganciclovir, which slows the replication of CMV, is a better candidate for CMV prophylaxis. At least one study has indicated that prophylactic ganciclovir can completely prevent CMV pneumonia in seropositive recipients or seropositive donors (37), but myelosuppression is the limiting toxicity for half of these patients. Therefore, recent approaches using ganciclovir when a positive CMV culture (blood, throat, urine, and bronchoalveolar lavage) is detected, or at day 30 in case of CMV in the bronchoalveolar lavage, are encouraging for seropositive patients or seronegative recipients with a seropositive donor (38,39).

More recently, the new antiviral drug, foscarnet, has gained interest because of its anticytomegalovirus activity by inhibition of CMV DNA polymerase. This drug has been shown to be effective in some cases of ganciclovir-resistant CMV and is less toxic to the marrow. This drug should be used with caution in patients with renal failure (40).

VI. GRAFT FAILURE

Graft failure can manifest itself as primary engraftment failure or as initial engraftment followed by secondary graft loss. Graft failure may or may not be associated with reappearance of recipient cells, but an active host response to the graft is often involved in allogeneic BMT (41). In the setting of autologous bone marrow, other causes are involved in the process of graft failure.

A definition of graft failure is not universally settled; however, when the granulocyte count is not sustained at $>200/\mu l$ by day 28, graft failure is thought to be present. Graft failure is confirmed when marrow biopsy reveals an empty or a poor marrow without myeloïd, erythroïd, or megakaryocytic precursors.

In the patient transplanted with HLA-identical donor, graft failure is mostly observed in patients with aplastic anemia who have been multiply transfused and are thus sensitized to minor histocompatibility antigens of the donor. Experience in patients who rejected their initial graft has indicated that cyclophosphamide (4×50 mg/kg) and ATG (3×30 mg/kg) allowed sustained engraftment. This approach is now applied for the first conditioning regimen, with very encouraging results.

Another approach to reduce graft failure is to increase the immunosuppression of the recipient by drug or irradiation (total-body or total-lymphoid irradiation). The best approach for the patient with aplastic anemia is to transplant early while still untransfused. When blood products are necessary, leukocyte depletion of the transfusion product reduces the risk of sensitization. Of note, recent reports on dogs suggest that irradiation of blood product with ultraviolet light could abrogate the sensitizing ability of the blood product (42). This observation deserves further investigation in the human.

In histoincompatible transplants, graft failure is more common even after TBI-containing regimens. These patients are more likely to develop severe GVHD, and aggressive attempts to prevent GVHD using T cell depletion have reduced the risk of GVHD but increased the incidence of graft failure. Other approaches to overcome this problem include the use of monoclonal antibodies (anti-HLA class II and anti-LFA 1) and ATG. However, although the engraftment is facilitated, the regimen-related toxicity is increased.

Autologous BMT is a successful therapeutic approach with increasing indications. Autologous marrow is often damaged by prior treatments and/or cryopreservation, and the rate of hematopoietic recovery appears to be dependent upon the number of colony-forming units (as determined in vitro by the colony-forming units–granulocyte-macrophage assay). In the "purged" marrow it is always recommended to store a second unmanipulated backup marrow for rescue.

To improve recovery after autologous BMT, several ongoing investigations are promising. Hematopoietic stem cells circulating in the peripheral blood have been shown to be capable of complete hematopoietic reconstitution, and data on humans demonstrate that recovery is faster than with marrow cells (43–45). This recovery is further accelerated if the patient is pretreated with recombinant myeloid growth factors before harvesting of the peripheral blood stem cells (46). Another interesting area of research is the "positive purging," or isolation of very early hematopoietic precursors characterized by CD34 antigen.

Late decreases in peripheral blood counts in patients following marrow transplant can be from a variety of causes. Suppression by co-trimoxazole (sulfamethoxazole-trimethoprim) may be one cause, and the drug should be avoided or combined with folinic acid. Cytomegalovirus infection often leads to a drop in blood counts, which is usually reversible after successful treatment of the CMV infection. Although rare, accidental administration of unirradiated blood products in the immunosuppressive posttransplant period can result in the establishment of transfusion-associated GVHD and consequent marrow aplasia. Isolated thrombocytopenia may occur in the setting of chronic GVHD, representing a poor risk factor.

Isolated anemia can be caused by renal dysfunction or persistent parvovirus B19 infection or the result of ABO-incompatible marrow graft. In this last situation, persistent host B lymphocytes can produce isoagglutinins that are reactive with donor red cells, leading to persistent hemolytic anemia.

VII. CYTOKINES

High-dose chemoradiation therapy used before autologous or allogenic BMT is intensively myelosuppressive and immunosuppressive and frequently results in severe and life-threatening infections. Hematopoietic growth factors (HGF) have the potential to accelerate hematopoietic recovery after BMT, and by shortening the period of pancytopenia, they are likely to reduce infections and bleeding complications. On the other hand, cytokines, particularly recombinant human interleukin-2, may have clinical application in the acceleration of immune recovery and some antitumoral benefit in malignant hemopathies.

A. Hematopoietic Growth Factors

Five HGF are currently available for clinical use: erythropoietin (Epo), granulocyte colony-stimulating factor (G-CSF), granulocyte-macrophage colony-stimulating factor (GM-CSF), macrophage colony-stimulating factor (M-CSF), and interleukin-3.

Several groups have reported increases in Epo levels parallel to hemoglobin levels in autologous BMT (47). In allogeneic BMT, several authors have shown impaired or deficient production of Epo, and an inappropriate response of Epo levels to anemia has been detected (48). An uncontrolled trial has shown that

Epo is capable of accelerating erythroid engraftment in allogeneic BMT, and this observation was confirmed by a recent randomized prospective study. An earlier appearance of reticulocytes and a diminished need for red blood cells transfusions were observed in patients treated with Epo (49). Of note, the treated group also received significantly fewer platelet transfusions, but this requires further studies to be confirmed.

Most of the studies with the four other HGF performed in the setting of BMT have been nonrandomized studies. Also, because there was a concern of provoking GVHD in allogeneic BMT, many of the studies have been conducted in autologous or syngeneic BMT (50). In a prospective placebo-controlled trial of GM-CSF after autologous BMT for lymphoid malignancies, Nemunaitis et al. (51) reported significantly fewer infections, days of fever, and days of antibiotics in patients receiving GM-CSF compared with the placebo controls. There was a trend toward earlier neutrophil recovery to $1000/mm^3$ in the GM-CSF-treated group. Red blood cell recovery was not different from that in the control group, but platelet recovery was accelerated, with fewer bleeding complications in the GM-CSF-treated group. Additionally, patients treated with GM-CSF had fewer days with mucositis and less interstitial pneumonia.

G-CSF has been extensively studied in the setting of high-dose chemotherapy, and a few series involved high-dose chemotherapy and autologous BMT. Using 5–10 μg/kg/day, neutrophil recovery was significantly accelerated in G-CSF-treated patients. These patients had fewer days of fever, antibiotic therapy, and oral mucositis. Recovery of platelets and erythroblasts was not different (52,53). G-CSF is better tolerated than GM-CSF, with only mild myalgia in some patients receiving >30 μg/kg/day.

Preliminary data are available for IL-3 and M-CSF after BMT. These suggest that the duration of severe granulocytopenia may be reduced by M-CSF (54) and platelet recovery may be accelerated by IL-3.

In the setting of allogeneic BMT, G-CSF and GM-CSF have been used with caution because of the potential stimulation of lymphocytes leading to an increased risk of GVHD and graft failure. However, preclinical observations in a canine model using DLA-identical littermates for allogeneic BMT did not demonstrate an increased incidence of GVHD or graft failure (55). G-CSF was thus administered after allogeneic transplantation in human beings, showing an accelerated recovery of neutrophils but not of erythrocytes, platelets, or monocytes. The incidence of GVHD and the relapse rate were similar to those in historical controls (56).

M-CSF was investigated after allogeneic BMT in a randomized placebo-controlled clinical study. Neutrophil recovery was significantly accelerated, and the incidence of graft failure was reduced.

HGF seem to accelerate hematopoietic recovery after autologous and allogeneic BMT without increasing the incidence of graft failure of GVHD.

However, controlled studies remain important to investigate further the impact on patient survival and the relapse rate.

B. Interleukin-2

The rationale for the use of IL-2 after marrow transplantation is based on several experimental observations. First, freshly isolated leukemia and lymphoma cells were previously shown to be sensitive to lysis by IL-2-induced lymphocyte-activated killer (LAK) cells in vitro. Moreover, IL-2-responsive LAK precursors (natural killer, NK, cells) have been identified in the peripheral blood of patients as early as 3 weeks after high-dose chemotherapy and marrow infusion. Soiffier and colleagues recently showed that IL-2 can be continuously administered for a prolonged period after autologous and allogeneic BMT (57). At low doses (2×10^5 U/m^2/day), all patients showed an increase in the number of NK cells in the peripheral blood. Moreover, the sensitivity of these NK cells to further activation by IL-2 in vitro was markedly enhanced while patients were receiving IL-2 in vivo. In this report toxicity was minimal, but the dose they used is generally one-tenth of the dose administered by others (58–60), who reported thrombocytopenia and capillary leak syndrome, for example. This lower dose allows a longer period of administration (>3 months). Another noteworthy feature is the absence of GVHD in the Soiffier series, although with higher dose Favrot et al. (58) reported a severe GVHD after allogeneic BMT. This can be explained by a specific stimulation of NK cells without a change in T cell number and also, in their cases, a T cell depletion of the marrow. Because NK cells are more likely to be involved in the graft-versus-leukemia effect of the marrow, this IL-2 stimulation of NK cells may be beneficial to patient in terms of relapse rate. In this setting large randomized studies are still warranted (61).

VIII. LONG-TERM FOLLOW-UP

Marrow transplantation is associated with a number of long-term complications that may not manifest themselves for months after the BMT. They result from immunological abnormalities, structural damage secondary to the conditioning regimen, and recurrence of underlying disease.

A. Infectious Problems and Vaccination Policy

Late infectious complications are more frequently seen in allogeneic BMT as opposed to autologous BMT and are far more frequent in patients with chronic GVHD. After discharge from the hospital, most patients are maintained on co-trimoxazole (sulfamethoxazole-trimethoprim) prophylaxis for 6–12 months, or as long as immunosuppressive treatment is needed. Both bacteria (such as encapsulated pyogenic cocci) and *Pneumocystis carinii* are effectively prevented by this prophylaxis, and in case of intolerance to sulfonamides, penicillin and inhaled pentamidine can be administered. In the setting of pneumococcal infection prevention, intravenous administration of high doses of immunoglobulins have proven useful.

After allogeneic BMT patients require revaccination, and because it is unlikely to have an adequate antibody and T cell immune response during the first year, it is generally recommended to revaccinate at 12 months with diphtheria and tetanus toxoid, 23-valent pneumococcal vaccine, 4-valent meningococcal vaccine, and HIB-protein conjugate vaccine. Tetanus toxoid antibody levels can be controlled 6–8 weeks after vaccination. Killed poliomyelitis (Salk) vaccine should also be administered 1–2 years after transplant. Measles, mumps, and rubella vaccines, which are live, should not be administered to allograft recipients with chronic GVHD. They can be given 2 years after transplant, but their necessity in the BMT setting is still debated. Booster vaccines for pneumococcal, meningococcal, and HIB antigens are recommended at 24 months (62).

Viral infections, generally caused by reactivation of latent endogenous virus in either the host or the donor cells, are very frequent; VZV recurrence may be expected in the majority of patients who were seropositive for VZV before transplant, generally occurring within the first 9 months after BMT but sometimes as late as 18–24 months. Such patients should be treated with acyclovir (10 mg/kg every 8 h for 10 days). HSV, CMV, and adenovirus infections generally occur within the first 4 months after transplant.

B. Hormonal Surveillance

Endocrine function is impaired in a significant number of patients following marrow transplant. Asymptomatic, well-compensated hypothyroidism occurs in up to two-thirds of patients after transplant. This complication appears to be primarily limited to patients who have received irradiation in their conditioning. It is reasonable to evaluate patients on a yearly basis with thyroid-stimulating hormone levels as well as routine thyroid function tests.

Growth retardation may be seen in children both because of a direct effect on the growth plates of the bone by radiation therapy and also, in some cases, because of growth hormone abnormalities induced by central nervous system irradiation.

Patients with total-body irradiation have a generally greater than 95% incidence of developing infertility secondary to ovarian failure or azoospermagenesis. Patients treated with chemotherapy alone may recover hormonal function, but this is particularly dependent upon age, the majority of women less than 25 years old having return of menstruation and normal follicle-stimulating hormone and luteinizing hormone levels. About two-thirds of men given chemotherapy alone recover sperm production.

C. Secondary Tumors

Secondary malignancies have been relatively infrequent (35 of 2000 patients in the Seattle experience). It is important to note that some secondary non-Hodgkin's lymphomas may arise in the setting of Epstein-Barr virus-associated lymphoproliferative disease. This complication, which can occur early after transplant, is most frequent in heavily immunosuppressed individuals, particularly those receiving T cell depletion of donor marrow or HLA-mismatched donors. Such B cell proliferations (oligo- or polyclonal) can be rapidly progressive and fatal. As in the solid organ transplant setting, reduction in or stopping the immunosuppression can result in spontaneous regression. Other therapeutic approaches, such as anti-B monoclonal antibodies, high-dose immunoglobulins, and interferon-α have been proposed but remain experimental.

REFERENCES

1. Braverman AC, Antin JH, Plappert MT, et al. Cyclophosphamide cardiotoxicity in bone marrow transplantation: a prospective evaluation of new dosing regimens. J Clin Oncol 1991; 9:1215–1223.
2. Atkinson K, Biggs JC, Golovsky D, et al. Bladder irrigation does not prevent haemorrhagic cystitis in bone marrow transplant recipients. Bone Marrow Transplant 1991; 7:351–354.
3. De la Camara R, Tomas JF, Figuera A, et al. High dose busulfan and seizures. Bone Marrow Transplant 1991; 7:363–364.
4. Bianco JA, Appelbaum FR, Nemunaitis J, et al. Phase I–II trial of phentoxifylline for the prevention of transplant-related toxicities following bone marrow transplantation. Blood 1991; 78:1205–1211.
5. Kletter Y, Riklis I, Shalit I, et al. Enhanced repopulation of murine hematopoietic organ in sublethally irradiated mice after treatment with ciprofloxacin. Blood 1991; 78:1685–1691.
6. Rabinowe SN, Soiffer RJ, Tarbell NJ, et al. Hemolytic-uremic syndrome following bone marrow transplantation in adults for hematologic malignancies. Blood 1991; 77:1837–1844.
7. Weysdorf D, Hakke R, Blazar B, et al. Risk factors for acute graft-versus-host disease in histocompatible donor bone marrow transplantation. Transplantation 1991; 5:1197–1203.
8. Jadus MR, Wepsic HT. The role of cytokines in graft-versus-host reactions and disease. Bone Marrow Transplant 1992; 10:1–14.
9. Aschan J, Ringden O, Sundberg B, et al. Methotrexate combined with cyclosporine A decreases graft-versus-host disease, but increases leukemic relapse compared to monotherapy. Bone Marrow Transplant 1991; 7:113–119.
10. Przepiorka D, Shapiro S, Schwinghammer TL, et al. Cyclosporine and methylprednisolone after allogeneic marrow transplantation: association between low cyclosporine concentration and risk of acute graft-versus-host disease. Bone Marrow Transplant 1991; 7:461–465.

11. Ringden O, Pihlstedt P, Markling L, et al. Prevention of graft-versus-host disease with T cell depletion or cyclosporine and methotrexate: a randomized trial in adult leukemic marrow recipients. Bone Marrow Transplant 1991; 7:221–226.
12. Blaise D, Olive D, Hirn M, et al. Prevention of acute GVHD by in vivo use of anti-interleukin-2 receptor monoclonal antibody (33B3.1): a feasibility trial in 15 patients. Bone Marrow Transplant 1991; 8:105–111.
13. Martin PJ, Schoch G, Fisher L, et al. A retrospective analysis of therapy for acute graft-versus-host disease: secondary treatment. Blood 1991; 77:1821–1828.
14. Tiberghien P, Racadot E, Lioure B, et al. Soluble CD8, IL-2 receptor, and tumor necrosis factor-alpha levels in steroid-resistant acute graft-versus-host-disease. Transplantation 1991; 52:475–481.
15. Sullivan KM, Agura E, Anasetti C, et al. Chronic graft-versus-host disease and other late complications of bone marrow transplantation. Semin Hematol 1991; 28:250–259.
16. Sullivan KM, Witherspoon RP, Storb R, et al. Alternating-day cyclosporine and prednisone for treatment of high-risk chronic graft-v-host disease. Blood 1988; 72:555–561.
17. Heney D, Norfolk DR, Wheeldon J, et al. Thalidomide treatment for chronic graft-versus-host disease. Br J Haematol 1991; 78:23–27.
18. Vogelsang GB, Farmer ER, Hess AD, et al. Thalidomide therapy of chronic graft versus host disease. N Engl J Med 1992; 326:1055–1058.
19. Eppinger T, Emninger G, Steinert M, et al. 8-Methoxypsoralen and UVA therapy for cutaneous GVHD. Transplantation 1990; 50:807–811.
20. Shulman HM, Hinterberger W. Hepatic veno-occlusive disease liver toxicity syndrome after bone marrow transplantation. Bone Marrow Transplant 1992; 10:197–214.
21. McDonald GB, Sharma P, Matthens DE, et al. Veno-occlusive disease of the liver after bone marrow transplantation: diagnosis, incidence and predisposing factors. Hematology 1984; 4:116–121.
22. Ozkaynak MF, Weinberg K, Kohn D, et al. Hepatic veno-occlusive disease post-bone marrow transplantation in children conditioned with busulfan and cyclophosphamide: incidence, risk factors, and clinical outcome. Bone Marrow Transplant 1991; 7:467–474.
23. Attal M, Huguet F, Rubie H, et al. Prevention of hepatic veno-occlusive disease after bone marrow transplantation by continuous infusion of low-dose heparin: a prospective, randomized trial. Blood 1992; 79:2834–2840.
24. Winston DJ, Gale RP. Prevention and treatment of cytomegalovirus infection and disease after bone marrow transplantation in the 1990s. Bone Marrow Transplant 1991; 8:7–11.
25. Verdonck LF, De Gast GC, Van Heugten HG, et al. Cytomegalovirus infection causes delayed platelet recovery after bone marrow transplantation. Blood 1991; 78:844–848.
26. Reusser P, Fisher LD, Buckner CD, et al. Cytomegalovirus infection after autologous bone marrow transplantation: occurrence of cytomegalovirus disease and effect on engraftment. Blood 1990; 75:1888–1894.
27. Wingard JR, Chen DY, Burns WH, et al. Cytomegalovirus infection after

autologous bone marrow transplantation with comparison to infection after allogeneic bone marrow transplantation. Blood 1988; 71:1432–1437.
28. Miller WJ, McCullough J, Balfour HH Jr, et al. Prevention of cytomegalovirus infection following bone marrow transplantation: a randomized trial of blood product screening. Bone Marrow Transplant 1991; 7:227–234.
29. Bowden RA, Slichter SJ, Sayers MH, et al. Use of leukocyte-depleted platelets and cytomegalovirus-seronegative red blood cells for prevention of primary cytomegalovirus infection after marrow transplant. Blood 1991; 78:246–250.
30. De Witte T, Schattenberg A, Van Dijk BA, et al. Preventing of primary cytomegalovirus infection after allogeneic bone marrow transplantation by using leukocyte-poor random blood products from cytomegalovirus-unscreened bloodbank donors. Transplantation 1990; 50:964–968.
31. Bron D, Klastersky J. Immunoprophylaxis of cytomegalovirus infections in transplanted patients. Eur J Cancer Clin Oncol 1989; 25(9):1365–1368.
32. Sullivan KM, Kopecky K, Jocom J, et al. Immunomodulatory and antimicrobial efficacy of intravenous immunoglobulin in bone marrow transplantation. N Engl J Med 1990; 323:705–712.
33. Bron D, Lagneaux L, Delforge A, et al. Prevention of CMV-induced myelosuppression by anti-CMV antibodies: an in vitro model. Exp Hematol 1991; 19:132–135.
34. Drobyski WR, Knox KK, Carrigan DR, et al. Foscarnet therapy of ganciclovir-resistant cytomegalovirus in marrow transplantation. Transplantation 1991; 52:155–157.
35. Reusser P, Riddell SR, Meyers JD, et al. Cytotoxic T-lymphocyte response to cytomegalovirus after human allogeneic bone marrow transplantation: pattern of recovery and correlation with cytomegalovirus infection and disease. Blood 1991; 78:1373–1380.
36. Meyers JD, Reed EC, Shepp DH, et al. Acyclovir for prevention of cytomegalovirus infection and disease after allogeneic marrow transplantation. N Engl J Med 1988; 318:70–75.
37. Atkinson K, Downs K, Golenia M, et al. Prophylactic use of ganciclovir in allogeneic bone marrow transplantation: absence of clinical cytomegalovirus infection. Br J Haematol 1991; 79:57–62.
38. Schmidt GM, Horak DA, Niland JC, et al. A randomized, controlled trial of prophylactic ganciclovir for cytomegalovirus pulmonary infection in recipients of allogeneic bone marrow transplants. N Engl J Med 1991; 325:1601–1607.
39. Goodrich J, Mori M, Gleaves C, et al. Early treatment with ganciclovir to prevent cytomegalovirus disease after allogeneic bone marrow transplantation. N Engl J Med 1991; 325:1601–1607.
40. Drobyski WR, Gottlieb M, Carrigan D, et al. Phase I study of safety and pharmacokinetics of a human anti-CMV monoclonal antibody in allogeneic bone marrow transplant recipients. Transplantation 1991; 51:1190–1196.
41. Klumpp TR. Immunohematologic complications of bone marrow transplantation. Bone Marrow Transplant 1991; 8:159–170.
42. Pamphilon DH, Alnaqdy AA, Wallington TB. Immunomodulation by ultraviolet light: clinical studies and biological effects. Immunol Today 1991; 12:119–123.
43. Gianni AM, Bregni M, Siena S, et al. Rapid and complete hemopoietic reconsti-

tution following combined transplantation of autologous blood and bone marrow cells: a changing role for high dose chemo-radiotherapy? Hematol Oncol 1989; 7:139–148.
44. Lopez M, Mortel O, Pouillart P, et al. Acceleration of hemopoietic recovery after autologous bone marrow transplantation by low doses of peripheral blood stem cells. Bone Marrow Transplant 1991; 7:173–181.
45. To LB, Roberts MM, Haylock DN, et al. Comparison of haematological recovery times and supportive care requirements of autologous recovery phase peripheral blood stem cell transplants, autologous bone marrow transplants and allogeneic bone marrow transplants. Bone Marrow Transplant 1992; 9:277–284.
46. Kotasek D, Sepherd KM, Sage RE, et al. Factors affecting blood stem cell collections following high-dose cyclophosphamide mobilization in lymphoma, myeloma and solid tumors. Bone Marrow Transplant 1992; 9:11–17.
47. Bosi A, Vannucchi AM, Grossi A, et al. Serum erythropoietin levels in patients undergoing autologous bone marrow transplantation. Bone Marrow Transplant 1991; 7:421–425.
48. Beguin Y, Clemons GK, Oris R, et al. Circulating erythropoietin levels after bone marrow transplantation: inappropriate response to anemia in allogeneic transplants. Blood 1991; 77:868–873.
49. Steegmann JL, Lopez J, Otero MJ, et al. Erythropoietin treatment in allogeneic BMT accelerates erythroid reconstitution: results of a prospective controlled randomized trial. Bone Marrow Transplant 1992; 10:541–546.
50. Brandt SJ, Peters WP, Atwater SK, et al. Effect of recombinant granulocyte-macrophage colony-stimulating factor on hematopoietic reconstitution after high-dose chemotherapy and autologous bone marrow transplantation. Blood 1988; 318:869–876.
51. Nemunaitis J, Rabinowe SN, Singer JW, et al. Recombinant granulocytes-macrophage colony-stimulating factor after autologous bone marrow transplantation for lymphoid cancer. N Engl J Med 1991; 324:1773–1778.
52. Sheridan WP, Wolf M, Lusk J, et al. Granulocyte colony-stimulating factor and neutrophil recovery after high-dose chemotherapy and autologous bone marrow transplantation. Lancet 1989; 2:891–895.
53. Taylor KMC, Jagannath S, Spitzer G, et al. Recombinant human granulocyte colony-stimulating factors hastens granulocyte recovery after high-dose chemotherapy and autologous bone marrow transplantation in Hodgkin's disease. J Clin Oncol 1989; 7:1791–1799.
54. Nemunaitis J, Meyers JD, Buckner CD, et al. Phase I trial of recombinant human macrophage colony-stimulating factor (rhM-CSF) in patients with invasive fungal infections. Blood 1991; 78:907–913.
55. Schuening FG, Storb R, Goehle S, et al. Recombinant human granulocyte colony-stimulating factor accelerated hematopoietic recovery after DLA-identical littermate marrow transplants in dogs. Blood 1990; 76:636–640.
56. Masaoka T, Takaku F, Kato S, et al. Recombinant human granulocyte colony-stimulating factor in allogeneic bone marrow transplantation. Exp Hematol 1989; 17:1047–1050.
57. Soiffier RJ, Murray C, Cochran K, et al. Clinical and immunological effects of

prolonged infusion of low-dose recombinant interleukin-2 after autologous and T-cell-depleted allogeneic bone marrow transplantation. Blood 1992; 79:517–526.
58. Favrot MC, Floret D, Negrier S, et al. Systemic interleukin-2 therapy in children with progressive neuroblastoma after high dose chemotherapy and bone marrow transplantation. Bone Marrow Transplant 1989; 4:499.
59. Blaise D, Olive D, Stoppa AM, et al. Hematologic and immunologic effects of the systemic administration of recombinant interleukin-2 after autologous bone marrow transplantation. Blood 1990; 76:1092–1099.
60. Higuchi CM, Thompson JA, Peterson FB. Toxicity of immunomodulatory effects of interleukin-2 after autologous bone marrow transplantation for hematologic malignancies. Blood 1991; 77:2561–2568.
61. Klingemann HG, Philipps GL. Immunotherapy after bone marrow transplantation. Bone Marrow Transplant 1991; 8:73–81.
62. Centers for Disease Control. Update and adult immunization: recommendations of the immunization Practices Advisory Committee. MMWR 1991; 40(RR-12):13–15.

22

Intensive Care

Jean-Paul Sculier
Institut Jules Bordet, Université Libre de Bruxelles, Brussels, Belgium

I. INTRODUCTION

Intensive care is becoming more and more important in the management of cancer patients, and major cancer hospitals have developed intensive therapy units not only for surgical patients but also for medical patients. However, there is limited information in the medical literature about intensive care in oncology, especially descriptions (1–3) of the types of patients admitted in such units.

II. DEFINITION OF THE MAIN INDICATIONS FOR INTENSIVE CARE IN ONCOLOGY

Admission of patients in an intensive care unit (ICU) is usually based on the following three principles (4). First, the patients must be "salvageable": patients whose chances of being cured or of going into remission are minimal should not be admitted to or should not stay in an intensive care unit (ICU). Second, the patient's "autonomy" must be respected: a patient who refuses intensive supportive therapy because he or she understands the potential poor prognosis of the underlying neoplastic disease should not be admitted to the ICU. Finally, because medical resources are limited, even in highly developed countries, "distribution justice" should be taken into account: patients with the best chances of benefiting from intensive therapy should be admitted in priority.

The assumption that patients with active malignant disease should not be admitted to an ICU often predominates in general hospitals and makes very difficult for oncologists a fruitful collaboration with intensive care specialists for the management of the critically ill cancer patients. This negative opinion is not supported by scientific data and results from a bias of many physicians, who refuse critical care to cancer patients although they are willing to provide it to patients with serious nonneoplastic diseases, such as advanced heart failure or liver cirrhosis, who do not have a better short- or long-term prognosis (5).

There are four main reasons to admit a cancer patient to the intensive care unit: (1) postoperative recovery (6,7) for advantages that are the same as those for any high-risk postoperative patient (availability of continuous hemodynamic monitoring, early identification of cardiovascular and respiratory disturbances, facilities for respiratory support, and constant skilled nursing care); (2) critical complications of the cancer disease and its treatment; these are various and can be very specific for oncology, and their management must always consider the presence of a severe chronic underlying disease; (3) intensive anticancer treatment administration and monitoring, useful in various situations, such as increased risk for treatment administration related to the patient's condition, administration of intensive chemotherapy requiring patient monitoring, treatment of unknown toxicity in phase I trials requiring optimal safety conditions of surveillance, and administration of treatment that frequently results in acute severe toxicity; and (4) acute disease (such as myocardial infarction or asthmatic crisis), possibly unrelated to the neoplastic disease or its treatment.

We focus in the present chapter only on the problems specific to oncological critical care; the reader can find more general information in textbooks devoted to critical care medicine.

III. PROGNOSIS OF THE CANCER PATIENT IN THE ICU AND MORTALITY

It has been reported that cancer patients who are admitted to an ICU have a higher mortality than those with other diseases: 55% (22 of 40) versus 17% (118 of 864) in the experience of a medical critical care unit (8) and 91% (20 of 22) versus 64% (37 of 58) in a series of patients with acute respiratory failure (9). These data must be considered cautiously, however, because of the small number of cancer patients in the series and because of the potential bias in referral of cancer patients to the ICU, the prejudice already discussed, making it possible that cancer patients have been at a more severe stage of the complication than noncancer patients. Moreover, in cancer centers, the ICU mortality is similar to that reported in general ICUs: 22% in a medical surgical unit (1) and 23 and 22% in two consecutive series in a medical critical care unit (2,3).

The combined impact of age and type of malignancy on ICU use and outcome was retrospectively studied at the Memorial Sloan-Kettering Cancer Center (10).

The care provided to all 1212 patients admitted over a 2 year period was reviewed with respect to use of total parenteral nutrition, mechanical ventilation, pulmonary artery catheterization, dialysis, and blood product transfusion. Also reviewed were mean length of stay in the ICU, primary diagnosis, outcome, and average daily severity of illness scores. Old patients (≥75 years) represented 14% of all intensive care unit patients, and younger (between 65 and 74 years) represented 28%. The ICU mortality of those two groups was significantly lower than that of the youngest (<65 years) patients (17, 27, and 30%, respectively). The use of nutritional support, pulmonary artery catheters, and dialysis was similar for all three groups, but older patients used less mechanical ventilation and needed fewer blood transfusions. The two older groups had more solid tumors, similar mean length of stay in the ICU, and lower average daily therapeutic intervention scoring system (TISS) scores compared with the younger cohort. Mortality was not significantly different between the three groups. This study suggests that age should not be considered a determining factor in the allocation of ICU beds to patients with malignancies; however, because of the retrospective nature of the investigation, patient selection bias cannot be excluded.

Scoring systems have been proposed to determine the prognosis in critically ill patients, such as APACHE II (acute physiological and chronic health evaluation), which consists of acute physiological measures, patient age, and chronic health status. A retrospective analysis of 451 ICU oncology admissions in a community hospital (11) was performed to determine the role of APACHE II as a predictor of outcome in critically ill cancer patients. A direct relationship between severity of physiological derangement and the risk of death was demonstrated. Patients with scores of 30 or greater had hospital mortality rates of 100% for postoperative and 92.6% for nonoperative conditions. In a small retrospective study performed in 52 patients with breast cancer at the M. D. Anderson Cancer Center (12), a higher APACHE II score was also found to be significantly associated with higher mortality. Other factors associated with a poorer outcome were the number of metastatic sites and the presence of respiratory failure. APACHE II has also been shown a successful prognostic score in granulocytopenic patients with hematological malignancies (13) in both ward and ICU settings. Of the 26 ICU patients, 6 survived with a mean APACHE II of 18 and 20 died with a mean score of 27.5. All 14 patients with APACHE II exceeding 27 on the day of maximal illness died.

More data are available for patients with hematological malignancies (14–19). In-ICU mortality ranged between 43 and 76%; 12–43% of the patients could be discharged alive from the hospital. Table 1 summarizes the underlying disease, the types of organ failure, the frequency of mechanical ventilation support, and the results. It should be noted that some of the reported series contain a few patients with aplastic anemia. The physiological score of the APACHE system

Table 1 Prognosis of Patients with Hematological Malignancies in ICU

	Schuster and Marion, 1985 (14)	Lloyd-Thomas et al., 1986 (15)	Butt et al., 1988 (16)	Torrecilla et al., 1988 (17)	Brunet et al., 1990 (18)	Yau et al., 1991 (19)
Number of patients	77	22	133[a]	25	260	92
Underlying disease						
Lymphoma	26	7	21	2	54	28
Leukemia	48	15	75	23	144	61
BMT[b]	—	—	—	25	?	—
Organ failure						
Respiratory	41	20	41	18	175	?
Renal	?	?	?	?	49	
Cardiac circulatory	15	?	36	12	106	
Bone marrow	?	15	?	8	123	
Cerebral	7	?	29	2	51	
Hepatic	?	?	?	2	?	
Septic shock, sepsis	14	?	28	12	235	?
Mechanical ventilation	52	17	67	16	111	?
Postoperative care, %	—	—	27	—	—	?
ICU mortality	59	55	48	76	43	65
Hospital mortality	80	82	?	88	57	77
Survivors, %	20	18	?	12	43	23

[a]Children
[b]Bone marrow transplant.

was found to be a significant predictor for short-term outcome (15,18). Brunet et al. reported (18) that survivors had a SAPS (simplified acute physiological score) calculated at admission of 11.2 ± 4.7; nonsurvivors had a SAPS of 16.1 ± 6.3. The number of organ failures was also found to be a significant predictor (15,17) for in-ICU mortality. However, there seems to be no relationship between the severity of the acute illness phase as assessed by the APACHE II and the duration of long-term survival after hospital discharge (19). The number of failed organs also appears to be not a good predictor of long-term prognosis (19).

Oncology pediatric patients admitted to the ICU have been evaluated for outcome (20). Severity of illness measured by the physiological stability index and quantity of care measured by the TISS were both predictors of in-ICU mortality, but the authors emphasized that these methods are not sufficient to decide withdrawal of support in individual cases. This point is also true of all the studies we have reported.

Causes of death were analyzed in a medical oncology ICU (21). Among 330 admissions, 55% were for a medical complication and 47 patients (28%) died in the ICU. Only 1 death was reported among the 150 patients admitted for monitoring during administration of an intensive or potentially toxic treatment. Autopsy was performed in 34 cases. The clinical diagnosis of the immediate cause of death was correct in only 41% of the cases, probably because uncomfortable investigations were often not performed when the survival estimation became very poor. Authors found an unexpected high frequency of pathological evidence of pulmonary edema (68% of the cases in which autopsies were done). No predictive factor for this phenomenon could be determined, but a tentative explanation was the existence of an enhanced immune response working on pulmonary capillaries sensitized by the metastatic process, making cancer patients more "fragile."

IV. CARDIOPULMONARY RESUSCITATION

Cardiopulmonary resuscitation (CPR) of the cancer patient is a controversial procedure, particularly if metastases are present. A review (22) of all the studies published from 1980 to 1989 dealing with survival after CPR showed that far fewer patients with cancer survived to discharge compared with patients with other diagnoses. Of nine studies of outcome after CPR, only two found patients with cancer who survived and were discharged (total of 7 patients of 243 resuscitated), and all these patients had localized disease; there were no survivors among patients with metastatic disease. These data, from which it could be recommended not to resuscitate metastatic cancer patients, are not supported by other experiences reported by intensive care specialists from cancer centers.

The effectiveness of cardiopulmonary resuscitation in medical and surgical cancer patients was evaluated at Memorial Sloan-Kettering Cancer Center in

New York (23). During a 3 year period, 750 patients suffered from cardiopulmonary arrest (1.53% of all admissions) and 114 were treated using resuscitative procedures because of their good general condition and the absence of a no-code status (not-for-resuscitation) order. Although 75 (66%) were successfully resuscitated, only 12 of these (16%), including patients with metastatic disease, survived long enough to be discharged from the hospital, after an average stay of 11.3 days in the ICU and with an overall mean survival after discharge of 223 days (median 150 days; range 3–350 days). A statistical analysis showed that performance status on admission was the single significant and independent factor that predicted the likelihood of being discharged alive before cardiopulmonary arrest and after successful CPR. Age, interval from diagnosis of cancer to the arrest, sex, underlying malignancy, and cause of arrest were not significant prognostic factors in the study.

A retrospective analysis of the patients admitted to a medical ICU was conducted at the Jules Bordet Institute in Brussels (24) to determine the effectiveness of and potential indications for CPR. During a 6 year period, cardiac arrest occurred in 49 nonsurgical cancer patients (Table 2). CPR was successful in 19 (39%), but only 5 (10%) were discharged alive from the hospital. CPR was successful in all 8 patients in whom cardiac arrest was the consequence of an acute cardiovascular drug toxicity, even if the cancer was metastatic and the purpose of the treatment not curative. Of these patients 5 could be discharged alive from the hospital. CPR was effective in only 25% of the patients in whom cardiac arrest was an ultimate complication of various problems, such as septic shock or respiratory failure complicating a neoplastic disease; none of these patients could be discharged alive from the hospital. The results of this study suggest that in cancer, as in other types of disease, CPR is mainly indicated when cardiac arrest is the consequence of an acute insult, as stated in the initial report in 1960 by Kouwenhoven et al. on closed-chest massage that was used with a high success rate to resuscitate victims of such insults as drowning, electrical shock, drug overdose, anesthetic accident, heart block, acute myocardial infarction, and surgery.

V. CRITICAL CARE OF PATIENTS WITH COMPLICATIONS CAUSED BY CANCER OR ITS TREATMENT

Complications of cancer and/or its treatment are multiple, as illustrated in Table 3 by data obtained during a 28 month period in the medical ICU at the Jules Bordet Institute in Brussels. These complications have specific characteristics related to their particular frequency (for example, coronary acute events are rare, but hypercalcemia is very frequent), to the occurrence of complications only seen in oncological patients (for example, acute tumoral lysis or leukostasis), and to

Table 2 Results of Cardiopulmonary Resuscitation According to Patients' Clinical Characteristics in a Medical Oncology ICU[a]

	Category			
	A	B	C	D
n	30	12	2	5
Mean age, years	50	56	57	52
Range	20–77	26–77	54–60	42–63
Type of tumour				
Solid	13	7	2	5
Locoregional	3	2	—	1
Metastatic	10	5	2	4
Hematological	17	5	—	—
Functional stage				
Diagnosis	2	—	—	—
Treatment for cure	14	4	—	—
Treatment for control	11	5	1	5
Candidate for palliative care	3	3	1	—
Cause of admission in ICU				
Cardiac arrest	5	5	2	2
Anticancer treatment	—	—	—	3
Medical complications	25	7	—	—
Cause of cardiac arrest				
Drug cardiovascular toxicity	—	2	1	5
Other causes	30	10	1	0

[a]Category A, patients who failed to respond to CPR; category B, patients who had a successful CPR but died later in the ICU; category C, patients who had a successful CPR but died in the hospital after discharge from the ICU; category D, patients who had a successful CPR and were discharged from the hospital.
Source: From Reference 24.

the presence of a severe underlying disease, that is, cancer. Management of the patient must take into account the underlying neoplastic disease making him or her more fragile because of the presence of immunosuppression, neutropenia, hemostatic disorders, metastatic process, and/or paraneoplastic syndromes. Treatment must integrate critical care support, anticancer therapy, and preventive or supportive care of toxic effects related to it. The toxicity of neoplastic drugs is often increased in critically ill cancer patients because of their poor general condition, a low performance status making them ineligible for regular cancer treatment protocols. In this section, we focus on points specific to intensive care,

Table 3 Types of Medical Complications Requiring Admission in a Medical ICU (Experience Obtained at the Jules Bordet Institute Between October 1989 and January 1992)

I.	Respiratory problems	58
	Upper failure	3
	Pleural effusion	10
	Pneumothorax	5
	Pneumonia	14
	Diffuse pneumonitis	8
	ARDS	4
	Various	14
II.	Cardiovascular problems	82
	Syncope	4
	Cardiac arrest	7
	Thromboembolic disease	15
	Arhythmias	26
	Cardiac failure	8
	Myocardial infarction	7
	Thoracic pain	4
	Pericardial disease	8
	Superior vena caval obstruction	3
III.	Renal and metabolic problems	58
	Acute renal failure	9
	Schwarz-Bartter syndrome	6
	Hypercalcemia	33
	Diabetes mellitus	2
	Tumoral lysis and/or leukostasis	8
IV.	Neurological problems	28
	Encephalopathies	5
	Infectious meningitis	1
	Neoplastic meningitis	1
	Intracranial hypertension	3
	Convulsions	8
	Paralysis and stroke	6
	Drug intoxication	4
V.	Digestive problems	13
	Acute abdomen	5
	Ascites	2
	Liver failure	3
	Digestive bleeding	3

VI. Infections, hematological, and shock problems	63
Fungal infections	2
Bacteremia	3
Febrile neutropenia	5
Septic shock	31
Hypovolemic shock	5
Other types of shock	2
Allergic reactions	2
Various types of bleeding	8
Coagulopathies	2
Severe anemia	3

other complications being discussed in more detail in other chapters in this book and in other books (25,26).

A. Respiratory Problems

Among all the potential complications of cancer or its treatment, respiratory problems are the only ones for which relatively consistent data are available from the point of view of critical care medicine, particularly concerning ARDS (adult respiratory distress syndrome), outcome of respiratory failure, and results of mechanical ventilation.

In addition to the usual causes, such as infections, ARDS can rarely be caused by specific complications of cancer. Initial presentation of cancer can be ARDS in solid tumors and lymphomas as well as in leukemia, as the result of a direct neoplastic infiltration of the lungs (27–29); it should be emphasized that this picture may be indistinguishable from ARDS from other causes. Anticancer treatment can also cause ARDS by various mechanisms; it can induce lung damage by tissue factors released from necrotic leukemic cells following chemotherapy (30). In the "retinoic acid syndrome," all-*trans*-retinoic acid induces a capillary leak syndrome, with fever, weight gain, and episodic hypotension and a respiratory failure syndrome caused by lung interstitial infiltration by maturing myeloid cells (31). Cytostatic drugs, cytokines, such as interleukin-2, and chest irradiation may also have a direct toxic effect on the lungs, leading to an increased alveolar capillary permeability and noncardiogenic pulmonary edema (32–34).

Neutropenia induced by chemotherapy does not protect the patients against ARDS (35); the frequency of neutropenia in bacteremic patients who had ARDS was compared with that in a control group who had bacteremia alone (36); 3 of 18 patients in the ARDS group were neutropenic, as opposed to 1 of 18 in the control group. Histological examination of the lungs from 2 of these patients with ARDS and neutropenia demonstrated the absence of neutrophils. A frequent cause of ARDS in febrile neutropenic patients treated it appropriate standard empirical antibiotic therapy is septicemia caused by streptococcal species, such as *Streptococcus mitis* (37).

Respiratory distress can also be caused by obstruction of the major airways by tumors involving the tracheobronchial tree. Because conventional treatment, such as radiation therapy and chemotherapy, is often too slow to reopen the airway, endoscopic neodymium:yttrium-aluminum-garnet (Nd:YAG) laser therapy should be used without delay and may allow very rapid relief of dyspnea (38). Another life-threatening emergency is massive hemoptysis, for which the etiology must be rapidly identified to provide appropriate treatment, such as surgery, endobronchial laser therapy, or bronchial artery embolization (39).

Table 4 summarizes the data available on the outcome of cancer patients with respiratory failure (14,15,17,18,40–44). All the studies except that by Snow et al. (40) were performed in patients with hematological malignancies or bone marrow transplantation. The vast majority of the patients (85–100%) were treated with mechanical ventilation. The causes of respiratory failure were often not explained, and the classifications used were heterogeneous, preventing the reader from achieving a good understanding of the frequency of the various complications requiring ventilation support. The in-ICU mortality ranged between 60 and 82%, with a rate of discharge from the hospital between 4 and 20%. The only study including patients with solid tumors (40) showed that patients with breast cancer treated by mechanical ventilation have a better survival than those with hematological or other solid malignancies. However, no multivariate analysis was made to confirm this observation. In the study performed in Seattle in 348 patients with respiratory failure complicating bone marrow transplantation and requiring artificial ventilation (44), 21% (72) were extubated and 4% (15) were discharged from the hospital, 10 (3%) surviving 6 months after transplantation. All the survivors were physically functional. Older age, active malignancy at the time of transplantation and donor-recipient marrow HLA nonidentity were found to be risk factors for subsequent respiratory failure in this population of 1482 patients, of whom 23% required mechanical ventilation.

B. Cardiovascular Problems

As shown in Table 3, the main cardiovascular problems requiring intensive care in cancer patients are arrhythmias and thromboembolic complications. As for other problems, such as myocardial infarction or cardiac failure, the treatment is basically the same as in nonneoplastic diseases. There is no study to support a more specific approach for cancer patients.

Intensive care specialists should be aware of the potential cardiotoxicity of a

Table 4 Outcome for Cancer Patients with Respiratory Failure[a]

	Snow et al. (40)	Schuster and Marion (14)	Estopa et al. (41)	Lloyd-Thomas et al. (15)	Torrecilla et al. (17)	Peters et al. (42)	Denardo et al. (43)	Brunet et al. (18)	Crawford and Petersen (44)
Number of patients	180	52	30	20	18	116	50	111	348
Patient selection	No	Hematological	Hematological	Hematological	BMT	Hematological	BMT	Hematological	BMT
Mechanical ventilation, %	100	100	87	87	89	100	88	100	100
Cause of respiratory failure, %									
ARDS	15			80					
Pneumonia	56		40	15					
Bleeding	16		13						
Postoperative	19								
Pleural effusion	29					16	18		
Pulmonary infiltrates						63	80		
Cardiorespiratory arrest						12			
In-ICU mortality, %	74	77	80	60	83		82	85	79
Hospital discharged, %		8	7	20		18	18	13	4
6 Months survival, %	7		7					79	66
Survivors MST						12 months	124 days		

[a]BMT, bone marrow transplantation; MST, median survival time.

series of anticancer drugs, including anthracyclines (doxorubicin), high-dose cyclophosphamide, amsacrine, fluorouracil, taxol, and interleukin-2 (45). High doses of cyclophosphamide, usually in the context of bone marrow transplantation, can induce particularly severe cardiac toxicity: myocardial necrosis with fatal failure, pericardial effusions with or without tamponade, life-threatening arhythmias, or conduction blocks. Total doses of more than 200 mg/kg should not be administered (46). This toxicity appears to be directly related to the dose expressed by body square meters (47) and to drug pharmacokinetics (48). Another commonly used cytostatic agent, fluorouracil, can cause various and frequent cardiac side effects: angina, supraventricular or ventricular tachycardia, congestive heart failure, reversible cardiomyopathy, myocardial infarction, and sudden death (49). The toxicity probably results from a direct toxic effect of the drug on the myocardial cell (50). Besides the hemodynamic consequences of the capillary leak syndrome, interleukin-2 can induce fatal noninfectious myocarditis or acute myocardial infarction (51).

Cardiac tamponade is a common cause of shock in the cancer patient. The diagnosis of pericardial effusion is performed by echography. Treatment requires drainage; intrapericardial sclerosis with tetracycline can avoid relapse (52). The superior vena caval obstruction syndrome, although spectacular in some cases, should no longer be considered an emergency for radiotherapy. With a careful surveillance, a work-up enabling a pathological diagnosis can be performed (53).

C. Renal and Metabolic Problems

Hypercalcemia is the most frequent metabolic complication of cancer (Table 3). Management has recently changed because of progress in therapy; rehydration and biphosphonates are today the standard treatment (54). Pamidronate (APD) seems the most effective biphosphonate today available (55). It is unclear, however, whether hypercalcemia is a direct cause of death in cancer patients or simply a marker of advanced disease. A retrospective study (56) of 126 consecutive patients with cancer-associated hypercalcemia attempted to answer this question. Despite effective antihypercalcemia treatment (mainly biphosphonates) that resulted in a very significant decrease in serum calcium levels and improvement in all symptoms (including renal and central nervous system manifestations) except pain, the overall median survival was very poor (30 days). Follow-up measurement of serum calcium was done in 40 patients until death; recurrent or persistent hypercalcemia was present in 11 and contributed to death in 7. These data suggest that hyperalcemia is a marker of advanced cancer rather than the actual cause of death in many cases. Moreover, the availability of specific anticancer treatment was an important prognostic indicator for survival. The median survival was 135 days for the 26 patients who were so treated, compared with 30 days in the remainder. From the critical care point of view, patients with severe hypercalcemia should probably not be admitted to an ICU if specific cancer therapy is not available.

Other metabolic emergencies include hyponatremia (often in the context of inappropriate secretion of antidiuretic hormone), ectopic adrenocorticotropic syndrome, adrenal failure, hypoglycemia, lactic acidosis, and tumoral lysis syndrome (57). Lactic acidosis may be a rare complication of extensive cancer, particularly metastatic hepatic lesions. Chemotherapy against the neoplastic disease is the only effective treatment of this type of lactic acidosis (58).

Tumor lysis syndrome is rarely spontaneous but it is often induced by chemotherapy. This clinical picture is composed of various metabolic derangements: hyperkalemia, hyperuricemia, and hyperphosphatemia resulting from massive cell lysis and a potential cause of severe renal failure. The release of several active enzymes by the lysed cells can induce lung damage and ARDS (59).

Renal failure can be caused in cancer patients by various etiologies: tumor invasion of the kidney or urinary tract (ureteral obstruction); the acute tumor lysis syndrome; nephrotoxic drugs, including high-dose methotrexate, cisplatin, and mitomycin; hypercalcemia; multiple myeloma; infections; and renal hypoperfusion. These aspects are discussed in Chapter 14.

D. Neurological Problems

Neurological complications are a less frequent source of admission of cancer patients to the ICU. This does not mean that neurological emergencies are rare, but they are usually not life threatening, such as epidural carcinomatosis. Encephalopathies, convulsions, and some paralytic presentations are the principal types of problems referred in our experience to intensive care. It should be noted that drug intoxication occurs rarely in the cancer patient population of a cancer hospital and is usually iatrogenic.

E. Digestive Problems

Digestive complications of cancer patients are not frequent in a medical ICU because many of them are treated in surgical ICUs. Acute abdomen, particularly in neutropenic patients, is a difficult problem. A retrospective analysis of 50 neutropenic patients (mainly with hematological malignancies) with abdominal pain (60) revealed that abdominal distension was the only sign associated with mortality. The study failed to find pivotal signs or symptoms for the decision for or against surgical intervention. Overall, 60% of the patients in this series died, confirming the results of prior reports. Care of patients with neutropenic enterocolitis (also called typhlitis) should be individualized (61): nonsurgical management with bowel rest, decompression, nutritional support, and broad-spectrum antibiotics is recommended initially. Surgery is indicated for those with perforation or those whose condition deteriorated clinically during close, frequent observation.

Hepatic venoocclusive disease (VOD) is a major complication of intensive therapy associated with bone marrow transplantation, with a potential high risk of death by liver insufficiency (62). Management of established VOD is essentially symptomatic, including careful monitoring of electrolyte balance.

F. Infectious, Hematological, and Shock Problems

Because of the effects of the neoplastic disease and/or its treatment, coagulation disorders, neutropenia, and immunosuppression are often present in the same patient, predisposing him or her to develop infections and septic or hypovolemic (by bleeding) shocks. As shown in Table 3 (and as expected), septic shock is a main cause of admission of cancer patients to the ICU. A retrospective analysis of causes of death in febrile granulocytopenic cancer patients receiving empirical antibiotic therapy (63) showed that infection was the main cause of death, two-thirds of the cases presenting with septic shock, followed by bleeding complications (diffuse or cerebromeningeal hemorrhage). Management of cancer patients with septic shock and other types of shock is standard, without critical care-specific measures, the choice of antibiotics being discussed in Chapter 1.

Allergic reactions to cytotoxic drugs are multiple and can be seen with many agents (64,65). Type I hypersensitivity reactions predominate. The drugs with the highest risk of such complications are L-asparaginase and taxol, followed by teniposide and etoposide, cisplatin and its analogs, and cytarabine. The exact mechanism by which a cytostatic drug induces an allergic reaction has rarely been investigated, and it is probable that ancillary drugs and excipients sometimes play an important role. When anaphylactic reactions are frequent, prophylaxis by antihistamines and corticosteroids may be administered and patients monitored in the ICU. In any case, these drugs should not be given in the absence of a physician.

VI. INTENSIVE CARE FOR ANTICANCER TREATMENT ADMINISTRATION AND SURVEILLANCE

Anticancer treatment administration and surveillance is a new activity for intensive care medicine resulting from the progress made by medical oncology requiring sophisticated support for some types of new therapies (2,3). Data about this indication are still very limited in the literature, and we illustrate this section by the experience we have acquired in our own ICU at the Jules Bordet Institute in Brussels. Today, this activity represents about 65% of the patient admissions in this unit: between October 1989 and January 1992, 667 patients were admitted for anticancer treatment but 302 were referred for serious medical complications, described in Table 3. As shown in Table 5, the types of indications for treatment administration and/or monitoring can be divided in four groups that we discuss separately.

A. Risk for Treatment Administration Related to the Patient's Condition

Anticancer treatment administration can be a special risk in some patients because their condition or the clinical situation. The problems to be managed are multiple, and when suspected, patients can be admitted to the ICU for the treatment surveillance. A severe risk of acute toxicity can be expected from drug interactions and from interactions between the patient and the treatment because of a patient's poor general condition or more specific problems, such as comorbidity or prior reactions to therapy. It should be noted that an anticancer treatment should be administered in such a patient only if the potential benefit to the patient is high and if he or she has given appropriate informed consent.

B. Administration of Intensive Chemotherapy Requiring Patient Monitoring

Intensive or high-dose chemotherapy, often performed in the context of bone marrow transplantation, can induce various severe nonhematological toxicities (66). Although with standard dose chemotherapy limiting toxicity is usually hematological (leukopenia and/or thrombopenia), in high-dose chemotherapy

Table 5 Types of Indications for Intensive Anticancer Treatment Administration and/or Monitoring (Experience Obtained at the Jules Bordet Institute Between October 1989 and January 1992)

Indication	Number of admissions
Risk for treatment administration related to the patient's condition	29
Administration of intensive chemotherapy requiring patient monitoring	83
Treatment of unknown toxicity in phase I trial requiring optimal safety conditions of surveillance	211
Administration of treatment frequently resulting in acute severe toxicity	344
Total	667

limiting toxicity can be multiple according to the drugs used: gastrointestinal (mucositis and diarrhea), cardiac (arhythmias, necrosis, and tamponade), pulmonary (fibrosis), neurological (encephalopathy, coma, and brain necrosis), renal (renal failure), urothelial (hemorrhagic cystitis), or hepatic (acute hepatitis and fibrosis).

The rigorous schedules for administering chemotherapy, infusion of large volumes of fluid, and management of the side effects may require close monitoring of the patient as optimally provided in an ICU. Two drugs can be particularly dangerous when given at high doses without appropriate expertise: methotrexate (67) and cyclophosphamide (46). The first can induce particularly severe renal failure and the second cardiac necrosis and arhythmias.

C. Treatment of Unknown Toxicity in Phase I Trials Requiring Optimal Safety Conditions of Surveillance

New phase I trials of anticancer drugs must be performed directly in patients with cancer because of their important carcinogenic properties. These drugs are usually given in patients who have good performance status and no other major disease but in whom cancer cannot be treated with effective curative or palliative antineoplastic treatment. If a severe toxic effect occurs, patients must be treated by adequate supportive care, including critical care techniques such as resuscitation. It is thus recommended that these new drugs be administered in optimal safety conditions like those present in ICUs. An example of the life-threatening complications that might occur during phase I trials is given by the potentiation of chemotherapy by drugs inhibiting the multiple-drug resistance expression in cancer cells, such as high-dose veraparamil, which has induced acute cardiac side effects, including heart block, that are appropriately managed by the ICU team (68).

D. Administration of Frequent Treatment Resulting in Acute Severe Toxicity

Administration of some anticancer treatments is regularly associated with a high risk of acute complications because of the immediate toxicity of the drug or the complexity of the care to be provided. It should thus preferably be managed in ICUs. Recent developments in medical oncology have produced two applications for this indication: chemotherapy with taxol and adoptive immunotherapy with interleukin-2 (IL-2).

Taxol is a new major antineoplastic agent derived from the bark of the western yew; it is able to induce irreversible aggregation of microtubules. It is associated with major toxic effects, mainly acute hypersensitivity reactions (69) requiring prophylactic administration of corticosteroids and antihistamines and cardiac arhythmias and conduction blocks (70), that seem particularly major when the drug is combined with cisplatin. It has been recommended that cardiac monitoring of the patients be performed during taxol infusions (45).

Interleukin-2 is the cytokine that has allowed a renewal of immunotherapy and is now part of the standard management of renal carcinoma. However, IL-2 is associated with complex and potentially severe toxicity, particularly when given at high doses (71). These side effects are mainly related to the occurrence of a capillary leak syndrome with a hemodynamic pattern similar to septic shock (72) that can evolve to a multiple organ failure syndrome (33). Patients treated by high-dose IL-2 require appropriate cardiac rate and rhythm, blood pressure, urinary output, body weight, respiratory rate, temperature, and consciousness and mental status surveillance. Treatment of complications may require critical care techniques, including vasopressors and mechanical ventilation.

VII. CRITICAL CARE TECHNIQUES IN CANCER PATIENTS

Critical care techniques performed in cancer patients are basically the same as in noncancer patients. We review some specific data and considerations that can be useful in the management of critically ill oncological patients.

A. Central Venous Catheters

Cancer patients, mainly those treated by chemotherapy, often have permanent central venous catheters. Totally implantable injection ports (73) are more and more used, and they appear to be safer than classic external indwelling catheters (74). Intensive care specialists should be aware of two important notions: these catheters cannot be used for correctly measuring central venous pressure, and in infection, the policy is to treat the patient through the catheter to try to maintain patency (in this situation, antibiotics should be administered through the suspect lumen). If the catheter is obstructed by a thrombus, low-dose urokinase can be used to restore its function (75). Streptokinase should not be used repetitively to avoid potential allergic reactions. Note also that the prolonged presence of a central venous catheter predisposes to the development of superior vena caval syndrome, a new iatrogenic entity (76).

Interleukin-2 induces defects in neutrophil chemotaxis, facilitating the occurrence of staphylococcal infections, with catheters as a common source. A randomized trial performed in 92 patients showed a significant reduction in triple-lumen catheter-related sepsis when prophylactic antibiotics were administered (77).

B. Invasive Monitoring and Right Cardiac Catherization

The risks of invasive procedures are likely to be high in cancer patients, particularly when they have neutropenia and/or thrombopenia. With appropriate management, including administration of platelets and fresh frozen plasma, however, these techniques can be performed without major complications (15) and can be helpful. In a series (18) of 54 patients with septic shock requiring right heart catheterization to adjust a treatment combining inotropic or vasoactive agents and volume expansion, 15 were discharged from the ICU (mortality 73%) and 4 were still alive 1 year later.

Intensive care specialists should be aware that a pulmonary artery catheter can be useful to obtain blood to perform pulmonary microvascular cytology and to contribute to the diagnosis of lymphangitis carcinomatosa (78).

C. Renal Replacement Therapy

Renal replacement therapy includes peritoneal dialysis, hemodialysis, and hemofiltration. In a series of 31 patients with hematological malignancy and acute renal failure (79), a combination of hemofiltration and hemodialysis was applied to 22 patients and recovery of renal function occurred in 6. In another study (18), hemodialysis was performed in 34 patients also with hematological malignancies for sepsis-related anuria (22 cases) or acute hydroelectrolytic disease (12 cases). Of these patients 11 were discharged from the ICU (mortality 67%) and 5 were still alive 1 year later. These results show that renal replacement therapy can be effective in critically ill cancer patients. For the cancer-associated hemolytic-uremic syndrome, immunoperfusion over staphylococcal A column appears to be the most successful treatment (80).

D. Respiratory Assistance and Mechanical Ventilation

In patients requiring respiratory assistance, continuous positive airway pressure (CPAP) by face mask can be a good means, in sufficiently compliant patients, of avoiding endotracheal intubation, particularly when respiratory failure is caused by diffuse pulmonary infiltrates, as in *Pneumocystis carinii* pneumonia (81,82). If tracheal intubation is necessary, the oral route is more advisable than the nasal to prevent infection of nasal sinuses.

If thrombocytopenia is associated with neutropenia, some authors recommend early tracheostomy to reduce the risk of occurrence of bleeding gums, nasal bleeding, and fungal infections of the oropharynx (83). Tracheostomy using electrocautery and careful technique can be performed without major complications in these patients. It also has the advantage of allowing easier tracheal aspirations, better oropharyngeal care, and more facile weaning (84).

The results of treatment of respiratory failure by mechanical failure have been reported in adult patients with solid tumors (40,85,86) and hematological malignancies (14,15,17,18,41–44) and in children (16,20). They are summarized in Table 6: survival rates (with extubation and ICU discharge) range between 0 and 35%. Some authors have reported that mechanical ventilation for more than

Table 6 Results Obtained in Cancer Patients with Respiratory Failure Treated by Mechanical Ventilation

Type of cancer	Number of patients	Survivors (%)	Reference
Any	180	26	Snow et al. (40)
Lung cancer	46	15	Ewer et al. (85)
Hematological malignancy	52	23	Schuster and Marion (14)
Hematological malignancy	26	7	Estopa et al. (41)
Hematological malignancy	17	35	Lloyd-Thomas et al. (15)
Hematological malignancy	16	6	Torrecilla et al. (17)
Hematological malignancy	116	18	Peters et al. (42)
BTM[a]	40	2.5	Denardo et al. (43)
Hematological malignancy	111	15	Bruent et al. (18)
BMT	348	21	Crawford and Petersen (44)
Children	15	0	Butt et al. (16)
Children	27	26	Sivan et al. (20)

[a]Bone marrow transplant.

5–7 days was associated with uniformly fatal prognosis (14,15,17), but this statement is not supported by the results of larger series (42,18) showing that long-term survival can be obtained after prolonged survival.

E. Multiple Life Support Techniques

The need for multiple life support techniques is associated with poor prognosis, as described by Brunet et al. (18). In their study, 62 patients had multiple life support techniques. Very few of those were discharged from the ICU: 4 of 31 requiring both mechanical ventilation and hemodynamic monitoring of shock, 1 of 8 requiring both ventilation and hemodialysis, and 1 of 12 requiring all three techniques.

VIII. CONSIDERATIONS OF ICU ORGANIZATION IN THE CONTEXT OF ONCOLOGY

The managememt of cancer patients may require adaptation in the ICU organization at the level of the facilities as well as the different components of the team. We give some specific recommendations in this section, the general management of intensive care being the subject of appropriate reviews (86).

The admission of neutropenic and immunosuppressed patients and of patients referred for anticancer treatment administration and surveillance impose adaptations of the ICU design. The first type of patient should be managed in single rooms with, particularly for autologous and allogeneic bone marrow transplant neutropenic recipients, a system for air handling, such as high-pressure, filtered air or laminar airflow (87). We believe that it is difficult not to provide these facilities to severely compromised patients, although they have not been validated in the ICU. The second type of patient requires critical care techniques in case of complications. Because they have, at admission and usually during the duration of their stay in the ICU, a very good performance status compatible with ambulatory activities, optimal privacy should be delivered in the room without compromising intensive surveillance. Figure 1 shows the ICU that we have designed at the Jules Bordet Institute in Brussels for medical cancer patients. The unit contains seven beds in five single rooms and one double-bed room. Protective isolation in one of the single rooms is possible for critical neutropenic patients, the bed being under a vertical laminar airflow hood. Each room has its own toilet. Cardiac monitoring is applied to each patient, and cardiac rhythms are centrally controlled at the nursing station by an arhythmia detector. Shades in the doors and walls allow a direct view of the patient if necessary. Critical care facilities, such as artificial ventilation and hemodynamic monitoring, are applicable at each bed level. Blood pressure can be measured by a noninvasive

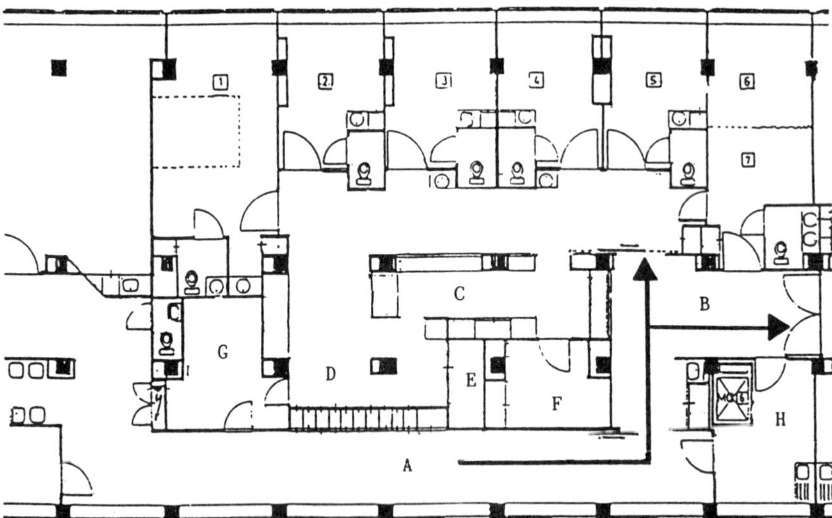

Figure 1 Plan of the ICU for medical cancer patients at Jules Bordet Institute in Brussels. A-hall; B-SAS; C-nurses' station; D-preparation place; E-pharmacy; F-material local; G-physician office; H-utility local; 1-laminar airflow room; 2–5-single-bed room; 6–7 double-bed room.

system incorporated in each monitor at the bedside. Supply is provided by a double-locker system, allowing reduction of personnel circulation into the unit. An air-conditioning system covers the whole ICU.

The ICU team should include a full-time medical director, attending physicians, a fulltime nursing director, and a nursing staff. The nurse-patient ratio should range between 1:1 and 1:3, depending on acuity, and 24 h in-house coverage is required by a physician, who may call, when necessary, the ICU director or other subspecialists, such as cardiologists or chest physicians. It is important that physicians and nurses have training in both critical care medicine and in oncology to provide to cancer patients optimally integrated care. As reported for the verapamil trial discussed earlier (88), critical care nurses may be uneasy about treating cancer patients in therapeutic protocols. In such a case, optimal nursing care can be provided if an appropriate educational program is designed. The redaction of adapted protocols for the internal use of the ICU staff appears to be successful. Those protocols should give a summary of the trial, the criteria of patient eligibility, the study plan, nursing considerations, a standard prescription plan, specific care descriptions, and management of the principal complications (89). It should be noted that if chemotherapy must be prepared in the ICU, special equipment is necessary to reduce the exposure of the nurses to potentially carcinogenic drugs.

IX. ETHICAL CONSIDERATIONS

The decision for admission of a cancer patient into an ICU depends not only on the prognosis of the complication requiring intensive care support but also and mainly on the prognosis of the underlying neoplastic disease function of the effective therapeutic possibilities, and on the role of an experimental therapy in the life-threatening complication requiring critical care. In the last situation, the critical care oncologist is confronted with a very difficult problem: he or she must provide intensive care to a patient with an initial good health status but with an incurable cancer who has received an investigational therapy resulting in a severe complication (4). This patient should receive appropriate treatment to avoid iatrogenic consequences, including toxic death, but his or her autonomy must be respected: the patient's agreement is necessary for performing critical care techniques.

To avoid unnecessary invasive resuscitation procedures, Australian authors (90) have proposed a staging system of the neoplastic disease to determine when resuscitation is appropriate in a given case: stage 1, or diagnosis, when the patient's disease is assessed and appropriate treatment goal and treatment are negotiated; stage 2, or potential cure, when the goal of treatment is cure with the risks of associated morbidity; stage 3, when disease is controllable but not curable, when a temporary remission that will significantly prolong life may be achievable; stage 4, when specific treatment aimed at cure or control has failed (this is the most critical point in the disease for many cancer patients); and stage 5, or palliative management. In these two latter stages, a not-for-resuscitation order should be given because the chances that a patient will benefit from cardiopulmonary resuscitation are minimal in such very rarely reversible situations, irrespective of the acute precipitating event, and cardiac arrest is usually the end result of generalized multisystem failure. For the same reasons, invasive life support methods, such as mechanical ventilation or hemodialysis, should not be performed, except in experimental therapy, as already mentioned.

If patient's salvageability and autonomy must be taken into account, distributive justice must also be considered because our resources are limited in terms of ICU bed availability. A difficult task for many physicians with these patients is to be free of prejudice. In a survey of physicians of different subspecialities with carefully designed clinical vignettes of patients with different chronic medical illnesses (91), decisions for resuscitation were less frequent for cancer vignettes than for vignettes of other chronic medical illnesses before and after mortality information was given. However, when looking at attitudes according to medical subspecialities, this difference was present in cardiologists, pulmonologists, and neurologists but not in hematologists or oncologists. Another study (5) performed in a general hospital showed that 47% of lung cancer patients had "do not resuscitate" orders compared with only 16% of those with cirrhosis and 4% of those with heart failure. In-hospital mortality was 14, 18, and 3%, respectively, 6 month survival estimate 54, 64, and 47%, and 5 year survival estimate 6.6, 21.9, and 11.1%. None of these differences were statistically significant! Physician judgment should be based on more scientific data, allowing appropriate decisions in a precise context.

X. PERSPECTIVES

Critical care medicine and oncology are at the beginning of a collaboration that should become more and more important in the future. Critical care medicine will more often be required to administer anticancer treatment and to support the complications. As in infectious diseases, therapy against cancer has as an objective the destruction of the pathological process with the intention to cure, even if this is not the case today for every patient. Treatment goals are thus not palliative as is the case for many degenerative diseases, such as cardiovascular disease or chronic obstructive pulmonary disease, in which the restoration of a normal healthy situation is practically impossible; they are etiological, and with the development of new therapies, more cancer patients will have the opportunity to receive curative treatment, a major reason to be actively managed in life-threatening situations. Distributive justice requires that these patients be admitted with a higher priority than those with incurable chronic degenerative diseases.

There is another reason for both medical disciplines to work together. In invasive cancer, as in multiple organ system failure (MOSF), a cascade of immune cells and cytokines is activated, in a more chronic way in the first disease. In fact, cancer induces during its development a kind of chronic MOSF syndrome. In both critical care medicine and oncology, a lot of research is performed to understand this immune cascade and to find tools to control its consequences. A better collaboration between researchers in both fields at the clinical as well at the laboratory levels would probably be beneficial to the progress of medicine.

SELECTED READING

Brunet F, Lanore JJ, Dhainaut JF, et al. Is intensive care justified for patients with haematological malignancies? Intensive Care Med 1990; 16:291–297. The authors reviewed their 4 year experience in the intensive care unit management of hematological malignancies. Among adults admitted, the overall mortality rates in the intensive care unit and in the hospital were 43 and 57%, respectively. Among survivors, 44% (35 patients) were still alive 1 year after admission. The impact of the life support techniques, such as hemodialysis or mechanical ventilation, was studied, and the authors conclude that such supportive therapies should be initiated for this type of patient.

Chevrolet JC, Jolliet P. An ethical look at intensive care for patients with malignancies. Eur J Cancer 1991; 27:210–212. Reflection on the intersections between oncology and intensive care. The first part is a review of the basic principles of patient admission to the intensive care unit: salvageability, respect of patient autonomy, and distributive justice. In the second part, the authors plead that a cancer patient should be considered as any other patient, because major progress has been made in both supportive and clinical cancer treatment.

Crawford SW, Petersen FB. Long-term survival from respiratory failure after marrow transplantation for malignancy. Am Rev Respir Dis 1992; 145:510–514. This study, performed at the Fred Hutchinson Cancer Research Center in Seattle, aimed to determine the effectiveness of assisted mechanical ventilation in patients with respiratory failure after marrow transplantation. Of 348 (23%) who required mechanical ventilation, 21% (72) were extubated and 4% (15) were discharged from the hospital with, 10 (3%) surviving 6 months after transplantation. All these survivors were physically functional. Older age, active malignancy at time of transplantation, and donor-recipient marrow HLA nonidentity were risk factors for subsequent respiratory failure.

Groeger JS. Critical Care of the Cancer Patient, 2nd ed. St. Louis: Mosby Year Book, The only textbook on critical care of cancer patient available in 1992. It reflects the practice at the Memorial Sloan-Kettering Cancer Center in New York. Chapters are mainly devoted to oncological emergencies. Some invasive procedures are discussed in the context of a neoplastic disease, as well as perioperative care, pain control, and sedation.

Sculier JP, Markiewicz E. Cardiopulmonary resuscitation in medical cancer patients: the experience of a medical intensive care unit of a cancer centre. Support Care Cancer 1993; 1:135–138. This retrospective study aimed to determine the effectiveness and potential indications of cardiopulmonary resuscitation (CPR) in medical cancer patients. During a 6 year period, cardiac arrest occurred in 49 cancer patients. CPR was successful in 19 (39%), but only 5 (10%) were discharged alive from the hospital. CPR was successful in all 8 patients in whom cardiac arrest was the consequence of an acute cardiovascular drug toxicity, even if the cancer was metastatic and the purpose of treatment not curative. It was effective in only 25% of those in whom cardiac arrest was an ultimate complication of various problems, such as septic shock or respiratory failure, complicating the neoplastic disease. The results suggest that in cancer, as in other types of disease, CPR is mainly indicated when cardiac arrest is the consequence of an acute insult.

REFERENCES

1. Turnbell A, Goldiner P, Silverman D, Howland W. The role of an intensive care unit in a cancer center. Cancer 1976; 37:82–84.
2. Sculier JP, Ries F, Verboven N, Coune A, Klastersky J. Role of intensive care unit in a medical oncology department. Eur J Cancer Clin Oncol 1988; 24:513–517.
3. Sculier JP, Markiewicz E. Medical cancer patients and intensive care. Anticancer Res 1991; 11:2171–2174.
4. Chevrolet JC, Jolliet P. An ethical look at intensive care for patients with malignancies. Eur J Cancer 1991; 27:210–212.
5. Wachter RM, Luce JM, Hearst N, Lo B. Decisions about resuscitation: inequities among patients with different diseases but similar prognoses. Ann Intern Med 1989; 111:525–532.
6. Filshie J, Robbie DS. Anaesthesia and Malignant Disease. London; Edward Arnold, 1989.
7. Howland WS, Rooney SM, Goldiner PL. Manual of Anesthesia in Cancer Patients. New York: Churchill Livingstone, 1986.
8. Hauser M, Tabak J, Baier H. Survival of patients with cancer in a medical critical care unit. Arch Intern Med 1982; 142:527–529.
9. Cox SC, Norwood SH, Duncan CA. Acute respiratory failure: mortality associated with underlying disease. Crit Care Med 1985; 13:1005–1008.
10. Chalfin DB, Carlon GC. Age and utilization of intensive care unit resources of critically ill cancer patients. Crit Care Med 1990; 18:694–698.
11. Abbott RR, Setter M, Chan S, Choi K. APACHE II: prediction of outcome of 451 ICU oncology admissions in a community hospital. Ann Oncol 1991; 2:571–574.
12. Headley J, Theriault R, Smith TL. Independent validation of APACHE II severity of illness score for predicting mortality in patients with breast cancer admitted to the intensive care unit. Cancer 1992; 70:497–503.
13. Johnson MH, Gordon PW, Fitzgerald FT. Stratification of prognosis in

granulocytopenic patients with hematologic malignancies using the APACHE-II severity of illness score. Crit Care Med 1986; 14:693–697.
14. Schuster DP, Marion JM. Precedents for meaningful recovery during treatment in a medical intensive care unit. Outcome in patients with hematologic malignancy. Am J Med 1983; 75:402–408.
15. Lloyd-Thomas AR, Dhaliwal HS, Lister TA, Hinds CJ. Intensive therapy for life-threatening medical complications of haematological malignancy. Intensive Care Med 1986; 12:317–324.
16. Butt W, Barker G, Walker C, Gillis J, Kilham H, Stevens M. Outcome of children with hematologic malignancy who are admitted to an intensive care unit. Crit Care Med 1988; 16:761–764.
17. Torrecilla C, Cortès JL, Chamorro C, Rubio JJ, Galdos P, Dominguez De Villota E. Prognostic assessment of the acute complications of bone marrow transplantation requiring intensive therapy. Intensive Care Med 1988; 14:393–398.
18. Brunet E, Lanore JJ, Dhainaut JF, et al. Is intensive care justified for patients with haematological malignancies? Intensive Care Med 1990; 16:291–297.
19. Yau E, Rohatiner AZS, Lister TA, Hinds CJ. Long term prognosis and quality of life following intensive care for life-threatening complications of haematological malignancy. Br J Cancer 1991; 64:938–942.
20. Sivan Y, Schwartz PH, Schonfeld T, Cohen IJ, Newth CJL. Outcome of oncology patients in the pediatric intensive care unit. Intensive Care Med 1991; 17:11–15.
21. Gerain J, Sculier JP, Malengreaux A, Rykaert C, Thémelin L. Causes of deaths in an oncologic intensive care unit: a clinical and pathological study of 34 patients. Eur J Cancer 1990; 26:377–381.
22. Faber-Langendoen K. Resuscitation of patients with metastatic cancer. Is transient benefit still futile? Arch Intern Med 1991; 151:235–239.
23. Vitelli CE, Cooper K, Rogatko A, Brennan MF. Cardiopulmonary resuscitation and the patient with cancer. J Clin Oncol 1991; 9:111–115.
24. Sculier JP, Markiewicz E. Cardiopulmonary resuscitation in medical cancer patients: the experience of a medical intensive care unit of a cancer centre. Support Care Cancer 1993; 1:135–138.
25. Dutcher JP, Wiernik PH. Handbook of Hematologic and Oncologic Emergencies. New York: Plenum Medical, 1987.
26. Groeger JS. Critical Care of the Cancer Patient, 2nd ed. St. Louis: Mosby Year Book, 1991.
27. McGowan MP, Pratter MR, Nash G. Primary testicular choriocarcinoma with pulmonary metastases presenting as ARDS. Chest 1990; 97:1258–1259.
28. Ravid M, Shapira J, Lang R, David R. Acute respiratory distress syndrome: a presenting syndrome of malignant lymphoma. JAMA 1979; 241:2191–2192.
29. Vernant JP, Brun B, Mannoni P, Dreyfus B. Respiratory distress of hyperleukocytic granulocytic leukemias. Cancer 1979; 44:264–268.
30. Hewlett RI, Wilson AF. Adult respiratory distress syndrome (ARDS) following aggressive management of extensive acute lymphoblastic leukemia. Cancer 1977; 39:2422–2425.
31. Frankel SR, Eardley A, Lauwers G, Weiss M, Warrell RP Jr. The "retinoic acid syndrome" in acute promyelocytic leukemia. Ann Intern Med 1992; 117:292–296.

32. Haupt HM, Hutchins GM, Moore GW. Ara-C lung: noncardiogenic pulmonary edema complicating cytosine arabinoside therapy of leukemia. Am J Med 1981; 70:256–261.
33. Sculier JP, Bron D, Verboven N, Klastersky J. Multiple organ failure during interleukin-2 administration and LAK cells infusion. Intensive Care Med 1988; 14:666–667.
34. Fulkerson WJ, McLendon RE, Prosnitz LR. Adult respiratory distress syndrome after limited thoracic radiotherapy. Cancer 1986; 57:1941–1946.
35. Ognibene FP, Martin SE, Parker MM, et al. Adult respiratory distress syndrome in patients with severe neutropenia. N Engl J Med 1986; 315:547–551.
36. Laufe MD, Simon RH, Flint A, Keller JB. Adult respiratory distress syndrome in neutropenic patients. Am J Med 1986; 80:1022–1026.
37. Arning M, Gehrt A, Aul C, Runde V, Hadding U, Schneider W. Septicemia due to *Streptococcus mitis* in neutropenic patients with acute leukemia. Blut 1990; 61:364–368.
38. Dedhia HV, Le Roy N, Jain PR, Thompson AB, Withers A. Endoscopic laser therapy for respiratory distress due to obstructive airway tumors. Crit Care Med 1985; 13:464–467.
39. Spain RC, Wittlesey D. Respiratory emergencies in patients with cancer. Semin Oncol 1989; 16:471–489.
40. Snow RM, Miller WC, Rice DL, Ali MK. Respiratory failure in cancer patients. JAMA 1979; 241:2039–2042.
41. Estopa R, Marti AT, Kastanos N, Rives A, Agusti-Vidal A, Rozman C. Acute respiratory failure in severe hematologic disorders. Crit Care Med 1984; 12:26–28.
42. Peters SG, Meadows JA III, Graley DR. Outcome of respiratory failure in hematologic malignancy. Chest 1988; 94:99–102.
43. Denardo SJ, Oye RK, Bellamy PE. Efficacy of intensive care for bone marrow transplant patients with respiratory failure. Crit Care Med 1989; 17:4–6.
44. Crawford SW, Petersen FB. Long-term survival from respiratory failure after marrow transplantation for malignancy. Am Rev Respir Dis 1992; 145:510–514.
45. Allen A. The cardiotoxicity of chemotherapeutic drugs. Semin Oncol 1992; 19:529–542.
46. Buckner CD, Rudolph RH, Fefer A, et al. High-dose cyclophosphamide therapy for malignant disease. Toxicity, tumor response, and the effects of stored autologous marrow. Cancer 1972; 29:357–365.
47. Goldberg MA, Antin JH, Guinan EC, Rappeport JM. Cyclophosphamide cardiotoxicity: an analysis of dosing as a risk factor. Blood 1986; 68:1114–1118.
48. Ayash LJ, Wright JE, Tretyakou O, et al. Cyclophosphamide pharmacokinetics: correlation with cardiac toxicity and tumor response. J Clin Oncol 1992; 10:995–1000.
49. Gradishar WJ, Vokes EE. 5-fluorouracil cardiotoxicity: a critical review. Ann Oncol 1990; 1:409–414.
50. De Forni M, Malet-Martino MC, Jaillais P, et al. Cardiotoxicity of high-dose continuous fluorouracil: a prospective clinical study. J Clin Oncol 1992; 10:1795–1801.
51. Kragel AH, Travis WD, Steis RG, Rosenberg SA, Roberts WC. Myocarditis or

acute myocardial infarction associated with interleukin-2 therapy for cancer. Cancer 1990; 66:1513–1516.

52. Davis S, Rambotti P, Grignani F. Intrapericardial tetracycline sclerosis in the treatment of malignant pericardial effusion: an analysis of thirty-three cases. J Clin Oncol 1984; 2:631–636.
53. Sculier JP, Feld R. Superior vena cava obstruction syndrome: recommendations for management. Cancer Treat Rev 1985; 12:209–218.
54. Bilezikian JP. Management of acute hypercalcemia. N Engl J Med 1992; 326:1196–1203.
55. Gucalp R, Ritch P, Wiernik PH, et al. Comparative study of pamidronate disodium and etidronate disodium in the treatment of cancer-related hypercalcemia. J Clin Oncol 1992; 10:134–142.
56. Ralston SH, Gallacher SJ, Patel V, Campbell J, Boyle IT. Cancer-associated hypercalcemia: morbidity and mortality. Ann Intern Med 1990; 112:499–504.
57. Ebie N, Ryan W, Harris J. Metabolic emergencies in cancer medicine. Med Clin North Am 1986; 70:1151–1166.
58. Sculier JP, Nicaise C, Klastersky J. Lactic acidosis: a metabolic complication of extensive metastatic cancer. Eur J Cancer Clin Oncol 1983; 19:597–601.
59. Tobias JD. Tumour lysis pneumopathy. Clin Intensive Care 1991; 2:305–308.
60. Wade DS, Douglass H Jr, Nava HR, Piedmonte M. Abdominal pain in neutropenic patients. Arch Surg 1990; 125:1119–1127.
61. Wade DS, Nava HR, Douglass HO Jr. Neutropenic enterocolitis. Clinical diagnosis and management. Cancer 1992; 69:17–23.
62. Shulman HM, Hinterberger W. Hepatic veno-occlusive disease-liver toxicity syndrome after bone marrow transplantation. Bone Marrow Transplant 1992; 10:197–214.
63. Sculier JP, Weerts, D. Klastersky J. Cause of death in febrile granulocytopenic cancer patients receiving empiric antibiotic therapy. Eur J Cancer Clin Oncol 1984; 20:55–60.
64. O'Brien MER, Souberbielle BE. Allergic reactions to cytotoxic drugs—an update. Ann Oncol 1992; 3:605–610.
65. Weiss RB. Hypersensitivity reactions. Semin Oncol 1992; 19:458–477.
66. Armitage JO, Antman KH. High-dose Cancer Therapy. Pharmacology, Hematopoietins, Stem Cells. Baltimore: Williams & Wilkins, 1992.
67. Ackland SP, Schilsky RL. High-dose methotrexate: a critical reappraisal. J Clin Oncol 1987; 5:2017–2031.
68. Pennock GD, Dalton WS, Roeske WR, et al. Systemic toxic effects associated with high-dose verapamil infusion and chemotherapy administration. J Natl Cancer Inst 1991; 83:105–110.
69. Weiss RB, Donehower RC, Wiernik PH, et al. Hypersensitivity reactions from taxol. J Clin Oncol 1990; 8:1263–1268.
70. Rowinsky EK, McGuire WP, Guarnieri T, Fisherman JS, Christian MC, Donehower RS. Cardiac disturbances during the administration of taxol. J Clin Oncol 1991; 9:1704–1712.
71. Siegel JP, Puri RK: Interleukin-2 toxicity. J Clin Oncol 1991; 9:694–704.
72. Diana D, Sculier JP. Haemodynamic effects induced by intravenous administration

of high doses of R-Met Hu IL-2 [ala-^{125}] in patients with advanced cancer. Intensive Care Med 1990; 16:167–170.
73. Gyves JW, Ensminger WD, Niederhuber JE, et al. A totally implanted injection port system for blood sampling and chemotherapy administration. JAMA 1989; 251:2538–2541.
74. Carde P, Cosset-Delaigne MF, Laplanche A, Chareau I. Classical external indwelling central venous catheter versus totally implanted venous access systems for chemotherapy administration: a randomized trial in 100 patients with solid tumors. Eur J Cancer Clin Oncol 1989; 25:939–944.
75. Haire WD, Liebermans RP, Lund GB, Edney J, Wieczorek BM. Obstructed central venous catheters. Restoring function with a 12-hour infusion of low-dose urokinase. Cancer 1990; 66:2279–2285.
76. Bertand M, Presant CA, Klein L, Scott E. Iatrogenic superior vena cava syndrome. A new entity. Cancer 1984; 54:376–378.
77. Bock SN, Lee RE, Fisher B, et al. A prospective randomized trial evaluating prophylactic antibiotics to prevent triple-lumen catheter-related sepsis in patients treated with immunotherapy. J Clin Oncol 1990; 8:161–169.
78. Masson BG, Krikorian J, Luki P, Evans GL, McGrath J. Pulmonary microvascular cytology in the diagnosis of lymphangitic carcinomatosis. N Engl J Med 1989; 321:71–76.
79. Harris KPG, Hattersley JM, Feehally J, Walls J. Acute renal failure associated with haematological malignancies: a review of 10 years experience. Eur J Haematol 1991; 47:119–122.
80. Lesesne JB, Rothschild N, Erickson B, et al. Cancer-associated hemolytic-uremic syndrome: analysis of 85 cases from a national registry. J Clin Oncol 1989; 7:781–789.
81. Schlemmer R, Dhainaut JF, Bons J, et al. Pneumopathies aiguës au cours des hémopathies malignes en aplasie: nouvelle approche nosologique et thérapeutique. Ann Med Intern 1982; 133:174–177.
82. Gregg RW, Friedman BC, Williams JF, McGrath BJ, Zimmerman JE. Continuous positive airway pressure by face mask in *Pneumocystis carinii* pneumonia. Crit Care Med 1990; 18:21–24.
83. Turnbull AD, Carlon G. Airway management in the thrombocytopenic cancer patient with acute respiratory failure. Crit Care Med 1979; 7:76–77.
84. Schlemmer B. Aplasie médullaire et ventilation artificielle. Rev Praticien 1990; 23:2152–2153.
85. Ewer MS, Ali MK, Atta MS, Morice RC, Balakrishnan PV. Outcome of lung cancer patients requiring mechanical ventilation for pulmonary failure. JAMA 1986; 256:3364–3366.
86. Miranda DR, Williams A, Loirat P. Management of Intensive Care. Guidelines for Better Use of Resources. Dordrecht: Kluwer Academic, 1990.
87. American Society of Clinical Oncology and American Society of Hematology. Recommended criteria for the performance of bone marrow transplantation. J Clin Oncol 1990; 8:563–564.
88. Dickinson MC. Education for staff who care for cancer patients in the critical care unit. J Nurs Staff Dev 1990; 6:202–203.

89. Sculier JP, Trillet V, Paesmans M, et al. Table ronde sur la méthodologie des essais cliniques. Rev Mal Respir 1992; 9:223–226.
90. Haines IE, Zalcberg J, Buchanan JD. Not for resuscitation orders in cancer patients—principles of decision-making. Med J Aust 1990; 153:225–229.
91. Lawrence VA, Clark GM. Cancer and resuscitation. Does the diagnosis affect the decision? Arch Intern Med 1987; 147:1637–1640.

23

Quality of Life as the End Point for Supportive Care Studies

David G. Warr and Ronald Feld
Ontario Cancer Institute, Princess Margaret Hospital, Toronto, Ontario, Canada

I. INTRODUCTION

Improved quality of life is an important goal of caring for patients with cancer (1). Enquiries about social and emotional well-being are a component of good patient care, but measures of these "soft" outcomes are infrequently used in clinical trials. Even in palliative care studies there are few examples of formal assessment of quality of life. Although one concern may be that these data are incapable of confirmation by other means, physicians readily accept as suitable outcomes other data that are also incapable of validation, such as patient self-report of treatment toxicity. A reluctance to embrace formal quality of life assessment must therefore also have another basis (see Table 1).

Most concerns about quality of life as an end point for clinical trials can be answered easily. Although no universally accepted measure of quality of life exists, there is agreement about the necessary attributes of these measures and a consensus that some attempts are reasonable approximations. An example is the functional living index, cancer (FLIC), which was derived from sound principles and correlates well with accepted measures of various quality of life domains, such as the Beck depression scale and Katz's activities of daily living index (2). The experience of the National Cancer Institute of Canada Clinical Trials Group suggests that concerns about patient acceptance, impact on resources, incomplete data collection, and potential impact on accrual are unnecessary (3). Although the analysis of repeated health measures with missing data is unfamiliar to most clinicians, there are methods that are appropriate from a statistical viewpoint (4).

Table 1 Potential Concerns About Quality of Life as an Outcome Measure

Unfamiliar jargon: reliability, validity, factor analysis, other
No gold standard for measurement of quality of life
Consumes finite resources
Imposition on patients?
Detrimental effect on patient accrual?
Attempts to collect data often unsuccessful
Uncertainty regarding how to analyze data
Benefits unclear

Perhaps the most difficult concern to allay is whether the yield of quality of life assessment will repay the effort, because thus far there have been few data upon which to make this judgment. This chapter presents the evidence supporting the contention that there has been useful information gained. In addition, we review when to use quality of life measures, the considerations that should guide the selection of a questionnaire, potential problems in data collection and interpretation, and the results in a few supportive care topics.

II. RATIONALE AS AN END POINT

In most supportive care studies, the intervention is designed to ameliorate a single problem, such as pain, emesis, or neutropenia. It is prudent to have a measure that focuses on an objective outcome, but there are benefits for also including an overall assessment of quality of life (see Table 2).

It is tempting in supportive care studies to assume that the adverse effects of treatment have such a minor impact on quality of life relative to the condition of primary interest that they can be discounted. However, there are studies in which appreciable numbers of patients refused a treatment that was superior in one outcome because of adverse effects, such as metoclopramide or tetrahydro-

Table 2 Potential Benefits of Quality of Life Assessment

Provide additional information on beneficial and adverse effects
More clearly outline impact of disease or symptom on overall quality of life
Allow choice of optimal therapy when survival is equivalent
Facilitate approval of new drugs
Provide prognostic information

cannabinol for emesis (5–7). The impact of drug toxicity on quality of life therefore cannot be ignored in supportive care trials.

In studies of antineoplastic agents, cooperative groups use toxicity scales to assess the frequency and maximum severity of adverse effects. With the exception of infrequently used daily diaries (8), there is no attempt to record duration of adverse effects. Because a severe but short-lived toxicity may be less troublesome than a mild but continuous adverse effect, the current approach loses potentially useful information. Multiple minor toxicities may also summate to create a major impact on function and/or satisfaction with life, and this cannot be estimated except with quality of life questionnaires.

In addition to more complete assessment of toxicities, quality of life assessment has the potential to record positive symptomatic benefits that would otherwise go unnoticed. In a study by Loprinzi et al. of megestrol acetate as an agent to minimize weight loss, it was noted that a smaller proportion of patients experienced nausea at the end of 30 days in the active treatment group (9). This raises the possibility that megestrol acetate might be useful for the gastrointestinal upset that is so frequent in advanced cancer. Although this benefit was detected by using standard toxicity recording, this was fortuitous because the placebo was more "toxic" than the active treatment. Favorable changes, such as mood elevation, improved energy, and better pain control, go unrecorded unless a more sophisticated approach is employed.

In some studies the intervention has potentially broad therapeutic advantages, for example prednisone for symptomatic prostatic cancer or admission to a palliative care program. In these circumstances a focus on a single outcome, such as pain, is inappropriate. The outcome measure should assess many areas and allow one to determine the overall effect on quality of life. Even when the key outcome is a single symptom, an ability to assess quality of life is crucial. Unlike chemotherapy trials, in which survival is usually viewed as the most important benefit, many supportive care studies have improved well-being as the goal. Demonstration of improvement in one symptom may be of biological interest, but if there is a diminished quality of life the treatment cannot be recommended as a way of improving well-being.

Quality of life data from supportive care studies may also be useful in facilitating approval of drugs for commercial use. The U.S. Food and Drug Administration has stated that quality of life considerations may be used to support an application for licensing (10). In some countries the costs of health care may be largely covered by public funding and decisions about treatment may be influenced by quality of life considerations. Two examples are cited. The Ministry of Health for the Government of Ontario funds erythropoietin in patients undergoing hemodialysis, and this decision was undoubtedly facilitated by its known favorable impact on quality of life. Although not yet operational, in Oregon there is an initiative for funding a number of health care interventions. The initial proposal stated that the improved quality of life (as measured by a scale of well-being) was one of the reasons for including a procedure on the list for funding (11), although more recently this criterion was removed because of concerns that it could discriminate against the disabled. As increasing attention is focused on the cost benefit of new health care interventions, it may be useful to have evidence for quantitative improvement in quality of life, as opposed to anecdote.

Perhaps the most compelling argument for obtaining quality of life data is the demonstration that it has changed clinical practice. With the limited amount of data from supportive care trials thus far, there are no available examples. However, two oncology studies challenged the existing beliefs of physicians. An early study by Sugarbaker et al. documented that patients who received limb-sparing treatment for sarcoma had poorer sexual function than those patients whose extremity was amputated (12). This study pointed out the need to improve the manner in which the radiation therapy was delivered if the potential benefits of limb-conserving surgery were to be realized. In a study by Coates et al. of patients with metastatic breast cancer, continuous chemotherapy was associated with better quality of life than intermittent therapy even in nonresponders (13). Although these results can be rationalized in retrospect, the authors state that they were not anticipated.

Another finding that was not anticipated was the prognostic value of quality of life data in chemotherapy trials. In a study of patients with nonmetastatic lung cancer by Ruckdeschel and Piantados (4) and a breast cancer study by Coates et al. (14), information on quality of life turned out to be a stronger predictor of survival than traditional factors. Experience with the prognostic ability of these questionnaires in supportive care studies is extremely limited. The Spitzer quality of life (Q-L) index was judged not to be a strong enough predictor of survival in terminally ill cancer patients to be clinically useful (15). Much more experience is required with a variety of instruments examining other end points, such as success in controlling pain, before the predictive value of these instruments can be assessed.

Although information attesting to the value of quality of life data in oncology research is still limited, it is compelling enough that the National Cancer Institute of Canada Clinical Trials Group now requires a statement in all phase III protocols that do not incorporate quality of life assessments to state the reason it is not being measured (16).

III. STUDY SELECTION FOR QUALITY OF LIFE ASSESSMENT

Quality of life is often a desirable end point, but it requires increased data collection, specific quality assurance efforts, and additional analyses. Because the resources of any clinical trials organization are finite, we now consider whether there are some supportive care topics and some study designs for which quality of life assessment is more relevant.

Quality of life data may not be helpful when differences between treatment groups in terms of toxicity and symptomatic benefit are unlikely. An example in supportive care is intravenous antibiotic studies for febrile neutropenic patients. In this circumstance, treatment recommendations are based upon considerations other than trivial differences in quality of life. It may be difficult, however, to predict accurately the degree to which well-being is affected. For example, although the use of blood products per se may seem to be of little interest, erythropoietin has been a topic for quality of life research in hemodialysis (17) and cancer patients (18) and granulocyte colony-stimulating factor demonstrated a measurable improvement in quality of life in patients with benign neutropenia (19). A reasonable conclusion is that most (but not all) supportive care topics can yield useful quality of life information and that there should be careful deliberation on a study-by-study basis

The design of a clinical trial has implications for the utility of quality of life assessment. Phase I studies that seek to define the maximum tolerable dose of a drug (e.g., a new antiemetic) are unlikely to yield useful quality of life data because of the small number of patients enrolled and the absence of any appropriate comparison group. An interesting exception is a study by Berdel et al. demonstrating that participation in phase I cytotoxic trials produced no measurable impairment in well-being, data that may be useful from an ethical perspective (20). In contrast, a large phase II or III dose-ranging study may be a very suitable design for a quality of life assessment, for example, a large parallel design study to establish the optimal dose of prednisone in improving well-being.

It has been suggested that collection of quality of life data be reserved for randomized trials because of the need for a comparison group (21). When quality of life rather than survival or tumor response is the end point, this need not be the case because the patient is sometimes used as his or her own control. In a single-arm study by Tannock et al. of patients receiving prednisone for prostatic carcinoma, a broadly based symptom assessment scale established that this was a palliative intervention worth considering (22). Two studies of laser therapy for upper and lower gastrointestinal obstruction are examples of clinical situations in which randomized trials will never be done because of the rarity of the situation, yet information was obtained that strongly supported the utility of the intervention (23,24). The absence of a parallel untreated group in these studies diminishes the certainty that observed improvements were a result of the treatment, but this may be the best available evidence upon which to base practice. Thus a randomized design is not a prerequisite for quality of life assessment in supportive care trials.

In summary, quality of life measures may be useful as a survey for toxicities or for benefits beyond those initially hypothesized. They should be used whenever inferences will be made about overall patient well-being.

IV. PITFALLS

A. Selection of Questionnaire

Although quality of life may be quantitated by utility assessment (25), this chapter focuses on the use of questionnaires in clinical trials to assess whether an intervention has produced a measurable impact on quality of life.

In theory, one could start from scratch and design a questionnaire that is appropriate for a study, but the labor-intensive nature of test construction precludes this approach for all but the most patient and dedicated investigators. When an instrument is created and used without documentation of validity, this poses problems in interpreting the results. A null result could mean either that there is no difference in quality of life or that the questionnaire was insensitive to change. A positive result may be suggestive but still requires some proof that the measure samples the relevant domains; for example, sampling only the physical domain and then calling this overall quality of life is inappropriate. Recognizing that established questionnaires may not sample all areas of interest in a given study, the European Organization for Research and Treatment of Cancer (EORTC) quality of life group has proposed that modules (groups of questions) that are disease or treatment specific could be added to a core questionnaire (26). This may seem attractive, but it does not obviate the need for the investigators to establish validity for any module that is devised.

Table 3 lists several considerations when selecting a quality of life measure for oncology trials. Gough suggested that a single question may be used to assess quality of life (27). Although these data are easy to obtain and may correlate well with more complex measures, they provide very little information. Most authors agree that a quality of life measure must assess more than a single

Table 3 Considerations in Selecting a Quality of Life Instrument

Does the questionnaire sample the necessary aspects of life (domains)?
Does the underlying construct of the questionnaire fit the study needs?
Is the questionnaire reliable?
Is the questionnaire valid?
Is the questionnaire sufficiently sensitive to changes in quality of life?
Has the questionnaire been tested in patients with cancer?
Is the questionnaire available in the appropriate language(s)?
Is the questionnaire feasible (e.g., self-administered, brief)?

outcome and at a minimum should include measures of the physical, emotional, and social domains (21,28–30). These multidimensional measures allow one to determine which aspects of life are most heavily affected, which in turn provides supportive evidence that any quantitative changes in overall quality of life are valid and provides a rationale for intervention in subsequent studies.

Although often ignored, the definition of quality of life used to construct the questionnaire may be important. If, for example, the investigator wishes to explore patient satisfaction, then FLIC, which defines quality of life in terms of function (2), is inappropriate, but one might consider the questionnaire devised by Ferrans and Powers (31). The underlying premise should be contained in the initial publication on questionnaire development, but it may be absent, leaving the reader to decide whether the approach taken is appropriate.

The initial article that presents a new questionnaire for consideration should provide evidence for reliability and validity. For example, the reader is referred to a recent article by Aaronson et al. on the development of a questionnaire by the EORTC (26). Reliability (the extent to which a measure is free of random error) is of critical importance, and evidence for reliability in the form of internal consistency (Cronbach's α) and test-retest correlations is frequently available. It is true that an unreliable measure is useless, but a reliable test is also useless if it does not measure that which is intended, that is, if it is not valid. An example of a test that is reliable but not valid is the use of Karnofsky performance status as the only measure of quality of life. This performance status measure has predictive validity for response and survival, but it is an inappropriate surrogate for a quality of life measure.

A common way of establishing validity is to correlate the various dimensions of the questionnaire with accepted measures. Investigators should look for evidence that the questionnaire can distinguish between groups of patients for whom there is a reason to believe that there are differences in quality of life, for example, patients with minimal versus marked symptoms caused by metastatic disease. For interventional (as opposed to predictive) studies, one wants evidence that the test is sensitive enough to detect clinically relevant changes, but this sensitivity to change data is generally lacking. A null result is therefore difficult to interpret because it could simply be caused by an inadequate questionnaire.

A questionnaire that is accepted as valid by some experts may still not be valid in the context of the proposed study. The measure should have been tested in an appropriate population, for example patients with cancer rather than psychiatric patients. Lest this seem somewhat strict, one should remember the example of measures of depression that regard weight loss and constipation as signs of depression: this may be true in the general population but not in the terminally ill.

Another problematical issue is the uncertain influence of language and culture. Even in countries that are largely English speaking, there may be a large enough immigrant population that an English version is a handicap to complete data collection. It is tempting simply to translate the questionnaire into another language, but this may not achieve the intended effect. Just as the slogan for a soft drink company was inadvertently translated from "Come alive! You're in the Pepsi generation" to "Pepsi brings your ancestors back from the grave!" the meaning of a quality of life questionnaire may be lost in the translation. At a minimum, any translated version should be retranslated into the language in which it was validated and compared with the original version. One cannot have absolute confidence, however, that the test will behave the same unless there is extensive cross-cultural validation, something that is being explored for the EORTC questionnaire but few others (26).

A critical consideration in selecting a questionnaire is the feasibility of administration given the time and personnel constraints. The sickness impact profile, which contains 136 items and is interviewer administered, is unlikely to be useful in cooperative group studies. As a rule of thumb for large studies, it is desirable that the test be self-administered and require less than 20 minutes for completion. Only when the supportive care study involves institutions in which there is a strong commitment to quality of life assessment is much more extensive evaluation likely to be feasible.

A final consideration is whether the questionnaire is answered by the patient or someone else. Most questionnaires are answered by the patient rather than a caregiver (family member or health care provider, such as a doctor or nurse). This is usually desirable because of the poor correlation between quality of life assessment by patients and others (32). However, there may be situations in which patient self-report is of questionable validity because of impaired cognition, as in hypercalcemia, and there may be circumstances in which the perspective of someone other than the patient is of primary interest to the investigator. The Spitzer Q-L index is an example of a questionnaire that can be completed by health care providers and for which there is evidence of validity (33). Nonetheless, many readers are sceptical about quality of life data reported by someone other than the patient, and the onus is on the investigator to corroborate the results by other means.

Instruments that have been used in oncology trials are reviewed by Cella and Tulsky (30), McMillen Moinpour et al. (21), and Osoba (28). Table 4 provides examples and a brief description of some questionnaires that have been use in supportive care studies.

B. Data Collection

Questionnaires may have demonstrable validity, but if data collection is incomplete or they are collected in a population with impaired cognition, the effort may be wasted. Some studies have reported that quality of life information

Table 4 Quality of Life Instruments Used in Supportive Care Studies[a]

Scale	Number of items and format	Comments	References
Functional living index, cancer	22 items focusing on actual performance; Likert scale/VAS format	Also created a version specifically for emesis (FLIE)	45
VAS, Priestman and Baum	25 items (physical, psychological, social, personal, quality of life); VAS format	Added all 25 item scores to get overall score	23, 24
VAS, Tannock	17 items (physical, emotional, social family sexual, employment); VAS format	Modified from a breast cancer questionnaire; used in conjunction with McGill pain questionnaire	48
Spitzer Q-L index	5 items (activity, daily living, health, support, outlook) rated 0, 1, or 2 and one visual analog scale for quality of life	Completed by patient, significant other, or health care provider	15, 23, 24
EORTC QLQ-C-30	30 items with 5 functional (physicial, role, cognitive, emotional, social) and 3 symptom (fatigue, nausea/emesis, pain) scales and a global health and quality of life scale; Likert format	Core questionnaire may be supplemented by disease- or treatment-specific module	34
Van Holten-Verzantvoort	4 items (mobility, gastrointestinal toxicity, bone pain, fatigue)	Called a quality of life questionnaire but very limited number of domains	49

[a]VAS,.

was available for less than one-half of the patients (34). Although claims have been made that sample size requirements may be smaller for the end point of quality of life as opposed to survival, power calculations are never provided. Even if the amount of information collected is sufficient for analysis, one still has the potential problem of bias. Failure to complete a questionnaire may be related to the patient's current quality of life; that is, missing data are more probable when the patient is sick (26). In recent years a major challenge has been for investigators to maximize the completeness of data collection.

Potential reasons for incomplete data collection are listed in Table 5. There have been very few investigations into which of these reasons are important. In a pilot study, Yancik et al. found that 14% of patients approached about quality of life refused to participate for a variety of reasons (35). Other investigators have not found refusal to be a major problem, however. Yancik et al. said that those responsible for collecting the data also believed that time constraints and lack of commitment by physicians contributed to incomplete data collection.

The Swiss Group for Clinical Cancer Research recently reported their experience with quality of life data collection in a phase III clinical trial of chemotherapy for small cell lung cancer (34). The only significant predictor of compliance was the institution at which the patient received treatment. Because compliance was lowest at baseline and did not correlate with tumor response, the conclusion was that the principal problems were not patient related and suggestions were made about questionnaire length and training of staff. A multivariate analysis by Ballatori et al. found that in a single-center study, level of education (higher is better) and age (younger is better) predicted for errors and missing data, whereas ECOG performance status was positive only in a univariate analysis (36). A multicountry study of the EORTC QLQ-30 found that increasing age, poorer performance status, and greater weight loss were associated with a lower frequency of repeat assessments (26). At present it seems reasonable to conclude that at baseline assessment much of the data collection problem is not patient related but that disease extent and possibly age may affect the ability to collect subsequent data.

Despite the difficulties in collecting quality of life data, there are examples

Table 5 Reasons for Incomplete Data Collection

Patient refusal
Patient too ill
Lack of commitment by data managers and investigators
Insufficient personnel in place to collect the data
No quality assurance program in place that audits completeness
Language barrier/reading level

of success. The National Cancer Institute of Canada Clinical Trials Group initially failed to collect enough quality of life data to allow analysis in a lung cancer trial of chemotherapy versus best supportive care (37), but more recent studies by the same group achieved more than 90% complete data collection (3). Whether this remarkable success can be achieved in patient populations with more advanced disease remains to be seen.

Another consideration in data collection is the frequency of assessment. Data must be collected at least twice (unless the study is of cross-sectional design). The possible conclusions with data collection at only two points in time may be limited, and the loss of data from one point in time means that the patient is unevaluable so that extreme care should be used to maximize completeness. No empirically derived guidelines for the frequency of data collection can be provided because this would vary with the instrument reliability and validity, the day-to-day variability in the health status, the sample size, and the magnitude of the difference regarded as clinically significant. As a rule of thumb, we believe it is unlikely that more than six appropriately timed assessments will be helpful. An exception might be the collection of a very limited amount of data, as in a daily diary card (8).

The expected temporal changes in well-being should dictate the timing of data collection. For example, in evaluating a new analgesic, several assessments during the first month might capture all the relevant data if there are no long-term adverse effects. On the other hand, the prophylactic effects of bisphosphonates for morbidity as a result of bone metastases are exerted over several months, and this should be reflected in the timing of any quality of life data collection.

C. Data Analysis and Interpretation

The data analysis for the quality of life endpoint is less straightforward than for survival. With survival data patients can be classified as alive or dead, whereas an almost continuous range of values is possible for quality of life, with the potential for swings in values rather than a continuous downward or upward trend. With quality of life data there will also always be some missing data, and unlike survival data these can never be recovered by even the most astute detective.

Although one could collapse the posttreatment data into a single statistic for comparison by taking the maximum or minimum results, it is preferable to make use of the data from multiple time points. The reader is referred to by Zee and Pater for a technical discussion on the use of analysis of variance (ANOVA), multivariate ANOVA, and growth curve models (4).

If possible, investigators should specify in the protocol the relationships that are of primary interest, for example, correlation between overall quality of life and mean severity of pain over the first month. It is tempting to examine all possible relationships and then report on "statistically significant" associations, but this dredging of the data will reveal multiple spurious relationships. As with subset analyses of chemotherapy trials for responding subgroups, this approach can only be regarded as hypothesis generating, that is, to be tested in future trials.

In cytotoxic studies it is not clear how to draw conclusions from quality of life data if differences in survival are in the opposite direction to quality of life. Survival differences in supportive care studies are possible (38) but infrequent, and the dilemma is more likely to be whether improvement in a specific symptom, such as pain in an analgesic trial, outweighs increased adverse effects, such as nausea, sedation, and constipation. It is in this situation that an item asking about overall quality of life may be very useful. If the objective of the trial is to improve patient well-being, then one can argue that the most important end point is the net change in quality of life.

V. RESULTS IN SELECTED SUPPORTIVE CARE AREAS

A. Pain

Because pain is a common problem in patients with advanced disease, it is surprising that little work has been done on the assessment of its impact on quality of life. This lack of investigation may be explained by several factors. First, the assessment may be seen as an imposition on the patient at a time when he or she is in distress. Second, as with supportive care studies in general, relatively few interventions are tested, compared with thousands of randomized trials conducted with antineoplastic agents. Third, there may be an understandable (but incorrect) assumption that any measure that improves pain will automatically improve quality of life.

The belief that pain has an adverse effect on quality of life is supported by two studies that show a correlation between pain intensity and impairment of quality of life (39,40). An alternative interpretation of these data may be that it was a higher opioid dose rather than the greater pain intensity that diminished quality of life. It would be of interest to analyze the relationship between pain intensity and quality of life adjusting for the opioid dose.

An analysis of the meaning of pain for individual patients has provided some interesting data. Although pain is not generally perceived as having any positive value, a survey by Padilla et al. indicated this may not be true for all patients (41). This observation plus the known adverse effects of analgesic therapy suggest that further exploration of the impact of current analgesic approaches on overall quality of life is prudent.

The adverse effects of opioids as well as advanced cancer on cognitive function have been documented by Bruera et al. (42). These findings raise the possibility that quality of life self-assessment by patients with more advanced disease or those who receive opioids may be inaccurate. It may be tempting to rely upon external raters in these situations, but this, too, may be misleading. In a small series of patients with cognitive failure who were agitated, some health care providers and family members interpreted the patients' behaviors as evidence of pain and significantly higher doses of opioids were used (43). When these patients recovered from their cognitive impairment, they had no memory of increased pain during the cognitive failure, suggesting that their pain intensity had been overestimated. No matter what perspective is used by investigators, there are potential problems with the validity of the data. A pragmatic approach is to exclude patients from self-assessment when there is moderate to severe impairment of cognitive function and to seek corroborative data whenever raters other than the patient must be used.

Further work evaluating quality of life in patients with pain may be helpful to underscore the importance of appropriately managing this problem and to determine more accurately the overall benefits of interventions that have appreciable toxicities, such as neurosurgery or opioids.

B. Emesis

Over the past 15 years there has been a marked improvement in the ability to prevent chemotherapy-induced emesis. The initial advances came about through the use of high-dose metoclopramide and derivatives of marijuana. These drugs had some limitation in their use, however, because of adverse effects. Refusal of treatment by patients, especially the young with metoclopramide use for multiple days (5) and the elderly with tetrahydrocannabinol (7). Quality of life was not an end point in these early studies. It is reasonable to assume that there was a net gain in quality of life for patients receiving cisplatin in whom severe emesis always occurred, but the risk-benefit tradeoff was not as clear for less emetogenic drugs, and as a consequence many patients may not have received the most effective antiemetic agents.

The newest generation of antiemetics, the serotonin receptor antagonists, have very few troublesome adverse effects but bring with them a new problem. They are substantially more expensive than some conventional alternatives, such as steroids and dopamine receptor antagonists. In systems in which health care is publicly funded by there has been no incremental funding, this antiemetic advance has economic consequences. To minimize the financial impact, institutional policies have been developed for the use of these new agents that restrict or prevent their use. In Canada, for example, the availability of ondansetron for in-hospital use in patients receiving doxorubicin ranges from standard practice to use only if there is severe emesis that the patient declares is unacceptable. This variability may be, in part, due to differences in perceptions about the importance of emesis as a determinant of quality of life.

There is a limited amount of data on the effects of postchemotherapy emesis on quality of life. Bliss et al. did not find that nausea and vomiting had a substantial impact on quality of life, but less than one-third of the patients were receiving chemotherapy and only four had treatment in the 24 h before completing the questionnaire (44). On the other hand, Lindley et al. demonstrated a relationship between quality of life as assessed by a modified FLIC (referred to as FLIE) and the severity of emesis (45). In fact, the difference in quality of life over a 1 week period following chemotherapy could be accounted for solely by the extent of problem with emesis. In a study by Soukop et al. comparing metoclopramide with ondansetron, the more efficacious treatment was associated with a less profound decrease in quality of life (5). This difference in self-rated well-being may not have been solely caused by differences in emesis because there was a higher dropout rate in the metoclopramide group because of the extrapyramidal effects. This difference in adverse effects underscores the caution that investigators should exercise in interpreting favorable differences in quality of life to changes in the outcome of principle interest (e.g., emesis) as opposed to differences in other drug effects.

These quality of life data support the results of a survey reported by Coates et al. that emesis is an important determinant of quality of life (46) and provide reassurance that the available measures are sensitive enough to pick up at least gross differences in quality of life.

C. Anorexia

Cachexia frequently occurs in the setting of advanced pancreatic or lung cancer. Although moderate-dose megestrol acetate has been demonstrated to increase appetite and body fat with little in the way of adverse effects, its use is still limited. There may be several reasons this drug is not more commonly used: profound weight loss may be relatively uncommon, it may not be a high priority for patients, physicians may not regard it as a high priority, or the cost of megestrol acetate may be perceived to outweigh the benefits. Quality of life research could be useful to define more clearly the beliefs of patients and physicians and to assess the impact of weight gain (or prevention of further weight loss) on quality of life.

One placebo-controlled study of megestrol acetate incorporating quality of life assessment was reported by Tchekmedyian et al. (47). No overall difference was observed in well-being, but a subset analysis of those patients who gained weight showed a marginal improvement. The results of the study are difficult to interpret because the authors chose to use a questionnaire of their own design and did not present any evidence for reliability and validity. This work should be repeated using an accepted measure.

D. Obstructive Symptoms

Symptoms caused by obstruction of the gastrointestinal tract are uncommon yet can be quite distressing and result in prolonged hospitalization. One approach advocated in palliative care units is the use of regular antiemetics and avoidance of nasogastric tubes (because they are uncomfortable) and surgery (because of the low success rate and morbidity). A recent development applicable to patients with primarily intraluminal tumor is laser surgery. This intervention is associated with apparently low morbidity and negligible mortality. Two studies have been carried out to assess the impact of laser surgery on quality of life, one for esophageal obstruction and the other for rectal obstruction. In both studies, serial assessments with a quality of life instrument showed evidence of enhanced health compared with baseline over a period of several months. Although these studies can be criticized because they were not randomized (not feasible because of the infrequency of the conditions), they give credence to statements that laser therapy is benefical. Similar studies are required for the more widely used application of laser surgery to relieve bronchial obstruction.

VI. SUMMARY AND PERSPECTIVES

It is feasible and conceptually desirable to use quality of life measures in most supportive care studies. Indeed, quality of life may sometimes be the most desirable end point. The limited experience thus far shows that these data may be useful in drawing conclusions and may lead to some unexpected dividends, such as improved prognostic ability.

In addition to expanding the number of supportive care studies incorporating quality of life as an end point, much additional work needs to be done on the questionnaires themselves. For example, there is a need for studies that compare some of the most widely used quality of life instruments, and the problem of cross-cultural validation has barely been examined. Incorporation of the principles that have facilitated more complete data collection will enhance this research effort (16).

SELECTED READING

Cella DF, Tulsky DS. Measuring quality of life today: methodological aspects. Oncology 1990; 4:29–38. An easy to read account of how one validates questionnaires and incorporates them into studies. Review of the contents of 23 measures used in cancer patients. One of twelve articles in an issue devoted to quality of life in patients with cancer.

McGowan I, Barr H, Krasner N. Palliative laser therapy for inoperable rectal cancer—does it work? A prospective study of quality of life. Cancer 1989; 63:967–969.

Barr H, Krasner N. Prospective quality-of-life analysis after palliative photoablation for the treatment of malignant dysphagia. Cancer 1991; 68:1660–1664. These references are good examples of how a single-arm study may benefit from quality of life assessment.

Osoba D. Measuring the effect of cancer on quality of life. In: Effect of Cancer on Quality of Life. Osoba D, Ed., Boca Raton, FL: CRC Press, 1991:25–40. An overview of why to measure quality of life, the barriers to assessment, and definitions of some basic terms use in test development. One of twenty-four chapters in a text devoted to the issue of assessing quality of life in patients with cancer.

Sadura A, Pater J, Osoba D, Levine M, Palmer M, Bennett K. Quality of life assessment: patient compliance with questionnaire completion. J Natl Cancer Inst 1992; 84:1023–1026. A report of what is achievable in terms of complete data collection within a cooperative group setting, including supportive care studies.

Schipper H, Clinch J, McMurray A, Levitt M. Measuring the quality of life of cancer patients: the Functional Living Index-Cancer: development and validation. J Clin Oncol 1984; 2:472–483. A good example of the processes involved in questionnaire development, including validation using accepted measures of various domains.

REFERENCES

1. Gough IR, Dalgleish LI. What value is given to quality of life assessment by health professionals considering response to palliative chemotherapy for advanced cancer. Cancer 1991; 68:220–225.
2. Schipper H, Clinch J, McMurray A, Levitt M. Measuring the quality of life of cancer patients: the Functional Living Index-Cancer: development and validation. J Clin Oncol 1984; 2:472–483.
3. Sadura A, Pater J, Osoba D, Levine M, Palmer M, Bennett K. Quality of life assessment: patient compliance with questionnaire completion. J Natl Cancer Inst 1992; 84:1023–1026.
4. Ruckdeschel JC, Piantodos S. Quality of life assessment in lung surgery for bronchogenic carcinoma. J Thorac Surg 1991; 6:201–205.
5. Soukop M, Hunter E, Kaye S, et al. Ondansetron compared with metoclopramide in the control of emesis and quality of life during repeated chemotherapy for breast cancer. Oncology 1992; 49:295–304.
6. Citron ML, Herman TS, Vreeland F, et al. Antiemetic efficacy of levonantradol compared to delta-9-tetrahydrocannabinol for chemotherapy-induced nausea and vomiting. Cancer Treat Rep 1985; 69:109–112.
7. Frytak S, Moertel CG, O'Fallon JR, et al. Delta-9-tetrahydrocannabinol as an antiemetic for patients receiving cancer chemotherapy. A comparison with prochlorperazine and a placebo. Ann Intern Med 1979; 91:825–830.
8. Geddes DM, Dones L, Hill E, et al. Quality of life during chemotherapy for small cell lung cancer: assessment using a daily diary card in a randomized trial. Eur J Cancer 1990; 26:484–492.
9. Loprinzi CL, Ellison NM, Schaid DJ, et al. Controlled trial of megestrol acetate for the treatment of cancer anorexia and cacchexia. J Natl Cancer Inst 1990; 82:1127–1132.
10. O'Shaughnessy JA, Wittes RE, Burke G, et al. Commentary concerning demonstration of safety and efficacy of investigational anticancer agents in clinical trials. J Clin Oncol 1991; 9:2225–2232.
11. Oregon Health Services Commission. Prioritization of health services. A report to the governor and legislature, 1993.
12. Sugarbaker PH, Barofsky I, Rosenberg SA, Gianola FJ. Quality of life assessment of patients in extremity sarcoma trials. Surgery 1982; 91:17–23.

13. Coates A, Gebski V, Stat M, et al. Improving the quality of life during chemotherapy for advanced breast cancer. A comparison of intermittent and continuous treatment strategies. N Engl J Med 1987; 317:1490–1495.
14. Coates A, Gebski V, Signorini D, et al. Prognostic value of quality-of-life scores during chemotherapy for advanced breast cancer. J Clin Oncol 1992; 10:1833–1838.
15. Addington-Hall JM, MacDonald LD, Anderson HR. Can the Spitzer quality of life index help to reduce prognostic uncertainty in terminal care? Br J Cancer 1990; 62:695–699.
16. Osoba D. The quality of life committee of the clinical trials group of the National Cancer Institute of Canada: organization and functions. Qual Life Res 1992; 1:211–218.
17. Laupacis A, Muirhead N, Keown P, Wong C. A disease-specific questionnaire for assessing quality of life in patients on hemodialysis. Nephron 1992; 60:302–306.
18. Abels RI. Use of recombinant human erythropoietin in the treatment of anemia in patients who have cancer. Semin Oncol 1992; 19(suppl 8):29–35.
19. Fazio MT, Glaspy JA. The impact of granulocyte colony-stimulating factor on quality of life in patients with severe chronic neutropenia. Oncol Nurs Forum 1991; 18:1411–1414.
20. Berdel WE, Knopf H, Fromm M, et al. Influence of phase I early clinical trials on the quality of life of cancer patients. A pilot study. Anticancer Res 1988, 8:313–321.
21. McMillen Moinpour C, Feigl P, Metch B, Hayden KA, Meyskens F Jr, Crowley J. Quality of life end points in cancer clinical trials: review and recommendations. Cancer 1989; 81:485–495.
22. Tannock I, Gospodarowicz M, Meakin W, Panzarella T, Stewart L, Rider W. Treatment of metastatic prostatic carcinoma with low-dose prednisone: evaluation of pain and quality of life as pragmatic indicators of response. J Clin Oncol 1989; 7:590–597.
23. McGowan I, Barr H, Krasner N. Palliative laser therapy for inoperable rectal cancer—does it work? A prospective study of quality of life. Cancer 1989; 63:967–969.
24. Barr H, Krasner N. Prospective quality-of-life analysis after palliative photoablation for the treatment of malignant dysphagia. Cancer 1991; 68:1660–1664.
25. Goodwin PJ. Economic evaluations of cancer care—incorporating quality of life issues: In: Osoba D, ed. Effect of Cancer on Quality of Life. Boca Raton, FL: CRC Press, 1991:125–136.
26. Aaronson NK, Ahmedzai S, Bergman B, et al. The European Organization for Research and Treatment of Cancer QLQ-C30: a quality-of-life instrument for use in international clinical trials in oncology. J Natl Cancer Inst 1993; 85:365–376.
27. Gough IR, Furnival CM, Schilder L, Grove W. Assessment of quality of life of patients with advanced cancer. Eur J Cancer Clin Oncol 1983; 19:1161–1165.
28. Osoba D. Measuring the effect of cancer on quality of life. In: Osoba D, ed. Effect of Cancer on Quality of Life. Boca Raton, FL: CRC Press, 1991:25–40.
29. Cook Gotay C, Korn EL, McCabe MS, Moore TD, Cheson BD. Quality of life assessment in cancer treatment protocols: research issues in protocol development. J Natl Cancer Inst 1992; 84:575–579.
30. Cella DF, Tulsky DS. Measuring quality of life today: methodological aspects. Oncology 1990; 4:29–38.

31. Ferrans CE, Powers MJ. Quality of life index: development and psychometric properties. Adv Nurs Sci 1985; 8:15–24.
32. Slevin ML, Plant H, Lynch D, Drinkwater J, Gregory WM. Who should measure quality of life, the doctor or the patient? Br J Cancer 1988; 57:109–112.
33. Wood-Dauphinee S, Williams JI. The Spitzer quality of life index: its performance as measure. In: Osoba D, ed. Effect of Cancer on Quality of Life. Boca Raton, FL: CRC Press, 1991:169–184.
34. Hurny C, Bernhard J, Joss R, et al. Feasibility of quality of life assessment in a randomized phase III trial of small cell lung cancer. Eur J Cancer 1992; 3:825–831.
35. Yancik R, Edwards BK, Yates JW. Assessing the quality of life of cancer patients: practical issues in study implementation. J Psychosoc Oncol 1989; 7:59–74.
36. Ballatori E, Roila F, Basurto C, et al. Reliability and validity of a quality of life questionnaire in cancer patients. Eur J Cancer 1993; 29A(suppl 1):S63–S69.
37. Rapp E, Pater JL, Willan A, et al. Can chemotherapy prolong survival in patients with advanced non-small-cell lung cancer—report of a Canadian multicenter randomized trial. J Clin Oncol 1988; 6:633–641.
38. Robustelli Della Cuna G, Pellegrini A, Piazzi M. Effect of methylprednisolone sodium succinate on quality of life in preterminal cancer patients: a placebo-controlled multicenter study. Eur J Cancer Clin Oncol 1990; 25:1817–1821.
39. Strang P, Qvarner H. Cancer-related pain and its influence on quality of life. Anticancer Res 1990; 10:109–112.
40. Ferrell BR, Wisdom C, Wenzl C. Quality of life as an outcome variable in the management of cancer pain. Cancer 1989; 63:2321–2327.
41. Padilla GV, Ferrell B, Grant MM, Rhiner M. Defining the content domain of quality of life for cancer patients with pain. Cancer Nurs 1990; 13:108–115.
42. Bruera E, Miller L, Macmillan K, Krefting L. Cognitive failure in patients with terminal cancer: a prospective study. J Pain Sympt Management 1992; 7:192–195.
43. Bruera E, Fainsinger RL, Miller MJ, Kuehn N. The assessment of pain intensity in patients with cognitive failure: a preliminary report. J Pain Sympt Management 1992; 7:267–270.
44. Bliss JM, Robertson B, Selby PJ. The impact of nausea and vomiting upon quality of life measures. Br J Cancer 1992; 66(suppl XIX):S14–S23.
45. Lindley CM, Hirsch JD, O'Neill CV, Transau MC, Gilbert CS, Osterhaus JT. Quality of life consequences of chemotherapy-induced emesis. Qual Life Res 1992; 1:331–340.
46. Coates A, Abraham S, Kaye SB, et al. On the receiving end—patient perception of the side-effects of cancer chemotherapy. Eur J Cancer Clin Oncol 1983; 19:203–208.
47. Tchekmedyian NS, Hickman M, Siau J, et al. Megestrol acetate in cancer anorexia and weight loss. Cancer 1992; 5:1268–1274.
48. Tannock I, Gospodarowicz M, Meakin W, Panzarello T, Stewart L, Rider W. Treatment of metastatic prostatic cancer with low-dose prednisone: evaluation of pain and quality of life as pragmatic indices of response. J Clin Oncol 1989; 7:590–597.
49. Van Holten-Verzantvoort AT, Zwinderman AH, Aaronson NK, et al. The effect of supportive pamidronate treatment on aspects of quality of life of patients with advanced breast cancer. Eur J Cancer 1991; 27:544–549.

24

Clinical Use of Hematopoietic Growth Factors

Arnold Ganser
Johann-Wolfgang Goethe University, Frankfurt, Germany

I. HEMATOPOIETIC SYSTEM

The constant need for mature cells in the peripheral blood and in the tissue is met by the proliferation, differentiation, and maturation within the progenitor cell pools in the bone marrow. Approximately 10 billion erythrocytes, granulocytes, and platelets are produced every hour, and this baseline production can be increased 10-fold in times of need. Once the erythrocytes have entered the bloodstream, their life span is about 120 days. Platelets circulate in the blood for approximately 8 days, but the half-life of neutrophils in the blood is only about 8 h.

The hematopoietic system is hierarchically organized. All the cellular elements of the blood originate from a common stem cell in the bone marrow. The totipotent stem cell with the capacity for giving rise to progenitor cells of both the lymphoid and the myeloid system and for repopulating lethally irradiated recipients is normally quiescent. Human pluripotent stem cells have been isolated. They can be cryopreserved and used for auto- and allotransplantation procedures in the treatment of cancer. In addition, they serve as targets for therapeutic gene transfer. With continuing differentiation the pluripotent progenitor cells become committed to a single cell lineage and further mature into the morphologically recognizable precursor cells of the bone marrow. The regulation of mature blood cell production mainly occurs within the morphologically identifiable bone marrow cell pools. The factors influencing differentiation and commitment are poorly understood, although the decision is thought to be stochastic. The microenvironment apparently plays an important role in this process by controlling self-replication, proliferation, and differentiation through the expression of certain adhesion molecules and the secretion of membrane-bound or soluble hormones, or cytokines.

The cytokines that predominantly regulate hematopoiesis are called hematopoietic growth factors (1). Hematopoietic growth factors are glycoprotein hormones that interact with hematopoietic cells at different levels of cell differentiation, from the multipotent progenitor to the circulating mature cell, through interaction with unique membrane-bound receptors. These factors are not only essential for the proliferation and differentiation of the progenitor cells, but they also act as survival factors for both the immature progenitor cells and the mature cells. Interleukin-1 (IL-1), IL-3, Steel factor (also called kit-ligand, stem cell factor, and mast cell growth factor) and the recently identified flt3-ligand stimulate proliferation and differentiation of the pluripotent progenitor cells (Table 1). Granulocyte-macrophage colony-stimulating factor (GM-CSF) stimulates the production of granulocytes. Macrophage CSF (M-CSF) stimulates macrophage proliferation and function. Erythrocyte formation is stimulated by erythropoietin. After considerable effort, a cytokine stimulating the events of platelet production has recently been identified (77–79). In addition, IL-1, IL-3, IL-6, IL-11, and GM-CSF act on the immature megakaryocytic progenitor cells, whereas erythropoietin stimulates late events (Fig. 1).

Besides the stimulatory cytokines, we now know a number of inhibitory cytokines that take part in the maintenance of the steady state but when overexpressed in disease can lead to cytopenia. The interferons, tumor necrosis factors (TNF), transforming growth factor β, and macrophage inhibitory protein 1α are involved in inhibition of hematopoiesis (2). Other molecules, such as IL-1,

Table 1 Hematopoietic Growth Factors and Their Target Cell Lineages

Cytokine	Stem cells	Granulopoiesis	Thrombopoiesis	Erythropoiesis	Monocytopoiesis
Steel factor[a]	+	+[b]	+[b]	+[b]	+[b]
Interleukin-3	+	+	+	+	+
GM-CSF	(+)	+	(+)	(+)	+
G-CSF	—	+	—	—	—
M-CSF	—	—	—	—	+
Erythropoietin	—	—	—	+	—
Meg-CSF	—	—	+	—	—

[a] *Synonyms*: stem cell factor, mast cell growth factor, kit-ligand.
[b] Strong synergism with lineage-specific growth factors.

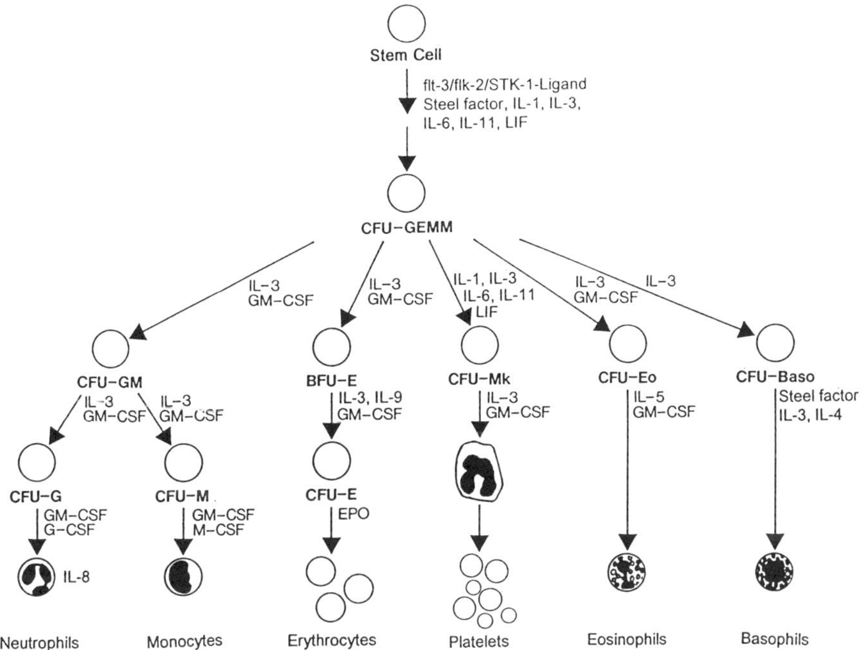

Figure 1

may be both stimulatory and inhibitory for hematopoietic cells. While stimulating early progenitor cells and granulopoiesis, IL-1 inhibits erythroid maturation. The in vivo effects of a given cytokine may be difficult to predict from in vitro experiments, because these cytokines form a network with a multitude of interactions at the level of both the immature progenitor cells and the functional end cells, which by themselves can be stimulated to secrete even more cytokines.

II. CLINICAL USE OF HEMATOPOIETIC GROWTH FACTORS

With the identification and recombinant production of the hematopoietic growth factors, these cytokines have been evaluated in the treatment of primary bone marrow failure states and after myelosuppressive chemotherapy or radiotherapy (1). In some areas, as in kidney failure patients with low endogenous erythropoietin levels, the substitution of a cytokine is already common practice, but in many other disease states the clinical value and best form of application of these cytokines are still under investigation (Table 2).

The formation of red blood cells is predominantly regulated by erythropoietin, a 30,400 D glycoprotein that is mainly (90%) produced in the peritubular interstitial

Table 2 Areas of Clinical Application of Hematopoietic Growth Factors

Reduction in chemotherapy- or radiotherapy-induced cytopenia
After conventional dose therapy
After dose escalation
After bone marrow transplantation
Stimulation of hematopoiesis in bone marrow failure states
Aplastic anemia
Chronic neutropenia
Agranulocytosis
Myelodysplastic syndromes
AIDS-associated neutropenia
Collection of hematopoietic progenitor cells
Mobilization of peripheral stem cells
Prestimulation of bone marrow progenitor cells
Replacement therapy for low or inadequate endogenous cytokine levels
Tumor-associated anemia
Chemotherapy-associated anemia
Stimulation of effector cell function in patients with
Infections
Burns
Disorders of leukocyte function
AIDS
Stimulation of antitumor activity

cells in the inner cortex of the kidneys (3). In adults, approximately 10% of erythropoietin is produced by hepatocytes. Hypoxia in the renal cortex is the major stimulus for erythropoietin production. Erythropoietin interacts with the receptor-bearing progenitor and precursor cells in the bone marrow. Erythropoietin is necessary for the replication and maturaton of the erythroid precursor cells to the mature erythrocyte. Under maximal erythropoietin stimulation this process can be expanded 10-fold. Under physiological conditions the response of the erythropoietin-secreting cells to hypoxemia is suboptimal, and in the anemia of chronic disease the plasma erythropoietin levels can be even lower relative to the degree of anemia. This suboptimal response implies that exogenous administration of pharmacological doses of erythropoietin will lead to expansion of erythropoiesis.

A. Tumor-Associated Anemia

Anemia is common in patients with advanced cancer. The etiology is multifactorial, including blood loss, hemolysis, nutritional deficiencies, bone marrow involvement by tumor, chemo- or radiotherapy, drug toxicity, hypersplenism, and the anemia of chronic disease. In patients with multiple myeloma, more than half of the patients and in the myelodysplastic syndromes nearly all patients have anemia at clinical onset. Depending on the pretreatment hemoglobin levels and the treatment used, about 20% of all patients with solid tumors in a regional cancer center require transfusions, with the highest rate of 34% in patients with lung cancer (4). In patients treated aggressively for acute leukemia, all patients require red blood cell transfusions. Some risks are associated with the transfusion of blood, however, including acute reactions of fever and chills, the risk of transmitting infections (hepatitis viruses and human immunodeficiency virus, HIV) and, possibly, immunosuppression.

The anemia of chronic disease (ACD), which is found in patients with chronic inflammatory, infectious, and neoplastic disorders, is one of the most frequently encountered anemias and is second in incidence to iron-deficiency anemia. Three features are characteristic of ACD: moderately shortened red blood cell survival, decreased iron reutilization in the bone marrow, and an erythropoietin response inadequate to the degree of anemia.

In patients with malignancies and in those undergoing bond marrow transplantation, the erythropoietin response to anemia is blunted, similar to patients with chronic infections. Several cytokines inhibit the production of erythropoietin, including IL-1 and TNF-α, but not interferon-γ (IFN-γ) (5). Also, various cytotoxic agents, including cisplatin and cyclosporin A, can inhibit erythropoietin production.

Because erythropoietin levels are even higher in patients with ACD than in nonanemic individuals, however, the decrease in the incremental response of erythropoietin to anemia cannot be regarded as the primary event. Cytokines that are elevated in patients with ACD-associated conditions and that inhibit erythroid progenitor cells colony-forming units–erythrocytes (CFU-E) include IL-1, TNF-α, IFN-α, IFN-β, and IFN-γ. The inhibition of CFU-E by IL-1 and TNF-α is indirect and mediated through induction of IFN-γ (6) and IFN-β (7), respectively. By interference with two levels of erythrocyte production, that is, by inhibition of erythropoietin production and marrow erythropoiesis, these cytokines may therefore amplify their effects on development of ACD.

B. Clinical Use of Erythropoietin

Indications for the use of erythropoietin in cancer patients include the prevention of homologous blood transfusion, with its immunosuppressive effects (8) and infectious risks, as well as the increased tissue oxygenation, which may improve the therapeutic effects of radiotherapy (9). It was previously established that erythropoietin treatment can correct anemia secondary to cancer in 40–50% of the patients (10–12), but higher response rates are seen in patients with multiple myeloma (10). The erythropoietin dosages needed in these patients are high, that is, 150–300 IU/kg/day, usually given as a subcutaneous bolus injection. Intravenous bolus injection is also possible but less effective. These erythropoietin dosages are well tolerated and are not associated with hypertensive reactions as long as the patient has no history of previous hypertension or atherosclerosis. In general, reversal of anemia is associated with an improved performance status.

Chemotherapy-induced anemia, that is, anemia following regimens with or without cisplatin, can also be ameliorated by treatment with erythropoietin, as demonstrated in several trials (10–14). As in patients with tumor-associated anemia, the erythropoietin dosage is high, that is, 150–300 IU/kg/day, usually given as a subcutaneous bolus injection. Erythropoietin has been given either after the end of the chemotherapy cycles or concomitantly if chemotherapy was not highly myelosuppressive. The increase in hematocrit and the improvement in quality of life in the erythropoietin-treated patients has been significant, and there was a trend for a reduction in the transfusion requirements in the large trials. Unfortunately, homologous blood transfusions cannot be avoided completely. Thus, besides the infectious risk, immunosuppression and a higher rate of tumor spread (8) associated with homologous blood transfusions still represent a potential risk that cannot be totally eliminated by the therapeutic use of erythropoietin.

The use of erythropoietin has also been evaluated in patients undergoing autologous or allogeneic bone marrow transplantation. In a large multicenter, placebo-controlled trial, high doses of erythropoietin were able to reduce the requirements for erythrocyte transfusions in patients undergoing allogeneic bone marrow transplantation who developed acute graft-versus-host disease (15). Furthermore, this reduction in erythrocyte transfusion needs was seen only after engraftment of the bone marrow, that is, in the fourth week after transplantation. No beneficial effect of erythropoietin was seen in patients undergoing autologous bone marrow transplantation. These findings can be explained by the increased production of IL-1β and TNF-α during the course of acute graft-verus-host disease. Both these cytokines not only are responsible for the blunted erythropoietin response to anemia but also suppress erythroid progenitor cell growth and maturation.

Prevention of radiotherapy-induced anemia by erythropoietin treatment has not yet been widely investigated, although improvements in therapeutic radiation by increased tissue oxygenation within the tumor and avoidance of the immunosuppressive effects of homologous blood could both result from the therapeutic use of erythropoietin (9). Initial results in patients with a variety of solid tumors indicate that the use of erythropoietin during supra- or infradiaphragmatic irradiation combined with oral iron supplementation leads to a significant increase in hematocrit (16,17). Whether the clinical results of irradiation will be improved as a result of increased tissue oxygenation must be the objective of future trials.

The response rates of patients who develop anemia as a result of primary disorders of the bone marrow are considerably lower than in patients suffering from ACD. The response rate is negligible in patients with acquired aplastic anemia, but the response rate to erythropoietin treatment ranges from 10 to 25% in patients with myelodysplastic syndromes (18). The erythropoietin dosages necessary for response are considerably higher than in patients with ACD. Instead of increasing the dosages, however, the combination of erythropoietin with other hematopoietic growth factors, such as granulocyte colony-stimulating factor (19,20) or granulocyte-macrophage colony-stimulating factor (21), apparently raises the response rate to 40–50%. Controlled, randomized trials are needed to confirm these promising initial results.

One of the problems of treatment with erythropoietin is the predictive value of laboratory parameters as to the likelihood of response in chronically anemic patients to an expensive treatment. In some but not all trials, the endogenous serum erythropoietin level was predictive, that is, the lower the endogenous level the higher the likelihood of a clinical response. In addition, the serum transferrin receptor level seems to be a useful indicator of erythropoietic expansion (22). As in the treatment of renal anemia, the presence of an active inflammatory process invariably prevents a response to treatment with erythropoietin.

C. Granulocyte Colony-Stimulating Factor and Granulocyte-Macrophage Colony-Stimulating Factor

G-CSF (23) is produced by activated monocytes and macrophages, neutrophils, fibroblasts, endothelial cells, and various tumor cell lines. The production is inducible by TNF-α, IL-1, GM-CSF, and endotoxin and inhibited by prostaglandin E_2. Natural G-CSF is an O-glycosylated monomeric glycoprotein. The sugar moiety is not necessary for the biological activity but prolongs the serum half-life. The gene for human G-CSF lies on chromosome 17. The biological activity of G-CSF is transduced through a high-affinity receptor.

The biological activity of G-CSF includes the stimulation of hematopoietic progenitor cells with an increased production of segmented neutrophils. In addition, the number of hematopoetic progenitor cells of all myeloid lineages in the peripheral blood is increased. G-CSF shortens the intramedullary maturation time within the neutrophilic lineage and accelerates the release of the neutrophils into the circulation. Treatment of undisturbed normal individual with an appropriate dose of G-CSF, such as 5 $\mu g/m^2$/day, results in a rapid release of the mature neutrophils from the bone marrow and marginal pools into the circulation, leading to a rise in neutrophil counts within hours. The increase in neutrophilic granulocytes observed during the following days results from a shortened maturation time and additional cell divisions at the promyelocyte and myelocyte levels. G-CSF also stimulates the phagocytosis and cytotoxicity of segmented neutrophils. Upon discontinuation of G-CSF treatment, the absolute neutrophil counts return to baseline levels within several days. In combination with earlier acting cytokines, such as Steel factor (kit-ligand), IL-3, or IL-6, G-CSF acts synergistically on progenitor cells. Myeloid but not lymphoid leukemias proliferate in response to G-CSF, as do some solid tumor cell lines.

GM-CSF (23) is produced and secreted by activated T lymphocytes, macrophages, and fibroblasts. The secretion is inducible by TNF-α, IL-1α, IL-2, interferons, and endotoxins, for example. GM-CSF is active as a monomer. Although glycosilated GM-CSF has a lower affinity to its receptor, both glycosylated and nonglycosylated forms are biologically active. Glycosylated GM-CSF has a longer serum half-life than the nonglycosylated molecule. The gene encoding GM-CSF is located on the long arm of human chromosome 5 in the vicinity of the gene for IL-3. The high-affinity GM-CSF receptor consists of an α and a β chain. The β chain is shared with the IL-3 and the IL-5 receptor.

The biological effects of GM-CSF include the stimulation of proliferation and differentiation of hematopoietic progenitor cells of the neutrophilic, monocytic, eosinophilic, early erythroid, and, partly, the megakaryocytic lineages. Additional effects are the functional stimulation of neutrophilic, eosinophilic, and basophilic granulocytes, as well as of monocyte-macrophages. Treatment with GM-CSF leads to an increase in the number of multilineage and lineage-committed progenitor cells. The half-life of neutrophilic granulocytes in the circulation is prolonged by GM-CSF from 7–8 h to more than 40 h. Myeloid but not lymphoid leukemic cells are stimulated upon exposure to GM-CSF. Some solid tumor cell lines respond to GM-CSF.

1. Tumor-Associated Neutropenia

Neutropenia in cancer patients usually results from treatment with myelosuppressive agents, including ionizing radiation. Apart from leukemia and disseminated lymphoma, it only rarely is the consequence of bone marrow involvement with tumor cells. Chemotherapy for cancer can lead to life-threatening neutropenia, which is the major cause of fever, infection morbidity, and mortality. In addition, neutropenia and neutropenia-associated infection are the major dose-limiting adverse effects of chemotherapy. The most important risk factor for infection is the severity and duration of neutropenia (24). With the advent of recombinant hematopoietic growth factors, especially G-CSF and GM-CSF, the management of cancer patients with treatment-induced neutropenia has therefore considerably changed.

2. Neutropenia After Cytotoxic Therapy

In general, hematopoietic growth factors, such as GM-CSF or G-CSF, can be used prophylactically, that is, to prevent infectious complications, or therapeutically at the time of febrile neutropenia, that is, when an infection is suspected.

The vast majority of the published trials have studied the effect of prophylactic treatment with either G-CSF or GM-CSF after chemotherapy or myeloablative chemotherapy with or without total-body irradiation followed by bone marrow transplantation. At the present time, neither GM-CSF nor G-CSF should be applied immediately before or concomitantly with chemotherapy or radiotherapy, because through stimulation into the cell cycle the sensitivity of normal hematopoietic progenitor cells toward the action of cytotoxic agents might be increased (25). Although sometimes observed in vitro (26–28), stimulation of tumor cell growth by GM-CSF or G-CSF has not been documented in the randomized trials apart from the myeloid leukemias.

Clinical trials with GM-CSF or G-CSF after standard chemotherapy protocols have clearly demonstrated that CSFs can reduce the treatment-associated myelosuppression by shortening the duration of neutropenia, reducing the nadir of neutrophil counts, and thereby allowing adherence to the chemotherapy regimens with improved dosing and scheduling (29–34). Depending on the aggressiveness of chemotherapy, alleviation of neutropenia with shortening of neutropenia by about 1 week results in a reduction in the rate of infections and use of antibiotics and a shorter stay in the hospital. G-CSF and GM-CSF are also successfully used in acquired immunodeficiency syndrome (AIDS) patients treated with chemotherapy for malignant lymphoma to reduce the severity and duration of neutropenia (35). However, GM-CSF treatment is associated with increased serum p24 antigen levels, indicating the induction of HIV-1 replication. The occurrence, severity, and duration of thrombocytopenia and anemia are not reduced by G-CSF or GM-CSF.

In randomized trials in patients with small cell lung cancer (29,32) and malignant lymphoma (31), postchemotherapeutic use of G-CSF resulted in less severe neutropenia and a reduction in the number of febrile neutropenic events. In some but not all trials, patients in the G-CSF-treated groups needed fewer antibiotics and were admitted to the hospital less frequently or were discharged from the hospital earlier. Although patients receiving G-CSF received a 10–15% higher average dosage of chemotherapy, no difference in the efficacy of chemotherapy, that is, in the remission rate, was noted. Similar observations were made with the use of GM-CSF (30,33,34). It therefore has been the criticism of the trials using G-CSF or GM-CSF after conventional dose chemotherapy that better adherence to the chemotherapy was not accompanied by a better response rate or survival of the patients. However, it must be remembered that the actual mortality rate of the trials in which both G-CSF and GM-CSF were tested was rather low.

Despite the lack of clear data that demonstrate that the use of G-CSF or GM-CSF had any major beneficial effect on the rate of treatment-related deaths or on the overall survival of the patients, there appear to be several settings in which the use of hematopoietic growth factors after conventional chemotherapy should be considered (Table 3). Since 6 days of grade IV neutropenia are

Table 3 Ways to Use G-CSF/GM-CSF After Moderately Myelosuppressive Chemotherapy

Primary prophylaxis:	G-CSF/GM-CSF given after each cycle of chemotherapy
Advantage:	most protection against febrile neutropenia
Disadvantage:	expensive since no selection
Secondary prophylaxis:	G-CSF/GM-CSF given only to patients with significant neutropenia during previous chemotherapy cycle
Advantage:	cytokine use restricted to those patients who have been shown to develop neutropenia (selection)
Disadvantage:	less protection against febrile neutropenia
Therapeutic use:	G-CSF/GM-CSF only given to patients with febrile neutropenia
Advantage:	cytokine use further restricted to those patients with suspected infection
Disadvantage:	lack of consistent evidence that cytokines in addition to antibiotics offer a major advantage in this situation

associated with more than a 50% incidence of fever and infection but a duration of grade IV neutropenia of only 3 days is significantly less risky (29), the prophylactic use of G-CSF or GM-CSF should be considered in any myelosuppressive chemotherapy regimens with a similar or higher risk of grade IV neutropenia. Similarly, in elderly patients with a higher risk of infectious complications or in those with concomitant diseases, the prophylactic use of cytokines should be considered. Another approach is the secondary prophylaxis: that is, individual patients with a significant myelosuppression to a normally less myelosuppressive chemotherapy regimen should be considered for receiving G-CSF or GM-CSF after the subsequent chemotherapy cycles. Using such an approach, it is still possible to adhere to the intended full-dose chemotherapy but not to reduce chemotherapy dosage or to delay treatment (29). Yet another approach would be the use of CSFs only in the case of suspected infection during neutropenia (36,37). A large multicenter trial on this interventional use in patients who develop febrile neutropenia after chemotherapy showed that subcutaneous G-CSF, 12 μg/kg/day, will be of moderate benefit (36).

Intravenous and subcutaneous administration of G-CSF is effective for elevating serum G-CSF concentrations (Table 4) (23). The recommended starting dose of G-CSF is 5 μg/kg/day given by subcutaneous bolus injection or intravenous infusion. Higher dosages up to 60 μg/kg have been applied in the phase I trials without reaching a dose-limiting toxicity. Administration of G-CSF is usually started 1 day after cessation of chemotherapy cycle to allow clearance

Table 4 Colony-Stimulating Factors Approved for Clinical Application

Cytokine	Generic name	Manufacturer	Dosage[a]	Route of application[b]
G-CSF	Filgrastim	Amgen/LaRoche	5–10 μg/kg	SC, IV
	Lenograstim	Chugai/Rhone Poulenc	150 μg/m^2	SC, IV
GM-CSF	Molgramostim	Schering/Sandoz	5–10 μg/kg	SC, IV
	Sargramostim	Immunex	150 μg/m^2	SC, IV

[a]Standard dose.
[b]SC, subcutaneous (bolus); IV, intravenous (continuous, short infusion, bolus).

of the cytotoxic drugs and continued until the recovery of the neutrophils above 5000/μl after the expected chemotherapy-induced nadir. There is usually a small drop in neutrophil counts after discontinuation of G-CSF, which should be of no concern, however. The interval between the end of chemotherapy and the start of G-CSF can be extended up to 4 days without losing the effect of G-CSF on neutrophil recovery.

GM-CSF is effective after both subcutaneous and intravenous administration (23). The usual dose is 5 μg/kg/day starting the day after the end of chemotherapy until the recovery of the granulocyte counts. It is not yet known whether the administration of GM-CSF can be delayed for several days without losing the effect on neutrophil recovery.

The use of G-CSF or GM-CSF after aggressive chemotherapy for myeloid malignancies (acute myeloid leukemia, AML, advanced myelodysplastic syndromes, and blast crisis of chronic myeloid leukemia) is still controversial. In a randomized trial, G-CSF started after the end of chemotherapy significantly enhanced neutrophil recovery and reduced the incidence of documented infections without promoting the regrowth of leukemic cells (38). In elderly patients with AML, use of GM-CSF seems to reduce the risk of early death (39). Sensitization of myeloid leukemic blast cells to chemotherapy by pretreatment and concomitant treatment with either GM-CSF or G-CSF is still experimental and until now has not proven advantage over conventional therapy. The use of G-CSF in parallel with chemotherapy in patients with acute lymphoblastic leukemia can reduce the duration and severity of neutropenia (40). However, the increased intensity of chemotherapy resulted in more pronounced thrombocytopenia and an increased need for platelet transfusions.

3. High-Dose Chemotherapy and the Use of G-CSF or GM-CSF

The rationale for dose intensification is the existence of a dose-response relationship for chemosensitive malignancies, not only for tumors in animal models (41) but also for chemosensitive human tumors. The steeper the dose-response curve, the more likely it is that dose intensification will be able to produce significant clinical benefits. Dose intensification may be achieved by increasing the dose of the individual drugs or by shortening the time interval between treatment cycles. By increasing the dosage of the drugs, it may even be possible not only to kill a higher fraction of sensitive tumor cells but also to overcome drug resistance.

Studies on dose intensification with the use of CSFs have shown that with allowances for greater toxicity during the hematological nadir, the doses of predominantly neutropenia-inducing agents, such as cyclophosphamide, taxol, mitoxantrone, and etoposide, can be increased 1.5- to 3-fold (42–47). The failure to counter the deep neutrophil nadirs, cumulative thrombocytopenia, increased need for erythrocyte transfusions, and extramyeloid toxicities associated with increased chemotherapy intensity limit the use of postchemotherapy G-CSF or GM-CSF. It must be stressed that at the present time intensification of the chemotherapy regimens by the use of CSFs has not resulted in improved survival rates. The use of earlier acting hematopoietic growth factors and/or the administration of CSF-mobilized peripheral blood progenitor cell populations will probably be necessary to provide sufficient myeloprotection.

4. Use of CSFs After Bone Marrow Transplantation (BMT)

High-dose chemotherapy followed by autologous bone marrow and/or peripheral blood stem cell transplantation represents the ultimate dose escalation (48,49). Prophylactic use of G-CSF or GM-CSF after autologous bone marrow transplantation for lymphomas and solid tumors results in a shortening of neutropenia by about 1 week, which is associated with a shorter duration of parenteral nutrition and time of hospitalization (50–55). Because the period of severe neutropenia, that is, $<100/\mu l$, is not shortened after autologous BMT, the rate of infections is not always clearly reduced. In allogeneic transplantation, the early neutrophil recovery is accelerated by the use of G-CSF or GM-CSF, without having an effect on the rate of febrile days or use of antibiotics (56,57). The incidence of graft-versus-host disease is not increased by either G-CSF or GM-CSF treatment. When GM-CSF is used in patients undergoing unrelated bone marrow transplantation, ANC recovery is accelerated without, however, affecting the incidence of bacteremia, graft-versus-host disease, or graft failure or the time to hospital discharge (58).

5. Autologous Transfusion of Circulating Hematopoietic Progenitor Cells

G-CSF and GM-CSF can be used to increase the number of circulating hematopoietic progenitor cells 5- to 15-fold (59–63). This increase in circulating progenitor cells can be achieved by cytokine treatment alone, that is, without prior chemotherapy, or in the rebound phase of chemotherapy during treatment with G-CSF/GM-CSF. The collection and readministration of these peripheral progenitor cells after myeloablative chemotherapy results not only in the rapid recovery of the neutrophils within a median period of about 10 days but also in the recovery of platelet counts within the same time period. Neither G-CSF nor GM-CSF given after the reinfusion of the peripheral progenitor cells results in further acceleration of hematopoietic recovery. This is not surprising, because it was shown that after myeloablative therapy the endogenous serum G-CSF concentrations are in the same range as can be achieved with therapeutic administration of the recombinant molecule.

For the planning of peripheral blood stem cell transfusions, it is important to know that patients who have received extensive prior chemotherapy and/or radiotherapy experience the smallest increase in circulating hematopoietic progenitor cells (64). Thus, in these patients, the collection of a sufficient number of progenitor cells can pose a problem. A possible solution to this problem of insufficient mobilization of progenitor cells could be the combined application of growth factors, for example an early-acting cytokine, such as Steel factor or IL-3, followed by a later acting factor, such as G-CSF or GM-CSF (64–66).

Besides a more rapid regeneration of platelet counts in comparison with the use of bone marrow cells, peripheral blood progenitor cells may be less contaminated with tumor cells, resulting in a lower relapse rate after autologous transplantation, for example, for non-Hodgkin's lymphoma (49). However, carefully controlled studies are needed in which the contamination of the autologous graft is monitored (67).

6. Adverse Effects of G-CSF and GM-CSF (23)

G-CSF is usually well tolerated, bone pain being the most frequent adverse effect but for which an analgesic is rarely needed. G-CSF does not affect the occurrence of adverse effects of cytostatic drugs on organ systems other than the bone marrow, mild bone pain being the only toxicity related directly to G-CSF (Table 5). Long-term administration of G-CSF in patients with chronic neutropenia can lead to clinically inapparent splenomegaly and, sometimes, thrombocytopenia. Other unusual adverse effects are cutaneous neutrophilic dermatitis (Sweet's syndrome) and the flaring of chronic inflammatory disorders, including vasculitis and rheumatoid arthritis. Alterations of laboratory parameters comprise an increase in serum alkaline phosphatase, serum lactate dehydrogenase, and uric acid. Tumor cells, with the exception of myeloid leukemias, are not usually stimulated by G-CSF.

Frequent side effects associated with glycosylated and nonglycosylated GM-CSF are predominantly fever and bone pain, which respond well to analgesics (Table 5). Erythema is frequent at the site of subcutaneous administration. At high dosages of 20–30 μg/kg/day, which are usually not used clinically, pericarditis and pleural effusions can occur. A "first-dose reaction" is

Table 5 Adverse Effects of G-CSF and GM-CSF

Grade	G-CSF	GM-CSF
Moderate	Bone pain, increase serum alkaline phosphatase, lactate dehydrogenase, γ-glutamyltransferase, uric acid	Bone pain, myalgia, lethargy, fever, exanthema, thrombophlebitis, "first-dose effect," decreased serum albumin and cholesterol, increased serum alkaline phosphatase and γ-glutamyltransferase
Dose limiting	Thrombocytopenia (rare), Sweet's syndrome (acute febrile neutrophilic dermatitis), vasculitis	Thrombocytopenia (rare), pericarditis, angioedema, capillary leakage syndrome

seen after the initial dose of nonglycosylated GM-CSF and is characterized by flushing, hypotension, transient hypoxia, and tachycardia. This reaction is not seen with continuing GM-CSF administration, but can recur after a 10 day GM-CSF-free interval. With glycosylated GM-CSF, a capillary leakage syndrome can occur at high dosages. Alterations in laboratory values include a hypoalbuminemia, a decrease in serum cholesterol levels, and an increase in serum alkaline phosphatase. Treatment with GM-CSF has been associated with transient thrombocytopenia. An idiopathic thrombocytopenic purpura can be reactivated, as can preexisting inflammatory disorders. The physiological basis for most of the adverse events seen during GM-CSF treatment appears to be the stimulation of monocytes-macrophages, which are primed to secrete increased amounts of IL-1, TNF-α, IL-6, and IL-8. Although some reports describe the stimulation of solid tumor cell lines and fresh tumor cell samples by GM-CSF, this has not been seen in the clinical trials when GM-CSF was used after chemotherapy. Exceptions are, of course, neoplasias of the myeloid system.

III. STIMULATION OF THROMBOCYTOPOIESIS

One of the major problems in the use of hematopoietic growth factors for acceleration of hematopoietic recovery after myelosuppressive therapy is the lack of a clinically tested cytokine that abrogates thrombocytopenia. Although some cytokines have already shown thrombopoietic activity in clinical trials, including IL-3 (68–70), IL-1 (71), and IL-6 (72), and others are being evaluated, such as IL-11 and leukemia inhibitory factor, these cytokines act at a relatively early stage of megakaryopoiesis (73). Therefore, the platelet response is delayed and in general marginal when these cytokines are used after chemotherapy. The search for and the recombinant production of a "thrombopoietin" with activity at late stages of megakaryocyte maturation and platelet production has recently been successful (77–79). Until such a factor has been tested clinically, the use of autologous peripheral stem cells could overcome the period of prolonged thrombocytopenia after highly aggressive chemo- or radiotherapy.

IV. COMBINATION OF SEVERAL GROWTH FACTORS

Although the majority of trials until now have studied the effect of single hematopoietic growth factors after myelosuppressive chemotherapy, the suppression of hematopoiesis most of the time is multilineage. Therefore, there is good reason for using growth factors that stimulate different cell lineages. These combinations include erythropoietin and either G-CSF or GM-CSF. From preliminary studies in patients with AIDS, we know that the combination of G-CSF and erythropoietin leads to an increase in both the hematocrit and neutrophil counts (74). In patients with myelodysplastic syndromes, the same growth factor combination or the combination of GM-CSF and erythropoietin acts somewhat synergistically on the increase in hematocrit, raising the response rate from 10–20% to 40% (19–21). Whether these growth factor combinations act additively or synergistically after myelosuppressive chemotherapy has not yet been established.

A different approach with regard to combinations of different hematopoietic growth factors is the combination of factors acting at different levels in the hematopoietic hierarchy, that is, the combination of early-acting and late-acting cytokines. This approach aims to induce synergistic activities, thereby potentiating the effect of the later acting cytokines or obtaining totally new hematopoietic effects not seen with single cytokines. Thus, the use of an early-acting cytokine could stimulate the proliferation of immature progenitor cells and thereby expand the number of cells susceptible to the action of late-acting cytokines. A different mechanism of action of early-acting cytokines could be an increase in the number of high-affinity receptors for the late-acting factors.

A combination that has been tested in this regard is IL-3 and GM-CSF (64–66,75); the combination of Steel factor and G-CSF is under evaluation. Because, until now, only a few combination schedules have been tested, it is not yet known whether these factors should be given sequentially or concomitantly. In addition, the adverse effects of the second cytokine can be aggravated by the use of the earlier acting cytokine. A comparable approach is the use of fusion proteins, such as PIXY 321, which contains both the IL-3 and the GM-CSF moiety (76).

The combinations of early- and late-acting cytokines in preliminary studies were able to increase substantially the number of circulating hematopoietic progenitor cells in patients who had not been pretreated with chemotherapy or in those patients recovering from antitumor therapy (64–66,75). It is not yet known, however, whether the progenitor cells harvested from the peripheral blood of patients receiving combinations of cytokines possess a higher repopulating capacity than those harvested after single cytokine treatment.

REFERENCES

1. Groopman JE, Molina JM, Scadden DT. Hematopoietic growth factors. Biology and clinical applications. N Engl J Med 1991; 321:1449–1459.
2. Moore MAS. Clinical implications of positive and negative hematopoietic stem cell regulators. Blood 1991; 78:1–19.
3. Krantz SB. Erythropoietin. Blood 1991; 77:419–434.
4. Skillings JR, Sridhar FG, Wong C, Peddock L. The frequency of red cell transfusion for anemia in patients receiving chemotherapy: a retrospective cohort study. Am J Clin Oncol Cancer Clin Trials 1993; 16:22–25.
5. Faquin WC, Schneider TJ, Goldberg MA. Effect of inflammatory cytokines on hypoxia-induced erythropoietin production. Blood 1992; 79:1987–1994.
6. Means RT, Dessypris EN, Krantz SB. Inhibition of human erythroid colony-forming units by interleukin-1 is mediated by gamma-interferon. J Cell Physiol 1992; 150:59–64.
7. Means RT, Krantz SB. Inhibition of human erythroid colony-forming units by tumor necrosis factor requires beta interferon. J Clin Invest 1993; 91:416–419.
8. Busch ORC, Hop WCJ, Hoynck van Papendrecht MAW, et al. Blood transfusions and prognosis in colorectal cancer. N Engl J Med 1993; 328:1372–1376.
9. Levine EA, Vijayakumar S. Blood transfusion in patients receiving radical radiotherapy: a reappraisal. Onkologie 1993; 16:79–87.
10. Ludwig H, Fritz E, Kotzmann H, et al. Erythropoietin treatment of anemia associated with multiple myeloma. N Engl J Med 1990; 322:1693–1699.
11. Oster W, Herrmann F, Gamm H, et al. Erythropoietin for the treatment of anemia of malignancy. J Clin Oncol 1990; 8:956–962.
12. Abels R, Larholt KM, Krantz KD, Bryant EC. Recombinant human erythropoietin (rHuEPO) for the treatment of the anemia of cancer. In: Murphy MJ, ed. Blood Cell Growth Factors: Their Present and Future Use in Hematology and Oncology. Dayton: AlphaMed Press, 1991:121–141.
13. Case DC, Bukowski RM, Carey RW, et al. Recombinant human erythropoietin therapy for anemic cancer patients on combination chemotherapy. J Natl Cancer Inst 1993; 85:801–806.
14. Markman M, Reichman B, Hakes T, et al. The use of recombinant human erythropoietin to prevent carboplatin-induced anemia. Gynecol Oncol 1993; 49:172–176.
15. Link H, Fauser A, Hübner G, et al. Recombinant human erythropoietin after bone marrow transplantation: a prospective placebo controlled trial in Europe. Blood 1993; 80(suppl 1):284A.
16. Vijayakumar S, Roach M, Wara W, et al. Effect of subcutaneous recombinant human erythropoietin in cancer patients receiving radiotherapy: preliminary results

of a randomized, open-labeled, phase II trial. Int J Radiat Oncol Biol Phys 1993; 26:721–729.

17. Lavey RS, Dempsey WH. Erythropoietin increases hemoglobin in cancer patients during radiation therapy. Int J Radiat Oncol Biol Phys 1993; 27:1147–1152.
18. Ganser A, Hoelzer D. Treatment of myelodysplastic syndromes with hematopoietic growth factors. Hematol Oncol Clin North Am 1992; 9:632–653.
19. Negrin RS, Stein R, Vardiman J, et al. Treatment of the anemia of myelodysplastic syndromes using recombinant human granulocyte colony-stimulating factor in combination with erythropoietin. Blood 1993; 82:737–743.
20. Hellström-Lindberg E, Birgegard G, Carlsson M, et al. A combination of granulocyte colony-stimulating factor and erythropoietin may synergistically improve the anaemia in patients with myelodysplastic syndromes. Leukemia Lymphoma 1993; 11:221–228.
21. Hansen PB, Johnsen HE, Hippe E, et al. Recombinant human granulocyte-macrophage colony-stimulating factor plus recombinant human erythropoietin may improve anemia in selected patients with myelodysplastic syndromes. Am J Hematol 1993; 44:229–236.
22. Beguin Y, Clemons GK, Pootrakul P, Fillet G. Quantitative assessment of erythropoiesis and functional classification of anemia based on measurements of serum transferrin receptor and erythropoietin. Blood 1993; 81:1067–1076.
23. Lieschke GJ, Burgess AW. Drug therapy: granulocyte colony-stimulating factor and granulocyte-macrophage colony-stimulating factor. N Engl J Med 1992; 327:28–35, 99–106.
24. Bodey GP, Buckley M, Sathe YS, Freireich EJ. Quantitative relationships between circulating leukocytes and infection in patients with acute leukemia. Ann Intern Med 1966; 64:328–340.
25. Momin F, Kraut M, Lattin P, Valdivieso M. Thrombocytopenia in patients receiving chemoradiotherapy and G-CSF for locally advanced non-small cell lung cancer (NSCLC) (abstract). Proc Am Soc Clin Oncol 1992; 11:294.
26. Park LS, Waldron PE, Friend D, et al. Interleukin-3, GM-CSF, and G-CSF receptor expression on cell lines and primary leukemia cells: receptor heterogeneity and relationship to growth factor responsiveness. Blood 1989; 74:56–65.
27. Berdel WE, Danhauser-Riedl S, Steinhauser G, Winton EF. Various human hematopoietin growth factors (interleukin-3, GM-CSF, G-CSF) stimulate clonal growth of non hematopoietic tumor cells. Blood 1989; 73:80–83.
28. Dippold WG, Klingel R, Kerlin M, et al. Stimulation of pancreatic and gastric carcinoma cell growth by interleukin 3 and granulocyte-macrophage colony-stimulating factor. Gastroenterology 1991; 100:1338–1344.
29. Crawford J, Ozer H, Stoller R, et al. Reduction by granulocyte colony-stimulating factor of fever and neutropenia induced by chemotherapy in patients with small cell lung cancer. N Engl J Med 1991; 325:164–170.
30. deVries EGE, Biesma B, Willemse PHB, et al. A double-blind placebo-controlled study of granulocyte-macrophage colony-stimulating factor during chemotherapy for ovarian carcinoma. Cancer Res 1991; 51:116–122.
31. Pettengell R, Gurney H, Radford JA, et al. Granulocyte colony-stimulating factor

to prevent dose-limiting neutropenia in non-Hodgkin's lymphoma: a randomized controlled trial. Blood 1992; 80:1430–1436.
32. Trillet-Lenoir V, Green J, Manegold C, et al. Recombinant granulocyte colony stimulating factor reduces the infectious complications of cytotoxic chemotherapy. Eur J Cancer 1993; 29A:319–324.
33. Hovgaard DJ, Nissen NI. Effect of recombinant granulocyte-macrophage colony-stimulating factor in patients with Hodgkin's disease—phase III trial. J Clin Oncol 1992; 10:390–397.
34. Gerhartz HH, Engelhard M, Meusers P, et al. Randomized, double-blind, placebo-controlled, phase III study of recombinant human granulocyte/macrophage colony stimulating factor as adjunct to induction-treatment of high-grade non-Hodgkin lymphomas. Blood 1993; 82:2329–2339.
35. Kaplan LD, Kahn JO, Crowe S, et al. Clinical and virological effects of human granulocyte-macrophage colony-stimulating factor in patients receiving chemotherapy for human immunodeficiency virus-associated non-Hodgkin's lymphoma—results of a randomized trial. J Clin Oncol 1991; 9:1329–1331.
36. Maher D, Green M, Bishop J, et al. Randomized, placebo-controlled trial of Filgrastim (r-metHuG-CSF) in patients with febrile neutropenia (FN) following chemotherapy (CT) (abstract). Proc Am Soc Clin Oncol 1993; 12:432.
37. Mayordomo JJ, Rivera F, Diaz-Puente, et al. Decreasing morbidity and cost of treating febrile neutropenia by adding G-CSF and GM-CSF to standard antibiotic therapy: results of a randomized trial (abstract). Proc Am Soc Clin Oncol 1993; 12:437.
38. Ohno R, Tomonaga M, Kobayashi T. Effect of granuöocyte colony-stimulating factor after intensive induction chemotherapy in relapsed or refractory acute leukemia. N Engl J Med 1990; 323:871–877.
39. Büchner T, Hiddemann W, Koenigsmann M, et al. Recombinant human granulocyte-macrophage colony-stimulating factor after chemotherapy in patients with acute myeloid leukemia at higher age of after relapse. 1991; 78:1190–1197.
40. Ottmann OG, Ganser A, Freund M, et al. Simultaneous administration of granulocyte colony-stimulating factor (filgrastim) and induction chemotherapy in acute lymphoblastic leukemia. Ann Hematol 1993; 67:161–167.
41. Skipper HE. Dose intensity versus total dose of chemotherapy: An experimental basis. In: DeVita VT, Hellman S, Rosenberg SA, eds. Important Advances in Oncology 1990. Philadelphia: J. B. Lippincott, 1990:43–64.
42. Bronchud MH, Howell A, Crowther D, et al. The use of granulocyte colony-stimulating factor to increase the intensity of treatment with doxorubicin in patients with advanced breast and ovarian cancer. Br J Cancer 1989; 60:120–125.
43. Steward WP, Verweij J, Somers R, et al. Granulocyte-macrophage colony-stimulating factor allows safe escalation of dose-intensity of chemotherapy in metastatic adult soft tissue sarcomas: a study of the European organization for research and treatment of cancer soft tissue and bone sarcoma group. J Clin Oncol 1993; 11:15–21.
44. Ajani JA, Roth JA, Ryan MB, et al. Intensive preoperative chemotherapy with colony-stimulating factor for resectable adenocarcinoma of the esophagus or gastroesophageal junction. J Clin Oncol 1993; 11:22–28.

45. Seidman AD, Scher HI, Gabrilove JL, et al. Dose-intensification of MVAC with recombinant granulocyte colony-stimulating factor as initial therapy in advanced urothelial cancer. J Clin Oncol 1993; 11:408–414.
46. Savarese DMF, Denicoff AM, Berg SL, et al. Phase I study of high-dose piroxantrone with granulocyte colony-stimulating factor. J Clin Oncol 1993; 11:1795–1803.
47. Rowinski EK, Chaudry V, Forastiere AA, et al. Phase I and pharmacologic study of paclitaxel and cisplatin with granulocyte colony-stimulating factor: neuromuscular toxicity in dose-limiting. J Clin Oncol 1993; 11:2010–2020.
48. Peters WP, Ross M, Vredenburgh JJ, et al. High-dose chemotherapy and autologous bone marrow support as consolidation after standard-dose adjuvant therapy for high-risk primary breast cancer. J Clin Oncol 1993; 11:1132–1143.
49. Vose JM, Anderson JR, Kessinger A, et al. High-dose chemotherapy and autologous hematopoietic stem-cell transplantation for aggressive non-Hodgkin's lymphoma. J Clin Oncol 1993; 11:1846–1851.
50. Brandt SJ, Peters WP, Atwater SJ, et al. Effect of recombinant human granulocyte-macrophage colony-stimulating factor on hematopoietic reconstitution after high-dose chemotherapy and autologous marrow transplantation. N Engl J Med 1988; 318:869–876.
51. Nemunaitis J, Rabinowe SN, Singer J, et al. Recombinant granulocyte-macrophage colony-stimulating factor after autologous bone marrow transplantation for lymphoid cancer. N Engl J Med 1991; 324:1773–1778.
52. Advani R, Chao NJ, Horning SJ, et al. Granulocyte-macrophage colony-stimulating factor (GM-CSF) as an adjunct to autologous hemopoietic stem cell transplantation for lymphoma. Ann Intern Med 1992; 116:183–189.
53. Gorin NC, Coiffier B, Hayat M, et al. Recombinant human granulocyte-macrophage colony-stimulating factor after high-dose chemotherapy and autologous bone marrow transplantation with unpurged and purged marrow in non-Hodgkin's lymphoma: a double-blind placebo-controlled trial. Blood 1992; 80:1149–1157.
54. Gulati SC, Bennett CL. Granulocyte-macrophage colony-stimulating factor (GM-CSF) as adjunct therapy in relapsed Hodgkin disease. Ann Intern Med 1992; 116:177–182.
55. Link H, Boogaerts MA, Carella AM, et al. A controlled trial of recombinant human granulocyte-macrophage colony-stimulating factor after total body irradiation, high-dose chemotherapy, and autologous bone marrow transplantation for acute lymphoblastic leukemia or malignant lymphoma. Blood 1992; 80:2188–2195.
56. Asano S, Masaoka T, Takaku F, Ogawa N. Placebo controlled double blind trial of recombinant human granulocyte colony-stimulating factor for bone marrow transplantation. Jpn J Med 1990; 3:317–324.
57. Powles R, Smith C, Milan S, et al. Human recombinant GM-CSF in allogenic bone-marrow transplantation for leukemia: double-blind, placebo-controlled trial. Lancet 1990; 336:1417–1420.
58. Appelbaum F. Personal communication 1994.
59. Gianni AM, Bregni M, Stern AC, et al. Granulocyte-macrophage colony-stimulating factor to harvest circulating haemopoietic stem cells for autotransplantation. Lancet 1989; 333:580–584.
60. Elias AD, Ayash L, Anderson KC, et al. Mobilization of peripheral blood progenitor

cells by chemotherapy and granulocyte-macrophage colony-stimulating factor for hematologic support after high-dose intensification for breast cancer. Blood 1992; 79:3036–3044.

61. Sheridan WP, Begley CG, Juttner CA, et al. Effect of peripheral-blood progenitor cells mobilised by filgrastim (G-CSF) on platelet recovery after high-dose chemotherapy. Lancet 1992; 339:640–644.
62. Shea TC, Mason JR, Storniolo AM, et al. Sequential cycles of high-dose carboplatin administration with recombinant human granulocyte-macrophage colony-stimulating factor and repeated infusions of autologous peripheral blood progenitor cells: a novel and effective method for delivering multiple courses of dose intensive therapy. J Clin Oncol 1992; 10:464–473.
63. Tepler I, Cannistra SA, Frei E, et al. Use of peripheral-blood progenitor cells abrogates the myelotoxicity of repetitive outpatient high-dose carboplatin and cyclophosphamide chemotherapy. J Clin Oncol 1993; 11:1583–1591.
64. Brugger W, Frisch J, Schulz G, et al. Sequential administration of interleukin-3 and granulocyte-macrophage colony-stimulating factor following standard-dose combination chemotherapy with etoposide, ifosfamide, and cisplatin. J Clin Oncol 1992; 10:1452–1459.
65. Brugger W, Bross K, Frisch J, et al. Mobilization of peripheral blood progenitor cells by sequential administration of interleukin-3 and granulocyte-macrophage colony-stimulating factor following polychemotherapy with etoposide, ifosfamide, and cisplatin. Blood 1992; 79:1193–1200.
66. Haas R, Ehrhardt R, Witt B, et al. Autografting with peripheral blood stem cells mobilized by sequential interleukin-3/granulocyte-macrophage colony-stimulating factor following high-dose chemotherapy in non-Hodgkin's lymphoma. Bone Marrow Transplant 1993; 12:643–649.
67. Moss TJ, Sandes DG, Lasky LC, Bostrom B. Contamination of peripheral blood stem cell harvests by circulating neuroblastoma cells. Blood 1990; 75:1879–1883.
68. Ganser A, Lindemann A, Seipelt G, et al. Effect of recombinant human interleukin-3 in patients with normal hematopoiesis and in patients with bone marrow failure. Blood 1990; 76:666–676.
69. Biesma B, Willemse PHB, Mulder NH, et al. Effects of interleukin-3 after chemotherapy for advanced ovarian cancer. Blood 1992; 80:1141–1148.
70. Postmus PE, Gietema JA, Damsma O, et al. Effects of recombinant human interleukin-3 in patients with relapsed small-cell lung cancer treated with chemotherapy: a dose-finding study. J Clin Oncol 1992; 10:1131–1140.
71. Smith JW, Longo DL, Alvord G, et al. The effects of treatment with interleukin-1alpha on platelet recovery after high-dose carboplatin. N Engl J Med 1993; 328:756–761.
72. Weber J, Yang JC, Topalian SL, et al. Phase I trial of subcutaneous interleukin-6 in patients with advance malignancies. J Clin Oncol 1993; 11:499–506.
73. Gordon MS, Hoffman R. Growth factors affecting human thrombopoiesis: potential agents for the treatment of thrombocytoenia. Blood 1992; 80:302–307.
74. Miles SA, Mitsyasu RT, Moreno J, et al. Combined therapy with recombinant granulocyte colony-stimulating factor and erythropoietin decreases hematologic toxicity from zidovudine. Blood 1991; 77:2109–2117.

75. Ganser A, Lindemann A, Seipelt G, et al. Sequential in vivo treatment with two recombinant hematopoietic growth factors (interleukin-3 and granulocyte-macrophage colony-stimulating factor) as a new therapeutic modality to stimulate hematopoiesis. Results of a phase I study. Blood 1992; 79:2583–2591.
76. Vadhan-Raj S, Papadopoulos N, Burgess A, et al. Effects of PIXY 321 a granulocyte-macrophage colony-stimulating factor/interleukin-3 fusion protein reduces chemotherapy-induced multilineage myelosuppression in patients with sarcoma. J Clin Oncol 1994; 12:715–724.
77. De Sauvage FJ, Hass PE, Spencer SD, et al. Stimulation of megakaryocytopoiesis and thrombopoiesis by the c-Mpl ligand. Nature 1994; 369:533–538.
78. Lok S, Kaushansky K, Holly RD, et al. Cloning and expression of murine thrombopoietin cDNA and stimulation of platelet production in vivo. Nature 1994; 369:565–568.
79. Bartley TD, Bogenberger J, Hunt P, et al. Identification and cloning of a megakaryocyte growth and development factor that is a ligand for the cytokine receptor Mpl. Cell 1994; 77:1117–1124.

Index

About the Editors

Jean Klastersky is Chief of the Department of Medicine and a Professor of Medicine, Medical Oncology, and Physical Diagnosis at the Institut Jules Bordet, Université Libre de Bruxelles, Belgium. The editor or coeditor of over 10 books and the author or coauthor of more than 340 professional papers, Dr. Klastersky is a member of the European Society for Medical Oncology, the European Society for Clinical Investigation, the American Society of Clinical Oncology, the American Association for Cancer Research, the American Society for Microbiology, and the Infectious Diseases Society of America, among others. He received the M.D. degree (1965) and the Ph.D. degree (1972) in medical sciences from the Université Libre de Bruxelles, Belgium.

Stephen C. Schimpff is Executive Vice President of, and a Professor of Medicine, Oncology, and Pharmacology in, the University of Maryland Medical System, Baltimore. Formerly, the Director of the University of Maryland Cancer Center, Baltimore, Dr. Schimpff is the author or coauthor of more than 170 professional papers in the fields of oncology and infectious diseases and the coeditor of several books. He serves on the editorial board of the *Journal of Supportive Care in Cancer* and is a reviewer for numerous other scientific journals. He is coeditor of the major oncology reference work *Comprehensive Textbook of Oncology*. Trained and certified in both medical oncology and infectious diseases, he is a Fellow of the American College of Physicians and the Infectious Diseases Society of America, as well as a member of the American Association for Cancer Research and the American Society of Clinical Oncology, among others. Dr. Schimpff received the B. A. degree (1963) in biological science from Rutgers University, New Brunswick, New Jersey, and the M. D. degree (1967) from Yale University Medical School, New Haven, Connecticut.

Hans-Jörg Senn is Chief of the Department of Medicine C (Onco-Hematology, Gastroenterology) and Chairman of the Interdisciplinary Oncology Center at the Kantonsspital, St. Gallen, Switzerland, as well as Associate Professor of Internal Medicine (especially Oncology) at Basel University Medical School, Switzerland. Dr. Senn is Chairman of the Scientific Audit Committee of the European Organization for Research and Treatment of Cancer in Brussels, Belgium, and Past President of the International Breast Cancer Study Group. He also serves as Editor-in-Chief of the *Journal of Supportive Care in Cancer* and of the series *Recent Results in Cancer Research*. A member of the American Society of Clinical Oncology as well as a board member of the European Society of Medical Oncology, he is author or editor of 11 oncology books and the author or coauthor of over 250 professional publications. Dr. Senn received his M.D. degree (1961) from Zurich University, Switzerland.